Research Methods in Family Therapy

Research Methods in Family Therapy

SECOND EDITION

Edited by
DOUGLAS H. SPRENKLE
FRED P. PIERCY

THE GUILFORD PRESS
New York   London

© 2005 The Guilford Press
A Division of Guilford Publications, Inc.
72 Spring Street, New York, NY 10012
www.guilford.com

Printed in the United States of America

This book is printed on acid-free paper.

Last digit is print number: 9   8   7   6   5   4   3   2   1

Library of Congress Cataloging-in-Publication Data
Research methods in family therapy / edited by Douglas H. Sprenkle, Fred P. Piercy.—2nd ed.
    p. cm.
  Includes bibliographical references and index.
  ISBN 1-57230-960-1 (hardcover)
  1. Family psychotherapy—Research—Methodology.   I. Sprenkle, Douglas H.   II. Piercy,
Fred P.
  RC488.5.R47 2005
  616.89'156'072—dc22

                                                                  2004025279

About the Editors

Douglas H. Sprenkle, PhD, is professor and director of the doctoral program in marriage and family therapy at Purdue University. He is a former editor of the *Journal of Marital and Family Therapy*. Dr. Sprenkle has received three major career honors from the American Association for Marriage and Family Therapy (AAMFT): the Cumulative Career Contribution in Family Therapy Research Award, the Training Award, and the Significant Contribution to Family Therapy Award. He has also received the Osborne Award for excellence in teaching from the National Council on Family Relations. Among his seven books, Dr. Sprenkle is the editor of *Effectiveness Research in Marriage and Family Therapy*, published by AAMFT in 2002.

Fred P. Piercy, PhD, is professor and head of the Department of Human Development at Virginia Polytechnic Institute and State University. He has served two times on the Board of Directors of AAMFT, and as the chair of the Commission on Accreditation for Marriage and Family Therapy Education. Dr. Piercy is also a member and fellow of both AAMFT and the American Psychological Association. He has written over 160 published articles, 5 books, and 35 funded grants. Most recently, he is the coeditor of the *Handbook of the Clinical Treatment of Infidelity* (with Katherine Hertlein and Joseph Wetchler; in press, Haworth Press) and coauthor of *Family Therapy Sourcebook* (2nd ed., with Douglas H. Sprenkle, Joseph L. Wetchler, and Associates; 1996, Guilford Press) and *Stop Marital Fights Before they Start* (with Norman Lobsenz; 1994, Berkley Press). Dr. Piercy has won both national and university teaching awards. He has also collaborated extensively with colleagues from the University of Indonesia and Atma Jaya University (in Jakarta, Indonesia) and was the principal investigator of a World AIDS Foundation-funded project in Indonesia.

Contributors

Katherine R. Allen, PhD, is Professor of Family Studies in the Department of Human Development and Adjunct Professor of Women's Studies at Virginia Polytechnic Institute and State University. Her academic interests are in family diversity over the life course, feminism and family studies, and qualitative research methods. Dr. Allen is coeditor of several books as well as author of numerous journal articles and book chapters. She serves on the editorial boards of *Journal of Marriage and the Family, Journal of Family Issues, Family Relations, Journal of Aging Studies,* and *Journal of GLBT Family Studies.* Dr. Allen is also a charter fellow of the National Council on Family Relations.

David D. Allred, BS, is a marriage and family therapy graduate student at Seattle Pacific University. He received his undergraduate degree in family, consumer, and human development from Utah State University.

Saliha Bava, PhD, is Associate Director of Houston Galveston Institute, an associate of the Taos Institute, on the core adjunct faculty for the master's psychology program at Our Lady of the Lake University in Houston, Texas, and on the online adjunct faculty for the Postgraduate Diploma in Discursive Therapies at Massey University in New Zealand. Dr. Bava's current areas of interest are collaborative learning, organizational consultation, postmodern/performative and hypertext discourses, research methodological discourses, and trauma and terrorism.

Pauline Boss, PhD, is Professor and American Association for Marriage and Family Therapy Supervisor in the doctoral training program at the University of Minnesota. She is currently the Visiting Moses Professor at the Hunter College School of Social Work in New York City and previously has been Visiting Professor at Harvard Medical School. Dr. Boss's research interests center on ambiguous loss, the unresolved grief experienced when loved ones go missing, physically or psychologically. Her latest book, *Trauma, Loss and Resilience: Therapeutic Work with Ambiguous Loss,* summarizes that work for clinicians and researchers.

Brent Bradley, PhD, is Assistant Professor and Director of the Marriage and Family Therapy Track in the Graduate Counseling Department at Indiana Wesleyan University. He is a licensed marriage and family therapist and a clinical member of the American Association for Marriage and Family Therapy. Dr. Bradley is a certified couple therapist and supervisor in emotionally focused therapy (EFT). An active writer, researcher, and presenter, he is currently working with colleagues on an EFT workbook for practitioners. Professional interests include process research on critical change elements in couple and family therapy, and working with affect and systems.

Linda M. Burton, PhD, is Director of the Center for Human Development and Family Research in Diverse Contexts and Professor of Human Development and Family Studies and Sociology at The Pennsylvania State University. She was a Spencer Foundation Fellow, Brookdale National Fellow, William T. Grant Faculty Scholar, and Fellow at the Center for Advanced Study in the Behavioral Sciences at Stanford University. Dr. Burton's research explores the relationship among community contexts, poverty, intergenerational family structure and processes, and developmental outcomes across the life course in ethnic/racial minority populations. She is currently one of six principal investigators involved in an extensive, longitudinal, multisite, multilevel study of the impact of welfare reform on families and children.

Dean M. Busby, PhD, is Professor and Chair of the Human Development and Family Studies Department at Texas Tech University. He received his doctorate in marriage and family therapy from Brigham Young University. Dr. Busby's research interests include couple assessment, premarital enrichment programs, premarital factors that lead to marital success, cultural identity, and Hispanic families. He has published books on family violence and on courtship and marriage. Dr. Busby has received state and federal grants for programs to help fathers from low-income families and to improve the quality of premarital relationships.

Ronald J. Chenail, PhD, is Professor of Family Therapy and Vice President for Research, Planning, and Governmental Affairs at Nova Southeastern University. In 2004, he became editor-elect of the *Journal of Marital and Family Therapy*, the flagship journal of the American Association for Marriage and Family Therapy, and is the founding editor of *The Qualitative Report*, one of the first online journals dedicated to qualitative inquiry. Dr. Chenail also serves on the editorial boards of *Qualitative Research in Psychology*, *Sistemas Familiares*, and *Journal of Systemic Therapies*. His books include *Medical Discourse and Systemic Frames of Comprehension*, *Practicing Therapy: Exercises for Growing Therapists*, and *The Talk of the Clinic: Explorations in the Analysis of Medical and Therapeutic Discourse*.

Carla M. Dahl, PhD, is Professor of Marriage and Family Studies, Director of the Marriage and Family Therapy training program, and Dean of the Center for Spiritual and Personal Formation at Bethel Seminary in St. Paul, Minnesota. She has been a psychotherapist and family life educator since 1981, and her research interests have included families and spirituality, spiritual and personal formation and change, grief and bereavement, perceptions of justice, boundary ambiguity, and clergy involvement with families.

Mary Dankoski, PhD, is Assistant Professor in the Department of Family Medicine at Indiana University. She received her doctorate in child development and family studies with a specialization in marriage and family therapy from Purdue University, where she also completed a graduate minor in women's studies. Dr. Dankoski's scholarly interests include behavioral science education for medical students and family medicine resident-physicians, medical family therapy, interpersonal violence, and feminist perspectives. She is a clinical member and approved supervisor of the American Association for Marriage and Family Therapy and is an active board member of the Indiana Association for Marriage and Family Therapy. Dr. Dankoski has published several articles and book chapters, and was the recipient of the 2002 AAMFT Dissertation Award.

William J. Doherty, PhD, is Professor and Director of the Marriage and Family Therapy Program at the University of Minnesota. He also directs the Families and Democracy Project. Dr. Doherty's principal current interest is in community-oriented projects that engage families as co-creators of initiatives and co-producers of health care and family education in their communities. In 2004 he began a federally funded action research project with unmarried new parents in urban communities.

Megan Dolbin-MacNab, PhD, is Assistant Professor in the Department of Human Development at Virginia Polytechnic Institute and State University. She received her doctorate in child development and family studies with a specialization in marriage and family therapy from Purdue University. Dr. Dolbin-MacNab's scholarly interests include affect regulation, attachment, grandparent-headed families, infertility, and longitudinal methods of data analysis.

Silvia Echevarria-Doan, PhD, is Associate Professor in the Department of Counselor Education at the University of Florida in Gainesville. She is a clinical member and approved supervisor of the American Association for Marriage and Family Therapy and a member of the American Family Therapy Association. Dr. Echevarria-Doan's scholarly work reflects her interest in strength-based family therapy and resilience, multicultural approaches in family therapy, qualitative research methodology, family therapy training, and family violence. She has presented internationally, nationally, and in state and local conferences on many of these topics and has received awards recognizing her research, teaching, and her focus on cultural diversity issues as an educator. Dr. Echevarria-Doan is also dually licensed as a marriage and family therapist and clinical social worker in the state of Florida.

Linda Stone Fish, PhD, is Professor in the Department of Marriage and Family Therapy at Syracuse University. Her scholarly interests include relationship development and family therapy with nontraditional populations. She is currently coauthoring a book with Rebecca Harvey, entitled *Nurturing Queer Youth: Family Therapy Transformed*, to be published by Norton.

Katherine M. Hertlein, PhD, received her doctorate in marriage and family therapy from the Department of Human Development at Virginia Polytechnic Institute and State University. She is a family therapist at Family Service of Roanoke Valley as well as a day treatment manager for a children's after-school treatment program in Roanoke, Virginia. Dr. Hertlein has published in and serves as a reviewer for several journals. Her areas of interest include research methodology and measurement, training and family therapy, and infidelity treatment.

Angela J. Huebner, PhD, is Assistant Professor in the Department of Human Development at Virginia Polytechnic Institute and State University. She received her doctorate from the University of Arizona. Her research interests include issues of risk and resiliency with adolescents. She has published in *Evaluation*, *Journal of Adolescent Health*, *Journal of Youth and Adolescence*, *Youth and Society*, and other journals.

Ebony Joy James, MFT, is currently a PhD student in the family therapy doctoral program at Virginia Polytechnic Institute and State University. She is a student member of the American Association for Marriage and Family Therapy (AAMFT) and a former staff member of the Commission on Accreditation for Marriage and Family Therapy Education of the AAMFT. Dr. James's current professional interests are in the areas of couple intimacy, sex therapy, and the mind–body connection.

Susan M. Johnson, EdD, is Professor in the Department of Psychology and Psychiatry at Ottawa University and Director of the Ottawa Couple and Family Institute. She is a registered psychologist and a member of the editorial boards of the *Journal of Marital and Family Therapy*, the *Journal of Couple and Relationship Therapy*, and the *Journal of Family Psychology*. Dr. Johnson is one of the originators and the main proponent of emotionally focused therapy (EFT), now one of the best-validated interventions for couples in North America. Always a proficient writer, researcher, and presenter, she is currently working with colleagues on developing a practitioner workbook for EFT.

Margaret K. Keiley, EdD, is Associate Professor in the Marriage and Family Therapy Program of the Department of Human Development and Family Studies at Auburn

University. She received her doctorate in human development and psychology from Harvard University. Dr. Keiley is a clinical member and approved supervisor of the American Association for Marriage and Family Therapy. Her scholarly interests include clinical research on emotinally focused therapy with incarcerated adolescents and their families; the development of affect regulation and attachment of individuals within the family context; the development of violence, sexual abuse, addiction, and externalizing–internalizing behaviors, and of treatments for these difficulties; and longitudinal data-analytic techniques (growth modeling and survival analysis). In 2003 Dr. Keiley was the recipient of the Distinguished Research Award in Human Development from Division E of the American Educational Research Association.

Ting Liu, PhD, is currently working as a clinician and Adjunct Assistant Professor in the Department of Human Development at Virginia Polytechnic Institute and State University. She received her doctorate in child development and family studies with a specialization in marriage and family therapy from Purdue University. Dr. Liu's scholarly interests include outcome research, attachment, affect regulation, therapist training, and working with minority clients. She has been conducting training workshops in emotionally focused therapy internationally for the past 4 years.

Kevin P. Lyness, PhD, is Associate Professor and Director of Research in the Marriage and Family Therapy Program within the Department of Applied Psychology at Antioch New England Graduate School. He was Assistant Professor in the Marriage and Family Therapy Program at Colorado State University for 5 years prior to moving to Antioch New England. Dr. Lyness is the former Assistant Editor of the *Journal of Marital and Family Therapy* and he serves on the editorial boards of the *Journal of Feminist Family Therapy* and the *Journal of Couple and Relationship Therapy*.

David P. Mackinnon, PhD, is a private-practice marital and family therapist at Heritage Professional Associates, Ltd., in Hinsdale, Illinois, and the founder and president of Lighthouse Coaching. He was formerly vice president and senior credit officer for Bank of America NT & SA. Lighthouse Coaching specializes in personal and executive coaching with owners of family- and closely held businesses and their management teams. Dr. Mackinnon's research interests are focused on incorporating systemic economic evaluations in marriage and family therapy outcome studies. He received his doctorate in marriage and family therapy from Purdue University. He is a clinical member of the American Association for Marriage and Family Therapy and serves on the editorial board of the *Journal of Couple and Relationship Therapy*.

Jay A. Mancini, PhD, is Professor in the Department of Human Development at Virginia Polytechnic Institute and State University. He received his doctorate from the University of North Carolina at Greensboro. Dr. Mancini's research has been published in numerous periodicals. His current research focuses on social organization and community capacity, and on sustaining community-based programs for families. He is a fellow of the National Council on Family Relations.

Laurel F. Mangrum, PhD, is a research scientist at the Center for Social Work Research at the University of Texas at Austin. She is involved in research funded by the Substance Abuse and Mental Health Services Administration concerning comorbid psychiatric and substance abuse disorders, screening and brief intervention techniques, and research-to-practice methods. Other areas of research include psychological assessment, diagnostic systems, psychometrics, and treatment outcome.

Lydia I. Marek, PhD, is a research scientist in the Department of Human Development at Virginia Polytechnic Institute and State University. She is also a licensed marriage and family therapist and a certified family life educator. She received her doctorate from Virginia Tech.

Dr. Marek has published articles in the *Journal of Community Practice, Journal of Family Psychotherapy, Family Therapy,* and other books and journals. Her research interests are in the areas of community-based program sustainability, community collaboration assessment, and effective program practices. She regularly presents at national conferences.

Nina C. Martin, EdD, is a Visiting Research Assistant Professor at the Institute of Juvenile Research in the Department of Psychiatry, University of Illinois at Chicago. She received her doctorate in human development and psychology from Harvard University. Dr. Martin's research interests include the relation between the family environment and adolescent internalizing and externalizing behaviors, the development of self-esteem during adolescence, and the application of longitudinal data-analytic methods to developmental phenomena.

Jennifer L. Matheson, MA, MS, is a doctoral candidate in the Department of Human Development at Virginia Polytechnic Institute and State University. Her dissertation is on the experiences of powerlessness among women who are in 12-step substance abuse recovery. She won the 2004 Outstanding Graduate Student Award in the College of Liberal Arts and Human Sciences at Virginia Tech, and she is the Student/Associate Representative for the Virginia Association for Marriage and Family Therapy. She is a former employee of RTI International, where she conducted social and health policy research. Her current scholarly interests include training, supervision, qualitative methods, substance abuse, and gender issues.

Eric E. McCollum, PhD, is Professor in the Department of Human Development at Virginia Polytechnic Institute and State University. He received his doctorate from Kansas State University. Dr. McCollum's research interests are in the family treatment of substance abuse and domestic violence. He has published in *Family Process, Journal of Marital and Family Therapy, American Journal of Drug and Alcohol Abuse,* and other journals. He regularly presents at national and international conferences.

Lenore M. McWey, PhD, is Assistant Professor in the Department of Child and Family Sciences at Florida State University. Her professional interests are in the areas of foster care and marital and family therapy research. Dr. McWey is an approved supervisor and clinical member of the American Association for Marriage and Family Therapy.

Tai J. Mendenhall, PhD, is Assistant Professor in the Department of Family Medicine and Community Health at the University of Minnesota Medical School. He is a clinical member and approved supervisor of the American Association for Marriage and Family Therapy, and works actively in behavioral health education with both graduate students in marriage and family therapy and medical residents in family practice. Dr. Mendenhall's research focuses on collaborative and participatory methods of engaging families and communities as active contributors to health care, with particular attention to those who are struggling with chronic illnesses.

Thorana S. Nelson, PhD, is Director of the accredited master's program in marriage and family therapy at Utah State University. Her research interests focus on various aspects of family therapy training and skills and she has published several articles on this topic. Dr. Nelson is also the author or coauthor of many articles and several books, including *101 Interventions in Family Therapy* and *101 More Interventions in Family Therapy,* which have been translated into Chinese.

Fred P. Piercy, PhD (see "About the Editors").

Alan Reifman, PhD, is Associate Professor in the Department of Human Development and Family Studies at Texas Tech University. His research interests include adolescent and young adult substance use, social networks, statistics, and methodology. His published meta-analyses focus on long-term correlates of attention-deficit/hyperactivity disorder (*Journal of*

Family and Consumer Sciences, 2003), children of divorce (*Journal of Divorce and Remarriage*, 2001), and Brazelton demonstrations with infants (*Journal of Pediatric Psychology*, 1996).

Julianne M. Serovich, PhD, is Professor in the Department of Human Development and Family Science at Ohio State University. Her research interests are in the areas of disclosure of HIV status to family members; family and child coping as a result of having an HIV-infected family member; and violence in gay, lesbian, bisexual, and transgendered relationships. Currently, Dr. Serovich is funded by the National Institute of Mental Health to study HIV disclosure by women and to develop an intervention to help HIV-positive persons disclose to their sexual partners.

Sara A. Smock, MS, is a doctoral student in marriage and family therapy at Virginia Polytechnic Institute and State University. Currently, she is the editorial assistant for *Family Relations*. She received the American Association for Marriage and Family Therapy's 2004 Dissertation/Thesis Award for her project entitled "Solution-Focused Group Therapy for Level 1 Substance Abusers." She is a member of the Solution-Focused Brief Therapy Association's founders group and has published and presented on solution-focused brief therapy.

Douglas K. Snyder, PhD, is Professor and Director of clinical psychology training at Texas A&M University. He has been recognized internationally for his programmatic research on couple therapy, is a coeditor of *Treating Difficult Couples* (2003, Guilford Press), and is the author of the widely used Marital Satisfaction Inventory. In 1992, the American Association for Marriage and Family Therapy honored Dr. Snyder with its Outstanding Research Award. A fellow of the American Psychological Association, he has served as associate editor of the *Journal of Consulting and Clinical Psychology* and the *Journal of Family Psychology*.

Douglas H. Sprenkle, PhD (see "About the Editors").

Carolyn Y. Tubbs, PhD, is Assistant Professor in the Couple and Family Therapy Program at the University of Guelph. She was a research scientist on Welfare, Children and Families: A Three City-Study and a Family Research Consortium III postdoctoral fellow. As part of her work, Dr. Tubbs has examined facilitators of family stability, family rituals, aging, and parenting in low-income families, as well as issues of shared parenting in couples with a history of intimate-partner violence.

Stephanie R. Walsh, PhD, is a postdoctoral fellow funded by a Department of Defense Behavioral Center of Excellence in Breast Cancer training grant to study quality of life among women with breast cancer. She is at Wake Forest University School of Medicine in the Department of Public Health Sciences. Dr. Walsh has been working specifically in the areas of sexuality after diagnosis and treatment, and couple and family relationships of younger women with breast cancer.

Karen S. Wampler, PhD, is C. R. and Virginia Hutcheson Professor and Chair of the Department of Applied and Professional Studies at Texas Tech University. She is also past editor of the *Journal of Marital and Family Therapy*. Dr. Wampler's primary interests are research methodology, including meta-analysis, and the development of observational measures of marriage and family process. Her current research focuses on couple interaction from an attachment theory perspective.

Preface

When my (D. H. S.) collaborator in the first edition of this volume, Sidney Moon, decided that working on a second edition was not compatible with her current position as an associate dean, my first choice to replace her was another administrator. Fully expecting Fred Piercy to say no, I was both shocked and delighted that he responded affirmatively—immediately and with no hesitation. Fred and I had worked together for 18 years in the Marriage and Family Therapy Program at Purdue University before he moved up to Department Head at Virginia Tech. He has a great reputation as a writer and editor and has been practicing and teaching qualitative research for years. This volume became another "excuse" for Fred and me to continue our fruitful professional relationship (and warm friendship) that had produced two editions of the *Family Therapy Sourcebook* as well as scores of journal articles. Fred was largely responsible for the qualitative section of this volume, which I believe is as rich as it is current. As was true for our prior collaborations, to work with Fred Piercy is to work with the consummate professional.

A lot has happened since the first edition of *Research Methods in Family Therapy* was published in 1996. Our first task was to make this volume as up to date as possible. Thirteen of the 21 chapters are totally new, while eight are substantial revisions of previous chapters.

The text reflects the sweeping changes that have occurred in qualitative, quantitative, and mixed methodologies in recent years. In an introductory chapter, we describe the significant changes in the research landscape and how the volume mirrors those changes. There is also a special new chapter written for graduate students who are novices in the research arena and may feel intimidated by it.

In the qualitative section, while there are updated chapters on more traditional methods like grounded theory, phenomenology, and focus groups, there are new chapters on contemporary developments like participatory research methods, feminist autoethnography, and performance methodology. This section also includes new chapters on qualitative data analysis software, how ethnography can be used to inform clinical practice, and future directions for qualitative methods.

In the quantitative section, we tried to capture the multiplicity and sophistication of contemporary methods. The previous chapter on experimental research was rewritten to emphasize randomized clinical trials, the new "gold standard" for evaluating interventions. There are updated treatments regarding meta-analysis and approaches to prediction research, including advanced techniques like canonical correlation, multiple discriminant analysis, and (new to this revision) cluster analysis. Also new to this edition are two chapters on advanced quantitative techniques at the cutting edge of family therapy research: multilevel growth modeling (sometimes called hierarchical linear modeling) and covariance structure analysis, including structural equation modeling. There is also a new chapter on economic evaluation methodology. Throughout the chapters, the authors highlight new software packages that support their work.

In the mixed-methods section, there are revised chapters on survey research (including the use of the Internet) and the Delphi method. There is a new chapter on task analysis, which applies this methodology to contemporary emotionally focused therapy. Finally, a new chapter on program evaluation demonstrates how researchers can use both quantitative and qualitative analysis to assess the effectiveness of current and future intervention programs.

We also wish to thank our editor, Jim Nageotte, of The Guilford Press, who encouraged us to do a second edition and has been both a cheerleader and helpful and friendly critic for this project all along the way.

Closer to home, I (F. P. P.) want to thank Susan Piercy, my wife, for reminding me to breathe, relax, and get away from my work from time to time. Without her I would be a dull guy, and not half as happy. Also, thanks, Doug, for asking me to be part of this project, and for the nice things you said at the beginning of this preface. I said yes so quickly partly because of our friendship and partly because of how well you do things. I admire your commitment to excellence. And, yes, we do make a great team.

Finally, I (D. H. S.) want to thank Sidney Moon, my collaborator on the first edition, who also happens to be my wife. Her steadfast love and support for all that I do is part of what makes ours a world-class marriage.

DOUGLAS H. SPRENKLE, PhD
FRED P. PIERCY, PhD

Contents

Contents

PART III. MIXED METHODS

PART IV. QUANTITATIVE METHODS

PART V. ADVANCED QUANTITATIVE METHODS

Research Methods in Family Therapy

PART I

INTRODUCTION

CHAPTER 1

Pluralism, Diversity, and Sophistication in Family Therapy Research

DOUGLAS H. SPRENKLE
FRED P. PIERCY

One of our main hopes in editing the second edition of *Research Methods in Family Therapy* is to enhance the status of research in the field, while also making the science of marriage and family therapy (MFT) more accessible to clinicians and students. Over the course of its history, the field of MFT has had an ambivalent relationship with research. On the one hand, the early family therapy pioneers considered themselves to be "researchers," and both Wynne (1983) and Haley (1978) claimed that in the early days there was no distinction between therapists and researchers. Such notables as Lyman Wynne, Murray Bowen, Theodore Litz, Gregory Bateson, Don Jackson, Jay Haley, and others came to family therapy though studying interactional patterns associated with problem families (Broderick & Schrader, 1981; Sprenkle & Moon, 1996). As the field has developed, it has always had an active (if small) research tradition—and, based on a thorough review of outcome research in the field (Sprenkle, 2002), one could make a case for the claim that some of the effectiveness research in MFT is among the most impressive in the clinical social sciences.

On the other hand, one can also make a case that although MFT is now more than 60 years old, the growth of the field has depended more on its intuitive appeal than on solid research evidence for its efficacy (Nichols & Schwartz, 1995). One explanation may be that the field's leaders were often highly charismatic individuals who were less interested in authenticating their claims than in building a following. Another explanation may be that the master's degree was established early (1970) as the minimal entry point into the field, and most master's-degree programs (with notable exceptions) have not offered rigorous research training. As the field grew, it also seemed to attract predominantly practically oriented clinicians who had neither the time nor the inclination for the laborious research enterprise. One study noted that over 80% of the members of the American Association for Marriage and Family Therapy (AAMFT) work in settings that can be considered predominantly clinical (Sprenkle, Bailey, Lyness, Ball, & Mills, 1997).

The result has been a research–practice gap, which, although it plagues all clinical fields, may be particularly prevalent in MFT:

> The culture [of MFT] does not support research. Ours remains a field where it is still possible for a highly charismatic individual to create a model of family therapy, become successful on the workshop circuit, and get lucrative book contracts to promulgate the model without offering evidence for its efficacy beyond personal testimonies. In many ways, rockstar status is accorded the clinical model developers and the "master therapists." Researchers, when contrasted with the "stars," are best warm-up acts, and at worst bit players. (Crane, Wampler, Sprenkle, Sandberg, & Hovestadt, 2002, p. 76)

Sprenkle (2003) has also argued that researchers have contributed to this chasm. They too often disdain clinicians or fail to heed the wisdom of good clinicians (cf. Piercy et al., in press). Furthermore, they often do not work very hard at making their work accessible to clinicians. The first deleterious consequence of this researcher–clinician gap is that research often gets dismissed as irrelevant, incomprehensible, or both. Consequently, research does not inform practice, and thus clinicians do not refine their practice. They keep doing what they've been doing. Second, the gap perpetuates a false dichotomy between clinical judgment and the scientific method—when, in fact, these are two overlapping ways of knowing, both to be valued and both to be questioned. The primary benefit of the science of therapy is that it forces us to use certain rules of evidence when making assertions about effectiveness. Although science is sometimes wrong (as is clinical wisdom), the strength of the scientific method is that it is more readily correctable. Third, the researcher–clinician gap challenges the status of MFT as an ethical profession. If we are sworn to advance the welfare of clients, how can we do so if we have insufficient evidence regarding which of our interventions are effective? Fourth, the gap diminishes the credibility of the profession to outside stakeholders such as policymakers and health care providers, who increasingly demand evidence-based claims. Fifth, the gap has contributed to the "outsourcing" of MFT research to those whose primary professional identity is something other than MFT (Sprenkle, 2003). We should be grateful to the psychologists and psychiatrists who have done the majority of MFT research, but as Crane and colleagues (2002) have put it,

> We have to take responsibility for setting the research agenda and training the requisite MFT researchers and stop depending on other disciplines to do it for us. . . . No one else will do research on MFT training. No one else will do research on matters that are uniquely important to [MFT practitioners]. (p. 78)

One of the major goals of the current volume, then, is to contribute to narrowing the divide between researchers and clinicians. Although the book is about research, we insisted that the chapter authors expend considerable effort demonstrating how the methods they describe are connected to the world of practice. While we think it unlikely that too many people will be able to lead professional lives where they are equally focused on the domains of research and practice, we hope at the very least that researchers and clinicians will each develop a mutual respect and appreciation for what the other group has to offer. Given the focus of the book, we especially hope that readers will come to value the varied, creative, and important ways in which researchers are trying to shed light on the therapeutic enterprise, and that many readers will be moved to choose "researcher" as at least one of their professional titles.

MEGATRENDS IN FAMILY THERAPY RESEARCH

In the opening chapter of the first edition of this book (Sprenkle & Moon, 1996), the editors identified four major trends in the history of family therapy research. In the first phase, the founders of the field, as noted above, were "researcher-clinicians" who focused on the impact of therapeutic interventions on clients and their families. They frequently reviewed audiotapes of their sessions, observed each other through one-way mirrors, and spent many hours discussing sessions and formulating hypotheses. Because hypotheses were developed, tested, altered, and retested in practice settings, research had direct clinical relevance (Sprenkle & Bischoff, 1995; Sprenkle & Moon, 1996; Wynne, 1983). However, what was then considered research would not be considered very rigorous by today's standards. Indeed, it might be labeled "soft" qualitative research, since it was impressionistic and there was not much effort to control for researcher bias.

In the second phase, the field moved from these impressionistic beginnings and started to emphasize quantitative and experimental research (Sprenkle & Bischoff, 1995). Family therapists began to operationalize some of their "fuzzy" concepts and were challenged to develop reliable and valid measures. There was a push toward outcome research to give credibility to this fledgling discipline. Some early studies compared family treatments to conventional treatments (often inpatient or individually oriented treatments) and found the family treatments to be superior to the conventional treatments on such important variables as recidivism (e.g., Langsley, Flomenhaft, & Machotka, 1969). Other outcome studies (e.g., Minuchin et al., 1975) applied a specific model of family treatment (in this case, structural family therapy) to a specific problem area (in this case, anorexia nervosa), and found the model to produce dramatic results. Even though the Minuchin and colleagues (1975) study had a major methodological limitation (no control group), the percentage of patients improving was dramatic and made the rest of the clinical world take notice.

At the same time, another group of early researchers pursued largely quantitative process research, which focused less on therapy outcomes and more on the processes occurring within therapy that contribute to the ultimate outcome (see Pinsof, 1981, for a summary of this early process research). This work would foreshadow the current emphasis on research that focuses on how and why change takes place, as opposed to just demonstrating that therapy "works" (see Bradley & Johnson, Chapter 14, this volume).

The third major trend was the qualitative revolution and the growing acceptance of methodologies that did not employ numbers (Moon, Dillon, & Sprenkle, 1990; Sprenkle & Bischoff, 1995). This movement grew out of powerful intellectual challenges to positivism (Anderson, 1990; Gergen, 1991) and the belief that quantitative research was often too "reductionistic" and linear. For example, Karl Tomm (1983) argued that attempts to operationalize circular and systemic concepts typically "kill the beast in an effort to understand him" (p. 39). Furthermore, qualitative researchers argued that family therapy had made its quantitative leap too soon and that concepts were operationalized before they were truly and deeply understood. They called for more attention to the context of "discovery," as opposed to the context of verification, and for descriptive research that would record in more detail the subtleties and complexities of therapy (Atkinson, Heath, & Chenail, 1991). Although these arguments were challenged by quantitative researchers (see Cavell & Snyder, 1991; Gurman, 1983), qualitative research has grown to become more acceptable and influential today.

The fourth major trend has been pluralism—a growing acceptance of a wide variety of research methods, both quantitative and qualitative. We, the current editors, welcome this trend. We live in a diverse country where political name calling and derision sometimes win out over respectful debate, tolerance, and civility. This can happen in the world of MFT research as well. We support a collaborative, learn-from-each-other stance toward MFT research methods, and have attempted to provide a sense of the richness and potential of our field's expanding methods in this edition of *Research Methods in Family Therapy*.

There are advantages, for example, in family therapy researchers' using both qualitative and quantitative methods, alone or in combination. As Acock, van Dulmen, Allen, and Piercy (2005) state, "Whether one uses numbers, narrative, poetry, drama, or photos as data, each points to a better understanding (or multiple understandings) of some phenomenon." In other words, multiple methods add to family therapy researchers' ability to capture and reflect change.

We believe that there is less tension today between quantitative and qualitative researchers. Both groups recognize that different research questions require different methods, and that different methods in turn give rise to different kinds of questions. For example, it is becoming increasingly common today for qualitative investigations to be embedded in the most rigorous quantitative clinical trials. Also, not only do qualitative insights often have clinical relevance in their own right, but they provide a richness that generates important research questions for quantitative investigation.

The fifth trend, which we believe is highlighted in the present volume, is the growing sophistication and multiplicity of family therapy methods. We discuss this trend in detail in the next section of this chapter, focusing on qualitative and quantitative (and mixed) methods separately.

SOPHISTICATION AND MULTIPLICITY

Qualitative Research

No longer can qualitative research be spoken of as one monolithic set of assumptions and methods (if it ever could). Today, qualitative research is evolving in many directions. For example, there are increasingly sophisticated, rigorous procedures mirroring quantitative methods that some qualitative researchers use to reflect participants' experiences. Many qualitative researchers, for example, use member checks, triangulation, persistent observation, audit trails, peer review, negative case analysis, and careful inductive analysis, to give their work credibility and trustworthiness.

Other evolving methods of qualitative research emphasize different goals, and should be judged by the degree to which they achieve these goals. For example, depending on their theoretical orientation, some qualitative researchers are interested in one or more of the following questions (Piercy & Benson, 2005):

- Is the research catalytic, liberating, transformative? Does it empower?
- Does the research bring findings to life? Is it evocative? Does it have a personal impact on the reader?
- Does the researcher locate him- or herself in the process of the research, and apply reflexivity to understand and interpret the data?
- Does the research have aesthetic merit? Does it employ the standards of good writing, art, or drama?
- Are important issues addressed? Is the research worth doing?
- Does the research have verisimilitude (the appearance of being true or real)?
- Does the research invite multiple interpretations? Does it involve the reader in the meaning-making process?

One could argue, of course, that most if not all of these questions should be applied to quantitative methods as well. Still, certain qualitative methods have focused primarily on one or more of these questions. Thus Patton (2002) contends that criteria for judging qualitative research flow directly from the theory and purposes of the research. For example, according to Piercy and Benson (2005),

> qualitative researchers who hold to a more realistic theoretical orientation (i.e., reality can be captured) detail elaborate methods for assuring the reliability and validity of their data (e.g., triangulation, audit trails, member checks, etc.). Social constructionist researchers, on the other hand, are more interested in interpretive methods and in assuring that their interpretations are credible and trustworthy. Critical theorists such as feminist family therapy researchers use research methods to critique society, raise consciousness, and bring about change. Qualitative researchers committed to the use of art, music, creative writing, and performance value affective as well as intellectual knowing. (p. 10)

Of course, distinctions such as these are not always this clear. For example, there is nothing to keep a feminist family therapy researcher from using aesthetic methods such as poetry, or more traditional qualitative procedures such as member checks. We embrace such complexity. After all, families are complex, and we need both qualitative and quantitative methods that capture this complexity.

In this second edition of *Research Methods in Family Therapy*, we have attempted to include a sampling of many evolving qualitative methods, and to underline the theoretical underpinnings, methodological procedures, and evaluation standards of each.

Quantitative Research

Quantitative research has burgeoned to the point where it was not possible to include all of the methods we would like to have seen represented in this volume. In order to include some new material, and to keep the book the same length, we had to make the painful decision to omit some of the topics covered in the first edition, even though these chapters remain valuable and worth reading. Some chapters were eliminated because they were redundant with new ones (Bischoff, McKeel, Moon, & Sprenkle, 1996; Greenberg, Heatherington, & Friedlander, 1996; Volk & Flori, 1996). Others, such as "Methods for Single-Case Experiments in Family Therapy" (Dickey, 1996), were eliminated because they described methods that are rarely used in family therapy research. Still others, such as "Methodological Issues and Strategies in Scale Develop-

ment" (Snyder & Rice, 1996), were omitted only because the principles of scale development are not unique to intervention research and can be found in various books on
methodology (see Nelson & Allred, Chapter 12, this volume, for references). An updated chapter on this theme would clearly have been included if space were not a premium.

    Virtually all forms of quantitative analysis appearing in leading social science
journals are now being applied to family therapy research. This volume covers family
therapy applications of such advanced techniques as canonical correlations, multiple-
discriminant-function analysis, cluster analysis, multilevel growth modeling (sometimes called "hierarchical linear modeling" or other names), and various forms of
covariance structure analysis (including path analysis and structural equation modeling). Some of the sophisticated software necessary to utilize these procedures is also
noted or described. Since the first edition of this book, there have been major advances
in the complexity and sophistication of procedures related to such methods as economic evaluation and meta-analysis. The quality and sophistication of clinical trials
using family therapy approaches has improved to the point where research on family
approaches to adolescent substance abuse, conduct disorder, major mental illnesses,
and adult alcoholism ranks with the best clinical research in any discipline (Sprenkle,
2002). If it ever were the case, it will no longer be possible for a single individual to become competent in all forms of family therapy research, and it will become increasingly challenging to teach family therapy research courses.

GOALS AND PURPOSES OF THIS VOLUME

The goals of this second edition are similar to those of the first edition, except that a
major purpose of the current volume is to offer a state-of-the-art description of research methods almost a decade later. In later sections, we note the specific chapters
that have been updated or replaced.

    As in the previous edition, we remain interested in promoting methodological plu-
ralism and demonstrating the advantages of being multimethodological. We also hope
that the reader will broaden his or her understanding of what constitutes "research."
Although white coats and number crunching may be aspects of the stereotypical vision
of research, this volume continues to offer a veritable smorgasbord of legitimate, rigorous research options that may not fit the reader's preconceptions. As noted above, we
also hope to add a few planks across the chasm that divides researchers and clinicians.
Finally, we hope that the reader will learn a lot about each of the methods described.
Each chapter is designed to be a complete introduction to a particular method, and
most of the chapters are structured similarly. They begin with a description of the assumptions and the historical development of the method, and also detail the types of
questions typically addressed. Then the authors provide information on the data collection and analysis procedures. The chapters conclude with a discussion of the kinds
of skills needed to use the method, the strengths and weaknesses of the approach, and
thoughts regarding how the method can be used to bridge research and practice.

    The guidelines for chapter authors are reproduced in Table 1.1. We gave authors
the freedom to deviate somewhat from the outline when a chapter's topic was less
amenable to this structure. We also encouraged the authors to address issues of style as
well as substance, in order to make most of the chapters accessible to persons with

TABLE 1.1. Guidelines for Authors

In the guidelines below, we indicate suggestions for developing the chapters. While authors should feel free to diverge from these guidelines somewhat, their purpose is to help create a consistent, coherent volume.

I. BACKGROUND
  A. Creative Introduction
     Provide a creative introduction to your chapter that will "hook" the reader into wanting to know more. Make your introduction concrete and accessible to clinicians who have little formal training in research.

  B. Philosophical Assumptions
     What assumptions underlie the methodology? How do these assumptions shape the research? Be brief here. Just hit the highlights.

  C. Historical Roots and Development
     How did the methodology develop both within and without the field of family therapy?

II. METHODOLOGY
   In this section, we would like each author to weave at least one concrete example of the method into the abstract description. Whenever possible, this example should be from the author's own work. If currently there are no good examples of the methodology in the family therapy research literature or the author's own research efforts, the author should invent a research example to weave into the description.

  A. Research Questions
     What family therapy research questions does this methodology answer?

  B. Sampling and Selection Procedures
     What is important to consider in selecting participants for family therapy studies conducted with this methodology? How is selection accomplished?

  C. Data Collection Procedures
     What data collection procedures do researchers usually use? What factors are important to consider in collecting the data? How do researchers assess systemic variables? How are the data recorded and stored?

  D. Data Analysis Procedures
     What methods do researchers use to analyze the data? Give concrete examples in nontechnical language.

  E. Reporting
     How do researchers report the findings? What does a typical research report look like? Where might it be likely to be published?

III. DISCUSSION
   A. Strengths and Weaknesses of the Methodology
      What are the strengths and weaknesses of the methodology when applied to family therapy research?

   B. Reliability and Validity
      Discuss the relevance of the concepts of reliability and validity to your tradition/method. Are reliability and validity addressed by the tradition/method? If so, how? If not, why not?

   C. Skills
      What special skills are needed to plan, execute, and interpret this kind of research? What are the implications for training clinicians? Researchers?

   D. Bridging Research and Practice
      In what ways might this methodology contribute to bridging the research and practice communities? How might clinicians best become involved in the methodology? How might the results be made more accessible to clinicians?

   E. Future Directions
      What future directions would you suggest for this methodology in our field?

   F. Exemplars
      List in American Psychological Association style up to five articles that can serve as models for the use of your method in family therapy research.

modest research training. In addition, we asked them to provide concrete examples of the methods, as opposed to presenting abstract accounts. An added feature of the guidelines for this edition was that we asked authors to list several published exemplars, so that interested readers could read excellent examples of studies employing the methods.

A SPECIAL CHAPTER FOR GRADUATE STUDENTS

As in the first edition of this book (Dickey, 1996), we have included a special chapter for graduate students. Research is a new topic for many graduate students. In Chapter 2, "A Graduate Student Guide to Conducting Research in Marriage and Family Therapy," Lenore M. McWey, Ebony Joy James, and Sara A. Smock provide a useful insider's guide for graduate students who are just becoming acquainted with the family therapy research process. Their chapter includes advice "from inception to defense" on such topics as authorship credit; seeking institutional review board approval; and issues related to selecting research questions, methodology, sampling, data collection, and analysis. The advice comes from the authors themselves, as well as from researchers across the country, who responded to questions that McWey and her colleagues posted on a listserv sponsored by the AAMFT. There is a lot of wisdom in this chapter. It should be a useful resource to orient new students to many of the issues and expectations they will face in their graduate research training.

QUALITATIVE METHODS IN THIS VOLUME
Qualitative Methods Updated from the First Edition

Several of the chapters on qualitative methods have been updated from the first edition. For example, Silvia Echevarria-Doan and Carolyn Y. Tubbs have updated the previous chapter on grounded theory in the current Chapter 3, "Let's Get Grounded: Family Therapy Research and Grounded Theory." In the chapter, they discuss some of the more recent debates concerning "objectivist" traditional views of grounded theory in contrast to developing "constructivist" views. (In line with our own thesis, they make the case that there is a place for both views in the field of family therapy research.) Similarly, they expand on the strengths and weaknesses of grounded theory methodology, ways in which grounded theory bridges research and practice, and possible future directions of grounded theory methodology in family therapy research. Finally, the authors discuss a recent study examining client strengths and resources, to illustrate how the family therapy researcher might apply grounded theory data analysis and reporting.

Similarly, in "The Use of Phenomenology for Family Therapy Research: The Search for Meaning" (Chapter 4), Carla M. Dahl and Pauline Boss elaborate both historically and in terms of present applications. Historically, they explain that their assumptions about phenomenology are less connected to the transcendental models of Husserl and Heidegger (himself a Nazi), and more to the models of these men's students and successors, who "survived Nazism but were not sullied by it." Their interpretive phenomenology is one that appreciates perceived and socially constructed knowledge. They describe well what phenomenology is and is not, and have added a fascinating section on ethics that addresses some of the sticky issues involved in studying personal experiences.

In Chapter 5, "Focus Groups in Family Therapy Research," Fred P. Piercy and Katherine M. Hertlein expand on the previous edition's focus group chapter by adding relevant current literature (the use of focus groups in academic journals has increased threefold in recent years) and attending to relevant ethical issues related to group interviewing. Focus group research, initially developed to tap the thinking of consumers, is a flexible qualitative method that family therapists can use for a wide range of purposes, including needs assessment, intervention material development, marketing, program design, strategic planning, and formative and summative evaluation. Although focus groups and family therapy are clearly different processes, many family therapists, by virtue of their work, already possess some of the requisite skills of focus group facilitation (e.g., comfort with group interaction, the ability to invite discussion).

Emphasizing Participation, Action, and Change: Action Research

The "gold standard" for some qualitative methods is the degree to which they empower participants to address problems and change oppressive systems. In action research, the researcher values collaboration and applying indigenous knowledge over strict experimental controls. In Chapter 6, "Action Research Methods in Family Therapy," Tai J. Mendenhall and William J. Doherty not only describe the theory and practice of action research methods, but provide plenty of excellent examples. They highlight the power of collaborative partnerships with community participants to generate useful knowledge and to solve local problems. Rather than the traditional goal of research (i.e., bringing incremental understanding to a problem that might eventually benefit a larger population), action research emphasizes the importance of understanding that can be applied to real problems here and now.

More Sophisticated Ways to Manage Data: Computer-Aided Qualitative Data Analysis Software

As anyone who has conducted qualitative research knows, qualitative methods can generate a mountain of data. In Chapter 7, "Computer-Aided Qualitative Data Analysis Software: General Issues for Family Therapy Researchers," Jennifer L. Matheson reviews the strengths and limitations of current computer-aided qualitative data analysis software (CAQDAS). She discusses how CAQDAS can help qualitative family therapy researchers manage their data before, during, and after their analyses. According to Matheson, qualitative software is no panacea. At the same time, technology has advanced to the point where analysis software is becoming more user-friendly, accessible, and robust; it provides a means for the qualitative researcher to manipulate words, film clips, audio interviews, photographs, client-generated art, and more.

The increased use of CAQDAS flies in the face of some people's view of qualitative research as necessarily less technologically sophisticated than traditional quantitative research methods. As qualitative analysis procedures become more refined, and as CAQDAS provides a technological means of managing large amounts of data, it will be difficult to pigeonhole all qualitative researchers as "low-tech" in their methods.

Applying Findings: Translation Research

Carolyn Y. Tubbs and Linda M. Burton describe how researchers can extend the findings of their research to the general public in Chapter 8, "Bridging Research: Using Ethnography to Inform Clinical Practice." Specifically, they discuss "translation research," in which a researcher takes the essential features of effective evidence based practices and applies them to nonresearch settings. Tubbs and Burton illustrate the iterative process of translation research by describing how findings from a large, multisite ethnographic study generated cultural insights that helped them refine a parent management training model. Their chapter not only represents the logical application of qualitative research findings, but is a good example of how qualitative and quantitative findings can enrich each other, and consequently the lives of those we serve.

Research that Emphasizes Reflexivity, Critical Theory, and Aesthetic Methods of Data Representation

In this edition, we have also included qualitative methods that grow out of both critical and postmodern theory, and that focus on evolving standards of reflexivity and evocative impact. For example, Katherine R. Allen and Fred P. Piercy's chapter, "Feminist Autoethnography" (Chapter 9), applies both a critical and a reflexive stance to understanding and addressing oppression in human relationships. A feminist lens helps the researcher identify inequities and the larger systems that maintain them. A more personal, autoethnographic lens allows the researcher to go back and forth between inner vulnerable experience and outward social, historical, and cultural aspects of life, searching for deeper connections and understanding. The combination of feminism and autoethnography, according to the authors, offers a more fully human method of inquiry. Allen, in her own sharing, demonstrates the power of this method to "touch the soul."

Similarly, in Chapter 10 ("Performance Methodology: Constructing Discourses and Discursive Practices in Family Therapy Research"), Saliha Bava describes performance methodologies and alternative forms of data representations (poetry, split dialogues, hypertext, interpretive writing, collages) that blur the boundaries among academic writing, literature, and art. These methods extend interpretive qualitative research to include an evocative process of performance, community meaning making, and shared generative inquiry. And, like Allen and Piercy, Bava "walks the walk." Her chapter is itself an example of a performance in discourse construction and discursive practices in research.

Allen, Piercy, and Bava all push the boundaries of traditional research, both qualitative and quantitative. Some will say that what they present is not research. Our view is that there are many ways to understand a phenomenon, and that performance and reflexive autoethnography have something to offer our field. According to Bava, "to diverge is to create," and although autoethnography and performance may not meet the traditional standards of research, they do (when well done) meet the evolving standards involving reflexivity, aesthetics, and evocative power that we mention above.

What Directions Will Qualitative Methods Take?

In Chapter 11, "Future Directions for Qualitative Methods," Ronald J. Chenail reflects on what he calls the scientific, artistic, and participatory styles of qualitative research, and possible future directions for each. His chapter serves to introduce the reader to the increased use of the Internet and other emerging methods, such as autoethnography, portraiture, recursive frame analysis, the Zaltman Metaphor Elicitation Technique, metasynthesis, appreciative inquiry, and narrative inquiry. In doing so, Chenail invites us to consider new ways to think about qualitative research.

Similarly, we hope that our collection invites the reader to view qualitative research as a rainbow of evolving methods, many with varying goals and specifications. With these new methods come new ways to conceptualize and carry out family therapy research.

MIXED METHODS IN THIS VOLUME

The methods described in Part III of this book are neither inherently qualitative nor quantitative. Mixed methods often incorporate dimensions of both approaches, and allow the researcher to capitalize on the synergistic interplay between quantitative and qualitative approaches. Of course, more "pure" qualitative and quantitative methods can also be combined within the same study, so the mixed methods are not the only way to achieve this synergy.

Survey Research

In Chapter 12, Thorana S. Nelson and David D. Allred present a revision of the first edition's chapter on "Survey Research in Marriage and Family Therapy." They define survey research as a "method of collecting data from or about a group of people and asking questions in some fashion about things of interest to the researcher for the purpose of generalizing to a population represented by the group or sample" (p. 211). The data the researcher seeks can be qualitative or quantitative, and this choice has a considerable influence on the kinds of sampling used, the nature of the questions asked, and the ways data are analyzed and reported. There is considerable new material in this chapter, including detailed attention to use of the Internet in survey research.

The most clear-cut mixed method is probably the one described by Linda Stone Fish and Dean M. Busby in Chapter 13, "The Delphi Method." In every case we have seen in the family therapy literature, this method has combined a qualitative analysis of a panel of experts' responses to a series of open-ended questions with a quantitative analysis of the same panel's responses to the researcher's summary of the open-ended responses. The Delphi methodology enables the researcher to formulate a consensus about an issue in the field without the expense of bringing experts together physically; it has the added advantages of confidentiality and freedom from peer pressure or the undue influence of outspoken panel members. The authors note a number of new studies utilizing this method, which has become popular with students because it does not demand large samples, advanced statistical expertise, or vast financial resources.

Intensive Research

There are several approaches that focus on intensive examination of individual units of analysis, and they may use both qualitative and quantitative methods of data collection and data analysis. The first edition included chapters on "Case Study Research"

(Moon & Trepper, 1996) and "Methods for Single-Case Experiments in Family Therapy" (Dickey, 1996).

In this second edition, Chapter 14 by Brent Bradley and Susan M. Johnson covers "Task Analysis of Couple and Family Change Events." Task analysis is a method for intensive study of therapist and client behaviors that lead to change in therapy. Although outcome research is important, this form of process research will probably become increasingly significant, since it addresses the very practical question of what specifically is helpful or unhelpful in therapy. Bradley and Johnson carefully examine the key tasks and steps of two important events in emotionally focused therapy—blamer softening and the resolution of attachment injuries. We expect that this chapter may be a favorite among clinicians, since the results give some clear direction regarding what to do (or not to do) within sessions.

Program Evaluation

In this age of accountability, family therapists must be able to identify clear intervention goals and to evaluate whether or not they have reached these goals. The field of program evaluation science can help. In Chapter 15, "Program Evaluation Science and Family Therapy," Jay A. Mancini, Angela J. Huebner, Eric E. McCollum, and Lydia I. Marek introduce family therapy researchers to program evaluation and its possible applications to family intervention programs. They provide two examples of intervention programs and then illustrate how to evaluate them systematically. They suggest the use of a logic model that links needs identification and analysis, desired results, measurable indicators, activities, monitoring, and resources. Their suggestions should be helpful to family therapists wishing to evaluate an intervention program.

QUANTITATIVE METHODS IN THIS VOLUME

Experimental Research

The chapter in the first edition on experimental research has been rewritten as "Clinical Trials in Marriage and Family Therapy Research" (Chapter 16), by Kevin P. Lyness, Stephanie R. Walsh, and Douglas H. Sprenkle. Clinical trials use the basic experimental paradigm, which calls for a clear manipulation of an independent or treatment variable, the random assignment of subjects to experimental and control groups, and careful attention to keeping the experimental and control groups similar in all ways other than on the treatment variables. The chapter talks about the stages of clinical trials, makes important distinctions (e.g., the difference between efficacy research and effectiveness research), and emphasizes the importance of making the interventions transportable to real-world settings. Although randomized clinical trials have been criticized, they have also become the "gold standard" for wider audiences such as the government and health care providers, and the field of MFT will probably be judged by its success or failure with this method.

In Chapter 17, "Meta-Analysis in Family Therapy Research," Karen S. Wampler, Alan Reifman, and Julianne M. Serovich note that meta-analysis is an empirical method for summarizing different quantitative research investigations. It also has many advantages over the traditional narrative review of the literature based on statistical significance. The researcher uses a common metric, known as an "effect size," to examine standard increments of change across a number of studies. Although it is not limited to experimental research, meta-analysis has been used most often in family therapy to summarize the effectiveness of interventions when grouped by such categories as model of therapy. In this revised chapter, the authors report on the proliferation of studies using this technique in the past decade, and note exciting new developments in this evolving method. Although the method is not without its critics, it has gained acceptance as one of the most useful methods for establishing treatment efficacy.

Another chapter on a method that is not limited to experimental research—Chapter 20, "Multilevel Growth Modeling in the Context of Family Research"—deserves mention here (see "Advanced Quantitative Methods in This Volume," below). Researchers can incorporate this advanced technique into clinical trial research to determine family members' trajectories of change, and to help ascertain why some members get better and some get worse.

Economic Evaluation Methodology

In Chapter 18, "Economic Evaluation Methodology for Family Therapy Outcome Research," David P. Mackinnon makes a strong case for the need to demonstrate the economic benefit as well as the effectiveness of treatments. In this extensive revision, he shows how cost-effectiveness research (the term that was used in the title of the chapter in the first edition) is only one aspect of a full economic evaluation of treatment. The new chapter also presents a more sophisticated methodology that is tailor-made for the target audience of the economic evaluation. In addition, the chapter shows the extent to which economic evaluations have been applied to many more family therapy studies in the past decade, even though the method is still underutilized. We support Mackinnon's belief that a major benefit of family therapy may be its economic advantages over other modalities.

Relational/Predictive Research

Relational/predictive research describes the relationships between/among variables and/or ways to predict variables from the knowledge of other variables. Analytical techniques used range from simple correlation and regression to such complex procedures as structural equation modeling.

In Chapter 19, "Approaches to Prediction: Correlation, Regression, and Classification Techniques," Douglas K. Snyder and Laurel F. Mangrum describe the use of correlation and related techniques to examine factors that contribute to marital stress and couples' responses to marital therapy. The presentation of methodology is divided into two major sections. The first, "Basic Techniques," describes correlation, regression, partial and semipartial correlations, and multiple regression. The second section, "Advanced Techniques," introduces the reader to canonical-correlation analysis, multiple-discriminant-function analysis, and (new to this revision) cluster analysis. The authors have also updated their citations of literature and have included references to new software packages.

Although included in the special section (Part V) on "Advanced Quantitative Methods" (see below), Chapter 21 on "Covariance Structure Analysis: From Path Analysis to Structural Equation Modeling" merits mention here, since it focuses on ways to study the complex relationships among multiple variables.

ADVANCED QUANTITATIVE METHODS IN THIS VOLUME

In this edition, we have included two chapters by Margaret K. Keiley and colleagues that focus exclusively on advanced quantitative techniques at the cutting edge of family therapy research. They are intended primarily for doctoral-level students and graduates, or for those trained at the master's level who have strong quantitative backgrounds and interests. Unlike most of the other chapters, they assume prior knowledge of intermediate statistical concepts. However, the authors have also used many concrete illustrations throughout their treatment of these methods to make the material come alive. If read slowly and carefully, these chapters, though challenging, will be rewarding. They are especially valuable for those readers who want a state-of-the-art understanding of where quantitative clinical science is going.

In Chapter 20, "Multilevel Growth Modeling in the Context of Family Research," Margaret K. Keiley, Nina C. Martin, Ting Liu, and Megan Dolbin-MacNab demonstrate how this method can be utilized to address how family members get better, get worse, or remain the same over time. Multilevel growth modeling also addresses the issues of why some family members grow differently and why some get better and some get worse. They illustrate the method though a careful analysis of the response to treatment of 123 women with drug addictions and their partners. Since this method is longitudinal, it should be of great value to a field with an inherent interest in the course of treatment results over time.

In Chapter 21, "Covariance Structure Analysis: From Path Analysis to Structural Equation Modeling," Margaret K. Keiley, Mary Dankoski, Megan Dolbin-MacNab, and Ting Liu describe one of the most powerful tools for answering the kinds of complex questions that arise in family research. Since family relationships are complex and multifaceted, the researcher needs complex statistical techniques to examine the relationships among variables and to determine the ways in which certain sets of variables predict other sets of variables. For example, do emotional support and sexual communication predict marital satisfaction, and to what extent are these predictor variables mediated by sexual satisfaction? This is but one of many concrete examples used by the authors to guide the reader through the different types of covariance structure analyses, such as path analysis, confirmatory factor analysis, and structural equation modeling. Although these methods are somewhat challenging to learn, they should have long-term payoffs for the MFT field, given our need to study the complex nature of family life.

SOME FINAL THOUGHTS ON APPROACHING THIS VOLUME

Although research can sometimes feel like a daunting enterprise, we hope that this book conveys the authors' enthusiasm and passion for these methods. We also hope that the book will help to demystify the research process somewhat. For students, we would certainly suggest beginning with Chapter 2 by McWey and colleagues; it is written in a way that is user-friendly and nonthreatening. For those new to quantitative research, Chapter 16 by Lyness and colleagues on clinical trials might be a good jumping-off point, followed by Chapter 17 by Wampler and colleagues on meta-analysis. For those new to qualitative research, a good entry point might be Chapter 5 by Piercy and Hertlein on focus groups, or Chapter 3 by Echevarria-Doan and Tubbs on grounded theory methods. These four chapters are especially clear exemplars of the quantitative and qualitative paradigms, respectively, and assume little prior knowledge. To get a feel for the mixed methods, we suggest Chapter 14 by Bradley and Johnson on task analysis, which is also clinician-friendly. Almost all of the chapters are self-contained, so we hope that readers will be guided by their interests rather than by the invariant order of our table of contents.

We hope that the book, approached in this way, will make the research enterprise more exciting for clinicians. There are really few questions a clinician might ask that are not amenable to research—provided that one allows for the kind of methodological pluralism set forth here. As promised, we have provided a smorgasbord of methodological options for doing family therapy research. We hope you will enjoy the feast!

REFERENCES

Acock, A., van Dulmen, M., Allen, K., & Piercy, F. (2005). Contemporary and emerging research methods in studying families. In V. Bengtson, K. Allen, A. Acock, P. Dilworth-Anderson, & D. Klein (Eds.), *Sourcebook of family theory and research* (pp. 59–85). Thousand Oaks, CA: Sage.

Anderson, W. T. (1990). *Reality isn't what it used to be*. New York: Harper & Row.

Atkinson, B., Heath, A., & Chenail, R. (1991). Qualitative research and the legitimization of knowledge. *Journal of Marital and Family Therapy, 17*, 161–166.

Bischoff, R. J., McKeel, A. J., Moon, S. M., & Sprenkle, D. H. (1996). Systematically developing therapeutic techniques: Applications of research and development. In D. H. Sprenkle & S. M. Moon (Eds.), *Research methods in family therapy* (pp. 429–443). New York: Guilford Press.

Broderick, C. B., & Schrader, S. S. (1981). The history of professional marriage and family therapy. In A. S. Gurman & D. P. Kniskern (Eds.), *Handbook of family therapy* (pp. 5–35). New York: Brunner/Mazel.

Cavell, T. A., &. Snyder, D. A. (1991). Iconoclasm versus innovation: Building a science of family therapy—comments on Moon, Dillon, and Sprenkle. *Journal of Marital and Family Therapy, 17*, 181–185.

Crane, D. R., Wampler, K. S., Sprenkle, D. H., Sandberg, J. G., & Hovestadt, A. J. (2002). The scientist-practitioner model in marriage and family therapy doctoral programs. *Journal of Marital and Family Therapy, 28*, 75–83.

Dickey, M. H. (1996). Methods for single-case experiments in family therapy. In D. H. Sprenkle & S. M. Moon (Eds.), *Research methods in family therapy* (pp. 264–285). New York: Guilford Press.

Gergen, K. (1991). *The saturated self: Dilemmas of identity in contemporary life*. New York: Basic Books.

Greenberg, L. S., Heatherington, L., & Friedlander, M. L. (1996). The events-based approach to couple and family therapy research. In D. H. Sprenkle & S. M. Moon (Eds.), *Research methods in family therapy* (pp. 411–428). New York: Guilford Press.

Gurman, A. S. (1983). Family therapy research and the "new epistemology." *Journal of Marital and Family Therapy, 9*, 227–234.

Haley, J. (1978). Ideas which handicap therapists. In M. M. Berger (Ed.), *Beyond the double bind: Communication and family systems, theories, and techniques with schizophrenics* (pp. 301–327). New York: Brunner/Mazel.

Langsley, D., Flomenhaft, K., & Machotka, P. (1969). Follow-up evaluation of family crisis therapy. *American Journal of Orthopsychiatry, 39*, 753–759.

Minuchin, S., Baker, L., Rosman, B., Liebman, R., Milman, L., & Todd, T. (1975). A conceptual model of psychosomatic illness in children. *Archives of General Psychiatry, 32,* 1031–1038.

Moon, S. M., Dillon, D. R., & Sprenkle, D. H. (1990). Family therapy and qualitative research. *Journal of Marital and Family Therapy, 16,* 357–373.

Moon, S. M., & Trepper, T. S. (1996). Case study research. In D. H. Sprenkle & S. M. Moon (Eds.), *Research methods in family therapy* (pp. 393–410). New York: Guilford Press.

Nichols, M. P., & Schwartz, R. C. (Eds.). (1995). *Family therapy: Concepts and methods* (3rd ed.). Boston: Allyn & Bacon.

Patton, M. (2002). *Qualitative research in evaluation methods* (3rd ed.). Thousand Oak, CA: Sage.

Piercy, F., & Benson, K. (in press). Aesthetic forms of data representation in qualitative family therapy research. *Journal of Marital and Family Therapy.*

Piercy, F., McWey, L., Tice, S., James, E., Morris, M., & Arthur, K. (in press). It was the best of times, it was the worst of times: Exploring graduate students' experiences of research training through alternative forms of data analysis. *Family Process.*

Pinsof, W. M. (1981). Family therapy process research. In A. S. Gurman & D. P. Kniskern (Eds.), *Handbook of family therapy* (pp. 699–741). New York: Brunner Mazel.

Snyder, D. K., & Rice, J. L. (1996). Methodological issues and strategies in scale development. In D. H. Sprenkle & S. M. Moon (Eds.), *Research methods in family therapy* (pp. 216–237). New York: Guilford Press.

Sprenkle, D. H. (Ed.). (2002). *Effectiveness research in marriage and family therapy.* Alexandria, VA: American Association for Marriage and Family Therapy.

Sprenkle, D. H. (2003). Effectiveness research in marriage and family therapy: Introduction. *Journal of Marital and Family Therapy, 29,* 85–96.

Sprenkle, D. H., Bailey, C. E., Lyness, K., Ball, D., & Mills, S. (1997). Submission patterns to the archival journal of the profession of MFT. *Journal of Marital and Family Therapy, 23,* 371–380.

Sprenkle, D. H., & Bischoff, R. J. (1995). Research in family therapy: Trends, issues, and recommendations. In M. P. Nichols &. R. C. Schwartz (Eds.), *Family therapy: Concepts and methods* (3rd ed., pp. 485–521). Boston: Allyn & Bacon.

Sprenkle, D. H., & Moon, S. M. (1996). Toward pluralism in family therapy research. In D. H. Sprenkle & S. M. Moon (Eds.), *Research methods in family therapy* (pp. 3–19). New York: Guilford Press.

Tomm, K. (1983, July–August). The old hat doesn't fit. *The Family Therapy Networker,* pp. 39–41.

Volk, R. J., & Flori, D. E. (1996). Structural equation modeling. In D. H. Sprenkle & S. M. Moon (Eds.), *Research methods in family therapy* (pp. 336–387). New York: Guilford Press.

Wynne, L. C. (1983). Family research and family therapy: A reunion? *Journal of Marital and Family Therapy, 9,* 113–117.

CHAPTER 2

A Graduate Student Guide
to Conducting Research in Marriage
and Family Therapy

LENORE M. McWEY
EBONY JOY JAMES
SARA A. SMOCK

When reflecting upon what it is like to be a graduate student researcher, one of us (EJJ) has said:

"When I think about it, I can't help but feel that I voluntarily got on one of the largest roller coasters in the world without meeting the height requirements. What better way to get my adrenalin pumping, or so I thought. I know where I started, but I don't know where I will end. Wait! 'Have a nice ride,' my advisor says. I am not so sure I am ready. Too late . . . the higher I go, the harder it is to see the people on the ground where I started, and all I can hear is the click, click, clicking of the roller coaster. It gets louder and louder the closer to the top I get. Then all of a sudden there is silence, and there is nothing else left to do but SCREAM. When asked to make research observations from a roller-coaster seat, I cannot help but focus on my own anxiety about the ride itself."

Sprenkle and colleagues (Sprenkle, 2002a) have charged our field with the task of engaging in research that would secure a spot for the field of marriage and family therapy (MFT) in the mental health profession. Although this charge may seem like an overwhelming task for a graduate student, research does not have to be as unpredictable as a roller coaster. The purpose of this chapter is to serve as a guide for MFT graduate students who conduct research. Other chapters throughout this book provide readers with specific information about a variety of research methodologies. However, in this chapter we share general suggestions for students to consider before they get on the research roller coaster. We surveyed researchers in MFT by posting a question on the American Association for Marriage and Family Therapy (AAMFT) research listserv. We asked for any advice that researchers would like to share with students embarking upon MFT research. We assured respondents that we would protect their anonymity; thus names are not associated with their statements. We have quoted many of their thoughts throughout this chapter. The chapter begins with a discussion about the background of MFT research and its methods. Then we present some "insiders' tips" for pursuing research, followed by a section on how to complete a thesis or dissertation. The chapter ends with a discussion about bridging the scientist–practitioner gap, as well as about the current state of research in the field of MFT.

BACKGROUND

Philosophical Assumptions and History

Olson (1976) wisely noted almost 30 years ago that in order to be truly systemic in our focus, we family therapists must be able to integrate research, theory, and clinical practice in everyday work. Nichols (1979) reported that the field of MFT seemed to demonstrate the largest deficit in the research arena, in comparison to theory and clinical practice. In order for the field to develop a solid identity, Nichols suggested that therapists strengthen and maintain the essential relationship between research and theory in the study and practice of MFT.

Several years later, a special issue of the *Journal of Marital and Family Therapy*, "The Effectiveness of Marital and Family Therapy" (Pinsof & Wynne, 1995a), provided the field with an inspection of the state of MFT research. This major compilation of research remains a landmark issue of the journal and holds a permanent place in the history of the MFT field. Conclusions derived from the collection of research suggested that generally MFT is better than no treatment at all, but that "there are no scientific data at this time to support the superiority of any particular form of marital or family therapy over any other" (Pinsof & Wynne, 1995b, p. 604). The special issue's editors went on to conclude:

> These positive conclusions must be tempered by a variety of methodological problems with the research. The body of scientific research underlying the field of marital and family therapy needs to continue to grow and improve methodologically and conceptually. (Pinsof & Wynne, 1995b, p. 610)

As we enter the 21st century, evidence-based practice has become more visible and widely practiced (Denton & Walsh, 2001). Managed care companies' requirements that services be effective and cost-efficient have assisted in the development of this trend, out of the emphasis on accountability and quality assurance for services to patients (Waehler, Kalodner, Wampold, & Lichtenberg, 2000). MFT practitioners must be informed and knowledgeable about practice standards and maintain a high level of competence, so that clients and third-party payers alike will find these services valuable and effective (Denton & Walsh, 2001).

MFT, as a field, has benefited from methodological advances as well. Over the past several years, there has been "a dramatic increase in the use of qualitative research methods" (Elliot, Fischer, & Rennie, 1999, p. 215). These advancements have lead some to conclude that researchers have moved beyond the quantitative–qualitative debate, to a recognition that both types of inquiry are useful in making meaningful contributions to our field (Ambert, Adler, Adler, & Detzner, 1995).

A further collection of effectiveness research in MFT has recently been published (Sprenkle, 2002a). Sprenkle (2002b) asserts, "To be sure, the evidence across all the arenas reviewed here is uneven and certain topics/approaches remain empirically underdeveloped. Nonetheless, the overall picture of regarding the science of MFT has, in my judgment, improved quite dramatically" (p. 9). However, Sprenkle (2002b) cautions us to recognize that the field of MFT must address a number of challenges "if we are serious about bridging the disastrous gap between researchers and clinicians that continues to plague the field" (p. 23). If MFT is going to be a viable mental health profession and compete for mental health resources, research—whether qualitative or quantitative—is necessary to document the current state of the field and to better understand the clinical practices of therapists and the clients they serve (Northey, 2002).

INSIDERS' TIPS FOR PURSUING RESEARCH

Getting Started

If you are an MFT graduate student who is unfamiliar with the research process, the first question that may enter your mind is "Well, even if I wanted to do research, how would I start?" You may want to consider a number of factors before electing to ride the research roller coaster. One MFT researcher shared that an important first step is to "learn how to be a good consumer (reader) of research." This includes being able to identify which studies have clear research questions, clear theories guiding the research, and clear procedures, as well as being able to distinguish between the different methodologies and epistemologies that guide research approaches. Another researcher advised, "Read a variety of journal articles and meet with others to discuss them." Reading and talking about good research will give you a sense of what good research looks like. It will also give you ideas for your own research questions and design.

A third tip a researcher shared was this: "Have students work with people doing research—either as a research assistant, or just to tag along with another faculty person and to interview that person about what he or she does." Yet another respondent suggested, "Help them learn about researchers' passions and motivations in doing research." As you think about working with a professor on his or her research, consider the following: Does the topic interest you? Does the study employ methods that you would like to learn more about? What will you gain by being a participant in the project? Whether or not you decide to work with someone already conducting research, you may want to identify a mentor to help guide you through the research process. Since faculty members are readily accessible to students, choosing a professor is a logical option. You may also decide to work with a peer who possesses more research experience than yourself. When choosing a mentor, you may want to consider the type of research the potential mentor conducts, as well as his or her topics of interest and work styles.

Authorship

If you decide to work with peers or faculty members on a research endeavor, be sure to address the question of authorship early in the process. Although this may be an awkward topic, discussing authorship at the beginning of a project may prevent misunderstandings, hurt feelings, or bigger problems down the road. According to the American

Psychological Association (APA, 2001, p. 6), "authorship is reserved for people who make a primary contribution to and hold primary responsibility for the data, concepts, and interpretation of results for a published work." In addition to discussing authorship, it may be helpful to discuss responsibilities. It is important to delineate specific expectations for different research team members. For example, if a research team designates a particular individual as first author, and if that individual neglects his or her responsibilities to the research team, be sure to discuss beforehand what you as a group are to do in that situation. For more specific ideas on determining authorship credit, see Fine and Kurdek (1993).

Research Questions

Defining research questions is an important first step in the research process. Try to conduct research on a topic that you find interesting. One MFT researcher commented, "If the research is interesting, it will make it easier for them [students] to get through the tough times." Thus it may be important to identify something about the project that will sustain you (e.g., "I'm learning how to do process research," "So this is what they mean by 'coding data,'" This should get me a good recommendation letter"). If you work with faculty members on their research, you may not be able to help choose the research topic. Thus, if you do not find the topic interesting, imagine the difficulty you may have completing a 6-month project you don't enjoy.

Dickey (1996) asserts that when you are trying to decide upon a research topic, you can ask yourself the following six questions to help guide you:

1. What is it you are interested in doing/finding out? What is the big question?
2. Why are you interested in doing this? What is so important about this topic/question?
3. How does your research relate to what is already known? What does the literature tell us?
4. How does this research differ from and/or extend previous research? What knowledge is likely to result?
5. How are you going to do this? What is the method and, possibly, the design?
6. What do you expect to find? What are the hypothesized results? (p. 193)

Chenail (1990) succinctly summarizes: "If you have a curiosity about research, scratch it" (p. 1).

Beyond an interesting question is the feasibility of the project. As one of our respondents put it, how "do-able" is the project that you envision? Make sure that your research question is one that can be answered. Asking, "Should therapists use evidence-based practice models in treatment?" is different from asking, "Is emotionally focused therapy (EFT) effective with families with truant teenagers?" The difference is that the first question is not easily answered and allows for value judgments, whereas the second question is researchable. As you think about your research interests, try to formulate a research question that is possible to answer. Additional things to think about as you formulate your research question include these: Does the question make a contribution to existing knowledge? Is the question clear? Is the question ethical? Is it important?

You may not be able to answer all of your questions in one study. That is okay. In fact, it is sometimes desirable to have one project be a springboard for future projects. If it seems that one endeavor may open possibilities for further research, ask yourself whether this is a research trajectory that you would like to pursue. Beginning to think about your research as "a vision of scholarship across one's career" (to quote another respondent) may help you think about how one project logically leads to another. This creates a knowledge base upon which you can continually build.

Theoretical Orientation

What theory or theories guide your research question? Attend to the interrelatedness of theory and the constructs in your study. How is theory captured in your research, and how will it be incorporated into your methods? For example, if you hypothesize that family therapy will be more effective than individual treatment in reducing depressive symptomatology, ask yourself, "What theory guides the interventions I will test?" Is it because you assume that differentiation is best achieved in the context of Bowenian family systems theory? Furthermore, consider the weaknesses of the theory or theories you use. For example, if you are using a Bowenian theoretical approach, attend to criticisms of the theory, such as the feminist critique of differentiation (Horne & Hicks, 2002; Knudson-Martin, 2002).

In addition, explore the existing literature on your research topic. What theory or theories have guided previous research? Discover what studies have already been conducted and areas that authors have suggested for future research. What are the deficiencies in the existing body of knowledge in your area of interest? Are there methodological deficiencies? Has all of the research been quantitative, or is some of it qualitative? In what ways can you contribute to what is already known?

Methodology

We ask that you please refer to the other chapters in this book for more information about specific methods. However, there are general methodological factors to consider as you navigate the research process. You can ask yourself whether you want to do a qualitative or quantitative project, or both, or neither. Chenail (1990, p. 1) asks, "Have you shopped the research market?", and asserts that there may be more research methods than there are researchers. Both quantitative and qualitative research are valued by the field of MFT (Faulkner, Klock, & Gale, 2002). So ask yourself which methodology you prefer, or which you want to learn more about. One MFT researcher recommended that students engage in both quantitative and qualitative research. She advised that a student conducting a survey use both closed- and open-ended questions.

Another researcher suggested that a different way to determine which approach to research you should take is to say, "This is a question that's important. What methodology would best address it?" Know what kind of question you are trying to answer. Quantitative research seeks to test hypotheses, make causal explanations, and generalize across samples (Elliot et al., 1999). Conversely, the intent of qualitative research is to understand the meaning of people's experiences (Ambert et al., 1995). Regardless of the methodology chosen, one MFT researcher stressed the importance of remembering that you should pay "careful attention to theory, design, sampling, measurement, [and] analysis," because each of these things affects the others.

If you are conducting a quantitative study, select a topic and identify your independent and dependent variables. Then try to operationalize terms within the research question. If, for example, your question is "Is EFT effective with families with truant teenagers?", what is meant by "EFT" for the purposes of this study? Does it mean therapy conducted by therapists trained by Dr. Susan Johnson in EFT, or does it mean therapy conducted by students who have had an EFT course? How will adherence to EFT be measured? Also, what is meant by the term "effective"? Does effectiveness mean lower scores on the Beck Depression Inventory? Does it mean clients' self-reports of improvement? How will you capture what it is you seek to discover? It is helpful to choose variables that are clear and measurable (e.g., if effectiveness is defined in terms of decreased depression, the Beck Depression Inventory can be used to measure this).

Ambert and colleagues (1995) assert that it is important to remember that qualitative research is not always a clear sequence of events, as quantitative research commonly is. However, Elliot and colleagues (1999) asserts that you should be careful to recognize a dangerous kind of qualitative research—the "no-method" type (p. 218). In other words, it is important to determine and be explicit about the type of qualitative research you will conduct and the procedures you will follow to guide you in the process (Ambert et al., 1995). One of our respondents recommended that you "have a working design," or a preliminary plan by which you hope to execute your study.

Hypotheses are not the same in qualitative research as they are in quantitative methods. In many instances, qualitative research may be cyclical as opposed to linear. You may start the research process with a general research question, then modify the hypothesis as data are collected. A strength of qualitative research is in the richness of the data and the ability to describe a phenomenon in great detail.

If the traditional quantitative or qualitative studies do not appeal to you, some researchers have suggested broadening how you view the research process. One researcher described an MFT program that has intentionally attempted to be more integrative in its approach to research:

> "We're talking to our students about considering research as a part of practice, rather than just kind of [an] adjunct set of skills or a way to do . . . research for a dissertation or how to read a research article. . . . So, given that, it makes more sense for us to think in terms of research being more of a participatory action type of research which involves studying something, and doing something immediately with it, rather than just adding to the repository of knowledge and wisdom. We want our students to approach research as an action step in the course of doing family therapy."

Another MFT researcher shared that she is excited about research she has been reviewing lately, because "in their methodology, people are experimenting, they're stretching, they're bending the rules." (Of course, it is important to remember that Picasso bent the rules of art only after he mastered those rules!) This researcher further asserted that creativity does not mean a lack of rigor; she stated that as a reviewer she is "very tough on the systematic part, and we're very dedicated to the rigor part."

Sampling and Selection Process

Before contacting potential participants, you must obtain approval from the appropriate authorities to conduct the study. If you are a graduate student, you will need to get approval from your university's institutional review board (IRB) for human subjects. If you are conducting your study at an agency, approval from the agency may also be required.

The sample for your study will have a major impact on your results and your ability to draw conclusions. Defining the population of interest for your study will determine your sampling frame. In quantitative research, you want to be able to make your sample truly representative of your population of interest. In order to do this, you will need to attend to the number of participants necessary to achieve the power to detect differences within your study. For example, if you are interested in the outcome of all truant high schoolers engaged in family therapy across the United States, your sample would then encompass a much broader range than if your population consisted of truant high school students in family therapy within a specific area of the country. Random sampling is generally considered the best sampling strategy, but this can be complicated, expensive, and sometimes impossible (e.g., if you want to study participants receiving a specific family therapy treatment). When random sampling is not feasible, other sampling strategies can be employed. For example, you can ask family therapists to refer clients to you for your study; you can consider using the facility where you are currently conducting therapy as a source for clients; or you can advertise in newspapers or other media.

If, however, you are interested in gaining a deeper understanding of a specific phenomenon, you will be more interested in spending longer periods of time with a smaller number of participants than in focusing on obtaining a large sample size (Ambert et al., 1995). For qualitative studies, "resources, time, depth, and purpose of the research place practical limitations on sample size requirements" (Ambert et al., 1995, p. 886). When you obtain saturation, or when trends in the data begin to recur, then you can stop adding new participants to their sample. In qualitative research, you want to capture the experiences of those whom you seek to understand. For example, if you are interested in understanding the impact of differing ethnicities upon the therapeutic relationship, then interviewing only Hispanics does not capture a range of differing ethnicities and does not allow you to understand what you sought to explore.

Measurement

Deciding how you are going to collect data is one of the most important aspects of conducting your study. If instruments are going to be used, then a number of factors must be considered. What instrument would be the best means of collecting data to answer the research question? Do previously developed measures exist? What are their psychometric properties, and upon what group or groups were they standardized? How expensive are the measures? If you plan to use observation to collect data, will there be more than one observer? How will interobserver agreement be reached?

After you have determined your measures, pilot-test your method for collecting data. When one of us (LMM, the "I" in this anecdote) was a student, I had the opportunity to engage in a large-scale research project. A peer, a faculty member, and I diligently prepared a survey to be sent to 800 potential respondents. The survey was disseminated via mail; therefore, we spent a great deal of money on postage. We felt great elation, both when we put the surveys in the mail and when we received our first response much sooner than we anticipated. However, our elation quickly turned to horror when we opened the envelope: The respondent indicated that she could not complete the survey because the items were aligned improperly, making it difficult for her to select responses. Although we had pilot-tested the survey, we had accidentally copied an earlier draft of the instrument. Needless to say, our response rate was low, and we remained at the mercy of the participants—who, to our embarrassment, had to draw arrows indicating which response went with which item. We promise that it is much better to have mistakes noticed during the pilot-testing phase than after the project is in full swing!

You may also want to seek advice from nonacademic clinicians. By doing so, you may be able to identify barriers to your research before you encounter them. For example, one student was interested in exploring the relationship between maternal depression and their children's cognitive capabilities. The student then received permission from the facility where she was planning to collect her data. But before launching the project, she met with the employees of the facility and discussed the idea and design of her research. In this meeting, the employees pointed out several important factors that she might want to consider before beginning her research. One suggestion regarded participant recruitment. The researcher had planned to recruit participants when they dropped their children off at the facility. However, the employees wisely noted that the parents seemed in a hurry to get to work when dropping off their children, and instead suggested that the researcher attend a parent–teacher group meeting to solicit participation. The suggestion made by the employees helped the student to recruit a sufficient sample size to proceed with her study. Discuss your plan with as many people as you can; by doing so, you may be able to avoid potential pitfalls.

Data Analysis

Although the approach to data analysis varies from method to method, several general aspects of such analysis must be considered. Generally speaking, data analysis "looks for patterns in what is observed" (Babbie, 1998, p. 24). But how these patterns are derived will differ, depending on the methods you use in your research.

If your study is a quantitative study, the measurement level of your data will dictate what you can and cannot do. For example, if you have nominal-level data, you will not be able to run regressions, correlations, and the like. If you have interval-level data, you will have more options in your statistical analyses. Don't be afraid to seek guidance in analysis. One particular reference that you may find helpful is Green and Salkind's (2003) user-friendly guide to conducting analyses in SPSS.

One MFT researcher stated, "If a student does qualitative research, an important point to remember is the reflexive position of the researcher, meaning that the biases and opinions of the researcher influence the research, no matter how objective the researcher tries to be." In qualitative analysis, bias can be introduced through the researcher. Revealing your perspective is an important way to enhance the credibility of your research (Ambert et al., 1995; Elliot et al., 1999). For example, if you are studying divorce and you have experienced a divorce in your own family, it will be important to be overt about the meanings you have made of divorce in relation to your personal experience, and to indicate how these may influence your interpretation of the data (Elliot et al., 1999).

Reliability and Validity

If you conduct a quantitative study, then "reliability" refers to the consistency of the data obtained, and "validity" means the accuracy of the findings. There are several different types of validity in quantitative research, including face validity, criterion-related validity, construct validity, and content validity, all of which influence the quality of your study (Babbie, 1998). One professor used to depict issues of reliability and validity through an example of a person's shoe size and reading level. The example was this: Dr. Smartypants sought to discover predictors of the ability to read, and found that shoe size was a strong correlate of reading level. The study proved to be reliable, in that every other researcher who replicated it found the very same thing. Yet the findings were spurious, because shoe size is more of an indicator of age than it is of reading level—and of course the older a person is, the better his or her reading level generally is. If Dr. Smartypants had controlled for age in his study, then the correlation between reading level and shoe size would probably disappear.

If you conduct a qualitative study, then issues of reliability and validity are quite different. Trustworthiness of the data in qualitative research approximates "reliability" in quantitative terms (Elliot et al., 1999). Explaining the context of the research, cycling between the interpretation and data, and grounding interpretations with examples all strengthen trustworthiness. "Validity" in qualitative research refers to the trustworthiness of the *interpretations* of the data made by the researchers. This type of trustworthiness equates with objectivity, dependability, credibility/authenticity, and transferability of the results. Efforts to compare the interpretations you make and participants' views, often called "triangulation," demonstrate validity in qualitative research (Ambert et al., 1995). This can be done through member checks, comparing data from different sources, and/or having multiple researchers code data.

Finding Funding

There are various funding possibilities for student research. Dissertation grants, federal funding, and foundations are all possible sources that you may explore. You can search the Internet for possibilities, or you can find out whether your institution has a funding database that you can search. When you search a database (such as Foundation Directory OnLine), try using a combination of terms including "dissertation," "thesis," and "student," but be aware that you may also be eligible for funding that is not specifically designated for student researchers. Therefore, try doing a general search with the keywords from your topic of interest (e.g., "domestic violence," "family counseling"), then explore the eligibility criteria related to any "hits" that you generate from your search. Don't be afraid to contact people at a potential funding source. By doing so, you may be able to get important answers, and you may also glean hints that might give you a better chance of funding. An idea that an MFT researcher shared with us is to "attend grant training workshops."

Regarding funding, another MFT researcher noted: "Quantitative research is more likely to be funded by federal funding agencies than qualitative research." We asked one team of qualitative researchers how they would suggest finding funding for qualitative projects. They responded:

"There are places where you can get funding for qualitative research, but that's a good question, because one of the dimensions of the kinds of research that we've been conducting in the community is that it's not done through funding from external sources. It's done with people in the local area, committing their time and efforts to work with the local people, so there may be some local funding—but these are by definition not large, nationwide survey-type things that require money. And we have to get smart about what happens after the funding stops . . .

just because you have a hot-shot grant from the federal government means nothing after the grant runs out to the local people."

Writing Up Your Study

As your project nears completion, authorship has (let's hope) been discussed, and you are ready to work toward submitting your work for publication. The first thing you may want to do is to determine your target journal. Then see whether any articles about a similar topic have been published in the journal in which you are hoping to publish. If so, you certainly want to cite them. Visit the target journal's website or refer to the journal itself for author instructions. Adhere to those instructions as you write your manuscript.

One error that many students make is in formatting tables. The APA publishes a book entitled *Presenting Your Findings: A Practical Guide to Creating Tables* (Nicol & Pexman, 1999), which provides examples of how to present data in APA format. Another common source of manuscript errors is the reference list. One professor, in order to check references, requires that manuscripts be submitted to her unbound. She then separates the reference list from the body of the manuscript; as she reads, she checks off the references on the list, ensuring that all references cited in the text are included in the list and are in APA format.

Although each journal is unique, generally when you submit your article to a peer-reviewed journal, the editor will first determine whether your submission is appropriate for the journal. If it is, the editor will then send copies of your manuscript to reviewers. The reviewers will not be provided with the names of the authors and will evaluate the study based on criteria established for the journal. Although the time for responses from editors varies from journal to journal, it will typically take at least 3 months before you hear about the fate of your manuscript. The decision is likely to take one of three forms: The manuscript is accepted with minor revisions, must be revised and resubmitted, or is rejected altogether. If when you get your decision letter your article's fate is "accepted with minor revisions," congratulate yourself and your research teammates, and go out to celebrate your accomplishment. If you receive a "revise and resubmit" letter, then you will be required to make the changes that the reviewers have identified and resubmit the manuscript, which will in turn be re-reviewed by the original reviewers. In addition, when you resubmit your article, you will need to enclose a letter specifying what changes have been made and where in the manuscript these changes are located. If the editorial decision is a rejection, however, you should study the reviewers' feedback to see how you might improve the article. You may also want to ask a trusted professor for honest feedback on the potential publishability of the article. Then, if you decide to do so, make the needed changes and try again by submitting your article to another journal—perhaps one with a higher acceptance rate.

HOW TO COMPLETE A THESIS OF DISSERTATION, FROM INCEPTION TO DEFENSE

"Thesis," "dissertation," and "all but dissertation (ABD)" are words that can cause any graduate student to have a panic attack. "What am I going to do?" and "How am I going to do it?" are commonly asked questions. In this section, we summarize steps in the thesis/dissertation process.

Take a Deep Breath and Relax

Writing a thesis or dissertation is a lot of work and will not be completed overnight. Accepting the inevitable fact that research is a lengthy developmental process will put everything into perspective. Though you may find it hard to believe at this point, writing a thesis or dissertation will probably be the best educational experience of your life—enjoy it.

Brainstorm Topics

Think about what you are interested in, and do some research on various related topics. Don't limit yourself too much in the beginning. Be open to a few different topics or areas. Sometimes the best thesis/dissertation ideas are discovered in the process of researching another topic. One person we know came up with his dissertation topic by reading articles that appealed to him in the top-tier journal in the field. He simply read and read, and subsequently got a variety of ideas for content, methodology, and measurement. He learned what the gaps were in a topic that interested him, and he translated that knowledge into a research topic.

Talk to Professors and Clinicians in the Field When Exploring Options

Although this statement seems elementary, neglecting to involve faculty members and other professionals can be detrimental. Some students try to pursue an idea that is not feasible and waste time because they do not confer with faculty members. One of our respondents called this "face time" and suggested that in the midst of the thesis/dissertation process, time spent with faculty members is time well spent.

Choose a Topic and Explore Potential Challenges

The best way to find out whether your topic will be appropriate is to try to "tear it apart." By this, we mean that you should try to think of any factors that would make your study unreasonable. Table 2.1 provides examples of questions that you may want to ask yourself. After asking these questions and any others that you think of, you may find that your topic has some potential weaknesses. If so, take these insights back to a professor and discuss them. If it seems as though the topic has too many challenges to be successful, choose another topic and repeat the questioning step. Once you have discovered a topic that "passes the test" (and that you are excited about), move to the next step.

Begin Finding Your Committee Members

It is important to find the chair of your committee first. This should be an individual who has some interest in your topic. You may have been talking with this person in the first few stages, but you must officially ask that individual to be the chair of your committee. You should choose someone who can be a mentor throughout the remainder of the process. Along with your chair, you will want to think of additional committee members. One faculty member among our respondents observed: "You want two kinds of committee persons—those who will help you, and those that will leave

---

TABLE 2.1. Questions to Consider in Choosing a Thesis/Dissertation Topic

Subjects
- Will I be able to recruit enough subjects? Is the study being conducted in an area where there is a large population of the group I want to study?
- How will I recruit participants? (Sometimes, due to the type of population being studied, there may be restrictions on advertising.)
- Will I have enough diversity among my subjects? (If you are doing research in a small, homogeneous community, you will have trouble generalizing your results.)
- If I am studying children, will I be able to get the necessary consent from their parents?

Measures
- What are the copyright laws on the measures I want to use? (Some scales are copyrighted and require the researcher to buy copyright privileges.)
- Can I find valid and reliable scales that measure what I want to measure? (Sometimes there aren't valid or reliable scales that will measure your dependent variable.)

Time
- What is my academic timeline? When do I hope or need to graduate?
- How long will it take for me to collect data? If I am going to work with a specific population, will I need a longer time period to complete my research?
- If I am planning to use a follow-up measure, will I have difficulty tracking my subjects?

---

you alone and let you do what you want to do." It is a good idea to consider the personalities of your committee members; this will ensure that they not only will be able to assist you, but can get along with one another as well. Finally, be sure that at least one person on your committee is familiar with the methodology that you plan to use.

Write Your Proposal and Set a Date to Present It to Your Committee

It is important to think ahead about your proposal. Some individuals become nervous about their proposal and procrastinate because they are unsure of what is expected of them. As a master's-degree candidate, one of us (SAS, the "I" in this discussion) also feared the unknown. The purpose of the proposal is to formally present your thesis/dissertation plan to your committee members. In most cases, you will need to have your final copy of your introduction, literature review, and methods sections written several weeks before you actually propose. You may seek the input of your committee members throughout this process. When writing my thesis, I was required to submit a copy of my proposal to my chair 3 weeks before my meeting date. Time periods may vary from program to program, so it is wise to check these issues out in advance. But it is important to set the date for your proposal in advance.

Write Your IRB and Informed Consent Forms

When approaching your thesis/dissertation proposal, you may want to begin thinking about compiling your IRB approval and informed consent forms. Although you cannot submit these forms until after you have obtained clearance from your committee at your proposal, it is a good idea to begin preparing these documents in advance. Ask your committee at, or before, your proposal meeting about the specific details concerning your university's IRB. If these forms are written before your proposal, you can have your committee members look them over while they are all assembled.

The Proposal Meeting

If possible, make a PowerPoint presentation of your literature review and methods sections to keep you on track during your proposal presentation. This does not need to be an extremely detailed presentation, but one that will aid in highlighting your major points. Remember, all of your committee members should have read your literature review and methods sections, so this presentation is a refresher for them. Also, dress professionally for your proposal. This meeting is an important step in the thesis/dissertation process and should be treated as such. In addition, be sure to leave time during your meeting for your committee to discuss questions or suggestions. Then, once all business is taken care of, your committee decides whether or not to give you the go-ahead with your research plan.

Expect to feel both relieved and overwhelmed after your proposal meeting. It is a wonderful feeling to know that you have completed a major step in the thesis/dissertation process, but you may also feel stress because of the corrections you need to complete. I (again, SAS) can remember coming home after my proposal and lying numb on my couch. I also remember shedding some tears, even though I don't consider myself an emotional individual. Take the emotional responses you feel as a sign that you have completed an important step in the process of finishing your project.

Making Corrections and Submitting Your IRB and Informed Consent Paperwork

Once your committee has given you approval to continue in the process, you will need to make the necessary revisions that they suggest. In addition, you will need to submit your IRB form and document to your IRB. Depending on the type of study you are conducting, your IRB approval may take days or weeks. This is something to keep in mind when you are planning for your project. For example, I (SAS) needed a full review for my thesis. The IRB committee met only once a month and required forms to be submitted several weeks before it met. Although not all theses/dissertations require a full review, it is important to give yourself enough time just in case.

Begin Data Collection

It is vital that you wait for IRB approval before conducting your research. Negative legal and ethical consequences can occur if you fail to wait for approval. Once you have IRB approval, you can begin to collect your data. As you continue with data collection, you may find that some aspects of your study have changed; if so, you must notify your IRB with the changes to your original submission. Usually this will require making corrections to the original document, along with writing a cover letter explaining your rationale.

Typically an IRB approval is only valid for 1 year, but in some cases the collection of your data may take more than a year. Thus, if this occurs, you must resubmit your IRB form for reapproval. When I (SAS) collected data, it took about 14 months to finish data collection. The IRB sent me a notice in the mail that I needed to resubmit my form for another year. The board did require making a few minor changes in my informed consent form. Most of the time, however, data collection for a thesis/dissertation can be completed within a year.

Analyze Your Data

Once you have obtained all your data, it is time to do analysis. Your committee members can be a tremendous help at this stage. In quantitative analysis, you will want to set up a database and codebook to enter your data. If you are doing a qualitative study, this may require transcription, coding, and so forth. Again, your committee members can guide you in this process.

Writing Your Results and Discussion Sections

Once your data are collected and analyzed, it is time to report on that information. Here are a few tips for writing this portion of your thesis/dissertation:

- Ask your committee members for their suggestions on how you should write up these sections.
- Find out whether some members have a specific writing style they will want you to use.
- You should also ask how many tables and charts to use.
- Look at completed theses/dissertations as examples.

Ask your chair to look at your work as you go along to save time and frustration. Since each thesis/dissertation is different, and each committee is different as well, it is always wise to seek counsel from others along the way.

Set a Date for Your Defense

As with the proposal, it is important to think ahead about setting your defense date. Many students find themselves in a pinch because they want to graduate at a certain time and have to squeeze in a defense date before that time. Again, planning ahead is very important. As with the proposal, you will need to get copies of your completed thesis/dissertation to your committee members several weeks before the defense date. It is also smart to check with them prior to the defense to see whether they have any major concerns. It helps to know about "red flags" before the actual defense.

Defend Your Thesis/Dissertation

This is it! You have finally reached the stage where you are ready to present your findings. Your defense will be similar to your proposal, but will include your results and the discussion of your findings. You will want to recap the literature review and methods sections of your thesis/dissertation briefly. The majority of your presentation will focus on your results and the discussion of your conclusions. Follow the same recommendations as for the proposal, and remember that you are almost finished!

You will probably have forms that need to be signed by your committee members on the day of your defense. Make sure you bring these with you. Since your committee will not formally meet again, it is important to get all members' signatures at that time.

Make Corrections

You will undoubtedly have some corrections to make before submitting your final copy. One set of corrections may involve formatting your thesis/dissertation to the standards required by your university. This can be a tedious process (although not difficult). Make sure to allow yourself adequate time for formatting and general corrections before the final copy is due.

Submit Your Final Copy

You will need to ask your institution about deadlines for submitting the final copy of your thesis/dissertation. Timing is important if you want to graduate in a particular semester. Again, planning for the amount of time this specific process will take is important. With hard work and determination, you will finish.

DISCUSSION

Strengths and Weaknesses in MFT Research

Several factors have been identified as sustaining the scientist–practitioner gap (Johnson, Sandberg, & Miller, 1999; Sandberg, Johnson, Robila, & Miller, 2002; Sprenkle, 2002b). For example, Pinsof and Wynne (1995b) assert that the field of MFT must develop a set of common measures from which outcome can be determined. Sprenkle (2002b) notes that challenges include the transportability of treatment models; differences among families in cultural adaptation levels and other characteristics, as well as differences among individual family members; the common-factors movement; clinical relevance; and resources. In addition, just because MFT practitioners receive research training, this does not mean that they will be any more likely to engage in clinical research (Johnson et al., 1999).

Yet there is some reason for optimism. Sprenkle (2002b) has noted that all of the quantitative research in the newest effectiveness book (Sprenkle, 2002a) involved randomized clinical trials, replicability of studies was being achieved, treatment adherence was noted in studies, and follow-up data were gathered. In addition, methodological developments in qualitative research in MFT have been observed. Studies have shown that qualitative analyses were virtually nonexistent for psychologists and researchers in medical settings; however, a substantial number of articles from members of the Commission on Accreditation for Marriage and Family Therapy Education, social workers, and therapists in private practice used qualitative methods, especially in studies focused on clinical processes (Hawley, Bailey, & Pennick, 2000). Faulkner and colleagues (2002) assert that in the 1990s there was a surge of encouragement for qualitative research in the field of MFT. In their review of two decades of publication trends, they have concluded that qualitative research is valued in the field of MFT. They assert that "we are now prepared to move to the next level, beyond the quantitative–qualitative debates and articles that promote the global benefits of qualitative research" (p. 74). Whether quantitative or qualitative, research in the field of MFT is growing stronger.

Bridging Research and Practice

One criticism of the scientist–practitioner gap in MFT is that the academics conducting research in universities do not relate to the obstacles that clinicians face in their practice. One researcher shared this observation with us: "If we get too far away from discussing their clinical issues, we're just taking ourselves right out of relevance, and they [students] just tell us immediately if they feel like we're drifting too far into the ivory tower." Yet, in a survey conducted regarding the demographics of authors in the *Journal of Marital and Family Therapy* over a 5-year span, the results showed the prototypical submitter to be a male PhD conducting research within an academic setting, whereas female clinicians are the prototypical AAMFT members (Sprenkle, Bailey, Lyness, Ball, & Mills, 1997). This finding suggests that a gap exists between research and practice in MFT. Discussing this issue with MFT graduate students serves as a possible means to narrow the gap.

Researchers in MFT are proposing that another evaluation criterion for MFT research should be "utility." One of our respondents told us:

> "Every study should be measured on the basis of whether or not at the time of the study . . . it has a purpose. Does it make anything better by it being done in the immediate sense? So a study that has good scores in terms of reliability and validity may fail the utility [criterion], in that it is just hollow knowledge that is just going to sit on the shelf and may never be used by anyone. So the utility element of rigor would kind of catch some of those kinds of studies that are just . . . armchair studies that really are not designed to do anything except probably get people dissertations and sit on the shelf in a lot of libraries."

Ask yourself whether your study can help advance knowledge in the field of MFT. Seeking to contribute to the foundation of knowledge in MFT has the potential to help propel our field forward.

Encouraging graduate students to choose topics that apply to clinicians is a way to bridge the gap. For example, as a master's-degree candidate, I (SAS) was challenged by a professor to pursue a research project that was applicable to MFT practitioners in the field. I chose to complete an outcome study that was directly connected to a popular model of clinical treatment. It was hard work, but it felt good to tackle an important, clinically relevant question.

Encouraging graduate students to bridge the gap by pairing up with clinicians in community agencies is another possibility. Most graduate students working on research projects only consult their professors, not clinicians in the community, when designing and conducting these projects. What if students paired up with community therapists to conduct research? This would be a great way to build a bridge between academics and practitioners. Some may argue that clinicians would not have the time or interest to do research. We would argue that clinicians are already doing research in an informal manner. Why not have graduate students formally study the issues that clinicians observe on a daily basis?

In a recent issue of the *Journal of Marital and Family Therapy*, McCollum and Stith (2002) discuss community agencies as potential resources for MFT research. Although this article aims at encouraging the entire MFT field to bridge the gap between research and practice, this movement must begin with graduate student research. One of the greatest reasons for partnering with agencies is developing treatment approaches with clinical effectiveness (Beutler & Howard, 1998). It is helpful to conduct research in an environment where actual clinicians treat actual clients. McCollum and Stith (2002) argue that if we researchers cannot demonstrate MFT's clinical usefulness and cost-effectiveness, we do an injustice to clinicians and clients alike.

As a graduate student, you may be wondering how you might complete your thesis/dissertation with the cooperation of a community agency. McCollum and Stith (2002) offer two suggestions for successfully conducting research in a community setting. First, they propose gaining access to an agency by building solid relationships with agency partners. They also recommend flexibility and perseverance when facing unanticipated challenges of conducting research in a community agency. Although I (SAS) did my outcome research in my program's clinic, I used an outside agency to recruit my subjects. It took a great deal of patience and persistence, but was successful in the end. Even though research collaboration with community agencies has its challenges, graduate students can benefit from the experience.

FUTURE DIRECTIONS OF MFT RESEARCH

The future of our field rests with MFT students, and there is no better time to engage in MFT research. It is no longer possible to be a superstar in the field if you do not have empirical data to support theoretical and clinical assertions. Accepting the challenge to bridge the gap between research and practice involves being trained to become not only a qualified therapist, but a seasoned researcher as well (Crane, Wampler, Sprenkle, Sandberg, & Hovestadt, 2002; McWey et al., 2002; Sprenkle, 2002b). The best way to understand the process of MFT research is to get involved with those who have already been on the roller-coaster ride a few times themselves. Research mentors are important to the new generation of MFT researchers. Hines (1996) surveyed 205 graduates of accredited MFT programs on how well they thought their programs had prepared them in several topic areas. Master's-level graduates, commenting on recommendations for programs to better prepare students for research, stated that training programs were staying "the same" in keeping the research component to one course. Doctoral graduates likewise felt that the research component needed to be "significantly increased" in MFT training programs. Crane and colleagues (2002) argue that students would become much more motivated and confident about research if research experiences were structured into MFT training programs to the same extent that clinical experiences are. By pursuing adequate training and (more important) significant experience and practice in research methods, you can enhance your ability and confidence in your own skills as a researcher (Johnson et al., 1999). By engaging in clinically significant research efforts, you also have the potential to improve the future of our field. Besides, you may even discover that you enjoy the roller-coaster ride.

ACKNOWLEDGMENT

We would like to extend our appreciation to all of the MFT researchers who shared their thoughts and suggestions with us.

A FEW HELPFUL RESOURCES FOR GRADUATE STUDENTS

Babbie, E. (1998). *The practice of social research* (8th ed.). Belmont, CA: Wadsworth.

Becker, H. (1986). *Writing for social scientists: How to start and finish your thesis, book, or article.* Chicago: University of Chicago Press.

Green, S. B., & Salkind, N. J. (2003). *Using SPSS for Windows and Macintosh: Analyzing and understanding data* (3rd ed.). Upper Saddle River, NJ: Prentice Hall.

Meloy, J. M. (2001). *Writing the qualitative dissertation: Understanding by doing* (2nd ed.). Mahwah, NJ: Erlbaum.

Nicol, A. A., & Pexman, P. M. (1999). *Presenting your findings: A practical guide for creating tables.* Washington, DC: American Psychological Association.

Roberts, C. M. (2004). *The dissertation journey: A practical and comprehensive guide to planning, writing, and defending your dissertation.* Thousand Oaks, CA: Sage.

Sprenkle, D. H. (Ed.). (2002). *Effectiveness research in marriage and family therapy.* Washington, DC: American Association for Marriage and Family Therapy.

REFERENCES

Ambert, A., Adler, P. A., Adler, P., & Detzner, D. F. (1995). Understanding and evaluating qualitative research. *Journal of Marriage and the Family, 57*(4), 879–893.

American Psychological Association (APA). (2001). *Publication manual of the American Psychological Association* (5th ed.). Washington, DC: Author.

Babbie, E. (1998). *The practice of social research* (8th ed.). Belmont, CA: Wadsworth.

Beutler, L. E., & Howard, K. I. (1998). Clinical utility research: An introduction. *Journal of Clinical Psychology, 54,* 297–301.

Chenail, R. J. (1990). Provocations for researching clinicians and clinical researchers. *The Qualitative Report, 1*(2–3). Retrieved from *http://www.nova.edu/ssss/QR/QR1-23/provocations.html*

Crane, R., Wampler, K. S., Sprenkle, D. H., Sandberg, J. G., & Hovestadt, A. J. (2002). The scientist-practitioner model in marriage and family therapy doctoral programs. *Journal of Marital and Family Therapy, 28*(1), 75–83.

Denton, W. H., & Walsh, S. R. (2001). Competence and integrity: Ethical challenges for today and the future. In R. H. Woody & J. D. Woody (Eds.), *Ethics in marriage and family therapy* (pp. 83–102). Alexandria, VA: American Association for Marriage and Family Therapy.

Dickey, M. H. (1996). Quantitative design in family therapy: Insider hints on getting started. In D. H. Sprenkle & S. M. Moon (Eds.), *Research methods in family therapy* (pp. 191–215). New York: Guilford Press.

Elliot, R., Fischer, C. T., & Rennie, D. L. (1999). Evolving guidelines for publication of qualitative research studies in psychology and related fields. *British Journal of Clinical Psychology, 38,* 215–229.

Faulkner, R. A., Klock, K., & Gale, J. (2002). Qualitative research in family therapy: Publication trends from 1980 to 1999. *Journal of Marital and Family Therapy, 28*(1), 69–74.

Fine, M., & Kurdek, L. (1993). Reflections on determining authorship credit and author order on faculty–student collaborations. *American Psychologist, 48*(11), 1141–1147.

Green, S. B., & Salkind, N. J. (2003). *Using SPSS for Windows and Macintosh: Analyzing and understanding data* (3rd ed.). Upper Saddle River, NJ: Prentice Hall.

Johnson, L. N., Sandberg, J. G., & Miller, R. B. (1999). Research practices among marriage and family therapists. *American Journal of Family Therapy, 27,* 239–249.

Hawley, D., Bailey, E. C., & Pennick, K. (2000). A content analysis of research in family therapy journals. *Journal of Marital and Family Therapy, 26*(1), 9–16.

Hines, M. (1996). Follow-up survey of graduates from accredited degree-granting marriage and family therapy training programs. *Journal of Marital and Family Therapy, 22,* 181–194.

Horne, K. B., & Hicks, M. W. (2002). All in the family: A belated response to Knudson-Martin's feminist revision of Bowen theory. *Journal of Marital and Family Therapy, 28*(1), 103–113.

Knudson-Martin, C. (2002). Expaning Bowen's legacy to family therapy: A response to Horne and Hicks. *Journal of Marital and Family Therapy, 28*(1), 115–120.

McCollum, E. E., & Stith, S. (2002). Leaving the ivory tower: An introduction to the special section on doing marriage and family therapy research in community agencies. *Journal of Marital and Family Therapy, 28*(1), 5–7.

McWey, L. M., Hernandez West, S., Ruble, N. M., Handy, A. K., Handy, D. G., Koshy, M., et al. (2002). The practice of clinical research in accredited marriage and family therapy programs. *Journal of Marital and Family Therapy, 28*(1), 85–102.

Nichols, W. (1979). Education of marriage and family therapists: Some trends and implications. *Journal of Marital and Family Therapy, 5,* 19–28.

Nicol, A. A., & Pexman, P. M. (1999). *Presenting your findings: A practical guide for creating tables.* Washington, DC: American Psychological Association.

Northey, W. F. (2002). Characteristics and clinical practices of marriage and family therapists: A national survey. *Journal of Marital and Family Therapy, 28,* 487–494.

Olson, D. (1976). Bridging research, theory, and application: The triple threat in science. In D. Olson (Ed.), *Treating relationships* (pp. 565–579). Lake Mills, IA: Graphic.

Pinsof, W. M., & Wynne, L. C. (Eds.). (1995a). The effectiveness of marital and family therapy [Special issue]. *Journal of Marital and Family Therapy, 21*(4).

Pinsof, W. M., & Wynne, L. C. (1995b). The efficacy of marital and family therapy: An empirical overview, conclusions, and recommendations. *Journal of Marital and Family Therapy, 21*(4), 585–613.

Sandberg, J. G., Johnson, L. N., Robila, M., & Miller, R. B. (2002). Clinician identified barriers to clinical research. *Journal of Marital and Family Therapy, 28*(1), 61–67.

Sprenkle, D. H. (Ed.). (2002a). *Effectiveness research in marriage and family therapy.* Alexandria, VA: American Association for Marriage and Family Therapy.

Sprenkle, D. H. (2002b). Effectiveness research in marriage and family therapy: Introduction. In D. H. Sprenkle (Ed.), *Effectiveness research in marriage and family therapy* (pp. 9–26). Alexandria, VA: American Association for Marriage and Family Therapy.

Sprenkle, D. H., Bailey, C. E., Lyness, K. P., Ball, D., & Mills, S. (1997). Submission patterns to the archival journal of the profession of MFT. *Journal of Marital and Family Therapy, 23*(4), 371–380.

Waehler, C. A., Kalodner, C. R., Wampold, B. E., & Lichtenberg, J. W. (2000). Empirically supported treatments (ESTs) in perspective: Implications for counseling psychology training. *The Counseling Psychologist, 28,* 657–671.

PART II
QUALITATIVE METHODS

CHAPTER 3

Let's Get Grounded

FAMILY THERAPY RESEARCH AND GROUNDED THEORY

SILVIA ECHEVARRIA-DOAN
CAROLYN Y. TUBBS

> The most potent obstacle to the recognition of family resources is the search for pathology.
>
> —KARPEL (1986)

BACKGROUND

The quote that opens this chapter was the catalyst that led one of us (SED, the "I" here) to the line of research that still holds my interest today. Well over a decade later, I am still holding the magnifying glass in search of more information about client strengths and resources in family therapy. This quote resonated with my thinking about resilience and its place in therapy. I was inspired to ask questions like: How do we get around this predominant "search for pathology" in therapy? How do we actually "recognize" family resources? How can we learn to do this as therapists? What are the implications of searching only for pathology? How often do we assume that families are not resourceful because of the problems they present with in therapy? Where do we hear about this in our coursework or training? If therapists do "recognize" family resources, how do they do this? Most importantly, how can we tap into these resources and use them in therapy? The other author (CYT) also took part in this initial research venture, which we discuss in this chapter.

Some of the questions inspired by our interest in focusing on resources in research were reflected in the research example presented in the first edition's chapter on grounded theory (Rafuls & Moon, 1996). Findings from that particular research study led to grounded theory on "resource-based consultation" (Rafuls, 1994). In practice, this has led to the development of "resource-based reflective consultation" (Echevarria-Doan, 2001)—an interventive, consultative method designed to elicit and

---

Silvia Echevarria-Doan was formerly known as Silvia Echevarria Rafuls.

promote resource-based language between client families and their therapists. This chapter highlights research that is also related to the set of guiding questions stated above. However, the research presented in this chapter was based on data collected from therapists who described how they actually went about accessing client strengths and resources during assessment. Findings from both of these studies contribute to a more substantive and perhaps formal theory related to how therapists recognize and use client resources and strengths in family therapy. At this point this is considered an evolving process, because we continue to collect data to better understand the process of searching for (and utilizing) strengths and resources in therapy. As Charmaz (2000) points out, in grounded theory "we revisit our ideas, and perhaps our data, and recreate them in new form in an evolving process" (p. 515).

The purpose of this chapter is to provide updated information about grounded theory methodology in general, and as it relates to family therapy research in particular. In terms of background, we discuss some of the more recent debates concerning "objectivist" traditional views of grounded theory, in contrast to developing "constructivist" views.. Throughout the chapter, we also discuss recent publications by Barney Glaser and the late Anselm Strauss, the founders of grounded theory (Glaser, 1998, 2002; Strauss & Corbin, 1998). We present in detail the research example mentioned earlier of therapists' ways of accessing client resources and strengths, to illustrate steps in data analysis and reporting in grounded theory methodology. In addition, we have updated parts of the discussion section to include more recent observations about the strengths and weaknesses of grounded theory methodology, ways in which grounded theory bridges research and practice, and future directions for this methodology in family therapy. We also have added five exemplars that serve as models of grounded theory methodology in family therapy research.

Philosophical Assumptions

Grounded theory is a methodology based on the development of theory from data that are collected and analyzed systematically and recursively. It is a way of thinking about or conceptualizing data as the essential elements from which theory evolves. At the heart of grounded theory is what is commonly known in qualitative research as the "constant comparative method" (Glaser & Strauss, 1967). This inductive analytical process involves a constant interplay between data collection and data analysis. Essentially, as data are collected, they are analyzed for emergent theoretical categories, which are systematically looped back into the collection of data and analyzed further for their interrelationships and meaning (Strauss & Corbin, 1998). This systematic and inductive process of data collection, analysis, further focused collection, and refined theoretical analyses leads to interpretations of the data that help build middle-range theoretical frameworks. Grounded theory emerges when theoretical saturation of meanings, patterns, and categories occurs (Glaser, 1978). Grounded theory procedure is useful to a researcher who wishes to generate inductive theory from data that are systematically collected and analyzed, whether these data are qualitative or quantitative.

Since the inception of grounded theory methodology, neither the theoretical perspectives nor the epistemological distinctions upon which it is based have been made explicit in its literature. In other words, epistemological and/or ideological frameworks were not specified (Glaser, 1978, 1992, 1998; Glaser & Strauss, 1967; Strauss &

Corbin, 1998), and this lack of specificity led to various sources of data collection in several disciplines for a multitude of purposes. Some would argue that there are problems in transferring a method among different theoretical perspectives and traditions, because of the lack of coherence in underlying assumptions, concepts, data collection methods, and the knowledge that the method produces (Bernard, 2002; Crotty, 1998; LeCompte & Preissle with Tesch, 1993; Williams, 2001).

In its earlier days, grounded theory was not tied to any one specific research tradition or research paradigm, but was considered theoretically consistent with several, both positivistic and nonpositivistic in nature. Yet even though grounded theory has usually been associated with nonpositivistic qualitative research, it could also plausibly be used for purposes of verification, which would make it consistent with positivistic tradition as well (Glaser, 1998; Glaser & Strauss, 1967).

Despite the unspecified nature of its theoretical and epistemological frameworks, some researchers have located grounded theory in phenomenology (Richardson, 1999), hermeneutics (Rennie, 1998, 2000), and social constructivism (Charmaz, 2000; Denzin, 1994). In some cases, this has led some "postmodern" and "poststructural" grounded theorists to categorize more traditional grounded theorists like Glaser, Strauss, and Corbin as positivists (Charmaz, 2000; Denzin, 1994). As Denzin (1994) points out, "Still some would contend that it [grounded theory] has yet to engage fully the new sensibilities flowing from the poststructural and postmodern perspectives" (p. 509). Generally, criticisms of grounded theory include the value- and theory-laden nature of its facts, ambiguities in incidence and categorical analysis, and its resounding commitment to "objective" methods and procedures for the sake of good science (Denzin, 1994).

In particular, Charmaz (2000) makes a case for what she calls "constructivist grounded theory." She asserts that the methods of Glaser, Strauss, and Corbin are filled with "objective underpinnings." More specifically, she aligns Glaser's (1978, 1992) work with positions that come close to "traditional positivism." Glaser responds to Charmaz in detail in his online treatise titled "Constructivist Grounded Theory?" (Glaser, 2002). In particular, he argues with the position Charmaz takes on data analysis, stating that "Data [are] discovered for conceptualization to be what it is—theory" (p. 1). He goes on to say, "Adding his or her interpretations would be an unwarranted intrusion of the researcher" (p. 2), which illustrates how strongly he believes in the constant comparative method and how reluctant he is to acknowledge subjectivity.

Charmaz (2000) refers to Strauss and Corbin's (1998) stance as one that assumes an "objective external reality." However, she goes on to say that their position moves into postpositivism, because they give voice to their respondents and recognize art as well as science in the analytic process and product. It is here that she introduces constructivist grounded theory, which takes a middle ground between postmodernism and positivism, and takes qualitative research into the 21st century. Charmaz claims that this can be done by forming a "revised, more open-ended practice of grounded theory that stresses its emergent, constructivist elements" by using "grounded theory methods as flexible, heuristic strategies, rather than as formulaic procedures" (p. 510).

Our interpretation of grounded theory remains consistent with nonpositivistic research traditions (Rafuls & Moon, 1996). Although we acknowledge that the rigor and systematized nature of grounded theory methodology, along with Glaser's (2002) elevated view of the method's "objectivity," can lead one to question this stance, we locate our view within earlier frameworks of "alternative" research paradigms. Our view of grounded theory is theoretically consistent with the alternative research paradigms presented by Hoshmand (1989) (i.e., naturalistic–ethnography, phenomenology, and cybernetic) and those presented by Guba (1990) (i.e., postpositivism, critical theory, and constructivism). Although "alternative" suggests marginalized positions, we view its use as simply a matter of descriptive convenience, not as a suggestion that these positions are less than, less central, or subordinate to more mainstream positivist traditions. In the broader sense, alternative research paradigms differ from the positivistic research traditions in three distinct ways: (1) ontologically, by not limiting a researcher to thinking of social reality as "out there" known only by "truths" that are driven by natural laws and arrived at only by controlled experimentation; (2) epistemologically, by not requiring the researcher to separate the subjective and objective aspects of knowledge and the value-ladenness of facts; and (3) methodologically, by not limiting the researcher to standards of precise measurement, operationalized concepts, or deductive practices of theory testing and verification alone (Guba, 1990; Hoshmand, 1989). Alternative paradigms offer researchers new ways of approaching knowledge that may be more conducive to the types of questions they are asking. In particular, discovery-oriented approaches offer the methodological options needed to address the diversity of clinical practice and families that we work with as family researchers. This offers us the notion that there is more than just one way of doing research, thus inviting those of us who perhaps might not have stepped into the research arena at all to participate.

Historical Roots and Development

The origin of grounded theory is credited to sociologists Barney Glaser and Anselm Strauss. Together, they wrote *The Discovery of Grounded Theory* in 1967. Grounded theory was created in order to "close the embarrassing gap between theory and empirical research" (p. viii), which Glaser and Strauss (1967) believed occurred because of the undue emphasis placed on verification of theory in sociological research at the time. Through grounded theory methodology, Glaser and Strauss set out to provide researchers with a formalized framework for generating theory from empirical data. Even though grounded theory was designed with the emphasis on generating theory, it was not intended to minimize the importance of verifying theory. As Glaser and Strauss (1967) saw it, generation and verification of theory were both necessary and complementary.

Even though much of the original research using grounded theory procedures was done in sociology, the methodology is not "discipline-bound" (Strauss & Corbin, 1990). Researchers in other fields (e.g., psychology, anthropology, nursing, education, social work, and even business management) have adopted grounded theory methods, and it undoubtedly will continue to spread into other fields (Strauss & Corbin, 1990).

Although not noted for their use of grounded theory methods, pioneering family therapists observed families in qualitatively oriented ways. As Gilgun (1992) points out, many of the early theorists in family therapy pursued their knowledge of families through direct client–therapist interaction and postsession reflection and analysis. Even though their qualitatively based observations formed the basis for many of the theories they developed in family therapy, it would be a stretch to consider these pioneering efforts to be grounded theory studies without having information about their methods of data collection and data analysis. Despite grounded theory's congruence with the practice of family therapy, our most recent review of grounded theory studies in family therapy found only a slight increase in such studies since the 1996 first edition of this book. Grounded theory was more notably represented in family therapy dissertations. Lack of greater representation of this methodology in family therapy research literature may be due to the time- and labor-intensive nature of theoretical sampling and theory development. Some researchers use it simply as a method of analysis, but with little effort to develop theory in the process. This may occur because researchers lack training in the development of theory using this method. It may also simply relate to time constraints, which keep researchers and clinicians alike from efforts to develop substantive theory.

After the inception of grounded theory in the mid-1960s, Glaser (1978, 1992) and Strauss (1987; Strauss & Corbin, 1998) developed diverging views of grounded theory methodology. The central issue in their debate was one of emphasis on different, yet (in our view) equally important, aspects of grounded theory methodology. Glaser emphasizes the "emergent" process of theory development, whereas until his death Strauss emphasized the "systematic" aspect of managing data analysis and synthesis. Glaser takes the position that grounded theory is to deal only with data that is relevant to the emerging theory, not data that are forced into a preconceived analytical framework by prescribing analysis according to certain conditions and consequences. These preconceived notions, he contends, may have nothing to do with those variables that are relevant to the emerging theory, and therefore are antithetical to the distinguishing feature of grounded theory as systematically emergent from data (Glaser, 1992).

Strauss (1987; Strauss & Corbin, 1998), on the other hand, believed that organization of the data is key to arriving at the emergent theory. As he put it, "the excellence of the research rests in large part on the excellence of the coding" (Strauss, 1987, p. 27). Strauss's emphasis on coding grew out of experiences in teaching students how to do grounded theory research (Gilgun, 1992; Strauss & Corbin, 1998). His formalized approach to coding data is especially helpful to beginning grounded theory researchers, because it helps reduce the ambiguity that generally goes along with grounded theory analysis.

Both Glaser and Strauss (and Corbin) have made significant contributions. We see this divergence in emphasis as a "both–and" issue, not an "either–or." In other words, we believe that there is room for both researcher creativity (as Glaser claims) and rigorous coding procedures (as Strauss claimed), rather than excluding either view of grounded theory. How to interpret and utilize specific procedures, as suggested by their differing perspectives, is best left up to the individual researcher and his or her research questions.

METHODOLOGY

Grounded theory methodology builds theory that emerges flexibly over time from data collection and analysis (Glaser, 1978; Glaser & Strauss, 1967; Strauss & Corbin, 1998). In grounded theory, the researcher becomes the primary instrument of data collection and analysis, and the researcher's theoretical sensitivity is what allows him or her to develop theory grounded in the data (Strauss & Corbin, 1998). A grounded theorist's awareness of the subtleties of meaning in data depends on personal qualities of insight, understanding, and the ability to make sense of what is pertinent.

The research study that serves as an example of grounded theory in this chapter is taken from data that were part of a survey conducted with therapists on their views of client resources and strengths in therapy. Electronic mail surveys were originally sent to randomly selected research participants from different disciplines (marriage and family therapists, clinical social workers, and mental health counselors) represented in listings obtained from professional organizations (the American Association for Marriage and Family Therapy, the American Family Therapy Academy, the National Association of Social Workers, and the American Counseling Association). The data used for the research example in this chapter were taken from responses to open-ended questions from those respondents who specified methods or ways in which they access client resources and strengths in therapy. Therefore, the sample we are using in this chapter constituted a criterion-based subsample of the entire group of survey respondents.

The purpose of the survey was to find out (1) whether participants thought it was important to assess for client resources and strengths; (2) if so, what were some of the ways they did this; (3) whether participants from specific theoretical orientations were more inclined to assess for client resources and strengths; (4) whether participants thought that assessing for strengths was theoretically consistent with their identified theoretical model(s); and (5) whether they had conducted research on any of their described methods.

The first section of the survey consisted of demographic items (age, gender, credentials, years of practice, primary setting, theoretical orientation, etc.). This section of the data was analyzed quantitatively, using means, percentages, and/or totals. The second section of the questionnaire included nine open-ended questions regarding assessment of client resources and strengths (mostly reflected in the points made earlier concerning the purpose of the survey). The responses to the open-ended questions were analyzed qualitatively using a constant comparative method. For the sake of keeping our research example within the guidelines of this chapter, we have chosen to focus specifically on data relevant to *how* client resources and strengths are accessed in therapy.

Research Questions

The research questions that are asked in a study ought to guide the research method that is used. In grounded theory, research questions are generally open-ended, flexible, and broad to begin with, and then become more focused and refined as analysis occurs. Research questions in grounded theory studies generally ask about concepts that have not yet been identified or explored, or whose relationships are poorly understood or conceptualized (Glaser & Strauss, 1967). Grounded theory questions also tend to be action- and process-oriented.

The two guiding questions that produced the data we analyzed for our research example in this chapter were these:

1. How do therapists assess for clients' resources and strengths in therapy?
2. What are the methods employed in their assessment process?

Sampling and Selection Procedures

Grounded theory is known for its emphasis on theoretical sampling. It is a way of "feeding into data for more induction" (Glaser, 1998, p. 157). Grounded theorists use theoretical sampling to refine and develop categories by going back to fill in conceptual gaps as a theory is developed. Theoretical sampling also helps to keep data collection to a minimum, because it leads researchers to relevant data based on emerging concepts. However, this does not indicate how to get started with sampling in the first place.

An initial sample is likely to be "selective." Selective sampling is based on a preconceived set of criteria that originates from the researcher's guiding assumptions and research questions. That is, selection is based on specific considerations that delineate appropriate units of analyses and participants, depending on what the researcher is setting out to discover. Criteria based on the research question(s) generally guide the researcher to one or more types of selection, or selection procedures. These include convenience selection, comprehensive selection, quota selection, extreme-case selection, typical-case selection, unique-case selection, and reputational-case selection (LeCompte et al., 1993). In grounded theory the term used is "theoretical sampling," because the researcher selects individuals who can contribute to an evolving theory.

For instance, in the study being highlighted for this chapter, a subsample of participants from a survey conducted by one of us (SED) was selected. In this case, participants were selected on the basis of details given in their description of how they assessed for client resources and strengths in therapy. This was based on the guiding questions stated earlier. If we were to look at this data set as part of the research agenda in a broader sense (i.e., the development of a substantive theory addressing how therapists access and use client resources and strengths), then we might argue that the selection of therapists for this study fits within the parameters of theoretical sampling. This is especially true if we consider one of the concluding remarks in the initial study (Rafuls, 1994):

> At this point it seems as though the development of a theory about Resource-based Consultation goes hand in hand with the development of procedures that will constitute its practice. In developing the theory further what might be necessary is to compare different groups across different types of families, in different settings, during different phases of treatment. (p. 104)

Initially, theoretical sampling is selective to the extent that the researcher searches for participants who might contribute to an evolving theory. Later, theoretical sampling is based on the data that informs the evolving theory. In terms of a priori views, even though naturalistic inquiry may keep a researcher from developing preconceived notions about the phenomenon being studied, it does mandate that the researcher be explicit about any such views from the beginning in the form of stated assumptions. Essentially, selective sampling allows researchers to develop their initial thoughts about a phenomenon in a manner that will ultimately drive theoretical sampling as data are analyzed. Furthermore, specific sampling procedures are important, given current review board and funding agency standards. It would be unlikely that researchers could get approval for their work without explicit criteria regarding the selection of participants and methodology to be implemented.

Data Collection Procedures

Data collection and data analysis in grounded theory are exceptionally intertwined, as analysis begins almost immediately after data are first collected. Data collection methods in grounded theory studies may include in-depth interviewing, participant and nonparticipant observation, and analysis of documents. Sources of data are numerous, including transcripts of interviews, audiotapes, videotapes, field notes, journals, theoretical and analytical memos, and other documents. Generally, the "trustworthiness" of findings in grounded theory study increases if multiple sources of data are utilized, if multiple methods of data collection and analysis are used, and if multiple investigators are involved (Lincoln & Guba, 1985). Because of the theory-guided, data-based nature of gathering information in grounded theory, data collection will not cease until theoretical saturation is reached (i.e., new data cease to yield new information). Before that point, coding and memoing, drawing on comparisons and contrasts, and arriving at analytical questions and hypotheses continue to generate additional questions for researchers that can potentially direct them to other valuable sources of data.

Data collection in qualitative research often calls for transcribing data. Grounded theory can give a researcher the freedom to opt out of transcribed interviews, because of the importance placed on the development of analytic schemes early on in the process. In other words, the process of transcription slows the researcher down, because data cannot be analyzed right away (until transcription is complete and is checked for accuracy) and because it provides too much unnecessary data (which may have nothing to do with the interchangeability of indices) (Glaser, 1998). In fact, Glaser (1998) advises against taping and transcribing if a researcher is working solo. In team situations, he recommends taping only for the sake of sharing interview data with those who did not conduct the interview. Although we have mostly relied on the standard practice of transcribing interview data, a happy medium—such as taking good field notes, along with taping for purposes of checking field notes or gaps of information— seems like a viable option.

In the study we are describing, the initial survey yielded 44 respondents. From this total, 20 were chosen because they responded in detail to questions related to how they assessed for client resources and strengths. At the time the subsample data were analyzed, a descriptive qualitative data analysis of the entire survey had been completed. Overall, the data yielded the following findings:

1. Eighty percent of participants (35) stated that assessing for client resources and strengths was an important part of assessment, in contrast to 55% (24) who stated that they conducted some form of assessment of resources and strengths with *all* of their clients.
2. Participants identified with a wide variety of theoretical models that they considered resource-based in terms of assessment. Although certain models generally perceived as more theoretically consistent with resource-based practice (e.g., solution-focused and narrative) were identified with greater frequency by participants, assessing for strengths was not exclusive to these models.
   - Responses indicated that this had more to do with the participants' interpretation of the models as resource-based.
   - Sixty-one percent reported consistency between their practice of assessing for strengths and their identified theoretical model(s).

3. Resource-based assessment was noted across models and disciplines, and was reflected in the following:
   - The assumption that clients have internal resources.
   - The search for solutions.
   - Review of past successes.
   - Future-focused questioning.
   - Active involvement of clients (e.g., experiential methods, written work).
   - Collaborative roles between therapists and clients.
4. Most methods were informal in nature and were conducted as part of the therapists' usual assessment processes (not specifically created to assess for strengths and resources separately).
5. Methods were based on assessment of both individual and systemic (family/community) resources, and were represented across disciplines/professional groups.
6. Research was not conducted by participants on their methods of assessment.

What was missing from these data was the information about the underlying processes—*how* therapists assessed for client strengths and resources. This was what led to the use of grounded theory methodology for this part of the analysis. Procedurally, all of the survey data (from the subsample of 20 respondents) related to how therapists assessed for strengths and resources were initially typed out verbatim on two-thirds of each page (left-hand side), leaving another third of the page on the right-hand side for coding.

Data Analysis Procedures

In grounded theory, data analysis begins as soon as a researcher begins to collect data. The constant comparative method of analysis for which grounded theory is known involves (as its name indicates) a continual process of categorization, sorting and resorting, and coding and recoding of data for emergent categories of meaning (Hoshmand, 1989; Strauss & Corbin, 1998). Dimensions and properties of these categories are compared with other emerging categories as the researcher keeps going back to the data. In order to develop theory, interrelationships between categories are analyzed until the researcher finds the one that is complete enough to encompass all that has been described in the story (Glaser & Strauss, 1967). This central phenomenon is at the heart of the integration process (Strauss & Corbin, 1998)—the core category that is related to all the other categories and is essentially the basic social process being studied.

In the sample study, data were first analyzed line by line, as is typically done in grounded theory. This initial line-by-line analysis allows a researcher to search for categories, properties, subcategories, actions, or events within the data (see the examples that follow). This is commonly known as "open coding" because of the questions the researcher asks to begin making meaning of the data. The idea is to be sure to ask questions of the data that help "[pinpoint] gaps and leads in it to focus on during subsequent data collection" (Charmaz, 2000, p. 515). The clear and thorough description of the constant comparative method given by Charmaz (2000) delineates the types of comparisons one might make in grounded theory analysis. She states:

> The constant comparative method of grounded theory means (a) comparing different peo-
> ple (such as their views, situations, actions, accounts, and experiences), (b) comparing data
> from the same individuals with themselves at different points in time, (c) comparing inci-
> dent with incident, (d) comparing data with category, and (e) comparing a category with
> the other category. . . . (Charmaz, 2000, p. 515)

A second level of coding, which often occurs concurrently with open coding is called "axial coding." Axial coding serves to make connections between categories and subcategories. As categories are developed, the researcher wants to be sure to draw comparisons between them and their subcategories. This is why this level of induction is referred to as "axial"—because the comparison of categories and subcategories oc-curs around the "axis" of a category (Strauss & Corbin, 1998). Essentially, the re-searcher makes use of a coding paradigm that identifies a central category emerging from the data and then explores the causal conditions influencing the phenomenon, along with the strategies or actions resulting from the phenomenon (Creswell, 1998). Context and intervening conditions that influence the strategies are identified, and consequences or outcomes of the strategies are also delineated (Strauss & Corbin, 1998).

Each phase of analysis in grounded theory raises the level of abstraction and con-ceptual level of the data being gathered. The next phase of analysis, "selective coding," involves coming up with a "story line" to integrate the categories that have emerged in axial coding. This leads to conditional propositions or hypthotheses about the phe-nomenon. In selective coding, the sorting of theoretical memos leads the researcher to an integrated theory. "Memos are the theorizing write-up of ideas about substantive codes and their theoretically coded relationships as they emerge during coding, collect-ing and analyzing data during memoing" (Glaser, 1998, p. 177). Therefore, theoretical memos play a key role in the write-up of a theory. They are often the only way one of us (SED, the "I" here) can keep ideas straight in terms of what the data is telling me or what I have arrived at in terms of my understanding of concepts up to a certain point (see examples below).

Memo writing can consist of a few words that let me know I need to get back to something, or a memo can turn out to be as lengthy as five pages when I "connect the dots" concerning a subcore or core category. A definite advantage is that once sorted, memos serve to help in the writing of your integrated concepts and/or theory. How-ever, this requires discipline and practice until memo writing becomes a natural part of the analytic process.

For our example, we would like to share excerpts from actual verbatim data taken from the survey (with comments pertaining to open coding on the right-hand side, as described earlier). These comments simply led to other questions, which helped form categories that were then compared for distinctions within and between each other. We are also including some sample memos, which led the researcher to the writing up of findings to this point of data collection. Below are responses from two respondents out of several that led us to the category "when assessment of client resources and strengths is conducted."

| CG7: "I do a very complete *intake* at the first session, because there *are questions you can ask* when you barely know a person that | • **Intake** (category)
• Early stages of therapy (property of intake) |

would be *almost foolish to ask later* and intrude on a different kind of relationship. If I take a case where someone else has done the intake, I look it over carefully and note any gaps so I can fill them in ASAP. I start with a *treatment contract* and we have to do those every 90 days, so that is another occasion to *talk with the client about what the problems are, and what resources are being applied. We include community resources* like AA, support groups, educational efforts, and use of state agencies in the treatment plans. I am *always listening for* helpful relationships, opportunities for referrals, and openings to invite family members or others to sessions."

- **Action—asking questions** (property of intake)

- **Timing** of assessment important in development of tx. contract (subcategory of intake)

- Focus on external resources (category)

- Action—**listening** (property of intake)

WG19: "In the initial interview, I *try to hear* how the client has dealt with *difficult situations in the past*, especially situations *similar to the presenting problem*. Sometimes I *give a client "homework"* to see if he/she can modify habitual behaviors. Sometimes *I see* whether the client has been thinking about a significant topic from the previous week's session or has repressed the topic.

I *ask* the client to describe the *presenting problem*. I may *ask* whether anything similar has happened to the client in *the past* and how he/she coped at that time. *I ask* about the family constellation and I ask the client to give me his/her view of each family member. In the next session, I see whether the client has thought about our topic over the week and how that thinking made him/her feel. I may give *homework* to see if the client can follow through on a task."

- Action—I **hear**
- Category (**past situation**)
- Property of situation

- Action—give HW
- Action—I **see**

- Category—client's view

- Action—I **ask**
- Category— **past event**

- Category—client's view
- Action—give homework

All of the verbatim excerpts from the survey that related to "when assessment of client resources and strengths is conducted" were condensed into the following statements:

Questions are asked at intake in order to make information about strengths part of the treatment contract (it would be foolish to ask later—CG7). (WP21)

Assessment is part of the initial interview when clients are asked about ways in which they have dealt with difficult situations in the past, esp. those similar to presenting problem. (WG19)

> [I] assess during beginning phases when information is gathered and throughout in terms of how recommendations are handled. (KD25)

> Assessing for [resources and strengths] is the "lodestar of each conversation" in terms of commitment and willingness to work in therapy. (CT 34)

These synthesized statements were further integrated theoretically in memo form.

Another category that emerged from the data was "types of questions asked by therapists."

The summary statements from all of the coded data that led to this category were as follows:

> I ask open-ended questions and focus on details that provide exceptions. (LB16)

> Use open-ended questions within the context of [developmental counseling and therapy and systemic cognitive–developmental therapy]. (KK24)

> Ask exception questions "when problem isn't" to find out about times that they were able to deal with the problem. (RB18)

> Ask exception questions (times when problem was not so bad and ask other members to describe clients' [strengths and resources]. (PC27)

> Ask direct questions about strengths, talents, and competencies (within and without)— INTERNAL AND EXTERNAL STRENGTHS distinguished. (LL26)

> Ask direct questions about different aspects of their lives (samples given). (TN32)

> Use combination of Michael White, [solution-focused], and narrative questions. . . . (CT34)

It was helpful to tie these thoughts together into a theoretical memo, as was done with all three main categories. The two categories described above ("when assessment of client resources and strengths is conducted" and "types of questions asked by therapists"), along with a third category ("past successes and future-oriented thinking in assessment"), led to the core category, "therapist tasks (when accessing client resources and strengths)."

To backtrack slighty, seven categories (assumptions; time frame; type of questions; temporal orientation—past, present, and future focus; steps/procedures; type of information sought; and format) initially emerged from the data. These seven categories were then collapsed into the three main categories when I (again, SED) made comparisons between similar and contrasting themes during axial coding. I made comparisons between respondents in terms of views, practices, situations, actions, and experiences. Comparisons were also made between incidents and between categories. Selective coding led to the core category that encompassed aspects of all three main categories as "therapist tasks" when I reached saturation by sorting memos—the final step in theory integration. In sorting memos, a researcher works his or her way to the highest level of conceptualization. Sorting also serves as a measure of how effective the choosing of a problem, collecting, coding, saturation, sampling, and memoing turned out to be (Glaser, 1998).

In the sample study, when I sorted all of the memos, I determined that the category "therapist tasks" had been established. This is what I wrote as a statement of theory at this point:

> Assumptions about clients' having resources, and having all that is needed within [themselves] for healing, leaning toward positive outcomes, and solutions, are consistent with resource-based assessment. Assessing for strengths and resources in the early phases of therapy allows therapists to make it part of treatment planning. As CG7 put it, "it would be foolish" to ask these questions later, because [a therapist] would not be able to consider strengths when the contract between client and therapist is being created. Gathering this type of information also helps therapists determine how difficult situations might have been handled in the past, in comparison to how current presenting problems have been handled. Analysis of verbal and nonverbal information is important within the scope of interviews, guided imagery, journaling, homework, role playing, field trips, [and] suggestive techniques like hypnotherapy (KD25) and reflecting teams (PC27).
>
> Questions that lend themselves to opening up details about exceptions (i.e., "when the problem isn't") help therapists discover ways in which clients have dealt with similar problems successfully. Questions about strengths, talents, and competencies can lead to both "internal and external" strengths and resources (i.e., those that are part of the client and those that have to do with his [or] her external support system). External strengths and resources can be assessed via "family constellation" questions, which have clients disclose their view of each of their family members (WG19), as well as through "community genograms" (KK24) and eco-maps (RF29). Listening for possible strengths [and] reflecting them back to the client, while the client considers how possible strengths could be used or might be noticed by others, can lead to interventions that assume [the] client's acquisition of strengths and resources.
>
> By using "self as exemplar," clients can revisit their past to find times when their presenting difficulty was not an issue or when other difficult situations were handled successfully. Therapists can tap client resources by working from "smallest to biggest success" and examining behaviors, attitudes, communication, and management of emotions associated with exceptional times (JM15). Sometimes clients reveal their strengths and resources in their presentation of self and their presentation of the issues in terms of how they have managed up to that point (KK24). In some cases, having clients take inventory of how past problems were solved in the past will help them eliminate methods they would not use again. Therapists can also use "others as exemplars" by having clients think of ways that others did (or would) go about solving similar problems. Further consideration may help clients find ways that might work better for them.
>
> Past successes can also be useful when clients need resources and strengths to process events they want to deal with in therapy (LH17). Future-oriented strategies, like "feed-forward" questions (RB18) or "future-emanated thinking" (JM15), help clients envision a future without the problem. The greater the descriptive detail elicited by the therapist, the better. For instance, therapists can ask clients "what would be different if they [clients] solved the problem" and work "step by step backwards from solution to problem" (TR30).

Implications of This Study

As mentioned earlier, grounded theory is known for its emphasis on theoretical sampling (based on analyzed data) that leads to further theory development. Some of the data in this study revealed concepts that hinted at other areas worthy of further investigation. For instance, various client-related attributes and actions contributed to the therapists' ability to access client resources. This leads us to think that, just as there are "therapist tasks," there may very well be client factors related to how they respond to therapists' search for their strengths and resources in therapy. In addition, some therapists referred to assumptions they held about strengths within individuals, which could also be investigated further. A third area for further inquiry is how deeply embedded the search for strengths and resources is in therapists' thinking (i.e., their theoretical orientations). All of these areas were derived from noticeable gaps in the data that were not saturated enough to be developed into categories. Besides these areas, a couple of other possibilities to explore further are (1) conducting in-depth interviews with therapists who had the most developed modes of assessing for client strengths and resources; and (2) comparing some of the findings from this study to those from previous resource-based studies (Echevarria-Doan, 2001; Rafuls, 1994; Rafuls & Moon, 1996). As grounded theory would have it, there are many "leads" to follow. It is no wonder I (SED) am still holding up that magnifying glass in search of all of the parts to a theory that will help us better understand the process of searching for and using strengths and resources in therapy.

Reporting

To report findings in grounded theory, the researcher does not need to wait for complete theoretical saturation of categories and/or testing of emergent hypotheses. Basically, the idea is to write up the sorted memos (generally called "sorts"), as demonstrated above in the final write-up of our research example (Glaser, 1998). However, because of the close connection between data collection and data analysis, reporting can begin from the time data are first collected. Initial reporting of emergent theory usually occurs during analysis in the form of informal discussions and/or presentations. We suggest, however, that reporting initial findings should go beyond personal communications and be published for reasons of exposure and critique. As Glaser (1978) asserts, grounded theory deserves publication for its rigor and value, and for the stake that grounded theorists have in affecting "wider publics" (p. 128) in order to make their theories count. Strauss and Corbin (1998) concur by suggesting that publication of grounded theory studies enhances collegial communication. Usually grounded theory research is written up as an integrated set of hypotheses rather than a report of findings. Although the degree of conceptualization involved in doing this requires integration of data, writing can also occur before integration occurs, for the specific purpose of working one's way out of the stumbling blocks of integration itself. This can be done by writing about the most relevant parts of one's theory and then analyzing them for their relationships (Glaser, 1978).

   Writing up grounded theory research has more to do with the relationship between concepts than it does with the description of people or phenomena. In contrast to ethnography and phenomenology, where description is paramount and low-inference descriptors substantiate credibility, description and illustration in grounded theory reporting are secondary to integrated conceptualization and are minimally utilized for support purposes, Glaser (1978) claims that the credibility of a grounded theory report is achieved by its integration and relevance and not by using illustrations as proof. Grounded theory research is written up so that the reader has an understanding of the conceptual work that goes into the analysis and its integration into a theoretical orientation (Glaser, 1978). This allows the reader to make reasonable judgments about the theory's "trustworthiness," which Lincoln and Guba (1985) define as the credibility and transferability of a study's findings. The trustworthiness of a study is influenced by the way that its findings are written (Lincoln & Guba, 1985). Grounded theory research can be reported in a paper, article, thesis, monograph, chapter, or book. Due to the approach's origin in sociology, writing has been often shaped by the style employed in sociological monographs and chapters (Glaser, 1978; Glaser & Strauss, 1967; Strauss & Corbin, 1998). This includes addressing the problem and core category derived from the use of grounded theory, the methodology, and a clear analytical story about the core category.

DISCUSSION

Strengths of the Methodology When Applied to Family Therapy Research

One of the strengths in using grounded theory methodology in family therapy research is that grounded theory is theoretically consistent with the practice of family therapy. This is especially important to clinicians, who are often discouraged by how irrelevant research is to their practice. The inductive nature of therapists' inquiry, their process with clients, and the hypothesis-driven conclusions they develop are very similar to steps taken by grounded theorists, as our example has described. Because the methodology requires skills paralleling those required of therapists, clinicians are more likely to turn to grounded theory methodology as a way to bridge clinical practice with areas of interest that they would like to investigate further. Therefore, when grounded theory methodology is applied in family therapy research, the kinship that exists between both processes is a definite strength.

The research questions that grounded theory can help family therapists answer constitute another strength, because of the compatibility that exists in the way that both processes ask questions. Often clinicians ask questions that can be answered in qualitative terms. Grounded theory, in particular, is applicable to questions therapists ask about the process of therapy or about clients in therapy, because such questions usually refer to meanings, perceptions, and understandings of clients. Therapists' questions are also related to sensitive topics dealt with in therapy, which are usually complex, qualified, ambivalent, situational, and/or changing over time. In addition, questions may relate to alternative perspectives, diversity, and uniqueness, all of which fit within the paradigm of grounded theory.

A final strength of grounded theory is its formulation as a general tool of inquiry (Glaser, 1992). That is, it serves well as the methodological component of paradigms whose epistemological and ontological positions define postpositivistic or constructivistic orientations. It is not exclusive to any particular paradigm; rather, it is a tool that facilitates analysis of data bounded by the epistemology and ontology of the paradigm of inquiry. Therefore, it can appropriately be used as an analytical tool in conjunction with other methodologies, such as phenomenology or ethnography (Lewis & Moon, 1997; Piercy, Moon, & Bischof, 1994).

Weaknesses of the Methodology When Applied to Family Therapy Research

Although grounded theory methodology is quite compatible with family therapy research, it does present some concerns associated with the recursive nature of theoretical sampling and theory development. Specifically, theoretical sampling and theory building in grounded theory studies may require considerable programmatic efforts; they can be time- and labor-intensive; it may be hard to delegate the analysis phase to research assistants; both sampling and theory development can be hard to do well; and some potential for role ambiguity and role conflict exists if research is conducted in a clinical setting. All of these concerns have implications for funding (related to the denial or depletion of resources) and for publication efforts (in terms of the extended time necessary to write up grounded theory studies in some cases).

Although we view the compatibility of the processes involved in clinical practice and grounded theory research as a strength, this complementarity also presents some concerns with regard to issues of informed consent and ethics. In other words, there is a good chance that grounded theory research in a clinical setting can have a therapeutic influence on its participants. Usually, any potential effects or influences of research are explained when informed consent is obtained. However, because therapeutic effects or influences are not predictable or known at the beginning of research, a discussion of these in specific terms is not possible during informed consent, thus raising ethical concerns as a weakness of the grounded theory design. For that matter, any design that is inductive and exploratory in nature (as grounded theory is) would raise this concern. Besides letting participants know that the possibility of influence on their therapy exists, there is little else a researcher is able to do in terms of informed consent as a way of addressing this concern. In addition, the exploratory nature of grounded theory methodology raises concerns when it comes to reviewing the literature one is to investigate. Glaser (1998), for instance, is vehemently against researchers' conducting literature reviews if true grounded theory is to take place. This is certainly problematic, given the proposal guidelines in many academic settings where grounded theory studies take place.

The philosophical and methodological differences between Glaser and Strauss concerning the tenets of grounded theory also continue to present challenges to researchers. The discord centered on two points: (1) the origin of research questions, and (2) the nature of the analytical process. Glaser suggests that research questions emerge from and are shaped by the data, whereas Strauss indicated that the researcher brings the question to the data and the data collection process. However, the differences between them over the nature of the analytical process have garnered the most attention. Glaser advocates methodological flexibility, to encourage emergence of theory from the data. On the other hand, Strauss supported adherence to the three-stage coding process, to ferret out theory about the phenomenon of interest (Babchuk, 1997; Glaser, 1992). As a result of these differing perspectives, two different approaches to grounded theory have evolved. Researchers must therefore ensure that the rationale and goal of their research designs are congruent with the grounded theory approach they utilize.

A fourth limitation to using grounded theory, particularly for family therapists with postmodernist leanings, is Glaser's firm assertion about the validity of constructivist explanations of the grounded theory process. He dismisses such explanations as unwarranted concerns with "data accuracy" and justifications of unacknowl-edged researcher bias (Charmaz, 2000; Glaser, 2001, 2002). Such assertions pose interesting, although not insurmountable, challenges for researchers who are comfort-able with the use and practice of grounded theory, but philosophically at odds with one of its creators.

Reliability and Validity

In the research world, the reliability and validity of a study serve as standards that de-termine how "good" research really is. This presents an epistemological problem when research paradigms digress from the positivistic traditions on which these criteria are based. Implicit in differing modes of discovery are different standards and procedures to arrive at "good science." In qualitative terms, we might say that the reliability and validity of a research study determine its credibility and trustworthiness (Lincoln & Guba, 1985). Although we could discuss reliability and validity as credibility and trustworthiness, we will stay (at the risk of being judged positivistic) within the lan-guage of research methodologists at large, but will discuss reliability and validity as they pertain to qualitative research.

In positivistic science, "reliability" is concerned with the replicability of findings, and "validity" is concerned with the accuracy of findings. Reliability is dependent on the resolution of both external and internal design problems (LeCompte et al., 1993). Validity is also assessed in terms of internal and external aspects of accuracy related to the findings.

"External reliability" refers to the likelihood that an independent researcher would find similar phenomena or generate the same constructs in the same or similar settings (LeCompte et al., 1993). The uniqueness or complexity of phenomena and in-dividuals, which is characteristically a part of naturalistic inquiry, presents some con-cerns with regard to this standard of reproducibility. However, steps can be taken to safeguard against threats to external reliability by providing readers with explicit de-tails regarding the researcher's theoretical perspective and the research methodology that was implemented in a study. The explication of data collection may include de-scriptions of the criteria for selecting participants, the interview guide questions, the researcher's role, and the methods of analysis (e.g., coding procedures and the devel-opment of categories and hypotheses). Under a similar set of conditions, it is feasible for another researcher to come up with a similar theoretical explanation about a given phenomenon. Glaser (1998, 2002) and Strauss and Corbin (1998) would argue that the very explicit nature of categorized steps in grounded theory research would pre-vent problems with external reliability, because they strongly believe that the process inherently allows for different observers to discover the world and describe it in simi-lar ways (Charmaz, 2000). Charmaz argues, "That's correct—to the extent that sub-jects have comparable experiences . . . and viewers bring similar questions, perspec-tives, methods, and subsequently, concepts to analyze those experiences" (p. 524).

"Internal reliability" refers to the degree to which another researcher would arrive at similar findings from the data that were collected in a previous study. Problems with internal reliability can be resolved by providing the reader with verbatim accounts or low-inference descriptors. Grounded theorists are faced with a dilemma, however: This supportive documentation should be kept to a minimum in grounded theory re-search, as emphasis is placed on depth of conceptualizations rather than on description. A more reasonable approach to remedying concerns related to internal reliability in grounded theory research may be to employ members of a given "culture" who can confirm, or disconfirm, a researcher's findings (LeCompte et al., 1993). Descriptions phrased as precisely and concretely as possible should help to remedy concerns about internal reliability. However, qualitative research approaches do not implement standardized interview protocols, because of their emphasis on discovery and open-ended interviewing. Instead, threats to internal reliability are remedied by employing differing methods of peer debriefing, and by providing readers with personal and professional information about the researcher that could have affected data collection, analysis, and interpretation.

"Internal validity" refers to the authenticity of representation—that is, the similarity between what researchers believe they observed and that which was actually observed (LeCompte et al., 1993). Use of multiple data sources, or what is known as "triangulation," is one way to address this concern (Denzin, 1978). In the research example used in the first edition (Rafuls, 1994; see Rafuls & Moon, 1996), the researcher dealt with internal validity in her study by interviewing families and therapists in progressive phases, which built on the participants' information and interpretation from one phase to another. Multiple data sources also included videotapes and audiotapes, transcript data, the researcher's notes and journal, and theoretical memos written by both the researcher and her assistant. Explication of her biases and assumptions as the researcher also exemplified a "disciplined subjectivity," which Erickson (1986) refers to as a way to control for observer effects. Here too, it is important to let the audience know about the researcher as a way of ensuring trustworthiness of findings and methods.

"External validity" refers to the generalizability of findings across groups. In grounded theory, the researcher is not interested in generalizations across populations, but in the transferability of theoretical abstractions. That is, grounded theorists are concerned with the analytical generalization and transferability of findings from case to case, rather than the generalizability of results from sample to population (Firestone, 1993). In grounded theory, this is achieved by maximizing comparisons across different groups of participants in differing contexts and situations through theoretical selection and saturation. The intentional sampling for theoretically relevant diversity that exists in grounded theory, and its analytically based process of theory building, are strengths in terms of external validity. A researcher's conceptualizations should be abstract enough that they can accommodate a variety of changing situations and can be readily understood, but not so abstract that they lose being able to relate to concepts (Glaser & Strauss, 1967). According to Lincoln and Guba (1985), the burden of proof for transferability lies less with the researcher than with the reader. It is the researcher's responsibility to provide sufficiently descriptive data—or, in the case of grounded theory, explanatory data—that will allow readers to make their own assessments of the validity of the analysis and its transferability to their own situation (Firestone, 1993).

Skills Required of the Researcher

Grounded theory researchers need to have both creative and critical thinking skills. They must also have excellent organizational and conceptual abilities, as well as good writing skills. In addition, grounded theory requires that researchers have good decision-making skills and an ability to deal with ambiguity. Great patience is also helpful when it comes to careful comparison of bits of data. As Glaser (1998) puts it, the tedious nature of constantly coding, collecting, and analyzing causes many researchers to "flip out with possibly non-patterned impressions and incident tripping or just default to conceptual description or pure description" (p. 151). He attributes this to a lack of tolerance for confusion and a need for immediate structure. Also, some researchers have preconceptions. Grounded theory is difficult for a "know-it-beforehand-for-sure" researcher.

Bridging Research and Practice

One of the strengths we have highlighted earlier is the compatibility that exists between family therapy practice and grounded theory research. This degree of compatibility also bridges the world of research and practice. It is especially important for clinicians who are skeptical, discouraged, or uninterested when they encounter research. No longer does research have to be associated with absolute truth, experimentation, quantification, and statistical significance alone. It is now also known as a creative, inductive, theory-building process that feels somewhat familiar and akin to the process of therapy.

The increased use of grounded theory in family therapy has only confirmed our belief in its utility for linking research to practice and vice versa (Christensen, Russell, Miller, & Peterson, 1998; Smith, Winton, & Yoshioka, 1992). A grounded theory approach facilitates and expedites the research-to-practice link, in that the categories, themes, and theory generated represent an "emic" (or insider's) perspective on the phenomenon of interest. Therefore, in reference to questions about family strengths and effective intervention strategies, the emergent theory identifies best practices based on the target population's lived experience, rather than on trial and error (Smith, Yoshioka, & Winton, 1993; Wiersma, 2003). The interplay between the constant comparative method and theoretical sampling inherent in grounded theory enhance the trustworthiness of best practices and decrease the potential for cultural inappropriate interventions, as well as for wasted time and resources.

Future Directions

Grounded theory is a methodology with widespread appeal and application to a number of fields of study in the social sciences. Family therapy is no different, as the exemplars presented at the end of this chapter demonstrate. The future of grounded theory methodology in family therapy research lies in its congruence with evolving, cutting-edge models of family therapy (i.e., constructivist, feminist, narrative, and collaborative language systems approaches). This is especially true if these models/approaches have not developed their own research methodology. Grounded theory is also useful alongside quantitative research in studies where a qualitative component complements the quantitative elements (e.g., as part of sampling selection, brief interviews, or follow-up studies). We want to emphasize, however, that grounded theory and qualitative research are not simply adjuncts or supplements to quantitative methods, but are equally important in understanding phenomena and generating theory. Grounded theory's flexibility, openness, process orientation, and collaborative tendencies also opens up possibilities for research that addresses lived experience in cross-cultural or gender-related research.

We believe it is healthy to promote the epistemological and methodological debates that have transpired recently in the research community (Charmaz, 2000; Glaser, 2002). Debates between grounded theorists are nothing new, given Glaser's (1978, 1992) and Strauss's (1987; Strauss & Corbin, 1998) public discourse disclosing their diverging views of the method itself. Arguments like those posed by Charmaz (2000) can only further define and enhance grounded theory's presence across numerous disciplines and epistemological camps. A "one-size-fits-all" mentality that stakes a claim of authority over this method would be of greater concern. Instead, our hope is that this debate in grounded theory will lead to rich methods and flexible thinking that can allow grounded theory to be incorporated into more interpretive and constructive paradigms, without fear of losing its strengths in the process.

EXEMPLARS

Coulehan, R., Friedlander, M. L., & Heatherington, L. (1998). Transforming narratives: A change event in constructivist family therapy. *Family Process, 37,* 17–33.—This study examined the behavioral antecedents of cognitive shifts occurring in constructivist family therapy. A grounded theory approach was used to analyze phenomenological data, which resulted in theory development and theory verification as the authors expanded Sluzki's model of transformation. Although the coding procedures are not articulated, the authors provide a strong explanation of their use of the constant comparative method.

Davey, M., Stone Fish, L., Askew, J., & Robila, M. (2003). Parenting practices and the transmission of ethnic identity. *Journal of Marital and Family Therapy, 29,* 151–164.—Davey and colleagues' study analyzed interview data to identify parenting practices that affect the transmission of ethnic identity to adolescents in white Jewish families from the Northeast. The authors provided extensive information not only about the three stages of coding (as articulated by Strauss and Corbin), but also about the trustworthiness of analysis. In addition, Davey and colleagues were explicit about the use of existent literature to inform the analysis.

Joanides, C., Mayhew, M., & Mamalakis, P. M. (2002). Investigating inter-Christian and intercultural couples associated with the Greek Orthodox Archdiocese of America: A qualitative research project. *American Journal of Family Therapy, 30,* 373–383.—The interfaith and intercultural marriages of Greek Orthodox individuals constituted the focus of this study. Focus group data were analyzed via the grounded theory methodology articulated by Strauss and Corbin, including the three stages of coding. Thirteen categories were identified. This article provides a clear, yet brief, overview of the major tenets of grounded theory.

Smith, T. E., Yoshioka, M., & Winton, M. (1993). A qualitative understanding of reflecting teams: I. Client perspectives. *Journal of Systemic Therapies, 12,* 28–43.—Smith and colleagues utilized the constant comparative method to analyze interview data in an initial step toward understanding clients' perspectives on the reflecting team process. The study focused on representative and unique responses obtained through theoretical sampling as the major strategy for grounding the findings. The strength of this article lies in the ample provision of verbatim excerpts, to allow the reader to draw his or her own inferences.

Wiersma, N. S. (2003). Partner awareness regarding the adult sequelae of childhood sexual abuse for primary and secondary survivors. *Journal of Marital and Family Therapy, 29,* 151–164.—This study utilized grounded theory to identify themes relevant to couples' awareness of the impact of childhood sexual abuse on one member of a couple. Wiersma clearly identified the three-stage coding process essential to the analysis (as articulated by Strauss and Corbin) and provided enough detail for the reader to follow the progression. The article also includes a helpful table that supported Wiersma's findings.

REFERENCES

Babchuk, W. A. (1997, October). *Glaser or Strauss?: Grounded theory and adult education.* Paper presented at the Midwest Research-to-Practice Conference in Adult, Continuing and Community Education, East Lansing, MI

Bernard, R. (2002). *Research methods in anthropology* (3rd ed.). Walnut Creek, CA: Altamira Press.

Charmaz, K. (2000). Grounded theory: Objectivist and constructivist methods. In N. K. Denzin & Y. S. Lincoln (Eds.), *Handbook of qualitative research* (2nd ed., pp. 509–535). Thousand Oaks, CA: Sage.

Coulehan, R., Friedlander, M. L., & Heatherington, L. (1998). Transforming narratives: A change event in constructivist family therapy. *Family Process, 37,* 17–33.

Creswell, J. W. (1998). *Qualitative inquiry and research design: Choosing among five traditions.* Thousand Oaks, CA: Sage.

Crotty, M. (1998). *The foundations of social research.* London: Sage.

Denzin, N. K. (1978). *Sociological methods: A sourcebook* (2nd ed.). New York: McGraw-Hill.

Denzin, N. K. (1994). The art and politics of interpretation. In N. K. Denzin & Y. S. Lincoln (Eds.), *Handbook of qualitative research* (pp. 500–515). Thousand Oaks, CA: Sage.

Echevarria-Doan, S. (2001). Resource-based reflective consultation: Accessing client resources through interviews and dialogue. *Journal of Marital and Family Therapy, 27,* 201–212.

Erickson, F. (1986). Qualitative methods in research on teaching. In M. C. Wittrock (Ed.), *Handbook of research on teaching* (3rd ed., pp. 119–161). New York: Macmillan.

Firestone, W. A. (1993). Alternative arguments for generalizing from data as applied to qualitative research. *Educational Researcher, 22*(4), 16–23.

Gilgun, J. F. (1992). Definitions, methodologies, and methods in qualitative family research. In J. F. Gilgun, K. Daly, & G. Handel (Eds.), *Qualitative methods in family research* (pp. 22–39). Newbury Park, CA: Sage.

Glaser, B. G. (1978). *Theoretical sensitivity: Advances in the methodology of grounded theory.* Mill Valley, CA: Sociology Press.

Glaser, B. G. (1992). *Basics of grounded theory analysis.* Mill Valley, CA: Sociology Press.

Glaser, B. G. (1998). *Doing grounded theory: Issues and discussions.* Mill Valley, CA: Sociology Press.

Glaser, B. G. (2001). *The grounded theory perspective: Conceptualization contrasted with description.* Mill Valley, CA: Sociology Press.

Glaser, B. G. (2002, September). Constructivist grounded theory? *Forum Qualitative Sozialforschung/Forum: Qualitative Social Research, 3*(3). Retrieved from *http://www.qualitative-research.net/fqs/fqs-eng.htm*

Glaser, B. G., & Strauss, A. L. (1967). *The discovery of grounded theory: Strategies for qualitative research.* Chicago: Aldine.

Guba, E. (Ed.). (1990). *The paradigm dialogue.* Newbury Park, CA: Sage.

Hoshmand, L. L. S. T. (1989). Alternative research paradigms: A review and teaching proposal. *The Counseling Psychologist, 17,* 3–101.

Karpel, M. (1986). *Family resources: The hidden partner in family therapy.* New York: Guilford Press.

LeCompte, M. D., & Preissle, J., with Tesch, R. (1993). *Ethnography and qualitative design in educational research* (2nd ed.). San Diego, CA: Academic Press.

Lewis, K. G., & Moon, S. M. (1997). Always single and single again women: A qualitative study. *Journal of Marital and Family Therapy, 23,* 115–134.

Lincoln, Y., & Guba, E. (1985). *Naturalistic inquiry.* Beverly Hills, CA: Sage.

Piercy, F. P., Moon, S. M., & Bischof, G. P. (1994). Difficult journal article rejections among prolific family therapists: A qualitative critical incident study. *Journal of Marital and Family Therapy, 20,* 231–245.

Rafuls, S. E. (1994). *Qualitative resource-based consultation: Resource-generative inquiry and reflective dialogue with four Latin American families and their therapists.* Unpublished doctoral dissertation, Purdue University.

Rafuls, S. E., & Moon, S. M. (1996). Grounded theory methodology in family therapy research. In D. H. Sprenkle & S. M. Moon (Eds.), *Research methods in family therapy* (pp. 64–80). New York: Guilford Press.

Rennie, D. (1998). Grounded theory methodology: The pressing need for a coherent logic of justification. *Theory and Psychology, 8,* 101–119.

Rennie, D. (2000). Grounded theory methodology as methodical hermeneutics. *Theory and Psychology, 10,* 481–502.

Richardson, J. (1999). The concepts and methods of phenomenographic research. *Review of Educational Research, 69,* 53–82.

Smith, T. E., Winton, M., & Yoshioka, M. (1992). A qualitative understanding of reflecting teams: II. Therapists' perspectives. *Contemporary Family Therapy, 14,* 419–432.

Smith, T. E., Yoshioka, M., & Winton, M. (1993). A qualitative understanding of reflecting teams: I. Client perspectives. *Journal of Systemic Therapies, 12,* 28–43.

Strauss, A. L. (1987). *Qualitative analysis for social scientists.* New York: Cambridge University Press.

Strauss, A. L., & Corbin, J. (1998). *Basics of qualitative research: Techniques and procedures for developing grounded theory* (2nd ed.). Thousand Oaks, CA: Sage.

Wiersma, N. S. (2003). Partner awareness regarding the adult sequelae of childhood sexual abuse for primary and secondary survivors. *Journal of Marital and Family Therapy, 29,* 151–164.

Williams, M. (2001). *Problems of knowledge: A critical introduction to epistemology.* Oxford: Oxford University Press.

CHAPTER 4

The Use of Phenomenology for Family Therapy Research

THE SEARCH FOR MEANING

CARLA M. DAHL
PAULINE BOSS

BACKGROUND

Are cows pink? "No," says the positivist, "they are black and white or brown—and sometimes combinations thereof." But those who have had direct experience with cows know they can be pink. We have seen them. At sunset, when the sky over a Wisconsin field is rosy and glowing, cows are pink. At that moment and in that particular context, the description of pink for cows is really true. This is phenomenology. True knowledge is relative.

We define a phenomenon—in this case, cows—by describing its essential impact on our immediate conscious experience (Becker, 1992). Artists, musicians, and poets have for ages recorded their interpretations of life by using the phenomenological approach. In this chapter, we focus on the phenomenology of everyday life—particularly marriage and family—to familiarize family therapists with a method of investigation and description that is compatible with their already developed skills of observation, creativity, intuition, empathic listening, and analysis.

What is clear is that the phenomenon of phenomenology itself has different meanings to different people. Deutscher (1973) refers to the term broadly as a tradition within the social sciences concerned with "understanding the social actor's frame of reference" (p. 12; see also Bruyn, 1966; Psathas, 1973). Others use the term more narrowly to refer to a European school of thought in philosophy (see, e.g., Schutz, 1960, 1967). Phenomenology has also been called the "microsociology of knowledge" by Berger and Kellner (1964; see also Kollock & O'Brien, 1994). Today many might argue that the original meaning of "phenomenology" has become ambiguous or has been lost altogether.

More critical, however, than one agreed-upon definition of phenomenology is what we believe about the world and the people in it, so our discussion (after a brief history) focuses on eight philosophical assumptions of phenomenology and the ways they shape research, as well as on what phenomenology is *not*. We then discuss the process of doing phenomenological research, including ethical issues that are particularly relevant.

Because marriage, family, and close relationships are such integral parts of everyday life, phenomenologists believe they should be studied as phenomena *in that context*—in the neighborhood, at home, at mealtime, during rituals and celebrations. To be sure, empirical findings have emerged from studying families in controlled laboratory settings or from large-sample surveys; however, phenomenologists believe that the phenomenon of interest, regardless of what it is, should be studied *where it naturally exists and from the actor's own perspective*. In family research, which has multiple perspectives, this means that we must either consider and describe diverse views, or explicitly label our work as restricted to one person's perspective of how a family or couple works. Either is acceptable, as long as it is labeled, because the phenomenologist's focus is on *whose* perspective is represented at that time and in that context.

Historical Roots and Development

Two theoretical perspectives are recommended for studying marital and family interactions: the symbolic interactionism of George Herbert Mead (1934) and the phenomenological analysis of the social structuring of reality, especially the work of Schutz (1960, 1962, 1967) and Merleau-Ponty (1945/1962). Although this chapter focuses on phenomenology, symbolic interactionism represents a compatible theoretical perspective.

Phenomenology originated well over 50 years ago in Europe; the University of Chicago subsequently became the initial base for U.S. consideration of this European tradition. Theoretical perspectives that therapists frequently associate with phenomenology are Erving Goffman's (1959) dramaturgical model and Berger and Luckmann's (1966) sociology of knowledge. Other perspectives are found in labeling theory, existential sociology, sociology of the absurd, symbolic interactionism, and ethnomethodology. Scholars disagree as to how much these perspectives differ from each other and in what ways.

In this chapter, we present phenomenology as interpretive inquiry and emphasize the cultural and political contexts that influence the interpretation of meanings. Also, we do not eschew positivism. This sets us apart from Martin Heidegger's phenomenology and places us more in line with his students and successors: Popper, Adorno, Mannheim, Freud, Klein, Arendt, Marcuse, Adorno, and Horkheimer. They survived Nazism but were not sullied by it, as was Heidegger. In 1945, he was tried as a collaborator with the Nazis and banned from teaching, but he continued to avoid taking responsibility for his complicity. The question for the critical reader is this: Can we separate this man's actions, or inaction, from his philosophy when that very philosophy is "being is doing"? For us, the *meaning* of Heidegger's philosophy cannot be separated from his Nazi affiliation in the *context* of the Holocaust (many of his colleagues—including his mentor, Husserl—were Jews). (See Collins, 2000; Philipse, 1998; Ree, 1999.)

Phenomenology survives primarily through Heidegger's uncompromised students and successors who left Germany to escape Fascism: Popper, Freud, and Klein ended up in London; Adorno and Mannheim at Princeton; Hannah Arendt and Karen

Horney in New York. The Frankfurt Institute reconvened on the American West Coast; in New York, the New School for Social Research became the center of thought with Levi-Strauss, Arendt, and Schutz (who linked Husserl's phenomenology to Weberian sociology).

During the postmodernism of the 1990s, phenomenology enjoyed a renaissance. Family researchers of both pre- and postmodern ilks became increasingly interested in how family members experience their everyday worlds and how their perceptions of what they experience lead to differing meanings. During this decade, researchers as well as therapists began increasingly to go into families' homes—into what Hess and Handel (1959) had earlier called the "family world." In this world, according to Hess and Handel, interactions between individuals in a family must be viewed in the context of how the individuals define one another as relevant objects. Today Gerald Handel is joined by Jane Gilgun, Judith Stacey, Linda Burton, and many others who reaffirm that people should be studied wherever they live their lives—in the home, in the neighborhood, in the car, at work, in school, in institutions, at the mall. To a phenomenologist, then, the important reality is what individuals, couples, or families perceive it to be; their "real" world is not likely to be found in the laboratory or clinic, but where they naturally interact in their daily lives.

Historically, this view for studying families represents the antithesis of logical positivism and empiricism; it challenges the assumption that the scientific method is *the* one way to accumulate truth and knowledge. Phenomenologists have criticized logical positivists in the areas of (1) verification (phenomenologists say that science needs common sense as well as method); (2) operationalism (phenomenologists recognize an inevitable gap between concepts and devices to measure those concepts); (3) invariance (phenomenologists see probabilistic conclusions as useful—even knowledge obtained without the scientific method is useful); (4) positive knowledge (negative findings are equally important, according to phenomenologists); and (5) lack of reflexivity (phenomenologists see a need to regularly examine their own feelings and perceptions—an idea akin to therapists' concerns regarding countertransference).

When we use a phenomenological approach, our a priori assumptions about how families work or do not work become the core of our inquiry, because no one method is prescribed in phenomenology. Our focus in this chapter, therefore, must necessarily be on assumptions shared by most phenomenologists. Any of the methods discussed in Part II of this volume could conceivably be used with a phenomenological approach, but *only* if the investigators accept certain assumptions.

Philosophical Assumptions of Phenomenological Family Therapy Researchers

The following list summarizes our basic assumptions as phenomenological family therapy researchers. Three assumptions relate to how we know, two to what we need to know, and three to where we locate ourselves in the research process.

How We Know

1. *Knowledge is socially constructed and therefore inherently tentative and incomplete.* Truth remains forever relative and elusive. The use of the scientific method, despite its apparent emphasis on conclusions, does not obviate this assumption.

2. Because knowledge is constructed, *objects, events, or situations can mean a variety of things to a variety of people in a family*. Chronic illness, for example, can mean "punishment from God" or "a challenge from God to show one's love in a new way"—both in the same family. Multiple perceptions of the same event or situation are therefore important to hear. Although we can observe and code family acts, "it is not appearance *per se*, but rather what appears to be that is critical. . . . Indeterminacy derives from varied interpretations, which in turn is constituted by and through language" (Gubrium & Holstein, 1993, p. 654).

Experiences, objects, events, or situations can mean different things to different family members (see, e.g., Boss, Beaulieu, Wieling, Turner, & LaCruz, 2003; Frankl, 1984). Just as family therapists do, phenomenological family researchers must elicit the perceptions and views of all family members to get the total picture of a particular family. Although this makes research more complicated, it realistically reflects the diversity of gender, generation, sexual orientation, ethnicity, and culture inherent in family life. Today, in this era of frequent divorce and remarriage, it can even be difficult to get agreement in couples' reports about existing child custody arrangements (Rettig & Dahl, 1993). Other, more intangible experiences are even more likely to be perceived in radically differing ways (e.g., Dahl, 1994; SmithBattle, 1996).

It is critically important, then, for us as family therapy researchers using the phenomenological approach to listen to and observe the "whole." We must not repeat the mistake of many researchers who interview mothers primarily (because they are most readily available) to gather data about children or families. We must attempt to hear the "family conversational voice" as a whole or to observe the "family world" as a whole. This cannot be done if we talk to only one family member (see, e.g., Boss et al., 2003; Garwick, Detzner, & Boss, 1994; Pollner & McDonald-Wikler, 1985/1994; Reiss, 1981/1994).

3. *We can know through both art and science.* We believe that important knowledge can be gained from folk stories, folk songs, and folk art. For example, richly detailed family-of-origin stories abound in the embroidery of Hmong refugee women in Minnesota, who, with needle and thread, have recorded their families' harrowing escapes from their homeland in Southeast Asia. Another example is Pablo Picasso's painting *Blue Family*, which shows parents and child in cold blue color, arms around only themselves, eyes all downward, no connection between family members. This painting depicts the same phenomenon described by David Reiss (1981/1994) as a "distance-sensitive family." Reiss, however, illustrated "distance" with an empirically based technical drawing of small separated circles, while Picasso painted on canvas what he felt were symbols of distance and a lack of familial connection. Both scientist and artist depicted the same phenomenon; both represented a reality of human families, but from their own experience, within their own discipline, and through their own mode of expression. Thus both depicted a form of true knowledge. Phenomenologists see their inquiries as both art and science.

What We Need to Know

4. *Common, everyday knowledge about family worlds is epistemologically important.* Phenomenologists are intensely curious about the "taken-for-granted" aspects of family life; everyday routines like bedtime are as interesting as life cycle rituals like weddings and funerals. The sacred and the mundane, the ordinary and the extraordi-

nary, are equally intriguing. Understanding everyday life is as necessary for comprehending how families work as is understanding the unique, spectacular, even catastrophic events families experience (e.g., Boss, 2002a, 2002b; Boss et al., 2003). If we investigators only gather data at special times of crisis or stress, our knowledge will be skewed. Family therapists most often witness family processes at times of stress or crisis. For research, it would be worthwhile to visit with families at times when they are not in need of professional help.

5. *Language and meaning of everyday life are significant.* Rather than referring to the science of linguistics, "the study of family discourse highlights how language serves to assign meaning to objects and social conditions" in everyday life (Gubrium & Holstein, 1993, p. 653). The family's language offers a source of information that is symbolically rich in meaning and information. The qualitative analysis of whole-family conversations for themes and patterns is therefore worthwhile (see Blumer, 1969; Garwick et al., 1994; Patterson & Garwick, 1994). Language remains the primary symbol of human interaction and needs to be studied where it takes place *naturally*. Neither the laboratory nor the therapy room is a natural setting, so we must get away from our offices to observe and interact with families in their natural settings (see, e.g., Burton, 1991, who actually spent time in high-risk neighborhoods researching child care; see also Henry, 1973; Liebow, 1967; Stacey, 1990).

Where We Locate Ourselves in the Research Process

6. *As researchers, we are not separate from the phenomena we study.* Social inquiry is influenced by our beliefs about how the world works. Our feelings, beliefs, values, and responses (about things like equality, patriarchy, matriarchy, mastery over nature, acceptance of nature, communitarianism, and individualism) influence the research questions we ask, as well as our interpretation of data. Subjectivity (rather than objectivity) is therefore recognized as our research reality and is paramount in the study of families and couples. A continuing and explicit process of self-reflexivity and self-questioning (preferably not in isolation) is therefore a necessary part of phenomenological inquiry and often leads to midstream changes in procedure if we believe that those changes would be more productive or ethical.

7. Because of the desire for understanding this range of family experiences, the phenomenological approach also assumes that *everyday knowledge is shared and held by researchers and participants alike.* There is little or no hierarchy about who is an expert. All persons—common and celebrated, researcher and participant, therapist and client—are considered epistemologists (Gubrium & Holstein, 1993). As researchers, we listen to stories, we observe interaction, we note feelings (theirs and ours); we ask questions because the families, not we ourselves, will accurately describe the phenomenon we are studying. For example, we could study the varying meanings of death or ambiguous loss in families by documenting their stories, just as Sedney, Baker, and Gross (1994) and Boss and colleagues (2003) used stories as an assessment device, as an initial intervention, and as a gauge of the progress of treatment in bereaved families.

The boundaries between when we are doing research and when we are doing therapy are more blurred in doing phenomenological inquiry than when we conduct positivist research. That is, the positivist roles of expert researcher and subject give way to a less hierarchical mindset in which phenomenological researcher and participant work together to gain meaning about a particular phenomenon. Although an inherent power differential may exist, as in therapy, we engage in a collaborative process that minimizes the impact of that power differential as much as possible. Caution must be used to protect families from our potential conflict of interest. While we are doing therapy, we cannot put the gathering of research data first; while we are doing research, we need to recognize that we are not doing therapy. The contract is different when the intent differs. This is an issue of ethics (Boss, 2003, 2005).

8. *Regardless of method, bias is inherent in all research and is not necessarily negative.* Bias must be made explicit at the beginning. Rather than pretending to be objective, we investigators should state, at the start of the project, what we believe in and value. The content of those beliefs and values, at least for purposes of research, is less important than our being open and straightforward. Alvin Gouldner, a sociologist of the rebellious 1960s, foreshadowed present postmodernism when he said that social sciences were not value-free and that traditional practices and assumptions of objectivity and neutrality were inconsistent with emerging social conditions. Gouldner called for a reflexive science that would be self-consciously self-critical. He insisted that scholars "raise their flag" early in their work to let others know explicitly their values and assumptions (Gouldner, 1970). We currently see this "raising of the flag" by clinical scholars using hermeneutics and critical theory (Goldner, Penn, Sheinberg, & Walker, 1990; Imber-Black & Roberts, 1992; Walters, Carter, Papp, & Silverstein, 1988; Welter-Enderlin, 1994; M. White, personal communication, March 1994).

Peeling Away the Onion: What Phenomenology Is Not

IS PHENOMENOLOGY DIFFERENT FROM DECONSTRUCTIONISM?

Although there are similarities, especially in rejecting the scientific method, phenomenology and deconstructionism are not the same. Both approaches recognize the indeterminacy of meaning, and many from both camps believe that regularity, order, and social organization exist—somewhere. For example, Gubrium and Holstein (1993) say, "The same meanings are not always attached to things, but there is regularity in the attachment process" (p. 654). Yet other phenomenologists, as well as deconstructionists, make no assumptions about regularity and order; nor are they interested in social organization. They are instead interested in patterns that connect through symbols of interaction. The phenomenon of interest to them is *meaning*, not object or structure.

In the end, the difference may be that deconstructionism allows the observer greater privilege because it is based on the *researcher's* reality, whereas phenomenology is a study of someone else's reality, albeit through the observer's eyes (P. C. Rosenblatt, personal communication, 1994). Also, in deconstructionism there is no emphasis on the need for self-reflection, as in phenomenology. *Feminist* deconstructionism, however, is an exception, because feminist scholarship requires self-reflection. The work of Rachel Hare-Mustin (1992, 1994) is an example.

IS PHENOMENOLOGY DIFFERENT FROM LOGICAL POSITIVISM?

Some say that phenomenology is theorizing with a sample of one. One person's perception is the truth for that person and in that context. "The appeal to context is more fundamental than the appeal to fact, for the context determines the significance of the facts" (Dreyfus, 1967, p. 43). In general, phenomenologists believe that reality is within a person's private perceptions—within his or her feelings, intentions, and essences. Most important, phenomenologists recognize a priori events. Fact and essence correlate. Edie (1967) summarizes the matter: "The 'essential' is thus what the human mind understands when it understands something in the flux of experience; what the mind adds to the world of fact is 'the necessary' or 'the essential'" (p. 9).

It becomes obvious that the quest for universal order is not as important to the phenomenologist as it is to the logical positivist. They are alike, however, in that both feel strongly about method, different though these methods are. *Instead of the scientific method of deduction, phenomenologists use the method of reduction.* The investigator begins with a generalization or a hunch, and peels layers away (like an onion) until he or she gets closer and closer to the essence of the phenomenon. The investigator keeps rejecting *what it is not* in order to get closer to *what it is.* This process of reduction, or "bracketing," continues as the researcher and the participant are in dialogue. They decide together when and how to "peel the onion."

It is apparent that reduction theorists (phenomenologists) and deduction theorists (positivists) represent two opposite points of view. There are relative strengths and weaknesses in both. Positivist researchers require theory building to be more empirically based. Parameters are clearly defined; concepts are operationalized; technical language is used. But what good is it to have a rigorous, tight methodology if an investigator is missing the point and busily, though methodically, going down a blind alley? Logical positivists' primary aim to generalize may make them miss critical individual differences. Generalizations or laws may be useful in the physical sciences, but they are less useful in family therapy research. The human mix is not as reliable as minerals and even more complex than chemicals.

IS PHENOMENOLOGY DIFFERENT FROM FEMINIST RESEARCH?

By itself, a researcher's choice of method cannot tell us whether or not the researcher is a feminist. Both positivism and phenomenology can be used for feminist inquiry; likewise, both can be used in ways that are biased against women or other disenfranchised groups. Rather than relying solely on method as the clue to a researcher's values and perspectives, we recommend looking critically at the researcher's stated (or unstated) assumptions regarding the context of the inquiry, the modes of inquiry, the questions asked, and the beneficiaries of the research. Simply concluding that feminists do only phenomenological study is incorrect. It is also incorrect to conclude that only feminists use this approach.

IS PHENOMENOLOGY DIFFERENT FROM CONTENT ANALYSIS?

Content analysis is a technique that allows a researcher to identify or "code" themes and patterns that emerge in qualitative data. Whereas phenomenological researchers *may* use content analysis, it is not necessarily their only approach to managing their data. Some, for example, may provide richly detailed accounts of their inquiry, known as "thick description," out of which only the reader draws conclusions. Some phenomenologists eschew any connection to techniques and refuse to talk of methodology. Conversely, some researchers who use content analysis techniques do so in nonphenomenological ways—in order to provide some kind of frequency count, for example, or to test hypotheses (Rosenblatt & Fischer, 1993).

METHODOLOGY

Within the phenomenological perspective, family therapy is perceived more as conversation than as intervention (Gubrium & Holstein, 1993). A phenomenological researcher who is also a family therapist extends the family's natural conversation, which is already taking place as the family and its individual members construct meaning and maintain that construction. Because family conversation takes place against a "taken-for-granted" backdrop within the everyday world, phenomenological inquiry—whether by a researcher or a therapist—involves making explicit and "reflectively bringing into nearness" (van Manen, 1990, p. 32) that which is implicit or obscured by its very taken-for-granted quality.

As with therapy, we might view the research process itself on two levels: one concerned with the principles by which the *family* has constructed its everyday world and with the contents of that everyday world, and one concerned with the principles by which the therapist-researcher and the family *co-construct* meaning and interpretations within whatever is taken for granted in the therapy setting. Gubrium and Holstein (1993) note that "family is a 'project' that is realized through discourse" (p. 655); family therapy research as well as family therapy can be similarly defined, providing two levels of inquiry for the phenomenological therapist-researcher.

In both research and therapy, the phenomenological inquirer is interested in stories. Defining therapy and research as storytelling and story listening changes the emphasis from problem solving to meaning construction. In this process, both the family and the therapist are brought into a deeper understanding of the nature and meaning of the everyday world and of that one family's lived experience. Thomas Moore (1992) notes that family therapy "might take the form of simply telling stories of family life, free of any concern for cause and effect or sociological influence. . . . We might imagine family therapy more as a process of exploring the complexity of our sense of life than of making it simple and intelligible" (pp. 28–29). These stories will often include paradox and contradiction. The phenomenological therapist or researcher does not need to "smooth out" discrepancies or inconsistencies, but rather looks for the meaning within them. What positivists call "anomalies" and statisticians call "outliers," phenomenologists call "reality," even though the sample size is small or the time spent together brief. Examples of this are the work on rituals developed by Imber-Black and Roberts (1992); the work of White and Epston (1990); and the work with New York families of persons missing after the World Trade Center attacks on September 11, 2001 (Boss, 2005; Boss et al., 2003).

Research Questions

Phenomenological research questions are questions of meaning designed to help the researcher understand the lived experience of the participant. For family therapists, these kinds of questions are familiar because they are often part of family therapy. Family therapists who wish to pursue phenomenological inquiry in a research mode might pursue any family phenomena of interest to them.

Generally, phenomenological researchers avoid questions that include such predetermined categories as "normal," "dysfunctional," "pathological," "deviant," and so on. They are more likely to ask participants to define the phenomenon in question than to define it for them. Positivists and phenomenologists take on different kinds of problems and seek different kinds of answers; thus their inquiry demands different methodologies. The positivist adopts a natural science model of research and searches for causes by using questionnaires, inventories, and scales to produce numerical data that can be statistically analyzed. In contrast, a phenomenologist seeks understanding through qualitative methods such as participant observation, in-depth interviewing, and other methods that yield descriptive data, and then works to extract the various truths and meanings from what Moore (1992) refers to as "the hard details of family history and memory" (p. 32). The phenomenologist looks for what Max Weber (1949, 1968) called *verstehen*, or "understanding." *Verstehen* refers to understanding "on a personal level the motives and beliefs behind people's actions" (Taylor & Bogdan, 1984, p. 2).

"Phenomenological questions are *meaning* questions" (van Manen, 1990, p. 23; emphasis in original). The therapist-researcher and the family members, by understanding the meaning of complex phenomena more deeply and fully, are enabled to act with greater awareness and consciousness. To put it another way, they are enabled to be more "thoughtful," which van Manen (1990) defines in the following way: "To be full of thought means not that we have a whole lot on our mind, but rather that we recognize our lot of minding the Whole—that which renders fullness or wholeness to life" (p. 31). Within this context, then, issues such as extramarital sexual behavior, deciding to divorce, providing care for an elderly parent, or choosing to have a baby or adopt a child become questions to be understood and lived, not "solved" and put away.

Two levels of phenomenological inquiry are available to a therapist-researcher: the dialogue *within* a family about a particular phenomenon, and the dialogue *between* the family and therapist-researcher about that phenomenon. At both levels, the "facts" of the situation take on far less importance than the *meaning* of that situation. Therapists who wish to pursue phenomenological inquiry at both levels find themselves in what van Manen (1990) calls the "attentive practice of thoughtfulness. . . . a heedful, mindful wondering about the project of life, of living, of what it means to live a life" (p. 12).

As phenomenological researchers, we have focused some of our work on questions that hold deep meaning for families: boundary ambiguity and ambiguous loss (Boss, 2002a, 2003, 2005), and the definition and expression of spirituality within families (Dahl, 1994). Our experiences as clinicians and researchers have both informed and invited further exploration in how families construct meaning in these areas.

Sampling and Selection Procedures

The phenomenological approach lends itself to small-N studies, in that it requires in-depth description of the experiences of each participant. The purposes are accurate understanding of meaning and establishment of possibilities, rather than generalization of findings. Randomness, therefore, is less important to a phenomenologist than to a positivist. A phenomenologist may develop a sample that is basically homogeneous, with the hope of amplifying differences that may exist, or one that is basically heterogeneous, with the hope of amplifying similarities that may exist.

For example, in Dahl's (1994) research on family spirituality, she wanted to understand the ways families construct meanings about spirituality, and so she developed the following criteria for a purposeful sample. A minimum of three persons were interviewed from each family system represented; when possible, at least one member of each of three generations was interviewed. At least one member had to have a child over the age of 5 years, so that there would be some element of the individual's past and present experiences of participating in rituals with the child, communicating about spirituality to the child, and co-constructing meaning with the child. The resulting subsample used for the final analysis consisted of three family systems, each from a different external demographic context.

Because of the likelihood of small samples and the deeply personal nature of meaning questions, confidentiality becomes an especially relevant issue in phenomenological research. Using pseudonyms, altering demographic details, and allowing participants to withdraw at any stage of the process, including the presentation of results, can provide participants some protection from uncomfortable or unwanted exposure.

Data Collection Procedures

What Are Considered Data?

All data are words about experiences and meanings. Data for the phenomenologist can therefore be obtained from family stories, family secrets, family rituals, ordinary dinner table conversations, behaviors, letters, diaries, photographs, and patterns in family behaviors or conversations. The primary focus of the researcher lies in the participants' meanings contained within the data. Creativity and intuition lead us to the phenomenon about which we are curious. In fact, for phenomenologists, intuition becomes an asset rather than something to suppress (Boss, 1987, 2005). But once there is a shift to what the researcher has observed, phenomenologists say that the focus is on the *researcher's reality*. Thus it becomes important to remain immersed in the *family's reality*.

What Procedures Are Considered Useful?

In phenomenological inquiry, any means of collecting information can be used that might allow the researcher access to the experience of another. These might include, for example, open-ended interviews; analysis of letters, diaries, oral histories, or narratives; or examination of photographs or videos. The methods phenomenological researchers use must adequately and accurately represent the "expressed daily life conditions, opinions, values, attitudes, beliefs, and knowledge base of the respondents" (Cicourel, 1986, p. 249). Phenomenological methods of data collection *allow participants to define phenomena for themselves*, and to describe the conditions, values, and attitudes they believe are relevant to that definition *for their own lives*. For example, Linda Coffey at the University of Chicago gave inexpensive disposable cameras to children in housing projects to record the relationships they believed were important to their well-being (L. Coffey, personal communication, June 1994).

An Example of Data Collection

With her family spirituality research sample, Dahl (1994) collected family stories about spirituality through the use of in-depth, focused interviews conducted at the participants' homes, in neutral locations, and in one case by telephone. Interviews ranged from 2½ to 4 hours in length, with an average length of just under 3 hours. She taped and transcribed the interviews, yielding 284 single-spaced pages. In addition, during the interviews she took notes of certain comments, self-reflection, and probes for further information.. These field notes totaled 108 pages after transcription. She also kept a journal throughout the study, noting her affective responses to the interviews and to the analysis process, thoughts about connections and linkages among and between families, and observations from her teaching and clinical practice that related to the study.

The Person of the Researcher as Instrument

If paper-and-pencil or other instruments are used at all for data collection in phenomenological inquiry, they must be carefully and thoughtfully chosen. Interview schedules must be developed in ways that allow participants to define the phenomenon being studied. But these means of collection are not the only instruments in a phenomenological study. We believe that the person of the researcher also becomes a major instrument in phenomenological research. Although the researcher is subject to stress, fatigue, confusion, and bias, the losses due to these factors are "more than offset by the flexibility, insight, and ability to build on tacit knowledge that is the peculiar province of the human instrument" (Guba & Lincoln, 1981, p. 113). We see similarity between this idea and Whitaker and Keith's (1981) ideas of "the person of the therapist" as central in family therapy.

The interpretations and theoretical links developed by phenomenological therapist-researchers are inevitably influenced by their own personal biography and family history. Clinicians call this "countertransference," a phenomenon that is not absent in phenomenological research (Boss, 1987). To increase awareness of the impact of the researcher as instrument, the therapist-researcher might keep a journal detailing experiences, emotions, insights, and questions resulting from the data collection process (see the description of Dahl's journal, above). Patton (2002) and Reinharz (1983) note that these are also legitimate and valuable parts of the data.

A prerequisite to "good" data collection is prior recognition of the content being discussed by respondents. According to Gergen and Gergen (1988), telling a story is the result of a mutually coordinated and supportive relationship between teller and listener. Furthermore, knowledge about the culture contained in a respondent's texts can only be expanded on when the researcher brings into the analysis what else is known about the participant and his or her circumstances (Mishler, 1986). This prior knowledge, however, must be evaluated against new learnings, just as new information must be integrated into prior knowledge. Otherwise, the researcher risks letting preconceptions guide and possibly obscure the process of discovering meaning in the moment.

DATA ANALYSIS PROCEDURES

A psychologist who turned to phenomenology to study human behavior, Amedeo Giorgi (1985), offers a data analysis method for those who insist on more structure. His method contains four essential aspects (the quotes are from Giorgi, 1985, p. 10):

1. *"Sense of the whole."* In this first step, the researcher reads the entire description of an observation or experience many times in order to gain a general sense of the whole.

2. *"Discrimination of meaning units within a psychological perspective and focus on the phenomenon being researched."* Once the sense of the whole has been grasped, the researcher goes back to the beginning and reads through the text once more, with the specific aim of discriminating "meaning units" from within a psychological perspective and with a focus on the phenomenon being studied. Meanings change as the interaction between narrative and reader progresses and the context changes; meaning units reflect these shifts and progressions. Researchers acknowledge that the selection of what stands out from the text depends on their own perspectives.

3. *"Transformation of subject's everyday expressions into psychological language with emphasis on the phenomenon being investigated."* Once meaning units have been delineated, the researcher goes through all the meaning units and expresses the psychological insight contained in them more directly. This is especially true of the meaning units most revelatory of the phenomenon under study.

4. *"Synthesis of transformed meaning units into a consistent statement of the structure of learning."* In this step, the researcher synthesizes all of the transformed meaning units into a consistent statement regarding the subject's experience. This step is usually referred to as the "structure of the experience" and can be expressed at a number of levels.

The purpose of analysis in phenomenological research is not to tie all loose ends together, but rather to describe and understand (as in *verstehen)* the experience of the participants. In this kind of phenomenological inquiry, data analysis and data collection go hand in hand (Patton, 2002; Reinharz, 1983; Rosenblatt & Fischer, 1993). Each informs the other in a dynamic, reciprocal, nonlinear process of questioning, reflecting, and interpreting. Hess and Handel (1959, 1967) describe this as a back-and-forth movement from one kind of data to another, from one participant's stories to another's, and from one family's themes to another's—all the while looking for *meanings that connect* and *meanings that differentiate*. The only rule of analysis is to remain vitally connected to individual and family conversations and stories.

Hess and Handel (1967) outline three assumptions regarding data gathered through phenomenological research. First, researchers must attempt to connect the data with useful ideas about the data. Although phenomenological researchers attempt not to impose *realities* on those of the participants, they definitely impose *structure* on them, which incorporates ideas that may be useful in accurately understanding them. Second, these data are to be taken at more than face value; they provide information about what specific meanings families give to reality and information about how they do that assigning. Third, individual family members' stories are accurately understood only within the family context and are illuminated by other stories in that context.

Accurate understanding of participants' experiences may come through a line-by-line analysis of a story or a frame-by-frame analysis of videos or photographs. It may come through conducting a search for significant words or phrases. It may come through gathering a more global impression of thoughts and themes that occur. The significant hallmark of phenomenological analysis is that the researcher makes every effort to stay connected to the experience of the participants. This may involve checking with the participants at several points in the collection, analysis, and reporting process, and letting them have input into the meaning being constructed by the researcher to see whether the interpretation is on target (Boss et al., 2003; Dahl, 1994).

In Dahl's (1994) analysis of data regarding family spirituality, immersion in the family stories happened through a series of listening experiences. She listened to the stories not only during the initial interviews, but also while transcribing them, reading the transcripts, and color-coding them to identify themes that began to emerge. Following Brown and Gilligan (1992), she listened first of all for the story itself, paying attention to metaphors, images, inconsistencies, and plot twists, as well as to her feelings about all of those. She listened again with attention to the family processes and dynamics described within the stories, and then again with attention to indicators of social or cultural context, especially those that might overpower or constrain a family's voice. The stories about family spirituality from each individual were analyzed for categories and themes; the stories of individuals within a given family system were analyzed with regard to one another; and the "meta-stories" of the three family systems were compared and contrasted.

This analysis resulted in a rich collection of stories. Some were extended ones describing death, loss, or particularly powerful experiences of spirituality as defined by a participant. Some were shorter, detailing an event or reporting a belief. And some were deceptively brief, simply a phrase or sentence holding much more than its size suggested: "My mother was a frequent flyer in the Catholic Church." "He died just when I started paying attention to him." "I left me."

In the end, Dahl's analysis of these stories reflected a number of intriguing ways families define and express spirituality. For example, families appear to be better able to sustain competing worldviews within their meaning-making processes than laboratory experiments have suggested they might be. Also, conversation and ritual are significant, reciprocally influential dimensions of family spirituality. In addition, contrary to the typical use of the word, "fundamentalism" can characterize a family's meaning-making process as well as any particular set of beliefs. And finally, as one participant concisely and confidently stated, "Families, whether they know it or not, come together to work out their spirituality." In phenomenological inquiry, these kinds of findings are not endpoints, but places to begin asking new questions.

The process of analyzing phenomenological data, regardless of type, must include immersion in the data to observe and define what is there and to notice what is not there; it must include incubation and reflection to allow intuitive awareness and understandings to emerge; and it must include creative synthesis that enables accurate and meaningful communication of the participants' experience (Patton, 2002; Rosenblatt & Fischer, 1993). The process must also include consideration of the researcher's intuition, because "discovery . . . happens not with the scientific method, by magic, or by luck, but through openness to heeding one's senses and responding to one's intuition. . . . We make ourselves discovery-prone by listening, being open to feelings, and recognizing apprehensions and emotions. This state does not happen by chance; it requires the willingness to open one's mind and feelings, to make oneself prone to discovery" (Boss, 1987, p. 154).

Brown and Gilligan (1992) refer to this openness as locating both the speaker and oneself as researcher in the narrative. Rather than a goal of "objectivity" during this listening, therapist-researchers pursue the goal of connection with an internal reality different from their own experience. It is precisely this *connection* that provides a "way of knowing, an opening between self and other that creates a channel for discovery, an avenue to knowledge" (Brown & Gilligan, 1992, p. 28; see also Allen & Walker, 1992).

Hare-Mustin (1994), however, raises a critical question: How does the researcher know that [his or her] mind and feelings are open? There is the problem that researchers may be imposing their own meanings and distorting rather than connecting. By pointing out that family therapists and researchers are influenced by the "dominant discourse of the time," or *zeitgeist*, Hare-Mustin draws our attention to the limitations of any one person's phenomenological view. As family therapist-researchers, we hope to be more reflexive and open to discourse than the average person; however, we must *always* be vigilant about what we bring to the research questions we ask and to our interpretations of the words and stories we hear. Human subjectivity is an important procedural item in data analysis and interpretation, and a critical point relating to "the person of the researcher" as previously discussed.

Ethical Issues in Phenomenological Inquiry

Given that the phenomenologist explores basic components of humanness and aspects of family, it is reasonable to assume that some participants will disclose information about sensitive issues. Survivors of sexual abuse, for example, may describe the effect that this experience has had on their experience of other aspects of life. The story of a participant's journey may include behaviors (past or present) that for him or her are shameful or embarrassing, or that may be considered illegal or immoral by others. Informed consent and confidentiality thus become important issues for both participant and researcher. For participants, assurance must be given that responses will be kept private and will be reported in a way that will not identify them. But Patton (2002) and Doherty and Boss (1991) also caution that interviewers must be clear about instances when breaches of confidentiality might be legally mandated (e.g., cases in which abuse of children or vulnerable adults is revealed during interviews).

LaRossa, Bennett, and Gelles (1981) delineate two broad categories of ethical concerns that are relevant for phenomenological research: informed consent and establishment of a risk–benefit equation. The first category of issues can be addressed by clearly explaining the participant's rights, both in the initial contact letter and consent form and at the time of the actual data collection. Because it is impossible to know in advance just where a participant's reflection may lead in any given interview (Doherty & Boss, 1991; LaRossa et al., 1981; Patton, 2002), explicit mention should be made of the right to withdraw from the project, to end the interview, or to ask that any form of taping stop at any time. Even with that option clearly established, phenomenological researchers need to be aware of the ambiguities inherent in the setting (often a participant's home) and the role (insider-outsider, therapist-researcher) (Gilgun, 1992; LaRossa et al., 1981; Olson, 1977). They should also be able to offer participants a selection of helping resources, should the interviewing process raise deeply unsettling issues (Boss, 1987; Gilgun, 1992).

Assessing potential risks and benefits is more complicated. LaRossa and colleagues (1981) encourage researchers to keep clearly in mind the potentially embarrassing nature of everything connected with family life, which is in our society considered "private business." Public exposure, then, can be disturbing for participants. Even if data are carefully disguised or not widely disseminated, an individual's *feeling* of self-exposure is another consideration. Family therapists who do phenomenological research are often already skilled in the development of rapport; supportive, empathically neutral responses throughout the interview; and postinterview debriefing—all of which can help alleviate this discomfort.

Phenomenological inquiry is useful to generate new hypotheses or new constructs, because its purpose is to gather understanding from patterns in the data. The research design is thus emergent. As investigators, we begin, like artists or novelists, with only preliminary ideas. As we proceed, things become clearer and new areas become subject to scrutiny. Here is where ethical dilemmas arise: Although the participants were informed and gave consent at the beginning of the study, this original consent may become invalid as new curiosities take us researchers in new directions. How can participants give informed consent when we keep changing method and focus? How can we as phenomenologists meet the criterion for informed consent when there is no allegiance to one method or goal?

When the general intent and scope of the research do not change, most human-subjects committees or local institutional review boards (IRBs) do not require a new informed consent procedure for every change in method or direction. Nevertheless, we recommend that researchers err on the conservative side and inform their IRB each time they change direction or sample to make sure that a new informed consent procedure is *not* needed. For each change, participants must know what is happening and that they can withdraw at any time, without prejudice.

We recommend obtaining such informed consent from all who participate in the study, regardless of their cognitive capacity. This may seem like a conservative position, but again, our goal is to do no harm. Patients with dementia have told us that they appreciate being asked about videotaping. So have children. We go beyond the legal requirements of obtaining consent from adults and those with power of attorney, and include everyone because it is more respectful. Everyone should be included in the process of informing and consenting.

This more conservative approach to informing and consenting is especially important in phenomenological studies, because this type of inquiry is by its very nature more personal. Investigator and participant get to know each other more closely than with positivist research. Usually even minors and other disenfranchised people want to know what is going on and why they should participate.

In phenomenological studies, issues of confidentiality also become more complicated. Researchers should always ask participants whether they agree with the plan for maintaining confidentiality. When one family was asked, they said they would give consent *only* if their full names were used in any reports of the study (Fravel & Boss, 1992). This was a couple whose three boys had been missing for more than 30 years. Both parents wanted their names used "just in case one of the boys was still out there somewhere." Betty and Kenny Klein of Monticello, Minnesota, taught the researchers never to take for granted what participants' perceptions are regarding confidentiality. A request for this amount of disclosure is rare, but it is not unusual to find families wanting varying degrees of confidentiality. Again, we recommend erring on the conservative side. That is, we recommend using strict confidentiality in studies of couples and families, because family members may not all agree on the need for it or may change their minds at a later date. There is less chance of doing harm as researchers if we proceed conservatively.

These ethical considerations must be part of a researcher's awareness. Patton (2002) describes the necessity of having "the utmost respect for these persons who are willing to share with you some of their time to help you understand their world" (p. 417). At the same time, however, researchers must also remember that in-depth interviews may have a therapeutic effect on families, and that the changes that may result may be desired by a family. "Our sensitivity to the costs should not obscure an equal sensitivity to the benefits that research may bring to the family as well as to us [the researchers]" (Boss, 1987, p. 152). As one participant in Dahl's study of family spirituality said, when asked what it was like to talk for several hours about her construction of meaning in times of great loss, "It's not often that I really get to talk like this. . . . and it's been finer [sic] than I thought it would be" (1994, p. 137). Asking families to share their stories also empowers them, because it indicates that we researchers value their knowledge and their potential contribution to the knowledge base of a larger system.

Reporting Findings

The descriptions of experience form the essence of phenomenological inquiry. In these descriptions, therapist-researchers present both patterns that are present and exceptions to those patterns. Consistent with the "onion-peeling" nature of this approach, the research report includes both what the phenomenon under study *is* and what it *is not*. For example, in the stories shared with Dahl (1994) about family spirituality, most participants were careful to distinguish between family "spirituality" and family "religiosity"—a distinction that proved important in both analyzing and reporting the findings.

In reporting and discussing the results of phenomenological research, therapists might follow the format suggested by Gilgun (1992). Supporting data for each pattern or exception are provided. The discussion is set in the context of previous research and theory. Such linkages enhance validity, as discussed previously. They also highlight ways in which findings "enhance previous knowledge, as correctives, as new knowledge, or both" (Gilgun, 1992, p. 26).

It is nearly impossible to describe a "typical" report of phenomenological inquiry. Because the nature of knowing is both artistic and scientific, we find that some reports comprise art, music, and literature that in the end describe the truth about people's experiences. Phenomenological inquiry, perhaps because of its respect for and valuing of stories, seems to hold a near-intuitive appeal for almost any audience. Phenomenological researchers may find receptive audiences among persons who have a particular interest in the phenomenon that was studied—scholars, students, professionals in larger systems (such as education, law, religion, or health care), policymakers, or community members.

The exemplars listed at the end of this chapter reflect other ways of reporting findings, perhaps more familiar to those accustomed to quantitative research reports. Despite the diversity of format, they illustrate two basic elements we consider characteristic of phenomenological research reports: the explicit location of the researcher in the work, and the explicit location of the participants in the data. The members of the audience—whether readers or viewers, one or many—are given direct access to the words of the participants, enabling them to engage in the coconstruction of meaning.

DISCUSSION

Reliability and Validity

In phenomenological inquiry, it does not make sense to search for traditional kinds of measurement reliability and validity. Rather, this approach makes subjective relevance and adequate description of greater concern (Daly, 1992; Gubrium & Holstein, 1993). Despite the tentativeness and openness inherent in phenomenological inquiry, such research must also be evaluated by the concept of "adequacy" (McLain & Weigert, 1979; Schutz, 1962). That is, readers or listeners must see in the description of the data the validity and applicability of any concepts presented by the researcher, and participants must also agree that the analysis is an accurate reflection of their perceptions. To foster this kind of validity, participants might be asked at the time of data collection whether they would be willing to be contacted subsequently to clarify meanings, comment on findings, or participate in further data collection.

A common challenge to this kind of research from more quantitative researchers involves the issues of representativeness and generalizability (Allen & Gilgun, 1987; Rosenblatt & Fischer, 1993). Given the complexity and diversity of a particular family's experience, phenomenological research is more interested in accurately reflecting a given family's experience than in generalizing about families. We must ask enough questions and involve enough family members to hear some differing perspectives, because in the microworld of even *one* family, there is always diversity in their gendered and generational perspectives—and often also differences in life experiences, socialization, class, beliefs, and values. Phenomenological research provides data that reflect this diversity, in addition to enabling identification of commonalities.

In order to ensure a greater degree of validity, the researcher must stay connected to those experiences of the participants and continue the back-and-forth movement between data collection and data analysis that is vitally important in phenomenological research. In addition, movement among present study, previous research, and theory development provides linkages that enhance validity (Boss, Kaplan, & Gordon, 1994; Fravel & Boss, 1992; Gilgun, 1992). Above all, the researcher must continue in dialogue with the individuals of interest. It would not be unusual for a phenomenological study to have the individuals of interest participate in the formation of questions, as well as in the interpretation of their answers. For example, Boss and colleagues (1994) asked Native American women to collaborate with them in formulating research questions and subsequently in interpreting answers and writing up results.

If, as a phenomenological researcher, you say you are studying families, whole families are what you must study. If you say you are studying couples (gay, lesbian, or heterosexual), those are precisely what you must study. If you say you are studying who looks after the children, you may have to look beyond the biological parents. In all cases, the issue is one of validity. We must study what we say we are studying.

In similar ways, traditional understandings of reliability are affected by the philosophical assumptions of phenomenologists. Whereas interrater reliability or test–retest reliability may matter in a particular way to a positivist researcher, phenomenologists would expect that different researchers—locating themselves differently in the process, given their unique sets of experiences, values, and personal meanings—may well explore somewhat different aspects of the same phenomenon and arrive at somewhat different descriptions of meaning. It is the explicit location of the researcher in the work that makes this possibility a strength, rather than a limitation. In addition, we would expect participants to find that phenomenological inquiry invites them to reflect on their own lived experiences by co-constructing meaning with one another and with the researcher. We would also expect that such reflection would result in new or different meanings at another time.

Bridging Research, Theory, and Practice

The goal of phenomenological inquiry is to produce a deep, clear, and accurate understanding of the experiences of participants and of the meanings found in or assigned to those experiences. Researcher and audience share a commitment to understand a phenomenon more clearly, often for a purpose such as personal, familial, institutional, or community change. To facilitate change, the presentation of phenomenological findings should be set in the context of previous research and theory. Such linkages enhance validity.

Polkinghorne (1989) summarizes the potential benefits of the clearer understanding derived from phenomenological research: increased sensitivity to the experiences of others, corrections and amplifications of empirically derived knowledge, and improved responsiveness of public policy to the realities described by participants. He encourages phenomenological researchers to maximize the effectiveness of these consequences by always including in their presentation of results the *implications* of those results for practitioners and policymakers. Here is where a therapist doing phenomenological inquiry can influence other therapists. A case in point is the work of the University of Minnesota's New York Ambiguous Loss Team working with families of missing labor union members after September 11, 2001 (Boss et al., 2003).

CONCLUSION

An old method of inquiry, phenomenology is enjoying a resurgence and has an intuitive appeal among family therapy researchers because it is the study of the phenomena of everyday family processes, both in good times and in bad times. In 1946, Edmund Husserl said that we should go back to the things themselves. The "things" were perceptions, feelings, memories, behaviors—in sum, the stuff of family life. Whether phenomenology becomes simply a place to start family therapy research or your continued research method of choice, rigor is necessary in how you proceed. Because that rigor depends much less on method than on philosophical assumptions, assumptions are the centerpiece of this chapter. They remain the essential guide for doing family therapy inquiry as a phenomenologist.

In the final analysis, we need both phenomenology and logical positivism. There is a place for the creativity of dreamers and storytellers, as well as for the methods of empiricists. Both have value, and both can produce information about family processes, but each needs the other. We still haven't finally defined families, let alone how they function and how they change across the life course. We need to ask new questions and ask old questions in a new way. This requires effort on our part to seek holistic, rather than microscopic, pictures of family life. In doing this, we should avoid static, noncontextual, and method-bound inquiries (Cowan, Field, Hansen, Skolnik, & Swanson, 1993). Phenomenological approaches can help.

The renaissance of phenomenology in family therapy research indicates a new acceptance of diversity in epistemology and methodology. Such acceptance is much needed, because diversity is increasing in family structures and functions to a point where we can no longer, with validity or fairness, claim a norm. Phenomenological inquiry helps us to see multiple ways that families can and do remain resilient despite increasing complexities.

EXEMPLARS

Arditti, J. A. (1999). Rethinking relationships between divorced mothers and their children: Capitalizing on family strengths. *Family Relations, 48*, 109–119.

Butcher, H. K., Holkup, P. A., & Buckwalter, K. C. (2001). The experience of caring for a family member with Alzheimer's disease. *Western Journal of Nursing Research, 23*(1), 33–55.

Garland, D. A. (2002). Faith narratives of congregants and their families. *Review of Religious Research, 44*(1), 68–92.

Gibson, P. A. (2002). Caregiving role affects family relationships of African American grandmothers as new mothers again: A phenomenological perspective. *Journal of Marital and Family Therapy, 28*(3), 341–353.

Hein, S. F., & Austin, W. J. (2001). Empirical and hermeneutic approaches to phenomenological research in psychology: A comparison. *Psychological Methods, 6*, 3–17.

SmithBattle, L. (1996). Intergenerational ethics of caring for adolescent mothers and their children. *Family Relations, 45*, 56–64.

ACKNOWLEDGMENTS

We wish to thank Lori Kaplan, PhD, for her contributions to an earlier version of this chapter, and Jessica Hulst and Heather Hanawalt for research assistance.

REFERENCES

Allen, K. R., & Gilgun, J. F. (1987, November). *Qualitative family research: Unanswered questions and proposed resolutions.* Paper presented at of the annual meeting of the National Council on Family Relations Theory Construction and Research Methodology Preconference, Atlanta, GA.

Allen, K. R., & Walker, A. J. (1992). A feminist analysis of interviews with elderly mothers and their daughters. In J. F. Gilgun, K. Daly, & G. Handel (Eds.), *Qualitative methods in family research* (pp. 198–214). Newbury Park, CA: Sage.

Becker, C. S. (1992). *Living and relating: An introduction to phenomenology.* Newbury Park, CA: Sage.

Berger, P. L., & Kellner, H. (1964). Marriage and the construction of reality: An exercise in the microsociology of knowledge. *Diogenes, 46*, 1–25.

Berger, P. L., & Luckmann, T. (1966). *The social construction of reality: A treatise in the sociology of knowledge.* Garden City, NY: Doubleday.

Blumer, H. (1969). *Symbolic interactionism: Perspective and method.* Englewood Cliffs, NJ: Prentice-Hall.

Boss, P. (1987). The role of intuition in family research. *Contemporary Family Therapy, 9*(1–2), 146–158.

Boss, P. (2002a). Ambiguous loss in families of the missing from war and terrorism. *Lancet*, *360*, 39–40.

Boss, P. (2002b). Working with families when there is no body to bury. *Family Process*, *41*, 14–17.

Boss, P. (2003). Ambiguous loss. In F. Walsh & M. McGoldrick (Eds.), *Living beyond loss: Death in the family* (2nd ed., pp. 164–175). New York: Norton.

Boss, P. (2005). *Loss, trauma, and resilience: Therapeutic work with ambiguous loss.* New York: Norton.

Boss, P., Beaulieu, L., Wieling, E., Turner, W., & LaCruz, S. (2003). Healing loss, ambiguity and trauma: A community-based intervention with families of union workers missing after the 9/11. *Journal of Marital and Family Therapy*, *29*(4), 455–467.

Boss, P., Kaplan, L., & Gordon, M. (1994, August). *The meaning of caregiving for Alzheimer's disease among Native American caregivers: Stories of spirituality, fatalism, and mastery.* Paper presented at the Fourth Annual International Conference on Alzheimer's Disease and Related Disorders, Minneapolis, MN.

Brown, L. M., & Gilligan, C. (1992). *Meeting at the crossroads: Women's psychology and girls' development.* Cambridge, MA: Harvard University Press.

Bruyn, S. T. (1966). *The human perspective in sociology: The methodology of participant observation.* Englewood Cliffs, NJ: Prentice-Hall.

Burton, L. (1991). Caring for children in high-risk neighborhoods. *American Enterprise*, *2*(3), 34–37.

Cicourel, A. V. (1986). Social measurement as the creation of expert systems. In D. W. Fiske & R. A. Sheveder (Eds.), *Metatheory in social science: Pluralisms and subjectivities* (pp. 246–270). Chicago: University of Chicago Press.

Collins, J. (2000). *Heidegger and the Nazis.* New York: Totem Books.

Cowan, P., Field, D., Hansen, D., Skolnik, A., & Swanson, G. (1993). *Family, self, and society: Toward a new agenda for family research.* Hillsdale, NJ: Erlbaum.

Dahl, C. M. (1994). *A phenomenological exploration of the definition and understanding of spirituality within families.* Unpublished doctoral dissertation, University of Minnesota.

Daly, K. (1992). Parenthood as problematic. In J. F. Gilgun, K. Daly, & G. Handel (Eds.), *Qualitative methods in family research* (pp. 103–125). Newbury Park, CA: Sage.

Deutscher, I. (1973). *What we say/what we do: Sentiments and acts.* Glenview, IL: Scott, Foresman.

Doherty, W. J., & Boss, P. G. (1991). Values and ethics in family therapy. In A. S. Gurman & D. P. Kniskern (Eds.), *Handbook of family therapy* (Vol. 2, pp. 606–637). New York: Brunner/Mazel.

Dreyfus, H. L. (1967). Phenomenology and artificial intelligence. In J. Edie (Ed.), *Phenomenology in America* (pp. 31–47). Chicago: Quadrangle Books.

Edie, J. (Ed.). (1967). *Phenomenology in America.* Chicago: Quadrangle Books.

Frankl, V. E. (1984). *Man's search for meaning* (3rd ed.). New York: Simon & Schuster.

Fravel, D. L., & Boss, P. G. (1992). An in-depth interview with the parents of missing children. In J. F. Gilgun, K. Daly, & G. Handel (Eds.), *Qualitative methods in family research* (pp. 126–145). Newbury Park, CA: Sage.

Garwick, A. W., Detzner, D., & Boss, P. (1994). Family perceptions of living with Alzheimer's disease. *Family Process*, *33*(3), 327–340.

Gergen, K., & Gergen, M. (1988). Narrative and the self as relationship. In L. Berkowitz (Ed.), *Advances in experimental social psychology* (Vol. 21, pp. 17–56). San Diego, CA: Academic Press.

Gilgun, J. F. (1992). Definition, methodologies, and methods in qualitative family research. In J. F. Gilgun, K. Daly, & G. Handel (Eds.), *Qualitative methods in family research* (pp. 22–39). Newbury Park, CA: Sage.

Giorgi, A. (Ed.). (1985). *Phenomenology and psychological research.* Pittsburgh, PA: Duquesne University Press.

Goffman, E. (1959). *The presentation of self in everyday life.* New York: Doubleday.

Goldner, V., Penn, P., Sheinberg, M., & Walker, G. (1990). Love and violence: Gender paradoxes in volatile attachments. *Family Process, 29,* 343–364.

Gouldner, A. W. (1970). *The coming crisis in Western sociology.* New York: Avon Books.

Guba, E. S., & Lincoln, Y. S. (1981). *Effective evaluation: Improving the usefulness of evaluation results through responsive and naturalistic approaches.* San Francisco: Jossey-Bass.

Gubrium, J. F., & Holstein, J. A. (1993). Phenomenology, ethnomethodology, and family discourse. In P. G. Boss, W. J. Doherty, R. LaRossa, W. R. Schumm, & S. K. Steinmetz (Eds.), *Sourcebook of family theories and methods: A contextual approach* (pp. 651–672). New York: Plenum Press.

Hare-Mustin, R. (1992, November). *On the need for second order change in family therapy research.* Plenary address presented at the Research/Clinical Conference of the American Family Therapy Academy, Captiva Island, FL.

Hare-Mustin, R. (1994). Discourses in the mirrored room: A postmodern analysis of therapy. *Family Process, 33,* 19–35.

Henry, J. (1973). *Pathways to madness.* New York: Vintage.

Hess, R. D., & Handel, G. (1959). *Family worlds: A psychosocial approach to family life.* Chicago: University of Chicago Press.

Hess, R. D., & Handel, G. (1967). The family as a psychosocial organization. In G. Handel (Ed.), *The psychosocial interior of the family* (pp. 10–29). Chicago: Aldine.

Husserl, E. (1946). Phenomenology. In *Encyclopedia Britannica* (14th ed., Vol. 17, pp. 699–702). Chicago: University of Chicago Press.

Imber-Black, E., & Roberts, J. (1992). *Rituals for our times.* New York: HarperCollins.

Kollock, P., & O'Brien, J. (Eds.). (1994). *The production of reality.* Thousand Oaks, CA: Pine Forge Press.

LaRossa, R., Bennett, L., & Gelles, R. (1981). Ethical dilemmas in the detailed study of families. *Journal of Marriage and the Family, 43,* 303–313.

Liebow, E. (1967). *Haley's corner.* Boston: Little, Brown.

McLain, R., & Weigert, A. (1979). Toward a phenomenological sociology of family. In W. R. Burr, R. Hill, F. I. Nye, & I. L. Reiss (Eds.), *Contemporary theories about the family* (Vol. 2, pp. 160–205). New York: Free Press.

Mead, G. H. (1934). *Mind, self and society.* Chicago: University of Chicago Press.

Merleau-Ponty, M. (1962). *The phenomenology of perception* (C. Smith, Trans.). New York: Humanities Press. (Original work published 1945)

Mishler, E. (1986). The analysis of interview-narratives. In T. Sarbin (Ed.), *Narrative psychology: The storied nature of human conduct* (pp. 233–255). New York: Prager.

Moore, T. (1992). *Care of the soul.* New York: HarperCollins.

Olson, D. (1977). "Insiders" and "outsiders" views of relationships: Research strategies. In G. Levinger & H. Rausch (Eds.), *Close relationships: Perspectives on the meaning of intimacy* (pp. 115–135). Amherst: University of Massachusetts Press.

Patterson, J., & Garwick, A. (1994). Levels of meaning in family stress theory. *Family Process, 33,* 287–303.

Patton, M. Q. (2002). *Qualitative research and evaluation methods* (3rd ed.). Thousand Oaks, CA: Sage.

Philipse, H. (1998). *Heidegger's philosophy of being: A critical interpretation.* Princeton, NJ: Princeton University Press.

Polkinghorne, D. E. (1989). Phenomenological research methods. In R. S. Valle & S. Haling (Eds.), *Existential–phenomenological perspectives in psychology* (pp. 41–60). New York: Plenum Press.

Pollner, M., & McDonald-Wikler, L. (1994). The social construction of unreality: A case study of a family's attribution of competence to a severely retarded child. In P. Kollock & J. O'Brien (Eds.), *The production of reality* (pp. 343–355). Thousand Oaks, CA: Pine Forge Press. (Original work published 1985)

Psathas, G. (1973). *Phenomenological sociology: Issues and applications.* New York: Wiley.

Ree, J. (1999). *Heidegger.* New York: Routledge.

Reinharz, S. (1983). Experiential analysis: A contribution to feminist research. In G. Bowers & R. Dueli Klein (Eds.), *Theories of women's studies* (pp. 162–191). Boston: Routledge & Kegan Paul.

Reiss, D. (1994). The social construction of reality: The passion within us all. In P. Kollock & J. O'Brien (Eds.), *The production of reality* (pp. 356–359). Thousand Oaks, CA: Pine Forge Press. (Original work published 1981)

Rettig, K. D., & Dahl, C. M. (1993). The impact of procedural factors on perceived justice in divorce settlements. *Social Justice Research, 6* (3), 301–324.

Rosenblatt, P. C., & Fischer, L. R. (1993). Qualitative family research. In P. G. Boss, W. J. Doherty, R. LaRossa, W. R. Schumm, & S. K. Steinmetz (Eds.), *Sourcebook of family theories and methods: A contextual approach* (pp. 167–177). New York: Plenum Press.

Schutz, A. (1960). *Der sinnhafte aujbau der sozialen welt.* Vienna: Springer Verlag.

Schutz, A. (1962). *Collected papers: Vol. 1. The problem of social reality* (1962–1966). The Hague: Nijhoff.

Schutz, A. (1967). *The phenomenology of the social world.* Evanston, IL: Northwestern University Press.

Sedney, M. A., Baker, J. E., & Gross, E. (1994). "The story" of a death: Therapeutic considerations with bereaved families. *Journal of Marital and Family Therapy, 20*(3), 287–296.

SmithBattle, L. (1996). Intergenerational ethics of caring for adolescent mothers and their children. *Family Relations, 45,* 56–64.

Stacey, J. (1990). *Brave new families: Stories of domestic upheaval in later twentieth-century America.* New York: Basic Books.

Taylor, S. J., & Bogdan, R. (1984). *Introduction to qualitative research methods: The search for meanings* (2nd ed.). New York: Wiley.

van Manen, M. (1990). *Researching lived experience: Human science for an action sensitive pedagogy.* Albany: State University of New York Press.

Walters, M., Carter, B., Papp, P., & Silverstein, O. (1988). *The invisible web: Gender patterns in family relationships.* New York: Guilford Press.

Weber, M. (1949). *The methodology of the social sciences.* New York: Free Press.

Weber, M. (1968). *Economy and society.* New York: Bedminster Press.

Welter-Enderlin, R. (1994). *Paare-Leidenschaft und Lange Weile [Couple passion over time].* Munich, Germany: Piper Verlag.

Whitaker, C., & Keith, D. (1981). Symbolic–experiential family therapy. In A. Gurman & D. Kniskern (Eds.), *Handbook of family therapy* (pp. 187–225). New York: Brunner/Mazel.

White, M., & Epston, D. (1990). *Narrative means to therapeutic ends.* New York: Norton.

CHAPTER 5

Focus Groups
in Family Therapy Research

FRED P. PIERCY
KATHERINE M. HERTLEIN

Dr. Stella Starr received a 4.9 overall rating (on a 5-point scale) for her workshop at the American Association for Marriage and Family Therapy (AAMFT) conference. Dr. David Dweeb, on the other hand, received a 2.1. The program committee considered Dr. Starr's ratings when they invited her back the following year to do a conference institute. She eventually wrote a book, appeared on *The Oprah Winfrey Show*, and now conducts workshops across the country. Dr. Dweeb, on the other hand, now shovels manure in a stable in the small town of Tumbleweed.

Such rating systems help program committees make gross distinctions between stars and dweebs. However, what kind of research might give us a clue as to why Dr. Starr received such high ratings? And, more important, what kind of research could help us learn from her success? One approach would be for the researcher to get groups of people together who attended one of Dr. Starr's presentations and ask them to talk about what they liked. A moderator could ask them questions that might encourage them to talk about what Dr. Starr said and did that made her workshop so popular. What about the workshop captured the participants' imagination? As one participant shares a thought, another could elaborate. This in turn might remind a third one about something else Dr. Starr did. The moderator would encourage a free discussion and would ask for specific examples of the qualities the participants identified.

Immediately after these group discussions, the moderator could jot down some of the preliminary themes that emerged. Later, a secretary could transcribe the audiotapes of the discussions. The research team could review the transcript for discrete behaviors and qualities of Dr. Starr, as well as illustrative examples of each. The team would put each on a separate 3″ × 5″ card and again inductively categorize them in terms of themes. The researcher then would write a research article in clear, practical language, including both themes and illustrations of workshop excellence. Dr. Dweeb, during a break at the Tumbleweed stable, could then read the article and learn to be a better presenter.

BACKGROUND

These kinds of small-group discussions and data analyses are what go on in focus group evaluation. Basically, a focus group involves an interactive group discussion on a particular topic within a permissive, nonthreatening environment (Krueger, 1988). Researchers use focus groups to understand participants' perspectives and views on a particular topic (Kitzinger & Barbour, 1999; Morgan, 1992). The open-response format and the synergistic, snowballing effect of group discussion often result in rich ideas that would be impossible to obtain through individual interviews or more quantitative methods (Edmunds, 1999). Focus group results are usually practical, and participants typically enjoy the focus group experience.

Philosophical Assumptions

Labels carry different connotations for different people. Depending on one's politics and ideology, one develops opinions, values, and prejudices about all kinds of labels— "conservative," "liberal," "Republican," "Democrat," "Baptist," "Amway distributor," and "telemarketer." Similarly, it is natural to judge a research procedure by the philosophical label associated with it. Labels such as "positivist," "postpositivist," and "social constructionist" all have their champions.

Focus group research methods, however, do not hold philosophical assumptions; focus group researchers do. For example, a positivist researcher, who assumes an objective reality, may use focus groups to generate ideas for quantitative items to measure that reality. A postpositivist, who believes both in an objective reality and in people's inability ever to know it fully, may still use focus group discussions to point toward or approximate that reality. Similarly, a social constructionist may discount objective reality altogether, but may still use focus groups to identify the subjective, mutually constructed community of beliefs surrounding certain topics.

In other words, there is no innate philosophical assumption attached to the use of focus groups. It is up to the researcher to clarify his or her philosophical assumptions and how he or she uses the focus group methodology consistent with those assumptions. Then the reader can evaluate the logic of the focus group methodology within the researcher's philosophical framework and inevitably make judgments about the framework itself.

Historical Roots and Development

Social science researchers have used various types of group interviews since the 1920s (Frey & Fontana, 1993). However, the precursor of today's focus group is usually considered to have originated in 1941, when Paul Lazarsfeld invited Robert Merton to assist him in evaluating audience response to radio programs at the Office of Radio Research at Columbia University (Kidd & Parshall, 2000). In their research, a studio audience listened to a radio program and pressed buttons on a polygraph-like device to indicate positive and negative responses to the program. Afterward, the researchers asked the audience members to explain their positive and negative reactions to the program; this was the beginning of what was then called the "focused group interview" (Merton, 1987).

In the midst of World War II, Merton used focused group interviews to analyze Army training and morale films for the Research Branch of the U.S. Army Information and Education Division. This experience resulted in a paper describing the methodology (Merton, 1946), and later in the book *The Focused Interview* (Merton, Fiske, & Kendall, 1956). Merton and his colleagues used their focus group research findings, both during the war and later at Columbia University, in writing their classic book on persuasion and the influence of the mass media, *Mass Persuasion* (Merton, Fiske, & Curtis, 1946).

Since that time, focus group interviewing has grown to be an important research tool, particularly in marketing. For example, focus groups are the most popular method among advertisers for evaluating television commercials. Similarly, movie studios frequently use focus groups to evaluate audience reactions to possible endings for new films. (The ending of *Fatal Attraction* was changed on the basis of focus group feedback.)

Focus group research is also becoming more popular in the academic literature, as evidenced by a threefold increase in the number of focus group studies in academic journals over recent years (Kitzinger & Barbour, 1999). Researchers are using focus groups in such other applied social science areas as program evaluation, public policy, social work, health care, and communication. Similarly, focus groups are beginning to be used in such diverse disciplines as family studies (e.g., Pramualratana, Havanon, & Knodel, 1985; Waugh & Bonner, 2002) and marriage and family therapy (e.g., Adams & Maynard, 2000; Polson, 1989; Polson & Piercy, 1993). Today, researchers are modifying focus group procedures to meet their own needs. For this reason, what is currently known as a "focus group" takes many different forms (Morgan, 1993) and does not necessarily follow all the procedures that Merton originally identified.

METHODOLOGY

Purposes and Research Questions

A research method should fit the purpose of an investigation, and research questions should flow logically from that purpose. Clearly, some purposes do not fit a focus group methodology. For example, if a researcher's purpose is to test for significant differences or to generalize with statistical precision to a population, the researcher should choose more quantitative procedures. However, if the researcher wants to understand a phenomenon from the point of view of a group of people who have experienced that phenomenon, focus groups may be helpful (Asbury, 1995).

The specific purposes of focus groups can vary widely. For example, they may be used to help quantitative social scientists develop questionnaires (Desvousges & Frey, 1989) or verify (i.e., triangulate) previous findings. Researchers may also use them to identify strengths and weaknesses of some concept or policy (Greenbaum, 1998). They can be used to generate theories and explanations (Morgan, 1993). Organizational administrators may use them to better understand what is going on in their organization, or the degree of consensus regarding a particular policy (Greenbaum, 1998). Cross-cultural researchers may use focus groups as a respectful way to understand participants who value oral communication and/or who cannot read. Other researchers may use them to raise sensitive topics (Zeller, 1993), to understand the needs of low-income minority populations (Jarrett, 1993), or to design AIDS prevention materials (Fetro, 1990).

Perhaps the most common reason for social scientists to use focus groups is for program evaluation (Edmunds, 1999; Krueger & Casey, 2000). Table 5.1 illustrates

TABLE 5.1. Uses of Focus Groups in Program Evaluation

<u>Focus groups before a project begins</u>

Needs assessment
- "What are the needs of the couples and families we want to serve? How can we meet these needs?"

Program material development
- "Does this brochure get information across in the most effective manner? If not, how could it be improved?"

Marketing
- "What are the best ways of reaching the group we want to serve? How can we best use media to get our message across? What kind of media?"
- "What media do persons who use intravenous drugs, and their families, read/see/hear? Where could we place information about our program so that these persons and/or their families might see it?"

Program design
- "What should be the components of our program? What components would best meet the needs of the people we want to serve? How should those components be organized?"

Strategic planning
- "What are the short- and long-term goals for our program? How can we best address these goals? Which goals should we address first? Why?"
- "What potential referral sources should we target? How should we contact these referral sources?"

<u>Focus groups during a program</u>

Ongoing program evaluation
- "Is our program doing what it should do? What do you like about the program? What do you dislike? How should we change the program to become more responsive to client needs?"

Reducing dropouts and no-shows
- "Why did you drop out of [or not show up at] our program? How could we have done a better job of encouraging you to stay involved?"

<u>Focus groups after a program</u>

Program evaluation
- "What did you like best about the program? What did you like least? What information were you most likely to use? How did you use it? What do you believe should be changed about the program for it to become more effective?"

Providing an organizational feedback loop
- "What is effective about the way this organization [leader/program/department] works? What should be changed? Why? How should it be changed?"

<u>Family-therapy-related focus group research questions: A few personal examples</u>

Stress among family therapy graduate students and their families
- "What stressors have been difficult to cope with in this graduate program? How have they affected your family? How have you coped with them? In what ways has your involvement in this program strengthened you individually and as a family? What suggestions do you have for future graduate students?" (Polson, 1989; Polson & Piercy, 1993).

Resiliency among families in Jakarta, Indonesia
- "What individual and family factors have allowed certain adolescents to stay out of trouble and to excel in school even though they live in high-crime, high-poverty areas of Jakarta, Indonesia?" (Piercy, 1993).

Evaluation of family therapy curricula for Indonesia
- "Are there any aspects of these curricula and learning activities that are not sensitive to the Indonesian culture? If so, what are they? How could they be changed?" (Limansubroto, 1993).

Resiliency among immigrant Hispanic families in therapy
- "Do you see your shared ethnicity to be a resource for your family? What aspects of your Hispanic culture have supported you through difficult times?" (Rafuls, 1994).
- [To family therapists, after they have viewed a videotape of Hispanic client families discussing strengths related to their culture:] "Does this information alter your initial impressions of your client family? Will any of the information you have gained be useful to you in work with other families?" (Rafuls, 1994).

purposes for which family therapists might use focus groups at the beginning, middle, and end of a project (Krueger, 1988), and examples of research questions that might logically flow from these purposes.

Sampling and Selection Procedures

Focus groups are usually composed of 6–12 people (Stewart & Shamdasani, 1990). Morgan and Krueger (1998) suggest using a smaller group when the intent is for each participant to contribute more in-depth information on a topic (e.g., an emotionally charged or controversial topic). Researchers should use a larger group when participants may have a lower level of involvement with the topic. If a group has fewer than 6 people, it is sometimes hard to generate a diversity of ideas. If the group has more than 12 people, not everyone gets a chance to talk and the moderator may find it difficult to keep the discussion focused on the research topic, or the discussion may be characterized by participants' taking turns to answer questions as opposed to interacting with one another (Green & Hart, 1999; Morgan, 1992). The ideal number of participants for general use is about 8. We usually invite 10, reasoning that 2 may drop out at the last minute.

Most focus group experts emphasize homogeneity among focus group members, as participants typically share more freely when they are with others from similar socioeconomic, educational, and cultural backgrounds (Morgan & Krueger, 1998). Even when a researcher wants to compare viewpoints of people from diverse categories, who thus may have different perspectives on a topic, Knodel (1993) suggests that it is better to hold separate focus groups—each homogeneous within itself, but differing on what he calls "break characteristics." A break characteristic is any characteristic that differentiates one group from another. For example, it might be important to evaluate teenagers' reactions to family therapy in groups different from their parents' groups, because the parents might inhibit the teenagers' discussion. Based on the purpose of the study, other possible break characteristics could include life stage, religion, socioeconomic status, residence (rural vs. urban), marital status, race, and gender (Diwan & Littell, 1996). Also, researchers sometimes base the selection of groups on certain break characteristics (e.g., economically disadvantaged rural women who have attended a parenting course at the local family service agency).

Participant selection is relatively easy when the purpose of a focus group study is clear. Krueger and Casey (2000) suggest that focus group researchers should seek out participants who are knowledgeable about the topic under investigation. Consider, for example, our initial illustration of wanting to understand what makes Dr. Stella Starr such a good workshop leader. First, we would choose participants from people who had actually attended one of Dr. Starr's workshops. Perhaps we would also like to restrict participants to those who attended Dr. Starr's AAMFT workshop last year. It might be less compelling to form focus groups by such break characteristics as residence, religion, or even gender.

As another example, one of us (FPP) supervised a series of focus groups to evaluate why some children living in high-crime, high-poverty areas of Jakarta, Indonesia excelled in school and stayed out of trouble. Given this premise, focus group participants were logically families living in these areas of Jakarta who had teens who excelled in school and stayed out of trouble. It also made sense for us to have separate focus groups for parents and teens, because the parents' presence would be likely to inhibit some teens from talking freely. We also decided to hold separate groups of male and female teens, because a mixed group of Indonesian teens would also probably inhibit discussion. (We wanted to avoid the "peacock effect"—i.e., the boys' showing off for girls—which our Indonesian colleagues said was likely to happen.)

A researcher may contact subjects through the mail or by telephone. When asking subjects to take part, the researcher should explain the purpose of the study, the time requirements (usually 2 hours), and the reason(s) why the participant was selected. Many focus group researchers offer incentives such as money or gifts to participants, and usually provide food and soft drinks at the focus group session itself. The day before the focus group session, the researcher should contact participants to remind them of the session and their previous commitment to take part.

Researchers must be creative in recruiting and accommodating hard-to-reach participants. This often involves going where the participants are. For example, we have held focus groups related to AIDS prevention in locations where sex workers congregate. It may also be important to provide babysitting services, transportation, or a central location. In some cases, researchers have also used teleconferencing to bring people together from different cities (Stewart & Shamdasani, 1990).

How many focus groups should be held for a particular research purpose? Krueger (1988) suggests that researchers should hold focus groups until the issues raised by the participants become repetitive and nonproductive. Morgan and Krueger (1998) state that researchers should consider the complexity of the topic as well as the goals of the project. They propose that those planning focus groups should plan to use more groups when there is a possibility of a diverse range of responses on the topic. This may mean scheduling four focus groups and canceling the last one if three seem sufficient. Depending on the purpose, however (e.g., "What do the administrators of this agency think should be its long-term goals?"), one focus group may be enough.

Data Collection Procedures

Role of the Moderator

Most focus group researchers use moderators to lead focus group discussions. The moderator should be familiar with the research topic and skilled in group dynamics. The moderator's job is to raise questions and guide the group back to the topic when it gets off track. The moderator should be a good listener and communicator who encourages shy participants to speak and is skilled at not letting dominant participants control the conversation (Edmunds, 1999; Greenbaum, 1998). He or she should be able to establish rapport, have a good sense of humor, be flexible, and use self-disclosure in a manner that encourages self-disclosure from the group (Morgan & Krueger, 1998). The moderator should also know when to pause and allow the group to process an issue, and when to probe for more information (e.g., "Would you explain what you mean by that?" or "Do you have an example?"). The moderator should try not to support some opinions (through nods of approval or such comments as "That's a great idea") while ignoring others. Finally, the moderator should be someone with good time management and organizational skills (Edmunds, 1999; Greenbaum, 1998).

There is little consensus as to the training necessary to become a focus group leader. Greenbaum (1998) presents three options for individuals interested in moderating training. First, interested individuals can apprentice themselves to or work for another focus group moderator. Second, the persons may participate in training courses. Finally, the individuals may seek a job in the marketing field. Moderators can be members of the research team, hired professionals, or even volunteers (Krueger, 1988). Krueger (1988) provides 12 hours of training for his volunteer moderators. We have found that we can use interpersonally skilled persons as moderators after we give them a thorough introduction to focus groups and opportunities to practice. We suggest that prospective moderators read either *Focus Groups: A Practical Guide for Applied Research* (Krueger, 1988) or the *Moderating Focus Groups* volume of *The Focus Group Kit* (Morgan & Krueger, 1998). Prospective moderators should subsequently observe an experienced moderator leading a focus group, and then lead a pilot focus group and receive feedback.

Krueger (1988; see also Morgan & Krueger, 1998) suggests that a focus group moderator work as a team with an assistant moderator. It is the assistant moderator's job to handle logistics (refreshments, lighting, seating), make sure that the tape recorder is working, and take comprehensive notes during the focus group. The assistant moderator may also wish to ask questions toward the end of the focus group and meet with the moderator at the end of the session for a postsession analysis of the major themes that were generated during the group.

The Interview Guide

The interview guide is the set of questions the moderator asks the focus group members. These questions should flow directly from the research questions being investigated in the study. The interview guide should include from 6 to 10 written questions, with possible subpoints within each question. The moderator should be familiar with the questions and use the list only as a reminder of upcoming questions (Krueger, 1988), as this enhances the natural flow of conversation from the participants (Edmunds, 1999).

The questions in the interview guide should be open-ended, clear, and conversational, and should encourage group discussion (Morgan & Krueger, 1998; Sharts-Hopko, 2001). It is often helpful to begin with a welcome, a statement of the purpose of the focus group, any ground rules, and an ice-breaking question that allows each member of the focus group to talk (Krueger, 1988). Following this opening question are introductory questions (ones that introduce the topic or issue that the group will discuss), transition questions (ones that link the introductory questions to larger questions), key questions (ones that drive the research), and ending questions (Morgan & Krueger, 1998).

Questions should be ordered by their relative importance to the research agenda from most to least important, beginning with the more general, less specific technical questions (Morgan & Krueger, 1998; Sharts-Hopko, 2001). Because a focus group discussion can take on a life of its own, it is important for the moderator to be flexible with the ordering of the questions and, when this is appropriate to the research topic, to follow the direction of the discussion. For example, if the discussion is yielding fruitful ideas in an unexpected direction, the moderator should probe the responses and add new questions as necessary (Stewart & Shamdasani, 1990). If more than one focus group interview is planned, the researcher may wish to consider using a "rolling interview guide" (Stewart & Shamdasani, 1990). That is, the experience of one focus group may lead the moderator to add or delete questions for the next focus group. Although this procedure has the advantage of adapting the learning from one focus group to the next one, it also has the disadvantage of lessening a researcher's ability to compare responses on the same questions across groups.

Specific Data Collection Procedures

Although some focus group researchers use videotaping, one-way mirrors, and even "focus meters" (small boxes that let participants indicate their positive or negative feelings), most focus group researchers favor more low-tech procedures. They reason that because the main data are the themes of the group discussions, the discussion itself is best captured verbatim for subsequent analysis. This is usually accomplished by audiotaping the focus group discussions and then transcribing them. The moderator and assistant moderator also typically maintain ongoing case notes during the focus group discussions and, immediately after the focus group, discuss and write summaries of their impressions and the themes they have noted.

Data Analyses

When Standard Data Analyses Are Not Necessary

The primary data source for most focus group analyses is the verbatim transcripts of the focus group sessions. However, because data analyses should be consistent with the purposes of the study, there are times when a brief written or even oral summary report may be all that is needed. In such cases, the comments of the moderator and assistant moderator may suffice. For example, one of us (FPP) held focus groups after each of a series of 5-day AIDS prevention workshops to learn about strengths and weaknesses of the workshop, so that our training team could improve the next workshop. For this purpose, all we really needed was a short written report and an oral summary.

There may be other times when the results of the focus group are so obvious that any additional analyses or write-up would be a waste of time and resources. For example, if the basic program evaluation question is "Are future family intervention programs like this needed?", the answer may become quite evident as the focus group proceeds. Similarly, if administrators and decision makers are the members of the focus group itself, they may not want any additional documentation.

Standard Cut-and-Paste Analyses

Most focus group analyses involve some variation of "code mapping" (Knodel, 1993) or cut-and-paste techniques (Stewart & Shamdasani, 1990). In code mapping, also known as "data indexing" (Frankland & Bloor, 1999), a researcher reads over the transcript of the focus group once to identify those sections that are meaningful to the research questions and to get an overall "feel" for possible categories under each of the research questions (Knodel, 1993, states that it is also acceptable to begin with hypothesized categories that can be confirmed, refuted, or added to on subsequent passes through the data.) On the second reading, the researcher marks initial category codes in the margins. The researcher may be coding words, sentences, interchanges, or conceptual units, and may pass through the data several times. This process is cyclical, and new codes and themes may emerge each time the researcher reads through the data (Frankland & Bloor, 1999). Once the coding is finished, the transcript is cut apart and sorted into meaningful categories under each of the research questions. These inductively derived categories provide the structure within which researchers will make their final interpretive analysis. Researchers typically use quotes from focus group members to illustrate the categories and assertions within the final report.

Computer software packages such as The Ethnograph (Seidel, Kjolseth, & Seymour, 1988), NVivo (Richards, 1999), and ATLAS.ti (Muhr, 1997) can be particularly helpful in coding and sorting categories (i.e., the "cut-and-paste" function). Also, researchers can use traditional word-processing software packages as alternatives to scissors, colored pencils, tape, and 5″ × 7″ cards. Although computer technology can help in indexing and cross-referencing, it is still up to the researcher to make sense of the data. To minimize researcher bias, we recommend that more than one researcher be involved in the data categorization and analysis. They can categorize the data independently and then come together to discuss and resolve differences.

Also, because researchers should be as familiar with the data as possible, we believe that it is helpful for them either to moderate the focus group themselves or at least to observe the group process. This is, of course, at variance with the objectivity usually emphasized in more quantitative procedures. However, because researchers sooner or later must analyze and make sense of the data, we believe that they should try to be as well acquainted with it as possible.

Content Analyses

Some focus group researchers discourage counting focus group data. Others have applied a wide range of content analysis procedures (see Krippendorf, 1980) to the transcripts of focus groups. The assumption driving the use of content analysis is that the analysis of language can provide a clue to the meanings participants ascribe to the subject of the focus group. The simplest content analysis is a finding–counting–sorting procedure that results in descriptive data such as counts of emotion-laden words, known as "semantic content analysis." Another type of content analysis, "pragmatic," centers on identifying cause-and-effect statements (Diwan & Littrell, 1996). The problem with such an analysis is that because words are used in context, the context of the subject should also be part of the content analysis.

One computer-assisted approach, available through most qualitative software, searches for keywords and lists each along with the surrounding text. The researcher can limit the surrounding text by specifying the number of words or letters surrounding the keyword and can subsequently categorize contexts as well as their relationship to keywords.

Reporting the Results

Focus group research can generate a tremendous number of data. It is not uncommon, for example, for one focus group session to generate 20 single-spaced pages of transcript. To report the results, researchers must look for statements that reflect themes, so that the trees can be seen in the midst of the forest. When the analysis of a focus group does not require a written report, the researcher can use a double-deck cassette player to find and record sections of the most meaningful quotes to supplement his or her oral report.

More frequently, though, data reduction and analysis occur through some form of cut-and-paste procedure. Whether the researcher uses a word processor, scissors, or

5″ × 7″ cards, the ultimate goal is to identify themes or trends, to use quotes to illustrate those trends, and to interpret these trends in the final report.

Morgan and Krueger (1998) suggest three types of final reports, each using the initial research questions as the primary outline or structure. The first method of presentation, the "raw data model," includes all participants' comments after a particular subject or research question. This involves little or no analysis by the researcher. The second method, the "descriptive model," includes summary comments regarding themes, followed by illustrative quotes by participants. The third method, the "interpretive model," includes summary descriptions followed by illustrative quotes and the researcher's interpretations.

Although Krueger's suggestions relate primarily to evaluation research, we also favor the interpretive model—use of summaries, illustrative quotes, and researcher interpretations—in writing up other focus group research studies. The appropriate journals for such reports will depend on what questions were addressed and whether the focus group was used alone or in concert with other quantitative or qualitative methods. We see no reason why rigorous, good focus group research cannot be published in such top family therapy journals as *Family Process* and the *Journal of Marital and Family Therapy.*

DISCUSSION

Strengths and Weaknesses of the Methodology

One international foundation funded 15 research projects related to women and AIDS. All 15 of these projects employed focus groups (International Center for Research on Women, 1992). Why are such organizations interested in focus group social science research? What do focus groups have to offer family therapy researchers? What are the weaknesses of such groups? Table 5.2 summarizes some of the advantages and disadvantages of focus group research.

Clearly, focus groups are not a panacea. Compared to other qualitative methods, focus groups do not allow for naturalistic observation as well as participant observation, and they do not allow for the same level of direct probing as individual interviews do (Morgan & Spanish, 1984). However, they do a better job of combining these two goals than either participant observation or individual interviews alone.

Moreover, focus groups seem to have several unique advantages. They are quick and inexpensive, and they capitalize on the synergistic, snowballing effects of group discussion. When facilitated well, they are respectful and tolerant of diverse opinions. They encourage phenomenological, context-sensitive understanding and are usually a positive experience for the participants. Furthermore, they can be catalytic, in that the group members may become motivated to take action regarding the topic they have discussed.

The limitations of focus groups center around their inability to provide quantitative hypothesis testing or probability estimates. Potential sources of bias are also inherent in focus group research (as they are in all forms of research). In focus group research, for example, we can never know for sure whether results are generalizable or whether a strong group member, unfamiliar surroundings, or the moderator may have somehow biased the results. On balance, however, if focus groups are used for appropriate purposes—such as understanding group opinion or generating theory—family

TABLE 5.2. Advantages and Disadvantages of Focus Groups

Advantages	Disadvantages
Format	

Advantages	Disadvantages
• The setting is more naturalistic than that of a controlled experiment.	• The setting is unnatural.
• The format allows the moderator to probe for more information.	• The procedures limit generalization.
• Synergistic group effect stimulates a wide variety of information.	• Participants' responses are not independent.
• Comments "snowball" or build on other comments to stimulate more creative ideas.	• The researcher has less control than in an individual interview.
• Can be used with children and other samples.	• The moderator may knowingly or unknowingly bias the data by verbal and nonverbal clues.
• The researcher may interact directly with the participants.	• Groups can vary considerably.
• The method is flexible.	• Focus groups may be difficult to assemble.
• The open-response format can generate a large number of rich data.	• The moderator must have special skills.
• The cost in both time and money is relatively low.	• Anonymity of participants may not be possible within the group.

Purpose	

Advantages	Disadvantages
• Can generate theory and/or explanations.	• Should not be used when statistical precision is a research goal.
• Can triangulate the results of other methods.	
• Can generate data on sensitive topics.	
• Can support community participation and ownership when used in strategic planning.	
• Can address a variety of questions.	
• Can provide a way for the researcher to increase the size of qualitative studies.	

Results	

Advantages	Disadvantages
• Serendipitous ideas often surface during the group discussion.	• The results may be affected by dominant or opinionated participants.
• Participants usually enjoy the experience.	• Traditional definitions of validity and reliability of data cannot be assured.
• The results have high face validity.	
• The results are available quickly.	
• The results can serve a catalytic function in motivating participants to action.	

Interpretation	

Advantages	Disadvantages
• The general results are usually easy to understand.	• The wealth of data may make summarization and interpretation difficult.

Note. Data from Hess (1968), Krueger (1988), and Stewart and Shamdasani (1990).

therapists should find them quite useful. Focus groups are robust, flexible, qualitative procedures that may be used on their own or in concert with other qualitative and quantitative procedures.

Ethical Considerations

Because focus group interviews take place in a group context, they are subject to a variety of unique ethical concerns. Participants should feel comfortable enough in the focus group setting to provide free and honest responses. A researcher should provide information about how the results will be used, describe all video and audio recording, and be sure to communicate each participant's right to decline the invitation to participate (Edmunds, 1999). Confidentiality is also an important consideration. Though the moderators can indicate that they will maintain the confidentiality of group members, there is no guarantee that other participants in the group will do likewise. Group members may disclose information that upsets other group members. Researchers can address some of these ethical issues by setting ground rules prior to the group, and by providing participants with opportunities to debrief after the group discussion (Kitzinger & Barbour, 1999).

Reliability and Validity

Reliability

You may have guessed that traditional notions of reliability are simply not that important in focus group research. Recall our initial example: We wanted to know why Dr. Starr was such a popular workshop presenter. To find out, we speculated about using focus groups of people who attended her highly rated AAMFT workshop and inductively deriving categories of effective workshop leader qualities that might emerge during the focus group discussion. Our results would be heuristic, in that they would raise possibilities of what might be effective for others, as well as future directions for more quantitative research on the subject. Our purpose in using the focus group format, however, would not be to determine whether the qualities that made Dr. Starr effective would also be the same for other presenters. All the same, Dr. Dweeb might still learn some useful presentation skills from reading our focus group results.

Reliability of procedures, on the other hand, *is* important in focus group research. Researchers should follow a standard, definable protocol for both running focus groups and analyzing focus group data. They should also summarize this protocol in published reports, so that the reader can follow the logic of the analysis. This consistency serves to make focus group procedures more accountable and trustworthy (Belgrave, Zablotsky, & Guadagno, 2002; Koch, 1994). Using multiple coders is yet another way to enhance reliability in focus group research (Kidd & Parshall, 2000).

Validity

Validity, at its most basic level, is the degree to which the data accurately reflect what the researcher intends to measure. Because researchers use focus groups to better understand participants' view on a topic, valid focus group data should be defined as those accurately reflecting the participants' views. Because the purpose of focus groups is to tap the perceived reality of participants, perceived reality is the reality against which the data must be considered. Do focus group data reflect perceived reality? They should, if the procedures we are advocating are followed closely.

A quantitative researcher once asked one of us (FPP) about how marketing companies, in all good conscience, can afford to make million-dollar decisions based on focus group results that the company cannot be absolutely sure will generalize to the entire population. This is a good question. It is up to each researcher and sponsoring agency to decide the degree to which they wish to make program decisions based on focus group data. In many cases, the richness of these data may indeed be more compelling than statistical analyses of decontextualized, reductionistic information. In other cases, this may not be true. When external validity is a concern, we believe that marketing researchers—and family therapy researchers—would do well to use multiple research methods. This is not an indictment of focus group data, which do exactly what they are intended to do. It is simply prudent to supplement such data with quantitative methods when a researcher desires statistical precision.

Several simple steps during or immediately after the focus group may enhance the credibility of the results. For example, researchers should use recording equipment that is sophisticated enough to record multiple participants and participants' talking at once without losing any individual participant's comments. Moderators or assistant moderators should also write down important statements and nonverbal behavior during the focus group. Finally, moderators may also conduct a brief member check at the close of the group, summarizing and getting feedback on what appeared to be important themes (Kidd & Parshall, 2000).

Bridging Research and Practice

As noted earlier, researchers can use focus groups to learn about a wide range of practice issues and can then use the focus group results to improve clinical services. For example, researchers can use focus groups to assess needs, understand problems, and evaluate services in order to improve them.

Broadly speaking, though, family therapists are always engaged in focus group research when they work with families or other client groups. With this chapter in mind, we suggest that you become a more purposeful focus group researcher the next time you review a videotape of one of your therapy sessions. You can do this alone, with colleagues, or in a supervision group. What themes do you notice in the session? What categories of problems, communication patterns, emotions, and interventions emerge as you watch and listen to the tape? How can you use this information to become more effective in your own work with clients? As you can see, the perceptual and executive skills of a focus group researcher may be useful to you as a practicing family therapist.

Future Directions

Family therapy researchers are just beginning to discover focus groups. For this reason, the future directions of focus group research are a little like the roads out of Chicago—they go off in all directions. One "road" points toward the use of focus groups for needs assessment, another toward their use for program evaluation, and still another toward their use for more holistic and culturally sensitive interpretation of quantitative results. There are, of course, many other roads to travel for the family therapy researcher interested in focus groups.

We are excited about the generative, humanizing potential that focus group research can bring to the field of family therapy. We hope you will consider traveling down some of the roads discussed in this chapter. The ride should be fun and the destinations worthwhile.

ACKNOWLEDGMENT

We wish to thank Vernon Nickerson for his contributions to an earlier version of this chapter.

REFERENCES

Adams, J. F., & Maynard, P. E. (2000). Evaluating training needs for home-based family therapy: A focus group approach. *American Journal of Family Therapy, 28*(1), 41–52.

Asbury, J. (1995). Overview of focus group research. *Qualitative Health Research, 5*(4), 414–420.

Belgrave, L., Zablotsky, D., & Guadagno, M. A. (2002). How do we talk to each other?: Writing qualitative research for quantitative readers, *Qualitative Health Research, 12*(10), 1427–1439.

Desvousges, W. H., & Frey, J. H. (1989). Integrating focus groups and surveys: Examples from environmental risk studies. *Journal of Official Statistics, 5*, 349–363.

Diwan, S., & Littrell, J. (1995). Impact of small group dynamics on focus group data: Implications for social work research. *Journal of Applied Social Sciences, 20*(2), 95–106.

Edmunds, H. (1999). *The focus group research handbook.* Chicago: NTC Business Books.

Fetro, J. (1990). Using focus group interviews to design materials. In A. C. Matielia (Ed.), *Getting the word out: A practical guide to AIDS materials development* (pp. 37–48). Santa Cruz, CA: ETR Associates.

Frankland, J., & Bloor, M. (1999). Some issues arising in the systemic analysis of focus group materials. In R. S. Barbour & J. Kitzinger (Eds.), *Developing focus group research* (pp. 144–155). Thousand Oaks, CA: Sage.

Frey, J., & Fontana, A. (1993). The group interview in social research. In D. Morgan (Ed.), *Successful focus groups: Advancing the state of the art* (pp. 20–34). Newbury Park, CA: Sage.

Green, J., & Hart, L. (1999). The impact of context on data. In R. S. Barbour & J. Kitzinger (Eds.), *Developing focus group research* (pp. 21–35). Thousand Oaks, CA: Sage.

Greenbaum, T. L. (1998). *The handbook for focus group research* (2nd ed.). Thousand Oaks, CA: Sage.

Hess, J. (1968). Group interviewing. In R. Ring (Ed.), *New science of planning.* Chicago: American Marketing Association.

International Center for Research on Women. (1992). *The women and AIDS research program* (Information Bulletin No. 1-3). Washington, DC: Author.

Jarrett, R. (1993). Focus group interviewing with low-income minority populations. In D. Morgan (Ed.), *Successful focus groups: Advancing the state of the art* (pp. 184–201). Newbury Park, CA: Sage.

Kidd, P., & Parshall, M. B. (2000). Getting the focus and the group: Enhancing analytic rigor in focus group research. *Qualitative Health Research, 10*(3), 293–308.

Kitzinger, J., & Barbour, R. S. (1999). Introduction: The challenge and promise of focus groups. In R. S. Barbour & J. Kitzinger (Eds.), *Developing focus group research* (pp. 1–20). Thousand Oaks, CA: Sage.

Knodel, J. (1993). The design and analysis of focus group studies: A practical approach. In D.

Morgan (Ed.), *Successful focus groups: Advances in the state of the art* (pp. 35–50). Newbury Park, CA: Sage.

Koch, T. (1994). Establishing rigour in qualitative research: The decision trail. *Journal of Advanced Nursing, 19,* 976–986.

Krippendorf, K. (1980). *Content analysis: An introduction to its methodology.* Beverly Hills, CA: Sage.

Krueger, R. A. (1988). *Focus groups: A practical guide for applied research.* Newbury Park, CA: Sage.

Krueger, R. A., & Casey, M. A. (2000). *Focus groups: A practical guide for applied research.* (3rd. ed.). Thousand Oaks, CA: Sage.

Limansubroto, D. W. (1993). *The compilation and organization of a family therapy teaching curriculum for Indonesian university students.* Unpublished master's thesis, Purdue University.

Merton, R. K. (1946). The focussed interview. *American Journal of Sociology, 51,* 541–557.

Merton, R. K. (1987). Focussed interviews and focus groups: Continuities and discontinuities. *Public Opinion Quarterly, 51,* 550–566.

Merton, R. K., Fiske, M., & Curtis, A. (1946). *Mass persuasion.* New York: Harper & Row.

Merton, R. K., Fiske, M., & Kendall, P. (1956). *The focused interview.* New York: Free Press.

Morgan, D. (1992). Designing focus group research. In M. Stewart, F. Tudiver, M. J. Bass, E. V. Dunn, & P. Norton (Eds.), *Tools for primary care research* (pp. 177–193). Newbury Park, CA: Sage.

Morgan, D. (Ed.). (1993). *Successful focus groups: Advancing the state of the art.* Newbury Park, CA: Sage.

Morgan, D., & Spanish, M. (1984). Focus groups: A new tool for qualitative research. *Qualitative Sociology, 7*(3), 253–270.

Morgan, D., & Krueger, R. A. (1998). *The focus group kit.* Thousand Oaks, CA: Sage.

Muhr, R. (1997). *ATLAS.ti—visual qualitative data analysis—management—model building* (Release 4.1, User's Manual, 1st ed.). Retrieved from *http://www.atlasti.de*

Piercy, F. P. (1993). *Final report of World AIDS Foundation Project, "AIDS prevention in Indonesia: Workshops for Health and Social Science Professionals."* Geneva, Switzerland: World AIDS Foundation.

Polson, M. (1989). *The exploration of program stress on trainee families in the Purdue Marriage and Family Therapy Program: A qualitatively oriented focus group study.* Unpublished master's thesis, Purdue University.

Polson, M., & Piercy, F. (1993). The impact of training stress on married family therapy trainees and their families: A focus group study. *Journal of Family Psychotherapy, 4*(1), 69–92.

Pramualratana, A., Havanon, N., & Knodel, J. (1985). Exploring the normative basis for age at marriage in Thailand: An example from focus group research. *Journal of Marriage and the Family, 47,* 303–310.

Rafuls, S. (1994). *Qualitative resource-based consultation: Resource-generative inquiry and reflective dialogue with four Latin American families and their therapists.* Unpublished doctoral dissertation, Purdue University.

Richards, L. (1999). *Using NVivo in qualitative research.* London: Sage.

Seidel, J., Kjolseth, R., & Seymour, E. (1988). *The Ethnograph: A user's guide.* Littleton, CO: Qualis Research Associates.

Sharts-Hopko, N. C. (2001). Focus group methodology: When and why? *Journal of the Association of Nurses in AIDS Care, 12*(4), 89–91.

Stewart, D., & Shamdasani, P. (1990). *Focus groups: Theory and practice.* Newbury Park, CA: Sage.

Waugh, F., & Bonner, M. (2002). Domestic violence and child protection: Issues in safety planning. *Child Abuse Review, 11*(5), 282–295.

Zeller, R. (1993). Focus group research on sensitive topics. In D. Morgan (Ed.), *Successful focus groups: Advancing the state of the art* (pp. 167–183). Newbury Park, CA: Sage.

CHAPTER 6

Action Research Methods in Family Therapy

TAI J. MENDENHALL
WILLIAM J. DOHERTY

"Action research" (AR) is a research paradigm that emphasizes close collaboration between researchers and community participants to generate knowledge that is useful for solving local problems. It originally emerged in social science in the 1940s, as a response to problems related to social structures that were seen as unfair and oppressive to minority and other marginalized groups (Corey, 1953; Hagey, 1997; Piercy & Thomas, 1998). Originally advanced by Kurt Lewin (1946), AR encompassed two principal areas of focus: (1) changing an oppressive system, and (2) acquiring critical knowledge about the system and its context. The democratic and participatory nature of AR processes (discussed below) was advanced as key, backed by the argument that those who directly experience a phenomenon are the best qualified to investigate it (DePoy, Hartman, & Haslett, 1999). Although AR's focus and visibility in contemporary times have extended beyond this original foundation into and across a wide range of health and human service fields, this method of investigative inquiry continues to be defined by central tenets related to a collaborative partnership between researchers and participants. Within this partnership, hierarchical differences are flattened, and all participants in the research process work together to create knowledge and effect change (Yoshihama & Carr, 2002).

Though it is still not widely practiced in marriage and family therapy (MFT) circles, AR has gained increased credibility in health care (e.g., medicine, nursing) since the early 1990s because of its potential to inform understanding of patients' experiences and to improve or generate the services provided to them (Fraser, 1999; Heslop, Elsom, & Parker, 2000; Kovacs, 2000; Tobin, 2000; Ward & Trigler, 2001). Similarly, its use is increasing in social work and family science because of its potential to inform understanding of clients' experiences and improve community outreach, education, and cultural awareness efforts (de Amorim & Cavalcante, 1992; Newfield, Kuehl, Joanning, & Quinn, 1991; Piercy & Thomas, 1998). As health care (broadly defined) moves forward in a state of constant change, the need for research strategies that permit analyses of change processes in real time (i.e., as change occurs) has become apparent (Hayes, 1996).

AR has been employed in a wide range of areas, including minority students' experiences in predominantly European American school environments, hospice access and use by African Americans, community-based organizations' response to the multiple needs of impoverished Hmong women, child care surveillance, health audits, dental and mouth care practices, management of preoperative fasting, patient problem-solving skills, maintenance of overall physical well-being, patient and practitioner satisfaction, patient and practitioner empowerment, patient–practitioner communication, and numerous other significant health care issues (Hampshire, Blair, Crown, Avery, & Williams, 1999; Herr, 1996; Hunt, 1987; Lindsey & McGuinness, 1998; McGarvey, 1993; McKibbin & Castle, 1996; Meyer, 2000; Reese, Ahern, Nair, O'Faire, & Warren, 1999; Yoshihama & Carr, 2002).

Authors of AR studies generally emphasize a core strength of the AR approach: Because it focuses on a problem within a specific site or community, the "local" practical problem is addressed directly and in context (Hambridge, 2000; McGarvey, 1993; Morrison & Lilford, 2001). Put simply, the immediate utility of AR projects to participants is high, unlike traditional interventions that apply general findings from research directed at larger populations to a specific context with its own unique features and attributes. Although this points to a potential weakness of AR in terms of generalizability on a broad scale (which is addressed in further detail in a later section of this chapter), most AR researchers argue that the relevance of knowledge generation and beneficial change for the community to which the work is directed is worth the tradeoff.

BACKGROUND

The ANGELS: An Example of Action Research in a Health Care Setting

We will provide the reader with an illustration of an AR project to illustrate several of the philosophical assumptions that are outlined below. What follows is a synopsis of an initiative carried out in a large hospital in a metropolitan community located in the Southern region of the United States. This project was facilitated by an MFT practitioner.

> Care providers in the Department of Pediatrics had been frustrated for some time with how things were going with their adolescent patients diagnosed with diabetes. Although some kids seemed to do okay—adhering (on their own or at their parents' insistence) to prescribed regimens of diet, physical activity, blood sugar monitoring, and insulin administration—a large proportion of patients were simply out of control in regard to their disease. Despite repeated efforts in conventionally teaching important components of diabetes management, hosting diabetes-related fairs and public forums, and providing persistent warnings about the long-term consequences of poor metabolic control, nothing was working. Adolescent patients continued to be brought in by their parents with poor physiological indicators (e.g., hemoglobin A1c levels and weight) and little apparent motivation to change. Parents complained about being "nags" to teenagers who wanted to be left alone. Patients complained about adults who would not "get off their backs" or allow them to have the same spontaneity and freedom as their

peers. Providers often felt triangulated into family conflicts right in the exam room, without any clear idea about what to do other than go over the same old information and warnings.

Initial conversations between the director of Pediatrics and one of us (TJM, an MFT practitioner who was situated in the Department of Psychiatry) identified new ideas for this old and increasing problem. Having recently been involved in the development of a democratic citizenship initiative oriented to adults with diabetes called Partners in Diabetes (Mendenhall & Doherty, 2003), the MFT practitioner suggested that an AR approach be applied to this problem because it would move efforts beyond the traditional top-down services that had already established themselves as ineffective. Not being familiar with flat-hierarchy interventions involving active patient and family participation, but maintaining an investment in addressing the problem aggressively and an openness to trying new solutions, the director mobilized other providers within the hospital to meet, learn about this approach, and decide whether and how to proceed.

Initial meetings with providers addressed how to engage patients as collaborators in the design of supplemental services to standard care. This would draw upon a variety of heretofore untapped resources, including patients' and families' lived experience and wisdom of living with diabetes on a day-to-day basis. The Families and Democracy Model (Doherty & Carroll, 2002b), which was designed purposely for professionals working with families in community settings, was introduced as a guiding framework for this effort. Through the lens of this model, providers are viewed as citizens with knowledge and skills who work actively with other citizens also possessing important knowledge and skills. Participants self-consciously and explicitly avoid conventional provider–consumer dynamics by recognizing and valuing all members' respective contributions to a common mission. Families are active producers and co-creators of action and change, and thus do not function in a conventional consumer/patient role.

Six families were invited to meet with providers and discuss ideas regarding the building of a citizenship initiative that would benefit adolescents and parents struggling with diabetes in the local community. The stage was set to work collaboratively, and a great deal of attention was given to discussing and understanding how these efforts would not follow the conventional provider-led approach. Adolescents and parents alike were enthusiastic about creating something new in democratic partnership with providers, with the larger vision of developing a model of care by and for its citizens with all participants functioning as stakeholders in the process. The group collaboratively identified key areas of concern, and developed solutions within the context of the hospital's and the surrounding community's resources. As adolescents, parents, and providers met over the following months, an exciting new program began to take root.

The ANGELS (A Neighbor Giving Encouragement, Love, and Support) initiative was designed and implemented as a supplement to standard care for families with an adolescent diagnosed with diabetes. In this program, adolescents and their parents who have lived experience with diabetes (called "support partners") are connected with other adolescents and parents (called "members") who are struggling with the illness. These efforts begin at the time of diagnosis, which occurs almost universally in the context of emergency hospitalization. It is during this time that the ANGELS support partners want to connect with members, because the motivation to adopt healthy lifestyles is the highest at a time of crisis. Support partners and members meet in a variety of combinations (e.g., adolescents with adolescents, parents with parents, families with families), and they continue to meet off hospital grounds (or via telephone or e-mail) after initial hospitalization. Sometimes members simply need a pep talk; other times ongoing support is offered for several months.

Outcomes following the implementation of the ANGELS program were originally assessed through dialogue among (1) providers directly involved in new patients' emergency hospitalization; (2) new patients and families receiving emergency services and ANGELS support; and (3) the patients, parents, and providers directly involved in the creation of the ANGELS initiative. Although most feedback was positive, some adjustments were made (e.g., efforts to synchronize standard care provision more closely with ANGELS meeting and support time, and to coordinate ongoing support following inpatient care more effectively). Researchers are now assessing changes in quantitative measures of patients' average metabolic control (hemoglobin A1c levels) in groups receiving support through the ANGELS program in addition to standard care versus groups receiving standard care exclusively. Anecdotal accounts suggest that the program's usefulness will be further validated as these evaluative efforts are advanced, but only time will tell.

Adolescents and parents in the ANGELS program worked democratically with providers throughout every stage of its development—initial brainstorming, the naming process, training design, public-visibility efforts, implementation, and ongoing problem solving and maintenance. Although the program functions under the auspices of an official hospital volunteer program, the ANGELS training reflects participants' viewpoints regarding the best ways to prepare for the role of a support partner, going far beyond basic provider-designed training about the generic volunteer role, general health issues, or diabetes-related topics. Intentionally relying on existing community resources, the ANGELS program has maintained its democratic character and ensured its long-term viability as a resource within its community. Initial efforts are now in process regarding the training of a new generation of support partners, many of whom at one time were members connected with this program during their own crises and early struggles with diabetes. Support partners' sense of personal ownership in the ANGELS program continues to be reflected in this progression, as they are assuming responsibility for components of this training and long-term vision.

Philosophical Assumptions of Action Research

As described above, AR involves active partnership and collaboration between researchers and subjects, in a manner wherein hierarchical differences are flattened and all participants in the research process work together to create knowledge and effect change. Although various investigatory approaches and methods exist, several key philosophical assumptions permeate AR initiatives. These are highlighted below.

Democratic Partnership

AR is explicitly participatory, insofar as it involves all project members (e.g., participants, community stakeholders, researchers) as collaborators at every stage in a cyclical process of knowledge development and change (Bradbury & Reason, 2003; DePoy et al., 1999). This participation is overtly democratic; all involved members are seen as equal contributors to the AR process and are expected to participate as such. The unique strengths, lived experience, knowledge, and wisdom of everyone involved are elicited and used (Casswell, 2000; Lindsey & McGuinness, 1998; Minkler, 2000). As researchers and other professionals contribute theoretical knowledge and a variety of specialized skills, layperson participants advance their local and real-world knowledge in synchrony. This collaboration can create a "whole" of knowledge and wisdom that is considerably more useful for improving the lives of a community (however defined) than the sum of the respective parts (Small, 1995).

Deep Investment in Change

AR aims at change. Indeed, its advocates maintain that change processes must occur before a group's endeavors can even be labeled as an AR initiative. This change can be defined in a myriad of ways unique to any individual research project, but it generally includes elements of challenging the status quo and somehow improving the lives of members in a community or a practice (Hambridge, 2000; Rolfe, 1996). As AR participants work together to generate new knowledge about a problem, they achieve an increased understanding of barriers and possible solutions (Reese et al., 1999). This newfound wisdom then informs newfound action for responding to troubles that the research participants are concerned about (DePoy et al., 1999; Hick, 1997).

Problem Solving in Context

As mentioned before, AR aims to generate knowledge and devise local-level solutions for specific problems within the parameters of a community's existing resources (McKibbin & Castle, 1996; Morrison & Lilford, 2001). Immediate relevancy is achieved through unique solutions that are identified and found to be effective. Because AR relies on existing resources within a community to solve a problem (e.g., persons, organizations, existing funding sources), effective solutions are not as apt to disappear in the future as they would be if they depended on external funds (e.g., a large research grant), which are most often temporary in nature and require a priori "deliverables" that are defined by whoever is providing the money.

A Cyclical Process of Action and Evaluation

Participants in AR initiatives go through a cyclical process of reflection and democratic action, in which (1) a problem is identified that is meaningful and important to all AR participants, and information is gathered regarding it; (2) solutions to address the problem are developed within the context of the community's existing (albeit often untapped) resources and refined; (3) interventions (broadly defined) are implemented to allay the problem; and (4) outcomes are evaluated according to what is essential in the eyes of the participants, and the intervention is modified in accordance to new information as necessary (Coghlan & Casey, 2001; Hambridge, 2000; Lindsey & McGuinness, 1998). This process repeats itself as many times as needed, as novel solutions are generated and refined to address practical problems (DePoy et al., 1999; Small, 1995).

Humility and High Adaptability to Change

AR researchers are self-evaluative and reflective on group processes and intervention outcomes. Participants maintain a high level of flexibility to accommodate changes as necessary across any part of a project (Morrison & Lilford, 2001; Razum, Gorgen, &

Diesfeld, 1997). This requires the ability to be humble as learning processes advance, and as problems are dealt with in what sometimes feels like a "trial-and-error" manner. Openness to new ideas and interventions is necessary as old and ineffective solutions are modified or cast out entirely (Hayes, 1996; Minkler, 2000).

A Slow and Messy Process

AR is generally a slow and messy process, especially during the initial phases of development. It takes a long time; setbacks, dead ends, and repeated experiences of "going back to the drawing board" are commonplace. No "cookbook" of methods exists, and the exact nature and sequence of steps will vary in each community and for each problem that AR participants choose to address (Hagey, 1997; Lindsey & McGuinness, 1998; Minkler, 2000).

ACTION RESEARCH METHODOLOGY

AR is more of a "style" of doing research than a particular "methodology" (Holter & Schwartz-Barcott, 1993; Meyer, 2000). The diversity of community settings in which AR has been employed further complicates efforts to outline clear-cut investigatory methods. Each researcher faces unique local problems, resources, customs, traditions, and language in each individual project. These unique issues determine what research strategies represent the best "fit" (Kondrat & Julia, 1998; Titchen & Binnie, 1994). In addition, most published accounts of AR focus more on the process and evolution of the initiatives than on the specific techniques that were used to gather and analyze data. This lack of detail often reduces the clarity of research reports, making it difficult to retrace the projects' steps (Healy, 2001; Kondrat & Julia, 1998).

With this said, it is important first to revisit the notion that AR is a *process* of research—a moving target—and that this necessitates flexibility in terms of what research methods (questions, types of data gathered, and means of evaluation) are most appropriate for any given research project at any given period of time. Second, it is important to reemphasize the collaborative nature of this research process between researchers and participants. This is research "with" people, not "on" people, and participants' lives are affected in profound ways through the research and its consequent changes. With this shared investment comes a shared ownership of the project; decisions made regarding the methods employed—and decisions made regarding how to gather and use outcome data (however defined)—are made collaboratively (Kondrat & Julia, 1998; Piercy & Thomas, 1998).

Research Questions

The research questions posed in AR begin with queries about purpose and with attention to the audience for whom the research is being conducted (Bradbury & Reason, 2003; Herr, 1996). Unlike in conventional research, these are important considerations in AR, because they reflect the comparatively higher complexity of stakeholders' being connected to and affected by the entire research enterprise. AR is not driven only by professionals' curiosity about a social topic or a particular group; it is also driven by a shared interest and commitment to a problem among multiple stakeholders who represent a variety of positions. This is where the first research questions are devised, and it represents the platform from which ensuing research questions evolve.

The cyclic process begins with the recognition of a problem that unites a community of professionals (researchers) and laypersons (participants) (Meyer, 2000; Minkler, 2000). If research efforts are pushed forward without active involvement with the community in defining this, then the research is by definition not AR. What concerns run deep in this community? What are members of this community struggling with, and what is seen as impeding change? What is the scope of the problem—that is, who does it affect, and how does it affect different members of this community in similar and different ways? What problem or problems are members of this community motivated to work toward resolving? What goal or focus will energize this community to unite and charge forward into the uncharted territory of change? Community dialogues regarding these questions can be held in a variety of contexts, ranging from one-on-one informal discussions to large public forums and town meetings. As community members come forward and join forces with researchers—each with important knowledge and wisdom to contribute—the first steps of AR are put into motion.

Research questions related to "the problem" (however defined), including its scope and its nature, are then followed by questions that solicit possible solutions (Casswell, 2000; Kondrat & Julia, 1998). What is important in this phase of the AR cycle is that community-based resources and wisdom are sought, and that community members' strengths and competencies are mobilized (Hagey, 1997; Minkler, 2000). This point warrants special emphasis because conventional modes of community outreach and problem solving do not do this. Instead, they typically involve a hierarchal sequence of service delivery that (1) is not usually well informed by its recipients; (2) places recipients in a passive stance that limits their influence to modify the service; (3) leaves untapped a variety of resources within the community that could be mobilized if the active participation of community members was fostered; and (4) creates a system of "helping" that is difficult to sustain, should outside funding or interest wane (Doherty & Carroll, 2002b; Mendenhall, 2002). By asking, "What resources [personal, tangible, relational, cultural, etc.] in this community can be tapped to address this problem?", participants in AR move outside the conventional "box" containing the notion that solutions to problems come from the top and move downward, or come from the outside and move inward.

Research questions related to the implementation of newfound solutions are remarkably varied in AR, because they must be made relevant to the specific problem and community context in which they are positioned (Kondrat & Julia, 1998; Meyer, 2000). Oriented in a general sense to the query "How did it work?", various foci are addressed: "What is the outcome of our efforts [subjective or objective]? What changes are most apparent and meaningful? What factors have most effectively contributed to the success of this intervention/solution? What has worked against us en route to our goals? What mistakes have we made? What have we learned that helps us refine this intervention/solution? What has worked especially well, and how can this be augmented or enhanced?" Answers to these investigatory queries serve the important function of refining applied solutions (or even going back to the drawing board) as participants endeavor to effectively align resources and strategies with the identified foci of intervention and attention.

It is important to note, too, that the research questions posed through the AR cycle of identifying problems, developing solutions, and assessing the outcome of solutions are put forth as part of an ongoing process of knowledge generation. This ensures immediate relevance to the participants across the research's course, and it fosters an ongoing sense of co-ownership in the work as everyone involved collaborates to identify (and answer) shared queries (Piercy & Thomas, 1998; Small, 1995).

Sampling and Selection Procedures

The sampling and selection procedures employed in AR are as diverse as the research questions outlined above, because the focus in this type of research is dynamic. It changes as attention shifts from problem identification, to the development of solutions and strategies, and to evaluating the success or failure of these solutions and strategies (Small, 1995).

Advocates of AR maintain a very open stance toward who participants are or might become. Involved members are not outlined in an a priori manner, because the process of engaging a community to unite against an identified problem and solve it tends to bring people "on board" at different stages across the research's course, and other members may drop out along the way (e.g., if they are not able to participate for any variety of reasons, or they do not share an invested stake or interest with the larger community). Regardless of the point in the AR cycle that an initiative has reached, however, participants' inclusion—whether they are laypersons or professionals—is generally defined by the experience of somehow being active stakeholders in the work (Mendenhall, 2002; Small, 1995). Whether the type of data that is actually collected is qualitative (e.g., in-depth interviews, focus group discussions) or quantitative (e.g., frequencies of a particular dependent-variable event or outcome, structured surveys), the persons sampled to provide these data tend to be those who are most affected by the process and evolution of the work itself (Bradbury & Reason, 2003; McNicoll, 1999; Small, 1995).

Data Collection and Analysis Procedures

Because researchers are often dealing with novel problems within the unique contexts of particular communities, they must be methodologically eclectic in order to match data collection efforts most closely with what is going on in the AR process (McNicoll, 1999). Researchers must be sensitive to the needs and viewpoints of multiple participants, and thereby must be careful to incorporate methods and measures that have high face validity and practical (and immediate) utility. For this reason, AR researchers tend to gravitate toward qualitative methods of data collection and analysis. Areas of focus in AR lend themselves well to methods that tap participants' subjective experiences. These foci include engaging communities and identifying concerns that run deep within them; monitoring intermember and intercommunity group processes as problems are identified and action is taken (via identifying solutions and democratically developing and implementing indicated interventions); and monitoring satisfaction and newfound experiences secondary to these said actions. Although objective measures of "success" can be created to assess a program's impact on a particular dependent variable (e.g., teen pregnancy rates in a particular school community), the majority of AR studies focus data collection on dynamic and evolutionary processes, which are better captured through the voices and observations of key participants.

Many different types of qualitative data in AR have been described in the literature: in-depth interviews (Lindsey & McGuinness, 1998; Razum et al., 1997); naturalistic case studies (Casswell, 2000); reflective journaling and meeting minutes (Hampshire et al., 1999; Nichols, 1995); thematic and content analysis of group process notes and publicly available documents (Nichols, 1995; Razum et al., 1997); focus groups (Small, 1995); participant observation (Lindsey & McGuinness, 1998; Maxwell, 1993); social network mapping (Bradbury & Reason, 2003); and oral histories and open-ended stories (Small, 1995). Gaining access to many of these types of data is generally not a tall order for researchers, because the very nature of AR necessitates their active participation in the investigatory activities that are being evaluated in the first place.

AR researchers have been especially vocal about using multiple methods, which enable the triangulation of different sources of data and increase confidence in the conclusions (Hagey, 1997; Lindsey & McGuinness, 1998; McKibbin & Castle, 1996; Nichols, 1995). Furthermore, the use of multiple methods better accommodates the diverse nature of AR participants, insofar as these methods capture multiple and representative viewpoints (Bradbury & Reason, 2003; McNicoll, 1999).

Whereas qualitative analyses (e.g., thematic analyses of transcribed in-depth interviews) are especially useful in helping researchers to understand participants' context, culture, beliefs, attitudes, community practices, and subjective experiences related to AR processes, quantitative measures are most usefully employed as part of the evaluation of an intervention's efficacy (Reese et al., 1999). Of course, consistent with the basic tenets of AR, it is important to involve participants in the selection of what is important to measure. For example, an AR initiative designed to improve diabetes care in a local community may or may not view patients' overall metabolic control (measured quantitatively by assessing hemoglobin A1c levels) as an important measure of "success." Instead, they may see the number of struggling patients in a community who connect with community services as a more important quantitative measure of "success." They may see this initial step as a stage setter for the improved subjective sense of self-efficacy and social support that will eventually help patients maintain better overall disease management (Mendenhall & Doherty, 2003).

Throughout the cyclical process of AR, the data that are collected and analyzed are presented back to the initiative's participants (Hambridge, 2000; Meyer, 2000; Nichols, 1995). This facilitates an active and purposeful dialogue between researchers and participants regarding the meaning and usefulness of data, which in turn helps generate action steps en route to identified goals. In the same manner that all participants were involved in the identification of a problem and the generation of solutions to address the problem, all participants maintain a sense of ownership in the results and are more engaged in subsequent decision making based on these results.

Reporting of Action Research Processes and Findings

Although the tide is beginning to shift, there is still little professional recognition of AR in mainstream refereed journals (Kondrat & Julia, 1998; McNicoll, 1999). There are many possible reasons for this. These may include AR's heavy reliance on qualitative methodologies with small samples (which are less impressive in mainstream academic circles than are large-sample quantitative studies); AR's reliance on local community resources versus large external funding sources; AR researchers' concern with direct application and social change versus more basic research; and/or AR research-ers' interest in interventions that change through iterative reflection–action–reflection cycles versus more standardized interventions.

AR is most commonly reported in written reports for AR participants; presenta-tions in community forums; books and book chapters; press conferences and press re-leases; and a variety of other civic and local government meetings (Healy, 2001; Kondrat & Julia, 1998; McNicoll, 1999). These types of reporting platforms are more consistent with the mission of AR efforts—to mobilize change in a community in a manner that benefits multiple members and stakeholders.

DISCUSSION

Strengths of Action Research

Below, we discuss a number of strengths inherent to AR. Each relates to its utility in improving practice (broadly defined) and benefiting the lives of a community's mem-bers.

Immediate Relevancy to Context

AR is carried out in the very context(s) that researchers seek to benefit. Members of the community define their concerns and play an active role in the research process. They develop and implement solutions to local-level problems with local-level re-sources. Although results from AR enterprises may not be generalizable on a broad scale, what is produced is immediately relevant and fine-tuned to the community where it was applied. This highly specific focus is considered by those involved as an advantage of AR (Hambridge, 2000; McKibbin & Castle, 1996; Meyer, 2000).

Use of Existing Resources

AR taps resources that already exist in a community, but that have heretofore been underutilized or entirely untapped. These resources can be personal (e.g., leadership skills, lived experience, and wisdom) or tangible (e.g., money, services), but they are not created through external funding. Although external funding has many advan-tages, a big disadvantage is the fact that externally funded services are often discontin-ued when these funds run out, or when funders' priorities change. Furthermore, by identifying and using participant resources, members gain an increased sense of owner-ship in solving the problem (Casswell, 2000; Hagey, 1997; Minkler, 2000).

Empowering Communities in Processes of Change

AR's forward-facing vision challenges the status quo, and its participants engage ac-tively in processes oriented toward improving the lives of those in a community. The democratic processes between professionals and laypersons facilitate a flat hierarchy, so that all work together to generate knowledge and effect change. Cohorts of commu-nity members who once felt disempowered become empowered as stakeholders in the AR process. As all develop a sense of co-ownership in identifying problems and solv-ing them, AR participants shift from being passive recipients of inadequate services to becoming active members of a team passionately invested in changing and improving the services (Hambridge, 2000; Piercy & Thomas, 1998).

Self-Reflection and High Adaptability to Change

AR researchers must be self-reflective and use their reflections to change course when necessary. If certain resources are not working out, what other resources are available? This reflective, humble, and flexible approach enables AR researchers to adjust and modify their approaches until they find the most effective means of addressing the problem (Hayes, 1996; Morrison & Lilford, 2001).

Forward-Facing Vision and "Thinking Outside the Box"

By definition, AR is a form of social inquiry that stands apart from conventional deductive research approaches, which are carried out "on" participants according to standard principles and sequences of hypothesis testing and variable measurement. AR researchers often find themselves in novel contexts with novel problems, and they must be open to learning from community members. They employ methodologically eclectic techniques that are sensitive to participants' perspectives and worldviews. AR researchers use a wide range of interventions, including oral histories, open-ended stories, creative arts, in-depth interviews, music, and focus groups. Although such methods may not be within the "toolbox" of conventional social science research, these and many others are routinely used in AR (Bradbury & Reason, 2003; Lindsey & McGuinness, 1998).

Weaknesses of Action Research

A number of weaknesses inherent to AR are also important to note. These limitations serve as warnings to those engaging in this type of inquiry, as well as challenges for those wishing to advance AR.

Incompatibility with Conventional Means of Professional Recognition

Because AR is oriented to solving immediate problems in small local communities, any given project is difficult to replicate on a larger scale or in other communities. Although community members benefiting from immediate community action applaud the fit of AR interventions to their community, mainstream social science does not tend to espouse this sentiment. Therefore, AR reports are comparatively difficult to publish or present in professional journals and forums, and this is an important issue for researchers to consider if they are positioned in academic contexts wherein they must publish to gain tenure and promotion. Relatedly (because AR focuses on small samples, deals with local problems, is not readily generalizable, and is difficult to publish or present professionally), it is also difficult to secure grant funding to support a researcher's time in the field while conducting this type of work. Tenure and promotion committees are not likely to be sympathetic to the facts that (1) AR is difficult to fund extramurally; and (2) a principal tenet of AR is that efforts to solve a community's problem should not rely on resources that originate from outside the community in question (Hampshire et al., 1999; Small, 1995).

The Slow and Messy Process

AR is marked by a series of trial-and-error movements through the cyclical process of identifying problems and generating solutions to improve the lives of a community (Hagey, 1997; Lindsey & McGuinness, 1998). It is common for participants in AR initiatives to see early efforts as completely or partially unsuccessful. Often researchers must return to the drawing board en route to accomplishing the initiative's shared goals. Unlike conventional research projects in which a timeline for participant recruitment, data collection, data analysis, and reporting of results can be tentatively outlined, AR can be entirely unpredictable. This can be frustrating to everyone participating in the AR process (especially when projects get "stuck" or are taking an unprecedented amount of time), and professional entities who are evaluating a researcher's productivity are not likely to be sensitive to this. Furthermore, the "endpoint" of AR is often not clear, for the reason that its cyclical process is, well, cyclical. The argument can be advanced—by anyone involved—that improvements can always be made, and that related problems can always be identified and focused on as old problems are addressed and solved.

Conventional Regulatory Bodies' Unfamiliarity with Action Research

Despite academia's unaccommodating stance to Action Research, an increasing number of researchers are investing their efforts in this type of investigative enterprise. Still problematic, though, are the questions of how AR is perceived by universities' institutional review boards, and how these regulatory bodies can be convinced that this type of research is acceptable in terms of participant safety and issues of confidentiality. Due to the ambiguity of what is ultimately going to transpire over the course of AR, as well as in terms of what is going to ultimately result from AR efforts, it is difficult to meet standard notions of what informed consent requires. Also, the public nature of AR initiatives makes it difficult to maintain participants' confidentiality. It is difficult to maintain anonymity in research write-ups, particularly since the participants are also the coresearchers. Anyone even peripherally involved in the investigation is likely to be able to identify participants when their statements are made as part of open community gatherings. There exist no easy answers to these questions as yet.

Issues of Reliability and Validity in Action Research

AR is oriented toward producing change in a local community composed of a unique and complex mix of contextual components that exist nowhere else in exactly the same manner. Thus there is inherent difficulty in generalizing findings. It is important, then, to seek standards of reliability and validity that go beyond conventional designs. Bradbury and Reason (2003) argue that

> the validity of the research is in some ways defined by the context of researchers/participants, as opposed to [a] (so-called) independent group of scientists. In this case, abstract generalizability, once assumed to be the quintessence of scientific value, is de-emphasized while other criteria such as the generation of usable knowledge that concretely generalizes to a growing proportion of an individual's or institution's life are offered in its place. (p. 172)

With this said, researchers involved in AR are highly invested in the process of generating knowledge with (not "on") participants. Participants are involved not only in the collection of data (however this is defined across AR's cycles), but also in the analysis and perusal of these data. Findings are regularly presented to participants, who give researchers feedback regarding the accuracy, usefulness, and implications of the findings. The immediate relevancy of these data are ascertained subjectively in this process by the group, and data are acted upon (or not) according to this collaborative, self-sensitive feedback process (Hambridge, 2000; Meyer, 2000).

Insider versus Outsider Positions of Researchers

Researchers' positions within AR are also important to consider, insofar as their standing as "insiders" or "outsiders" permits or restricts closeness to a group's internal processes and functioning. Insider investigators (e.g., hospital personnel working with patients who are invested in improving local health care in a concerned community) tend to possess familiarity with interpersonal and interdepartmental dynamics and politics, and are generally well suited to access and be accepted by a range of research participants (Coghlan & Casey, 2001; Razum et al., 1997).

Primary Source Data

Whether originally "insiders" or not, researchers in AR generally work actively with participants across an investigation's evolution and development. This enables them to observe group processes firsthand, record process notes, and interview people with whom they have already worked closely. The data they derive and analyze are therefore explicitly "primary source data." Adams and Schvaneveldt (1991) maintain that "the best research is done with primary sources since they originated via eyewitnesses or participants in the situation [that is being researched]" (p. 305).

Use of Multiple Methods

As described above, many different types of data and methods are described in the AR literature (e.g., in-depth interviews; naturalistic case studies; reflective journaling; thematic and content analysis of group process notes and publicly available documents; focus groups; and participant observation). To augment the validity of any of these methods' findings, researchers in AR are especially vocal about the utility of using multiple methods, because this enables a triangulation of data and increases confidence in the ultimate conclusions (Hagey, 1997; Nichols, 1995).

Requisite Skills for Investigators Involved in Action Research

A number of skills and personal attributes are helpful in negotiating the terrain of AR, and they are important to highlight here.

Charismatic, and Then Collaborative, Leadership

Researchers tend to function in leadership positions throughout an AR investigation's evolution, but the nature of this leadership is not a static one. Instead, it is remarkably dynamic—changing from a very active and often charismatic leadership role during the early stages of AR, to equal participation in and facilitation of group processes in later stages (Lindsey & McGuinness, 1998; Mendenhall, 2002). During the early phases of AR, the leaders are highly engaged in eliciting potential members' participation through bringing groups together to identify and channel their shared investments en route to creating change (however change is defined). This is often facilitated through an energetic and inspiring persona, and is evident in leaders' public speaking ability, affability, and comfort in new social contexts. However, leaders in AR projects must also be able to hand leadership over to the group as group ownership develops. This is not always easy for charismatic persons who enjoy being the center of attention. It is key to balance charisma with a collaborative style and sense of teamwork.

Group Facilitation Skills

Throughout AR, leaders must be able to effectively facilitate group processes (Hagey, 1997; Lindsey & McGuinness, 1998). In early stages, this may take the form of eliciting equal participation and input from involved participants in sharing personal concerns and negotiating common worries. Group processes also include identifying group missions and conferring necessary tasks in information gathering and resource tapping, as well as educating participants and discussing how AR initiatives are different from conventional initiatives. Later on, group facilitation skills can include processing information relevant to implemented changes or interventions, negotiating changes that the group believes are important, reflecting about intergroup processes that are working for or against broader goals, and pacing meetings and ensuring that all agenda items identified by members as important to address are given attention.

Humility

AR professionals must shift away from conventional ways of working that define their roles as that of "experts"—those who know most of the answers, direct group decisions, and shape group evolution (Hambridge, 2000; Minkler, 2000). Because most professionals are socialized through their training to function in an expert role, they sometimes find it difficult in AR to resist being a group's problem solver, or to deflect participants' attempts (especially early on) to gain knowledge or advice in a conventional top-down fashion. Professionals must be able to say, "I don't know," when they do not know the answer to something (and sometimes even when they do know the answer). They also must be able to roll up their sleeves and work with participants in the processes of knowledge generation in a collaborative manner, in which they function as any other member of the group—each with important knowledge and skills to offer, and each aware of (and embracing) the knowledge and skills of everyone else (Mendenhall, 2002; Mendenhall & Doherty, 2003).

Patience, Flexibility, and a High Tolerance for Ambiguity

As we have emphasized throughout this chapter, AR is slow and messy work, and it is marked by a series of trial-and-error movements along a path that is rarely straightforward from beginning to end. Professionals who require set protocols, timelines, and schedules are likely to be uncomfortable in AR. Ambiguity in time, steps, and tasks is more the rule than it is the exception. As AR participants come together to address a problem, it is not known beforehand how the problem's scope will be defined, what resources and strategies within a community are extant (or how they will be tapped and integrated into any kind of intervention), or what decisions regarding action will be made. Although AR can sometimes feel energizing to its members as problems are addressed and progress is made, it can also feel extremely frustrating as an initiative's pace is outmatched by its participants' enthusiasm to make something happen. Also, solutions may not always work, and the group may find itself back at the drawing board. Leaders must be patient over the course of these processes, and remain able to facilitate discussions about related frustrations. They must also be highly tolerant of the ambiguous nature of the uncharted territory that always lies before those engaged in AR (Mendenhall & Doherty, 2003).

Bridging Research and Practice

The purpose of creating knowledge through AR is to effect change, and the ongoing process of AR's cyclical course within an immediate context commands this (Coghlan & Casey, 2001; Greenwood, 1994; Piercy & Thomas, 1998). Instead of having to move research into the "real world" through practice and application, AR is conducted *in* the real world and involves both investigation and action as inseparable facets of its overall course.

Future Directions

AR is here to stay, as evidenced by its increasing visibility in social science and health care circles, despite institutional recognition and award systems that work against it. As our efforts to improve community problems and practice move forward, so has our need to employ research strategies that permit analyses of information and the incorporation of change processes in real time (Greenwood, 1994; Hampshire et al., 1999; Meyer, 2000). While these efforts proceed and we continue to work together to improve communities through any variety of actions, the following points are important to consider.

Increased Multidisciplinary Collaboration

AR efforts must identify resources within communities to address real problems of focus, and thus must recognize the many valuable types of knowledge and wisdom that multiple participants bring to the table. Many AR projects, however, do not involve professionals from a variety of disciplines (i.e., they rely on a few select professionals who represent a limited specialty area). As professionals from more and more fields (e.g., medicine, nursing, social work, family science, MFT, anthropology) employ AR, efforts to collaborate across disciplines are not only practical but sensible, insofar as they combine one discipline's strengths with those of others around the table (Mendenhall & Doherty, 2003; Small, 1995).

Increased Visibility in Graduate Education

AR has not yet received a great deal of attention in graduate research courses across social science and health care fields, and students' and young professionals' exposure to this type of work is limited as a consequence (McNicoll, 1999; Small, 1995). Increasing AR's visibility in graduate education will better prepare our next generation of researchers and practitioners to engage in investigative efforts that are designed to immediately benefit the communities where they live. A challenge to this call rests in the likelihood that many of the professionals who are teaching graduate research are not themselves familiar with this approach. Current-generation educators therefore have the responsibility to learn about AR, so that they can facilitate students' exposure to, and encourage their interest in, this type of work.

Increased Visibility in Professional Arenas

Consistent with the preceding argument that we need to increase AR's visibility in graduate education, we must continue to increase AR's visibility on a larger scale across professional arenas. This may take the form of publication in mainstream refereed journals (e.g., *Journal of Marital and Family Therapy, Family Process, Social Work*); the introduction of new journals that are oriented specifically toward AR (e.g., *Action Research International, Journal of Action Research in Education*); or increased attention in national and international forums through public presentations, posters, or discussion groups. All such efforts that facilitate widespread familiarity and exposure to AR will serve to augment and stabilize its position as an accepted research practice in family therapy and health care science. Its potential will only be realized when AR becomes a common way of working with communities to improve the lives of those within them.

CLOSING THOUGHTS

As AR researchers committed to advocating the use of AR in MFT research, we end this chapter by noting two significant obstacles that will have to be overcome for this approach to have a home in our field. The first issue is whether MFT researchers can find outlets for their work in peer-reviewed, academic journals. Without these outlets, untenured faculty members risk professional suicide if they focus their careers around AR. We are optimistic that journal editors in our field will be open to well-conducted AR studies, just as they have been open to qualitative studies and to effectiveness outcome studies operating within other methodological parameters than those of traditional empirical research. The journal *Family Process*, for example, has explicitly invited AR studies in the area of "family-centered community building" (Doherty & Carroll, 2002a).

More difficult will be the challenge for doctoral students whose faculty advisors are unfamiliar with AR. One solution may be to create an AR interest group for both students and faculty with interests in this kind of research, for the purposes of mutual support and feedback. Interest groups could be formed at the program, department, university, community, and/or national levels. A similar interest group was successful in the National Council on Family Relations in the early 1980s. Specifically, the Qualitative Family Interest Group began an ongoing process of mutual education of students and junior faculty. A core group of seasoned qualitative family researchers served as mentors to promote this kind of research with families. Leaders in the MFT field could create an AR Interest Group that would operate online during the year and meet face to face at the American Association for Marriage and Family Therapy's annual conference. Since its origins in the 1950s, the MFT field has been open to radical new approaches; we are confident that AR can flourish in MFT if we undertake our work with creativity, rigor, and passion.

EXEMPLARS

The following are five exemplars of AR that demonstrate the utility of this investigative approach across a wide variety of social concerns.

Exemplar 1. Gallagher and Scott (1997) describe the STEPS Project (Seniors and Persons with Disabilities Task Force for Environments Which Promote Safety) as an AR initiative oriented to identifying and rectifying factors that contribute to injurious falls experienced by elderly and disabled persons in public places. Participants included seniors, disabled persons, health care practitioners, and research partners situated in a local community. Their efforts facilitated gathering data relevant to the most common locations of falls, environmental problems causing the falls, and demographics of persons who had fallen. The group then hosted a symposium of community providers, engineers, city planners, and politicians to make recommendations leading to the repair of hazardous surfaces, removal of unsafe obstacles, and establishment of effective means to report hazards as they are recognized by members of the community.

Exemplar 2. Stevens and Hall (1998) describe an AR project involving the efforts of providers at a local women's health organization to address risky sexual behavior in lesbian and bisexual women. Providers collaborated with lesbian and bisexual women (who served in the capacity of peer educators) in gathering extensive data about the sexual practices of the target community. These data informed both individualized and large-scale education related to safer sex practices. Several positive outcomes were recognized as a consequence of these efforts, including increased intent to change risky behaviors, improved ability to discuss and negotiate safer sex with partners, and early changes in community conventions regarding sexual practices and expectations.

Exemplar 3. Whitmore and McKee (2001) describe an AR initiative mobilized to evaluate the services of a local center oriented toward street-involved youth. This project involved an active collaboration between center staff and youth, and engaged multiple facets of the local community (e.g., youth, agency staff, the business community, and police) in the identification of ways to improve service delivery to youth and their effective integration into the community. AR efforts were effective in activating the redesign of the agency's management structure, the founding of a youth advisory committee, improved relations with the business and law enforcement community, and overall youth–staff relations within the center itself.

Exemplar 4. Barrett (2001) describes the MARG (Midwives Action Research Group) as an initiative highly invested in generating, implementing, and evaluating changes in health care practices related to new mothers and to midwifery practice in a local hospital community. Participants worked collaboratively to identify concerns regarding women's experiences during hospitalization and their access to informed choices. Changes in practice were made in response to these efforts. For example, the institution responded to the group's expressed need for time and space for women to meet and talk with each other for the purposes of fellowship and support. This change reflected MARG's earned credibility in this system, and helped the initiative develop a permanent presence within the system.

Exemplar 5. Kondrat and Julia (1998) describe an AR project in south India that was used to help rural communities improve systems of care and rehabilitation for children with disabilities. Rehabilitative service professionals worked in partnership with parents of disabled children to engage with disabled persons, families, community leaders, and indigenous health workers, and to identify specific needs and resources in local areas relevant to this problem. The group developed and implemented training and education outreach initiatives as a result of these efforts. Ongoing evaluative strategies focused on individual children's progress and overall program effectiveness.

REFERENCES

Adams, G. R., & Schvaneveldt, J. D. (1991). *Understanding research methods* (2nd ed.). New York: Longman.

Barrett, P. A. (2001). The Early Mothering Project: What happened when the words "action research" came to life for a group of midwives. In P. Reason & H. Bradbury (Eds.), *Handbook of action research: Participative inquiry and practice* (pp. 294–300). London: Sage.

Bradbury, H., & Reason, P. (2003). Action research: An opportunity for revitalizing research purpose and practices. *Qualitative Social Work, 2,* 155–175.

Casswell, S. (2000). A decade of community action research. *Substance Use and Abuse, 35,* 55–74.

Coghlan, D., & Casey, M. (2001). Action research from the inside: Issues and challenges in doing action research in your own hospital. *Journal of Advanced Nursing, 35,* 674–682.

Corey, S. (1953). *Action research to improve school practices.* New York: Teachers College, Columbia University.

DePoy, E., Hartman, A., & Haslett, D. (1999). Critical action research: A model for social work knowing. *Social Work, 44,* 560–569.

de Amorim, A. C., & Cavalcante, F. G. (1992). Narrations of the self: Video production in a marginalized subculture. In S. McNamee & K. J. Gergen (Eds.), *Therapy as social construction* (pp. 149–165). London: Sage.

Doherty, W. J., & Carroll, J. S. (2002a). The citizen therapist and family-centered community building: Introduction to a new section of the journal. *Family Process, 41,* 561–568.

Doherty, W. J., & Carroll, J. S. (2002b). The Families and Democracy Project. *Family Process, 41,* 579–590.

Fraser, D. M. (1999). Delphi technique: One cycle of an action research project to improve the pre-registration midwifery curriculum. *Nurse Education Today, 19,* 495–501.

Gallagher, E. M., & Scott, V. J. (1997). The STEPS Project: Participatory action research to reduce falls in public places among seniors and persons with disabilities. *Canadian Journal of Public Health, 88,* 129–133.

Greenwood, J. (1994). Action research: A few details, a caution and something new. *Journal of Advanced Nursing, 20,* 13–18.

Hagey, R. S. (1997). The use and abuse of participatory action research. *Chronic Diseases in Canada, 18,* 1–4.

Hambridge, K. (2000). Action research. *Professional Nurse, 15,* 598–601.

Hampshire, A., Blair, M., Crown, N., Avery, A., & Williams, I. (1999). Action research: A useful method of promoting change in primary health care? *Family Practice, 16,* 305–311.

Hayes, P. (1996). Is there a place for action research? *Clinical Nursing Research, 5,* 3–5.

Healy, K. (2001). Participatory action research and social work: A critical appraisal. *International Social Work, 44,* 93–105.

Herr, K. (1996). Action research as empowering practice. *Journal of Progressive Human Services, 6,* 45–58.

Heslop, L., Elsom, S., & Parker, N. (2000). Improving continuity of care across psychiatric and emergency services: Combining patient data within a participatory action research framework. *Journal of Advanced Nursing, 31,* 135–143.

Hick, S. (1997). Participatory research: An approach for structural social workers. *Journal of Progressive Human Services, 8,* 63–78.

Holter, I., & Schwartz-Barcott, D. (1993). Action research: What is it? How has it been used and how can it be used in nursing? *Journal of Advance Nursing, 18,* 298–304.

Hunt, M. (1987). The process of translating research findings into nursing practice. *Journal of Advanced Nursing, 12,* 101–110.

Kondrat, M. E., & Julia, M. (1998). Democratizing knowledge for human social development: Case studies in the use of participatory action research to enhance people's choice and well-being. *Social Development Issues, 20,* 1–20.

Kovacs, P. (2000). Participatory action research and hospice: A good fit. *Hospice Journal, 15,* 55–62.

Lewin, K. (1946). Action research and minority problems. *Journal of Social Issues, 2,* 34–46.

Lindsey, E., & McGuinness, L. (1998). Significant elements of community involvement in participatory action research: Evidence from a community project. *Journal of Advanced Nursing, 28,* 1106–1114.

Maxwell, L. (1993). Action research: A useful strategy for combining action and research in nursing? *Canadian Journal of Clinical Nursing, 4,* 19–20.

McGarvey, H. E. (1993). Participation in the research process: Action research in nursing. *Professional Nurse, 8,* 372–376.

McKibbin, E. C., & Castle, P. J. (1996). Nurses in action: An introduction to action research in nursing. *Curationis, 19,* 35–39.

McNicoll, P. (1999). Issues in teaching participatory action research. *Journal of Social Work Education, 35,* 51–62.

Mendenhall, T. J. (2002). *Partners in Diabetes: The process and evolution of a democratic citizenship initiative in a medical context.* Unpublished doctoral dissertation, University of Minnesota.

Mendenhall, T. J., & Doherty, W. J. (2003). Partners in Diabetes: A collaborative, democratic initiative in primary care. *Families, Systems and Health, 21,* 329–335.

Meyer, J. (2000). Using qualitative methods in health related action research. *British Medical Journal, 320,* 178–181.

Minkler, M. (2000). Using participatory action research to build healthy communities. *Public Health Reports, 115,* 191–197.

Morrison, B., & Lilford, R. (2001). How can action research apply to health sciences? *Qualitative Health Research, 11,* 436–449.

Newfield, N. A., Kuehl, B. P., Joanning, H., & Quinn, W. H. (1991). We can tell you about psychos and shrinks: An ethnography of the family therapy of adolescent substance abuse. In T. C. Todd & M. D. Selekman (Eds.), *Family therapy approaches with adolescent substance abusers* (pp. 277–310). Boston: Allyn & Bacon.

Nichols, B. (1995). Action research: A method for practitioners. *Nursing Connections, 8,* 5–11.

Piercy, F. P., & Thomas, V. (1998). Participatory evaluation research: An introduction for family therapists. *Journal of Marital and Family Therapy, 24,* 165–176.

Razum, O., Gorgen, R., & Diesfeld, H. J. (1997). Action research in health programs. *World Health Forum, 18,* 54–55.

Reese, D. J., Ahern, R. E., Nair, S., O'Faire, J. D., & Warren, C. (1999). Hospice access and use by African Americans: Addressing cultural and institutional barriers through participatory action research. *Social Work, 44,* 549–559.

Rolfe, G. (1996). Going to extremes: Action research, grounded practice and the theory–practice gap in nursing. *Journal of Advanced Nursing, 24,* 1315–1320.

Small, S. A. (1995). Action-oriented research: Models and methods. *Journal of Marriage and the Family, 57,* 941–955.

Stevens, P. E., & Hall, J. M. (1998). Participatory action research for sustaining individual and community change: A model of HIV prevention education. *AIDS Education and Prevention, 10,* 387–402.

Titchen, A., & Binnie, A. (1994). Action research: A strategy for theory generation and testing. *International Journal of Nursing Studies, 31,* 1–12.

Tobin, M. (2000). Developing mental health rehabilitation services in a culturally appropriate context: An action research project. *Australian Health Review, 23,* 177–184.

Ward, K., & Trigler, J. (2001). Reflections on participatory action research with people who have developmental disabilities. *Mental Retardation, 39,* 57–59.

Whitmore, E., & McKee, C. (2001). Six street youth who could. In P. Reason & H. Bradbury (Eds.), *Handbook of action research: Participative inquiry and practice* (pp. 396–402). London: Sage.

Yoshihama, M., & Carr, E. S. (2002). Community participation reconsidered: Feminist participatory action research with Hmong women. *Journal of Community Practice, 10,* 85–103.

CHAPTER 7

Computer-Aided Qualitative Data Analysis Software

GENERAL ISSUES FOR FAMILY THERAPY RESEARCHERS

JENNIFER L. MATHESON

BACKGROUND

I was not always comfortable using software for analyzing qualitative data, but I was thrust into it during my 11 years at a major research organization and over the course of three graduate programs, including two in family therapy. In each of those settings, I learned and practiced the science and art of qualitative research, including developing skills in the use of "computer-aided qualitative data analysis software" (CAQDAS). I used early CAQDAS packages for basic data management purposes, such as to manage interview data and qualitative responses to questionnaires; I then applied to them the most basic nonhierarchical coding schemes and printed the results for report writing. This is the way perhaps 60% of users take advantage of CAQDAS: as an electronic file cabinet utilizing only the most basic frequency counts of codes (Fielding, 2000).

As a graduate student in marriage and family therapy, I have used CAQDAS in a more sophisticated manner to manage large quantities of interview data, develop hierarchical coding trees, and use the powerful search and theory-building components of the software. I have gone to at least two formal CAQDAS training sessions (specifically, for NVivo and NUD*IST) and taken a graduate-level course on the use of CAQDAS in dissertation research. I have worked on dozens of projects using CAQDAS, both on my own and with large research teams, and I have provided informal training for graduate students interested in using the software for their own research. Although I do not feel like an expert on CAQDAS, I have had enough experience in using it to be able to empathize with and provide some direction to family therapy researchers who are struggling to make sense of it and are curious about what it offers.

As both a student and a professional, I have worked with people who are enthusiastic about using CAQDAS, as well as people who are not. Some even consider the use of CAQDAS a separate kind of analysis, like grounded theory or content analysis

(Fielding, 2000). This chapter is for anyone curious about how CAQDAS has evolved and how it can be used in family therapy research, because even those who choose not to use CAQDAS should be familiar with a range of available options. Among other things, I describe the history of CAQDAS, some of the similar and unique features of the currently used software packages, and some of the ways family therapy researchers can use CAQDAS. I share some of my own experiences throughout to illustrate my points. It is helpful for a novice to approach CAQDAS with a spirit of openness, realizing that none of the software packages are flawless, that none will be all things to all people, and that all have the potential to be used in as flexible a way as the researcher's creativity will allow.

Assumptions and Biases

In order to be reasonably transparent as both a CAQDAS user and the author of this chapter, I lay out some of my assumptions and biases here. Just as computer users have a bias toward the operating system to which they are most accustomed (e.g., IBM vs. Apple), and certain software packages are beloved by those who have used them, so I have a bias toward the CAQDAS packages I have used the most. I have used packages such as The Ethnograph, AskSam, NVivo, ATLAS.ti, and NUD*IST in the past. I am currently partial to NVivo and ATLAS.ti, because these are the ones I have used the most, have had training in, and are being used by the others with whom I have recently worked on qualitative research teams. All of the other CAQDAS products may be excellent, but my bias is toward those I have used. I have tried to present a balanced view of this technology and do not consider any one package to be superior to all others, but the reader will undoubtedly sense my deeper knowledge of some packages.

It is important to note early in this chapter that CAQDAS is simply a tool to aid qualitative researchers in managing their data before, during, and after analysis. CAQDAS does not teach people how to analyze qualitative data, nor should it be used as such a teaching tool. I assume that people who will be using this chapter to help them decide whether or not to use CAQDAS in family therapy research already have some experience and training in analyzing qualitative data without software. I am not an advocate for using CAQDAS as a substitute for learning the intricate and important processes involved in high-quality qualitative analysis, but for learning and using it as one of many research tools.

This chapter does not represent a "how-to" for CAQDAS. The individual instruction manuals and online tutorials for each CAQDAS package are charged with that goal. Nor is this chapter meant to be an extensive review of all of the packages that have been available during the history of CAQDAS. For more extensive reviews of specific software packages, please see the excellent reviews by Weitzman and Miles (1995) and Tesch (1990). Instead, I describe the basic history of CAQDAS; the types of CAQDAS packages currently available, as well as the common and unique elements users will find; strengths and criticisms of CAQDAS; and ways in which it can be used by family therapy researchers.

History of CAQDAS

Qualitative data are non-numeric and unstructured pieces of information, such as interview responses, participant observation, life histories (Mangabiera, 1995), focus group transcripts, or photographs. The first known use of computers to aid in qualitative data analysis was in the 1960s, when content analysis was being automated by a few researchers, though few people took it seriously. Early efforts to use computers were as word processors and as ways to store, organize, and manipulate large amounts of textual data. Weitzman and Miles (1995) noted that in the 1980s, "most qualitative researchers were typing up their handwritten field notes, making photocopies, marking them with pencil or colored pens, cutting them up, sorting them, pasting them on file cards, shuffling cards, and typing their analyses" (p. 4). It was at this same time that the formal development of CAQDAS first occurred (Fielding, 2000), and the refinement of various software packages to aid in qualitative research analysis has continued ever since. CAQDAS took the cutting-and-piling method to a new level, helping to organize, store, and retrieve data in a neater, more secure, and more flexible way. CAQDAS eliminated the need for multiple copies of transcripts, use of index cards, and pasting or piling data-filled scraps of paper all over the office floors and walls. According to Kelle (1997),

> The development of software for textual data management did not start before qualitative researchers who were also ambitious computer users discovered the great possibilities for text storage and retrieval offered by computer technology. This did not take place before the advent of the Personal Computer which led to a shift from the prominent paradigm of computer use from "computers as number crunchers" to "computers as devices for the intelligent management of data," incorporating facilities for the complex and convenient storage and retrieval of text. Consequently, the newly developed software programs for computer-aided textual analysis became tools for data storage and retrieval rather than tools for "data analysis." (p. 2)

Another historical factor leading to more widespread use of CAQDAS was the analysis of focus group data in market and social research (Fielding, 2000). The increased use of multiple-method studies, where an efficient way of analyzing qualitative data is necessary to justify the place of qualitative methods in the overall research design, also helped promote CAQDAS.

The earliest CAQDAS packages were rudimentary and mostly provided simple storage, management, and retrieval of data by use of basic search functions. Words or phrases could be searched if they were previously coded, and multiple codes could be put on various parts of the documents. Since then, dozens of other packages have arrived that are continually built upon to meet the diverse needs of researchers. Some of these are reviewed and highlighted in this chapter.

THE CURRENT GENERATION OF CAQDAS PACKAGES

There are qualitative researchers who are leery of the use of computers in qualitative analysis. According to Tesch (1990), qualitative researchers vary in how they analyze their data, but they agree that the analysis "is the process of making sense of narrative data" (p. 4). The use of computers and CAQDAS takes this one step further by organizing qualitative data, giving the researcher added flexibility in how to handle the stores of data, and neatening the cutting-and-piling process. In the following discussion, I provide a general overview of the features researchers can expect to find when they investigate whether to use CAQDAS for their qualitative research needs and which software packages to consider. The information is based on a number of excellent books and articles on the topic (see the References section), as well as my own experience. This chapter updates some of the previous findings, due to the advances that have been made in the development and use of CAQDAS; it also explores the unique ways in which family therapy researchers are starting to use CAQDAS and may use it in the future.

There are no best CAQDAS packages for use by all social scientists (Fielding, 1995b). Just as for other software packages that are developed for specific audiences or purposes, the individual researcher must investigate those packages that are currently available to determine which is best for a specific project. In addition, most software packages will be regularly upgraded—not only to resolve software "bugs," but also to provide new and improved features for the user. In order to provide increasing convenience, all of the CAQDAS software products highlighted in this chapter are supported by information and documentation for their own websites. Many provide test versions of their software for those shopping around for products, so that they can benefit from some hands-on experience with the software before buying.

The overall trend in the beginning of the 21st century is toward greater support and enthusiasm for the use of CAQDAS in the social sciences. Although some researchers continue to be skeptical and uncertain of the use of computers for qualitative research (Weitzman & Miles, 1995), others believe that the use of computer techniques strengthens and sometimes legitimates the analysis of "soft" or unstructured data (Richards & Richards, 1991). CAQDAS is likely to be in more and more demand because of its ability to handle and analyze more data than ever before. It can help to improve the reliability of data, in that more data potentially provide more evidence, and it can handle more data than human memory alone. In addition, new "third waves" of CAQDAS, such as NVivo and ATLAS.ti, have been developed; these allow researchers to analyze and organize not just text documents, but hyperlinks to audio, visual, digital, and Internet data. Pictures and videoclips can be linked to text, as well as sound bites from interviews. Newspaper clippings can be analyzed, along with other external text documents. What follows is a description of the general types of CAQDAS packages in use today, as well as some of their common and unique features.

General Types of CAQDAS Packages

Many myths abound about what CAQDAS packages can do. The main purpose and utility of CAQDAS is to facilitate analysis. The software cannot analyze data; it can only help the researcher through the process of data management and analysis (Fielding, 1994; Weitzman & Miles, 1995). Expectations for CAQDAS packages are often greater than the reality of what they can do, and researchers sometimes take it for granted that the computer can perform many analysis tasks for them (Richards & Richards, 1991). Many CAQDAS experts caution against this and consider this to be one of the major hazards to the use of CAQDAS for serious research.

There are several different types of CAQDAS, though the types tend to overlap and are not mutually exclusive. In addition, the higher-level software usually includes features of the less sophisticated ones, but not in all cases. For a careful review of many of the most widely used CAQDAS packages as of the mid-1990s, please see the sourcebook on CAQDAS written by Weitzman and Miles (1995).

Although the number of different types and the exact definitions may vary, the core types of CAQDAS include word processors, text retrievers, textbase managers, code-and-retrieve packages, theory builders, and conceptual network builders (Fielding, 1994; Richards & Richards, 1994; Weitzman & Miles, 1995). Word processors, text retrievers, and textbase managers were not necessarily developed explicitly for qualitative researchers (Weitzman & Miles, 1995), but have become important tools for simple organizational and retrieval needs. Text retrievers allow the researcher to recover the data pertaining to each category based on keywords that appear in the data (Fielding, 1994). So, for example, if "social class" is a code, every time the term "socieconomic status" appears in the text, the software will pull it out. The software can also search for that term as a code instead of as just text in the document, so that if the respondent did not use the words "social class," the researcher may assign that phrase as a code to a part of the document that indicates that concept. Examples of this type of CAQDAS package include Metamorph, Orbis, The Text Collector, WordCruncher, ZyINDEX, and Sonar Professional (Fielding, 1994; Weitzman & Miles, 1995). These packages specialize in finding all the instances of words, phrases, character strings, and combinations of these in any number of files. They can also find words that are misspelled, sound alike, are synonymous, or have a given pattern (i.e., any two letters, a hyphen, three pairs of numbers). After the search is complete, these packages can sort or mark the located text into new files or hyperlink memos to the original document at a given point. Some allow for content analysis activities, including counting the occurrences of a given word or string, displaying words as they appear in the data, creating lists of words, and organizing lists of all words and phrases in their contexts.

Textbase managers are a variant of text retrievers and do the more sophisticated jobs of organizing, sorting, and making subsets of text followed by search and retrieval capabilities (Fielding, 1994; Weitzman & Miles, 1995). Some deal with highly structured text organized into "records" or specific cases; some deal with fields or numerical/text information appearing for each case; and some can handle quantitative information. Some of the packages available that fall into the category of textbase managers include AskSam, Folio VIEWS, Tabletop, and winMAX. These differ from the other text retrievers in their specialized capabilities for managing and organizing data, and for creating different sets or subsets of data for further analysis. In addition, they search for and retrieve various combinations of words, phrases, coded segments, codes, memos, or other material (e.g., pictures, audio recordings, or video recordings). Some of these packages also have advanced hypertext, annotation, memoing, and coding functions. Both the basic text retrievers and the more sophisticated textbase managers are fast and can recover the required instances of text almost instantly.

Code-and-retrieve packages specialize in dividing text into segments or chunks, attaching codes to the chunks, and then finding and displaying all the chunks with a given code (or combination of codes). These CAQDAS packages were often developed by qualitative researchers (Weitzman & Miles, 1995), and they manage the kinds of marking-up, cutting, sorting, reorganizing, and collecting tasks that qualitative researchers have traditionally done via the "cut-up-and-put-in-folders" or "file-card" approaches (Bogdan & Biklen, 1982). Most provide the capability to search for character strings (e.g., "*movies") or codes (e.g., "horror movies"). Examples of code-and-retrieve packages include Martin, HyperQual, QUALPRO, Kwalitan, and The Ethnograph. Code-and-retrieve software allows a researcher to recover data that relate to a given code, such as "social class," but in which the words "social class" do not necessarily appear. The researcher uses highlighted blocks or type in symbols like "***" to indicate the beginning and end of the segment that is thought to relate to "social class." The researcher can then retrieve all the data that pertains to that theme, otherwise known as a "single sort." Some packages also permit the retrieval of data where one category is discussed in relation to another (e.g., all instances where there is talk about the relationship between "gender" and "social class"). This is known as a "multiple sort." Code-and-retrieve packages often allow for writing memos in support of the analysis, although not all link these memos directly to the text or code(s) they represent. They may provide some hypertext capability, though it is probably limited in comparison to the textbase packages mentioned above.

The CAQDAS packages known as "theory builders" have mostly been developed by qualitative researchers and contain most of the features of the text retrievers, code-and-retrieve packages, and textbase managers. Although they do not analyze data for the researcher, nor do they actually build theory, they include special features that improve the researcher's ability to make connections between codes, formulate propositions about the data in a conceptually structured manner, and test those propositions to see how they work (Weitzman & Miles, 1995). Some of those include NUD*IST, NVivo, ATLAS.ti, HyperRESEARCH, QCA, and AQUAD. They are more sophisticated in their ability to search for codes and strings, including the ability to search using a predefined set of "attributes." Some of these might include attributes given to a particular interview, such as the gender of the respondent and interviewer, the type of interview, or the interviewee's religious affiliation. Many of these packages support the analysis of nontext data, such as audio, digital, video, or photographic data. The demand for these kinds of capabilities in the past decade have led to improvements in managing and analyzing this kind of data, and it is likely that the more qualitative researchers use these functions, the more they will need these and other higher-level functions to be developed.

Common Features of CAQDAS Packages

In general, there are certain features common to all CAQDAS packages, and others that only a subset can boast. The following list outlines some of the features researchers should expect to see in the most current and widely used CAQDAS packages:

- They support some level of text data. All allow text files to be imported, and many allow data to be entered straight into the software.
- They provide some ability to code text and keep track of those codes.
- They provide the opportunity to include researchers' memos as part of the data (though they differ in how those memos are inserted, how much coding can be done on them, and how searchable they are).
- All packages have some searching capability—from something as rudimentary as the "find" function in a word processor, to something as sophisticated as searching strings of terms and coded segments linked to certain attributes given to each file of data.
- All packages allow for output of the data and analyses, whether in printed form, or electronically through downloads and import–export functions.

Although this seems like a small list of common features, it seems as though the current generation of CAQDAS are quite similar in general, but vary on either how they approach these functions or contain a few specialized functions they call their own. The following section highlights some of the differences among packages one might consider when deciding which to use.

Unique Features of Some CAQDAS Packages

As well as common features among CAQDAS packages, there are some differences that should be understood before a CAQDAS package is selected for qualitative research. Because each product has some unique features, and none are right for all researchers, I recommend a careful exploration of the software websites (see Table 7.2, later in the chapter) to learn more about each package. Some of the ways in which CAQDAS packages are different are listed below.

- Some allow data entry and editing in the software package itself, while others require that the files be saved as a certain file type and read into the package.
- Coding capabilities vary. Whereas packages such as winMAX, MAXqda, NVivo, NUD*IST, and ATLAS.ti allow the researcher to code during the analysis, others may require setting up codes ahead of time and importing them into the system.
- How codes are applied to text varies somewhat. Whereas some packages require that codes apply to entire sentences or full lines of text, others such as NVivo or ATLAS.ti allow any portion of any document to be coded, from one letter of one word to an entire document.
- Packages such as NVivo, ATLAS.ti, and C-I-SAID incorporate the technology of hypertext. Sound bites, video clips, images, and database data can all be linked anywhere in a document, or any document or node can be hyperlinked to any number of other documents or nodes, building webs of ideas. The researcher creates multidimensional data with these features.
- Though all CAQDAS allow for the inclusion of memos and journal entries, some go one step further and permit those to be entered as hypertext in exactly the location of each document that the researcher deems fit. In NVivo and ATLAS.ti, for example, if the researcher has an idea about one part of one interview, he or she can enter a memo in that exact location, and that memo can be coded and searched in exactly the same way as the text and codes in the document itself. In this way, memos are linked theoretically and conceptually as well as operationally (Fielding, 1995a).
- Some packages allow only text data, while others support a wide range of inputs, such as text, electronic documents, quantitative data, pictures, audio sound bites, news clips, websites, and videotapes of interactions (Fielding, 1995b). ATLAS.ti is the only package explicitly stating that it supports the analysis of digital data. Although some packages handle videotaped data, what they actually do is catalog where an item of data is located based on typed input, such as "in drawer three of the filing cabinet" (Fielding, 1995b).
- C-I-SAID is the only package that is sophisticated in its ability to work with audio data. Its primary goal is to help manage and analyze audio data bites as opposed to text alone. It can record audio data, help the researcher analyze segments of this data, and transcribe the audio data. Voice recognition software that is used to accomplish this transcription, however, is still rather simple. Although one person can "train" the software to recognize his or her voice, no software connected to CAQDAS can as yet recognize more than one voice (e.g., an interviewer and interviewee).
- A number of packages such as NVivo, NUD*IST Version 6 (also called N6),

and ATLAS.ti contain a merge function, so that the same projects being worked on by multiple people on separate machines can be brought together to ease the collaborative cross-coding process. These may be the same project on different computers (e.g., one at home, one at the office, and a laptop) or different versions of the same project being coded by separate research team members. Unfortunately, early reviews of this feature are negative, citing the errors and complications often caused by the use of this addition (Plass & Schetsche, 2000).

• Some packages such as NVivo use spreadsheet-like technology to store lists of attributes of documents or codes, or they can import that information from statistics packages or spreadsheets. This allows the researcher not only to organize and describe the data and documents more effectively, but also to search all documents by certain attributes. Attributes might include variables such as gender, age, relationship status, interviewer's name, and so forth. The attributes table is a flexible and helpful way to increase the amount and quality of information stored and searchable in each document.

• NVivo is one of the first CAQDAS packages to support and integrate the benefits of rich text as opposed to plain text format. Now a number of others have followed suit. The researcher can use color, boldface, highlighting, underlining, and various font sizes to make data stand out or to organize information in groups.

• Colored coding stripes in the margin of the text documents in packages such as NVivo and ATLAS.ti allow the researcher to see patterns of coding at a glance. All codes assigned to any part of the document can be seen simultaneously without taking the codes out of the context of the larger document. These colored coding stripes can also be printed with the text, as long as a color printer is used.

• Although most forms of CAQDAS provide some search capabilities, the "third-generation" theory-building CAQDAS packages (such as NVivo and ATLAS.ti) have more advanced search capabilities than earlier forms do. The researcher can search text, coding, and hypertext. The search tool is designed for a range of qualitative questions, from preliminary exploration to rigorous hypothesis testing. Simple searches, Boolean searches, or proximity searches can be chosen and tailored to any research question. Researchers can "scope" the search as accurately as they wish, filtering and selecting just the material needed to be searched. It is easy with NVivo's search function to explore and refine questions, asking the same question of a new scope or a new question of the same material. The results of searches are even coded separately, so that a researcher can build on each search in order to ask future questions.

• Packages such as NVivo and ATLAS.ti can draw and modify visual models of data elements, concepts, relationships, and other thinking. Documents, codes, attributes, and other ideas can be dropped into a model, and they can be linked and layered to represent increasing levels of understanding, complexity, structures, or processes being analyzed and tested. Models can be used at any stage of the project in order to aid visualization and documenting of the research process. In addition, documents, nodes, and attributes are "live" in the model in Nvivo, in that the researcher can click on their icons to inspect their data or properties.

A final difference among various CAQDAS packages is that most of them use different words to describe their functions, even though many of their functions are the same or similar across packages. For example, whereas most packages call the word or phrase assigned to a meaningful text unit a "code," NVivo and NUD*IST call this same feature a "node." In addition, NUD*IST and NVivo call the entire set of documents, codes, and search activities a "project," while ATLAS.ti refers to them as a "hermeneutic unit." Such differences in language can create confusion and frustration for the researcher trying to find and use the most user-friendly package. In addition, it can be difficult for the researcher who has never used a CAQDAS package to understand clearly which ones perform the needed functions if the phraseology used to describe basic functions is stylized and used for marketing or to create a sense of specialization and uniqueness. Ideally, future CAQDAS developers should agree on a standard terminology that reflects the common language of most qualitative researchers. This will help limit the intimidation and frustration that many potential CAQDAS users feel, and it should increase the user-friendliness of the technology.

Table 7.1 is a chart outlining which currently used CAQDAS packages feature various key functions, so that researchers can quickly compare the various packages in use by social scientists today. Included too is a comparison of the prices of various versions and upgrades of these software packages. I based the inclusion of those CAQDAS packages in Table 7.1 on two primary factors. First, if I was able to find literature describing the use of the software package in the past 10 years, I considered it for inclusion. Second, I chose those packages that had active, updated websites to provide support for the software and the user. "Support" means some online documentation to describe the packages as well as information on how to order the software. As a further aid, Table 7.2 provides a list of many of the currently used CAQDAS products and their websites, so that researchers may investigate the promise of each package for their own particular needs.

DISCUSSION

Criticisms of the Use of CAQDAS

The growing literature on CAQDAS reflects both hopes and fears for its use. I agree with Barry (1998), who says, "I think it is quite possible that some of these fears about CAQDAS do originate from those who have not worked with it very much if at all" (p. 3). She describes these as the main fears: (1) that CAQDAS will distance people from their data; (2) that it will lead to the quantitative analysis of qualitative data; (3) that it will lead to increasing homogeneity in methods of data analysis; and (4) that it may "hijack" the analysis (i.e., rigorous analysis procedures will be discarded in favor of simplistic search-and-retrieve functions). Although it is clear that the CAQDAS packages provide a range of interesting and potentially useful features to aid researchers in qualitative data management and analysis, the following is a summary of some of the criticisms found in recently published literature in the social sciences.

• By focusing so closely on the parts or segments of a document, researchers lose the larger contextual view of the data (Seidel, 1998). One response to this criticism is that in order to find those small bits of data, the researchers have to have processed the larger set of information in context. The trick, therefore, is to avoid intensive coding in the early analysis.

• Researchers may be alienated from their research, the data, and the analysis when using CAQDAS. A response to this criticism is that the use of CAQDAS is not what distances people from their research; it is the delegation of many of the functions

TABLE 7.1. Comparison of CAQDAS Products

Features	ATLAS.ti	Ethnograph	NUD*IST (N6)	NVivo	winMAX	MAXqda	AnSWR	C-I-SAID	HyperRESEARCH
Rich text				√		√	√		
Type/edit on screen	√		√ (limited)	√		√	√		
Code in text	√	√	√	√	√	√	√	√	√
Hierarchical codes	√	√	√	√	√	√	√		
In vivo coding	√		√	√		√			
Search	√	√	√	√	√	√		√	√
Hypertext	√			√				√	√
Graphic visualization	√		√ (external)	√					√
Theory building	√		√	√	√				√
Merge	√	√	√	√		√			
Nontext/numeric	√		√	√	√		√	√	√
Automating processes	√		√	√	√				√

Attributes									
Audio record	√	√			√	√		√	√
Transcription					√	√		√	√
Spell-check				√			√	√	√
Memos	√	√	√	√	√	√	√	√	√
PC or Mac	PC or Mac	PC	PC	PC or Mac	PC	PC	PC	PC	PC or Mac
Cost									
Standard/(Upgrade)	$950/($428)	—	$560/($260)	$735/($455)	$368	$745	Free	$99	$370/($145)
Student/(Upgrade)	$190	$200/($118)	$150	—	$113	$190		$99	—
Education/(Upgrade)	$470/($212)	$295/($118)	$340/($160)	$445/($170)	$283	$445		$99	$370/($145)

Note. The data provided in this table are drawn from the information that the software companies have published as marketing materials on the Internet. The accuracy of the information, therefore, is dependent on the quality of the information provided from the distributors on their websites as of February 1, 2004.

TABLE 7.2. Contact Information for Major CAQDAS Packages

Software name	Official website
AnSWR	*http://www.cdc.gov/hiv/software/answr.htm*
ATLAS.ti	*http://www.atlasti.de*
C-I-SAID	*http://www.code-a-text.co.uk*
The Ethnograph	*http://www.qualisresearch.com*
HyperRESEARCH	*http://www.researchware.com/#HyperRESEARCH*
MAXqda	*http://www.scolari.co.uk*
NUD*IST (or N6)	*http://www.qsr.com.au*
NVivo	*http://www.qsr.com.au*
winMAX	*http://www.scolari.co.uk*

once conducted by the key researchers. Researchers who are computer-shy often prefer to delegate some of the CAQDAS tasks to more computer-savvy team members, thereby eliminating themselves from tasks they once felt comfortable doing by hand. No matter how easy the functions of analysis become through the use of CAQDAS, key researchers should be the ones to conduct each step of their analysis in order to remain as close as possible to the data. Although it is an unpopular view, this even means transcribing some if not all of the data, instead of delegating this task to junior members of the research team (or outsourcing all data to professional transcriptionists).

• Formatting and editing documents to enter into the CAQDAS software can be time-consuming.

• Because of ease of use and functionality, some fear that CAQDAS will attract individuals with no formalized social science training, who may not understand how to conduct rigorous qualitative research (Fielding, 2000).

• CAQDAS packages can be cost-prohibitive. Individual licenses are commonly in the $500 range, and updates cost about half that much. Shared licenses are equally expensive.

• Formal training is often expensive, can be difficult to find, and may require significant travel. Many independent contractors now provide training, and although this is well executed and is often tailored to the individual needs of research teams, it is costly. In addition, written literature beyond the user's manual can be difficult to obtain.

Benefits of the Use of CAQDAS

The benefits to using CAQDAS are numerous. Although many of the criticisms listed above have some validity, there are also great hopes for CAQDAS packages. Some of the hopes cited by Barry (1998) are that CAQDAS will (1) automate, speed up, and liven up the coding process; (2) provide more complex ways of seeing the relationships in the data; (3) provide a formal structure for writing and storing memos to assist in the analysis; and (4) help to develop more conceptual and theoretical thinking about the data. The researcher who chooses to use CAQDAS can also expect it to help do the following:

- Accommodate both computer and "by-hand" work interchangeably.
- Provide availability of online support and discussion groups to help resolve computing and analysis problems.
- Observe the coding in the data documents to provide a contextual picture not available with the "cut-up-and-put-in-folder" approach. This helps identify the landscape or topography of the data.
- Print or view on screen the full hierarchical structure of the coding scheme. These codes can also be manipulated, changed, reworked, deleted, and improved in the documents or away from them in their own context.
- Search all data, codes, attributes, and memos in the project (by word, phrase, sentence, section, paragraph, code, etc.). Output from each search parameter is provided in various ways for portability of data and results.
- Provide great flexibility in coding. Codes can be predetermined by the researcher in the form of a "template" of codes, and/or developed during analysis.
- Automate some functions, such as assigning codes to certain questions or each response to a question of interest.
- Maintain a record of all searches and store those in a way that makes accessing them again simple.

Practical Use of CAQDAS

Researchers who have a sizeable number of "soft" data, such as field notes, minutes from meetings, press reports, and interviews, can benefit from the use of computers to help them manage their analysis (Fisher, 1995). I am often asked by researchers whether or not to use CAQDAS, in what cases it would be prudent to use it, and whether it is worth the time and money to use it. In keeping with Weitzman and Miles (1995), I tell them "This depends on what your data are like, how you like to approach them, and how you would like to analyze them."

As I see it, there are two main groups of CAQDAS users, with two sets of issues they should consider when deciding whether or not to use CAQDAS: novices and experienced users. Novice users should ponder the amount of time they have to devote to learning the software, as well as the cost of the software if they do not already own it. More experienced users (and the novices, once they decide on the previous two issues) will need to think of how they plan to analyze and report on the data, as well as the quantity of data they will be managing and analyzing. This section briefly outlines some of the ways researchers might approach these key issues in considering whether or not to use CAQDAS for a given research project.

Sophistication of Analysis

Whether I use CAQDAS or not in a particular piece of research often depends on what my intended results will look like. This takes into account the purpose of the research and the audience. If I am conducting focus groups simply to inform the development of a questionnaire, or to report to a third party on the general sense people have of a phenomenon of interest, I probably will not use CAQDAS. In these cases, my analysis will not require theory building as much as it will inform the wording I might use when developing questionnaire items, so the use of CAQDAS may not be prudent. I have also conducted case studies that require in-depth description of one case. I personally have never used CAQDAS in these cases, because one of the most useful attributes of the software is the capability to do advanced searches across many data sources. On the other hand, if I am conducting research where the aim is to explore meaning making or people's experiences with a particular phenomenon, and where the purpose of my research is to examine a multitude of theories and possible assumptions, I will use CAQDAS.

Number of Data

Besides the type of research analysis, another issue to think about is the number of data you will be managing. I am in no way rigid about the amount of data I think is appropriate for CAQDAS, but I have noticed that the more data I have, the more I lean toward using CAQDAS. If I am analyzing qualitative interviews and hope to write descriptive results, I will use CAQDAS if I have more about 50 pages of text to analyze. It takes considerable time and resources to enter the data, code, perform searches, and print out the results. For fewer than 50 pages of text, it may be more expeditious simply to read and reread the documents and create a simple coding scheme on paper that can be used to develop the analysis and results. On the other hand, for a researcher who is just beginning to learn how to use CAQDAS, a small number of short cases is exactly the type of project with which to start. Learning to use the software is easier if there are fewer documents to manipulate.

Time and Cost to Learn the Software

There are few courses available in the United States to students and professionals in family therapy that focus exclusively on the analysis of qualitative data. Students often get a class period or less on how to analyze qualitative data while the rest of the content focuses on methods. Researchers must rely on themselves and the few resources available to learn to use CAQDAS effectively. As noted earlier, formal training by professionals who are expert in the use of a particular CAQDAS package is expensive and can be cost-prohibitive, especially for students. I was trained twice during my master's program by grant money that was used to support large qualitative studies led by my professors. Any opportunity students and professionals have to attend CAQDAS training or to work on a team where CAQDAS is being used would be helpful as an introduction to the software. Equally as important is continuing to use the software over time to maintain newly learned skills. Nowhere is the phrase "use it or lose it" more applicable than in learning to use CAQDAS.

In addition to the issues listed above, using CAQDAS is practical in contemporary qualitative research for both general use and more specific circumstances. In general, CAQDAS is compatible with many of the qualitative methods in frequent use throughout the social sciences. Some of these methods include grounded theory, phenomenology, ethnography, case studies, focus group research, and discourse analysis. Various data representations, such as aesthetic methods and performance texts, are also good candidates for the use of CAQDAS.

More specifically, CAQDAS is practically applied in the ever-increasing use of multimethod studies, where efficient analyses of data are needed to justify the use of qualitative methods in the overall research design (Fielding, 2000). Internet-based research is another place where CAQDAS is being practically used. CAQDAS is easily applied when data are already in text format and can be seamlessly downloaded into the software, managed, and analyzed (Fielding, 2000). In my own research on how faculty members in marriage and family therapy balance their work and personal lives, I collected preliminary data by use of an Internet-based questionnaire that included both quantitative and qualitative questions (Matheson & Rosen, 2002). I was able to import the respondents' qualitative data directly into NVivo in order to analyze the responses to those questions. This allowed me to skip an entire step of the data preparation process that I would have had to complete first, had I chosen to use a pen-and-pencil questionnaire as opposed to the Internet-based interface. These are only a few of the practical ways in which CAQDAS is being applied in qualitative research, and some of the issues most researchers must face when deciding whether and when to use this software.

Future Directions for CAQDAS in Family Therapy Research

Since the mid-1980s, the number of journal articles, journals, books, and conferences on the topic of CAQDAS has been increasing (Weitzman & Miles, 1995), though there is barely more than anecdotal evidence that family therapy researchers have been using CAQDAS software in their research. Some university researchers in family therapy are beginning to use CAQDAS for analyzing interviews and other qualitative data from their clinical research. Graduate students in family therapy are also developing CAQDAS skills in their academic programs and taking those skills into their future work, thereby expanding the number of people who are using the software and the ways in which it is used.

My review of the published literature between 1990 and 2003 found few articles on the use of CAQDAS in family therapy research. Although we know anecdotally that family therapy researchers are using CAQDAS in their qualitative research, they are either not publishing the results or not being explicit enough in their methods and analysis sections to fully describe the use of this technology. Clearly, this is an area full of possibilities for family therapy researchers to publish their studies and write articles describing the use of this research tool. The future holds great promise for the ways in which this software will continue to be used in our field and other social science disciplines.

Although most (perhaps as many as 80%) of those using CAQDAS are in academia (Fielding & Lee, 1991), software packages are becoming more user-friendly and more accessible to clinicians and researchers outside of academia. Clinicians can begin using this software to organize qualitative data collected in their practices, so that they can easily query the data over time to learn more about trends in their practice. Interviews and qualitative responses on intake or feedback forms can all be entered into CAQDAS to aid in long-term management, storage, and analysis of data. The possibilities are encouraging when we look at how successfully CAQDAS has been used in research to this point and where it may lead those of us who view ourselves as practitioner-researchers.

The future of CAQDAS is exciting and full of promise for those who want to explore various ways of managing qualitative data. Each year more is written on the topic of CAQDAS, and the number of articles that include the results of qualitative research using CAQDAS is increasing. Table 7.3 provides a list of recently published ar-

TABLE 7.3. Examples of Published Social Science Research Using CAQDAS

Crowley, C., Hallam, S., Harre, R., & Lunt, I. (2001). Study support for young people with same-sex attraction: Views and experiences from a pioneering peer support initiative in the north of England. *Educational and Child Psychology*, *18*(1), 108–124.

Lutenbacher, M., Cohen, A., & Mitzel, J. (2003). Do we really help?: Perspectives of abused women. *Public Health Nursing*, *20*(1), 56–64.

Okamoto, S. K. (2003). The function of professional boundaries in the therapeutic relationship between male practitioners and female youth clients. *Child and Adolescent Social Work Journal*, *20*(4), 303–313.

Perrott, K., Morris, E., Martin, J., & Romans, S. (1998). Cognitive coping styles of women sexually abused in childhood: A qualitative study. *Child Abuse and Neglect*, *22*(11), 1135–1149.

Richter, K. P., & Bammer, G. (2000). A hierarchy of strategies heroin-using mothers employ to reduce harm to their children. *Journal of Substance Abuse Treatment*, *19*(4), 403–413.

Rosen, K. H., Matheson, J. L., Stith, S., McCollum, E. E., & Locke, L. D. (2003). Negotiated time-out: A de-escalation tool for couples. *Journal of Marital and Family Therapy*, *29*(3), 291–298.

Spring, B., Rosen, K. H., & Matheson, J. L. (2002). How parents experience a transition to adolescence: A qualitative study. *Journal of Child and Family Studies*, *11*(4), 411–425.

ticles from peer-reviewed journals that illustrate the use of CAQDAS in qualitative research in the social sciences. Each article includes some details about the process of qualitative analysis using the chosen software. These articles are also helpful in illustrating how some researchers write up the results of qualitative data that are managed using CAQDAS.

SUMMARY

Although it is true that there are several valid criticisms of the use of CAQDAS in the social sciences, there are many benefits that draw people into using these software packages for their qualitative research needs. No package is right for all researchers, but developers since the 1980s have created a wide and varied set of new software packages that have consistently been revised to fit the needs of qualitative researchers. Innovations continue to occur in the development of CAQDAS, and the future appears bright for their continued use in all social science disciplines, including family therapy research.

REFERENCES

Barry, C. A. (1998). Choosing qualitative data analysis software: ATLAS.ti and NUD*IST compared. *Sociological Research Online*, *3*(3), 1–20. Retrieved from *http://www.socresonline. org.uk/home.html*

Bogdan, R. C., & Biklen, S. K. (1982). *Qualitative research for education: An introduction to theory and methods*. Boston: Allyn & Bacon.

Fielding, N. G. (1994, September). *CAQDAS networking project: Getting into computer-aided qualitative data analysis* (ESRC Data Archive Bulletin). Retrieved from *http://caqdas. soc.surrey.ac.uk*

Fielding, N. G. (1995a). *CAQDAS networking project: Choosing the right qualitative software package* (ESRC Data Archive Bulletin No. 58). Retrieved from *http://caqdas.soc.surrey. ac.uk*

Fielding, N. G. (1995b). *CAQDAS networking project: Fitting packages to projects* (ESRC Data Archive Bulletin No. 59). Retrieved from http://caqdas.soc.surrey.ac.uk

Fielding, N. G. (2000). The shared fate of two innovations in qualitative methodology: The relationship of qualitative software and secondary analysis of archived qualitative data. *Forum: Qualitative Social Research*, *1*(3). Retrieved from *http://qualitativeresearch.net/fqs/ fqs-eng.htm*

Fielding, N. G., & Lee, R. M. (1991). *Using computers in qualitative research*. Newbury Park, CA: Sage.

Fisher, M. (1995). Desktop tools for the social scientist. In R. M. Lee (Ed.), *Information technology for the social scientist* (pp. 14–32). London: UCL Press.

Kelle, U. (1997). Theory building in qualitative research and computer programs for the management of textual data. *Sociological Research Online*, *2*(2). Retrieved from *http:// www.socresonline.org.uk/socresonline/2/2/1.html*

Mangabeira, W. (1995). Qualitative analysis and microcomputer software: Some reflections on a new trend in sociological research. *Studies in Qualitative Methodology*, *5*, 43–62.

Matheson, J. L., & Rosen, K. H. (2002). *How MFT faculty balance their work and personal lives: A qualitative study*. Unpublished master's thesis, Virginia Polytechnic Institute and State University, Northern Virginia Graduate Center.

Plass, C., & Schetsche, M. (2000). The analysis of heterogeneous text documents with the help of the computer program NUD*IST4. *Forum: Qualitative Social Research*, *1*(3), 1–7. Retrieved from *http:www.qualitative-research.net/fqs-texte/3-00/3-00plassschetsche-e.pdf*

Richards, L., & Richards, T. (1991). Computing in qualitative analysis: A healthy development? *Qualitative Computing*, *1*(2), 234–262.

Richards, T. J., & Richards, L. (1994). Using computers in qualitative research. In N. K. Denzin & Y. S. Lincoln (Eds.), *Handbook of qualitative research* (pp. 445–462). Thousand Oaks, CA: Sage.

Seidel, J. (1998). Qualitative data analysis. *Qualis Research*. Retrieved from *http://www. qualisresearch.com*

Tesch, R. (1990). *Qualitative research: Analysis types and software tools*. New York: Falmer Press.

Weitzman, E. A., & Miles, M. B. (1995). *Computer programs for qualitative data analysis: A software sourcebook*. Thousand Oaks, CA: Sage.

Yuen, H.-K., & Richards, T. J. (1994). Knowledge representation for grounded theory construction in qualitative data analysis. *Journal of Mathematical Sociology*, *19*(4), 279–298.

CHAPTER 8

Bridging Research

USING ETHNOGRAPHY TO INFORM CLINICAL PRACTICE

CAROLYN Y. TUBBS
LINDA M. BURTON

BACKGROUND

In a recent public service announcement, *The Enforcer*, aired on national television, a 30-something African American mother uses a hard glare and firm tone to keep her teenage son in check. Her son laments to a friend on the telephone, "I don't know why she is tripping. It was only weed. I only tried it once." She then appears in his bedroom door and states, "You are grounded! That means no phone!" Her demeanor throughout the short vignette conveys that she means what she says, and she says what she means: "No weed!" A disembodied announcer's voice states, "She doesn't love being tough. She's tough because she loves." The exasperated teen grimaces each time she reminds him with the "No weed!" mantra that he is incorrectly engaging in privileges (e.g., playing video games) that have been removed. "She is the Enforcer, and she knows that she can make a difference," the announcer asserts. Her vigilance and comments indicate that she is serious about enforcing the parameters of his grounding. Unbeknownst to the mother, the fruit of her determined parenting presence manifests itself when her son, standing near bleachers in an empty high school stadium with peers, flatly refuses an offer of a marijuana cigarette while citing his grounding as the reason. His familiar grimace and abrupt refusal highlight the lesson he has learned from his dealings with *the Enforcer*. The announcer's voice summarizes the primary message of the vignette. "The Enforcer: She's more than a hero—she's a good mom. You are more powerful than you know" (Office of National Drug Control Policy, 2003a).

The seeds of this message were sowed in a survey conducted by the Partnership Attitude Tracking Study (Office of National Drug Control Policy, 2003b). The results of the study indicated that non-substance-abusing adolescents who listened to their parents' antidrug messages were less likely to engage in substance use than those who did not listen. The results also indicated that mothers were more likely than fathers to deliver antidrug messages. Just as the antidrug coalition transformed this finding into a

136

compelling media message, so have grant-funding agencies prioritized moving research findings from the realm of the academy to the real world (National Institute of Mental Health [NIMH], 1999, 2002). This practice, defined as "translation research," identifies evidence-based practices in basic and applied research and attempts to maximize their benefits in nonresearch settings in as little time as possible (NIMH, 2002).

Using the fruits of research to benefit the lives of laypersons is not new. Evidence from several venues, including telecommunications and law enforcement, indicates that innovations in these fields were the results of technological advances originating in military, aerospace, and psychological research (Blau, 2003; Childers & Delany, 1994; Gudjonsson & Haward, 1998; McLaughlin, 1997; National Aeronautics and Space Administration, n.d.; Ubelaker, 2000). Similarly, new pharmacological treatments regularly result from "off-label" research with drugs approved for other uses (Center for Rural Health, 2001; Serradell & Patwell, 1991; U.S. Pharmacopeial Convention, 2003).

In the social sciences, findings from survey research have been the most likely candidates for translation research, because they emphasize generalizability and replicability (Frank et al., 2002). However, we believe that qualitative research— specifically, ethnographic research—also has value in bridging research and practice, because the observations about behavior that ethnography produces reveal more detail about the nuances and mechanisms of the phenomenon of interest.

This chapter discusses a specific type of translation research, one that utilizes basic ethnography to inform clinical research and practice. First, we define translation research and review ethnography as a research method. We then discuss the strategy that we have utilized for employing ethnography; we draw on a multisite ethnographic study (*Welfare, Children, and Families: A Three-City Study*) for examples to illustrate our points. Specifically, we examine parenting issues in low-income, urban families, with a particular focus on families of color. Our intent is to illustrate ethnography's ability to provide cultural insights that can inform an intervention (for a specific population) prior to its being tested.

Translation Research

According to Frank and colleagues (2002), translation research spans a continuum from "basic science to development of new treatments, from treatment development to clinical trials, and from clinical trials to practice. The goal of translation research is to merge and create a network of knowledge: from basic science, to clinical trials, to patient care" (p. 633). Creating new interventions or treatments from existing treatments or knowledge meets this goal. Findings from basic research on change processes in both nonclinical and clinical populations form the pool of existing knowledge from which applied researchers draw. "Evidence-based" practices or "best" practices that have emerged from new or modified treatments based on basic research have been tested successfully in applied research. The final phase of translation research occurs when evidence-based practices are used in clinical trials to ascertain their effectiveness in various populations and settings (Frank et al., 2002).

Donoghue and Hyla (2001) suggest that generative knowledge produced by empirical research has only a limited impact on the decision-making behavior of researchers and funders. This disconnection between research and practice results in "[a] disparity between treatments selected and carried out in clinical trials and those selected and carried out in 'real world' (i.e., primary care and specialty practice) settings [and] has led to considerable tension between clinical researchers and practitioners and between clinical trials or 'efficacy' and 'effectiveness' researchers" (Frank et al., 2002, p. 632). Translation research is one effort to address this disparity. Its primary goal is to design methods that will "translate" basic research from the controlled, artificial, and ideal conditions of the laboratory to the variegated, unpredictable, and uncontrolled settings of life.

Educational and medical researchers lead in translating best practices into classroom and community-oriented interventions based on best practices, while mental health research lags behind (Cabana, Rushton, & Rush, 2002; Reddy, Taylor, & Sifunda, 2002). In education, translation research has focused on literacy instructional strategies (O'Boyle & Gill, 1998). In medicine, evidence-based practices for chronic illnesses, such as diabetes and asthma, have been parlayed into primary and secondary forms of intervention (Satariano & McAuley, 2003). "Primary" intervention focuses on disease prevention, whereas "secondary" intervention centers on the interruption or resolution of a disease (Edelson, 2000; Mrazek & Haggerty, 1994). Although translation research for physical health concerns continue to grow, an NIMH report concluded that translation research for mental health problems is lacking: "All too often, clinical practices and service system innovations that are validated by research are not fully adopted in treatment settings and service systems for individuals with mental illness" (cited in Frank et al., 2002, p. 631).

What is the cost of not engaging in translation research? As noted earlier, translation research entails not only moving basic and applied research into nonresearch settings, but also shaping interventions so that they are effective, in terms of problem resolution and cost, in various settings and with different subpopulations (Frank et al., 2002). When this does not occur, the intrinsic value of research is diminished, its service component is lost, and clients' lives are not improved. As Brosseau (2003) states, "Research shows us what works, and when that research is not applied, or translated, to clinical practice, it is wasted."

The model of translation research articulated by Frank and colleagues (2002) outlines four successive phases that must be completed in order to accomplish translation: (1) Basic research occurs; (2) its findings are operationalized into specific interventions; (3) clinical trials are conducted to determine effectiveness; and finally (4) emergent best practices (or interventions) are incorporated into the practice setting (see Figure 8.1). The model identifies a clear progression from explaining a phenomenon to finding ways to effectively address the problematic aspect of the phenomenon in as many settings and populations as possible.

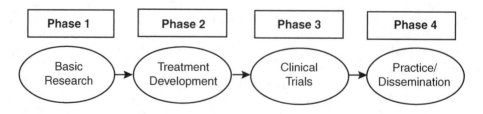

FIGURE 8.1. Translation research model. Data from Frank et al. (2002).

Bridging Ethnography and Family Therapy

Ethnography, as a scientific method, focuses on the "inferential keys to culture"—that is, the social and verbal interactions, habits, and meanings generated by a particular group (Miles & Huberman, 1994). In seeking to find patterns of regularity in the complexity of human interactions, ethnography moves from descriptive reporting to cultural interpretation (Van Maanen, 1995). It accomplishes this goal through analysis of detailed descriptions of contexts, events, behaviors, and conversations. Wolcott (1995) defines "ethnography" as a commitment "to looking at, and attempting to make sense of human social behavior in terms of cultural patterning . . . to understand how culture influences specific aspects of some human group in particular" (pp. 83–84). As the study of symbols and meanings, ethnography is inherently holistic, naturalistic, and nonreductionistic.

Few studies or practices have linked findings from existent ethnographic research and family therapy, when in fact there is a natural marriage between the two. The hegemonic influence of systems theory in family social science makes the study of the family, and family therapy by extension, perfect candidates for ethnography. Family therapy researchers have long been interested in the antecedents and consequences of interactional sequencing (i.e., the spatial and temporal aspects of relationships and critical events, and the rules that govern interactions), and in the meanings generated and guiding the interactional process. These cultural meanings underscore systems theory's germaneness to ethnographic methodology.

There are important issues to consider in the bridging process. The long-term and naturalistically based type of contact inherent to traditional ethnography has not been the norm in mental health research generally, and marriage and family therapy research specifically. It is difficult to use ethnographic methodology in family therapy research, for four reasons. First, clinical researchers are helpers before they are researchers; therefore, they are bound by the implicit and explicit expectations of mental health practice. The moral, ethical, and legal mandates governing their behavior are more stringent (and punitive) than those governing the behavior of nonclinical, sociological ethnographers (Schein, 1987). Hence the transition from the role of helper to that of researcher is not easily accomplished. A second issue is that family therapy occurs almost exclusively in settings that are artificial for a family. Professional helping, for the most part, distinguishes itself from informal forms of helping by contextualizing itself outside the family's naturalistic setting (i.e., the home). Therefore, naturalistic forms of inquiry about the family are often left to nonclinical family scholars. Third, the economic reality of mental health settings renders it difficult, if not impossible, for mental health researchers to work and conduct participant observation research in the same setting, especially with the recent emphasis on managed care. Finally, funders and research review boards express concerns about ethical issues involving permeable boundaries and relationship duality, both of which are inherent to ethnographic research. Again, the preeminence of the helper role leaves duty-to-warn and do-no-harm mandates intact even while research is being conducted. Hence, for these reasons, family therapy researchers are reluctant to attempt the more traditional forms of ethnographic research (i.e., long-term immersion with interview *and* participant observation). Modified forms of ethnography, such as ethnoscience, which utilize formalized interviews as ethnographic data and postulate that language (even more than behavior) provides the raw data from which culture can be interpreted, are more appropriately suited to these constraints (Schwandt, 1994; Sells, Smith, Coe, Yoshioka, & Robbins, 1994).

Why Use Ethnographic Data to Inform Clinical Practices?

Schein (1987), however, believes that the gaps between the traditional ethnographer and the clinical researcher are less difficult to bridge, and that the two roles manifest many parallels. In an excellent monograph, *The Clinical Perspective in Fieldwork*, he articulates the dialectic between the roles of clinician and ethnographer for the clinical ethnographer. He asserts that both the clinician and the ethnographer have "research" agendas attendant to their work. If basic research seeks to explain a phenomenon, applied research generates potential solutions to human and social problems, and action research engages solution seekers in the problem-solving process, then the clinician inherently enters the helping situation with an action research orientation (Patton, 2001). That is, the clinician's primary goal is to engage solution seekers (clients) in the process of solving their "problems." On the other hand, the ethnographer engages the cultural space, artifacts, and participants in the process of understanding the culture.

We agree with Schein that these two roles complement each other in the translation research process, because, as indicated earlier, basic research informs applied research as the clinical ethnographer moves from one role to the other. In the type of translation research we undertook, which we call "bridging research," we took findings from basic research (traditional ethnography) to begin the process of informing the development and dissemination of the applied research (clinical interventions) (see Figure 8.1).

In Figure 8.2, we outline our model, which elaborates on the translation process. In our model, Phase 1 (basic research) has been renamed "informing research," and we include applied research as a potential source of informing research. Interventions from applied research that need to be refined reenter the translation model as informing research if they are ineffective in Phase 3 (see Figure 8.1). Phase 2 of the translation research model—treatment development—has remained the same. The bridging research described in the remainder of this chapter focused on the intervening step between informing research and treatment development, and this is the component we have added. In this model, bridging research consists of a comparative analysis, the goal of which is to tighten the ensuing treatments prior to pilot testing. (Note: Although in our later discussion we refer to phases of the bridging process, the reader should not confuse these "phases"with those presented in the translation research model in Figure 8.1. In an effort to clarify the distinction, we use arabic numbers [i.e., 1, 2, 3] in Figure 8.1 and below to connote the "phases" described in Frank et al., and roman numerals [i.e., I, II, III] to identify the "phases" that we used in our bridging research process.)

The unique nature of our particular endeavor stemmed from our use of research that embraced the complexity of the context in which the research was conducted (i.e., its unpredictability, uncontrollability, and variegatedness), and thereby provided nuanced insight into the perspectives of the target population on the phenomenon of interest. The study (described later in this chapter) examined ethnographic field notes and qualitative interviews to understand parenting practices in a sample of low-income, urban-dwelling mothers. Ethnographic data provided both "emic" and "etic" perspectives simultaneously, hence capturing a rich, panoramic, and longitudinal view of the target population. Informal and formal interviews provided information from

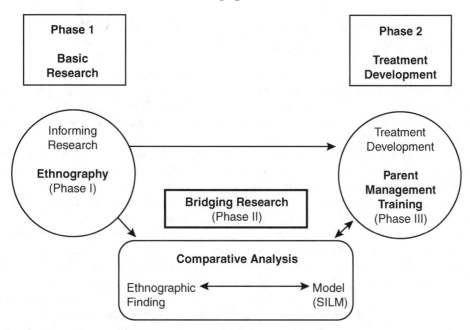

FIGURE 8.2. Bridging process within the translation process.

those who have been shaped by and are shaping the culture (the emic view), while participant observation information revealed an outsider's perspective (the etic view).

The type of bridging research we utilized drew on ethnographic data to enrich understandings of clinical issues and to expedite the translation process. The example we provide here focused on parenting practices in low-income families. Bridging research occurred between Phase 1 and Phase 2 of the translation research model (Figure 8.1). First, we analyzed ethnographic data to understand parenting practices in a population whose parenting is highly vulnerable to its residential, ethnic, and economic locations in the social strata. The goal of the analysis was to identify the cultural rules that shaped and defined parenting in the population, as well as the way these rules were influenced by broader social forces. The dynamic nature of the ethnographic data permitted a panoramic view of parenting dimensions (as opposed to a snapshot), in terms of both the evolution of parenting over time and the multiple impacts of individual parenting behaviors on various members of the family (Rosier, 2000). Second, we compared these findings with the constructs in a behaviorally based model of parenting that incorporated evidence-based practices in its intervention component. The results of the comparative analysis were then examined in order to propose changes to the model's intervention component, which in turn would allow for both clinical research of the model's effectiveness in the target population and for effective dissemination. These two steps constituted the bridging research process. Finally, we made the transition to Phase 3 of the translation research model by preparing a document that informed modification of the intervention model and its existent interventions, in order to enhance service delivery and accessibility.

In the next section, we detail the constituent components that were utilized in our bridging research. Afterward, we describe how the components interfaced in the bridging process.

BRIDGING RESEARCH: THE CONSTITUENT COMPONENTS

Social Interaction Learning Model

The "social interaction learning model" (SILM) specifies risk contexts (e.g., divorce and poverty) as disruptors of parenting practices, and disrupted parenting practices as proximal mechanisms for child adjustment (Forgatch & DeGarmo, 2002; Patterson, 1986, 1997). Its intervention component, "parent management training" (PMT), has been found to be effective in teaching parents, across the income spectrum, skills that decrease negative child behavior (Forgatch & DeGarmo, 2002). The SILM posits that there are two types of parenting practices. First, there are coercive parenting practices in which parents fail to discipline children effectively, resulting in increased negative exchanges between parents and their children (Patterson, Reid, & Dishion, 1992; Snyder & Huntley, 1990). As children become more unresponsive, they become more difficult to discipline, and parents tend to use more aversive disciplinary tactics (Patterson, 1986). In contrast, effective parenting practices emphasize social processes involving mutual expectations, shared goals, and coregulation of behavior (Kuczynski & Hilderbrandt, 1997; Kuczynski, Marshall, & Schell, 1997; Maccoby & Martin, 1983). Parental responsiveness to children's bids for attention, and children's readiness to comply, positively influence the overall harmony of the relationship (Parpal & Maccoby, 1985; Shaw, Keenan, & Vondra, 1994). These two types of parenting practices—effective parenting practices and coercive parenting practices—and their constructs are important to understanding the SILM and originate from extensive outcome research on it (Forgatch & DeGarmo, 1999, 2002; Forgatch & Martinez, 1999).

Coercive Parenting Practices

Three negative interactional patterns, which contribute to the development and maintenance of oppositional child behavior, are particularly relevant to the SILM. "Negative reciprocity" is a series of negative practices exchanged between the parent and the child (although not all are of the same degree or intensity) until a major unfavorable reaction or incident occurs. The second negative interactional pattern is "escalation" (e.g., from shouting to humiliation, hitting, or another intense behavior). Escalation involves aversive exchanges between parent and child that increase in intensity. Finally, "negative reinforcement"—that is, or rewarding aversive behaviors used to escape or avoid undesirable situations, such as letting a child out of time out even though the time is not up—is the third coercive parenting practice.

The SILM draws from the ecological and family systems theoretical traditions and has been refined with data from European American families across economically diverse groups (Forgatch & DeGarmo, 2002). Its clinical application, PMT, has been tested with low-income populations; however, the effectiveness of PMT has not been clinically researched in low-income, urban populations of color. Its clinical use as both a prevention and an intervention program provided us with a natural framework from which to begin the process of translating findings from ethnographic research.

Effective Parenting Practices

Five behaviors constitute effective practices that contribute to healthy child adjustment and parent–child interaction. First, "skill encouragement" entails the ways in which parents promote children's' competencies by using positive reinforcement contingent on prosocial behavior. Second, "discipline" (also called "limit setting") involves the establishment of appropriate rules with age- and incident-appropriate sanctions. "Monitoring" (also called "supervision") consists of the ways parents keep track of their children's whereabouts and activities. Fourth, "problem solving" incorporates skills that facilitate resolution of disagreements, negotiation of rules, and the establishment of agreements about positive consequences for following the rules (e.g., allowance, extra privileges) and sanctions for violating the rules (e.g., work chores, privilege removal). Finally, "positive involvement" includes the many ways parents provide youngsters with loving attention.

Ethnographic Data

Three-City Study

The data on mothers' parenting practices featured in this chapter came from the ethnographic component of a larger research project, Welfare, Children, and Families: A Three-City Study. The study was carried out over a period of 4 years in Boston, Chicago, and San Antonio. The purpose of the project was to monitor the consequences of welfare reform for the well-being of children and families. The study comprised three interrelated components: (1) a longitudinal in-person survey of approximately 2,400 families with children ages 0–4 and 10–14 in low-income neighborhoods, about 40% of whom were receiving cash welfare payments when they were first interviewed in 1999; (2) an embedded developmental study of a subsample of about 630 children ages 2–4 in 1999 and their caregivers; and (3) an ethnographic study of 256 families, residing in the same neighborhoods as the survey families and recruited according to the same family income criteria, who were followed intensively until the project ended in August 2003. In all three components and in all three cities, African American, Hispanic, and non-Hispanic European American families were represented. A detailed description of the Three-City Study and a series of reports are available at *http:// www.jhu.edu/~welfare*.

Ethnographic Component

Families were recruited into the ethnographic component of the project at formal child care settings (e.g., Head Start centers, WIC, neighborhood community centers, local welfare offices, churches, and other public assistance agencies) between June 1999 and December 2000. Of the 256 families participating in the ethnography, 44 were recruited specifically because they had a child ages 0–8 years with a moderate or severe disability.

An ethnographic approach allowed for a longitudinal exploration of the day-to-day activities and experiences of specific group over time, through close observation and in-depth interviewing. It resulted in holistic insight into the complexities of respondents' daily lives, as well as their cognitions and behaviors. The goals of the ethnography were to learn how the decisions of low-income families were influenced by the welfare system, and to describe the interaction of welfare policies, family behaviors, and child development (Winston et al., 1999).

All families participating in the ethnography had household incomes not exceeding 200% of the federal poverty line (U.S. Dept. of Health and Human Services,

2002). The majority of the participants (42%) were of Hispanic ethnicity (e.g., Puerto Ricans, Mexican Americans, and Central Americans). Of the remaining participants, 38% were African Americans and 20% were non-Hispanic European Americans. Over half of the mothers were age 29 or younger, and a majority of the respondents had a high school diploma or a general equivalency diploma (GED), or attended trade school or college. Forty-nine percent of the families were receiving welfare (Temporary Assistance for Needy Families, or TANF) when they entered the study; one-third of these, in compliance with welfare regulations, were also working. Fifty-one percent of the sample was not receiving welfare (TANF) benefits, and the primary earners in the household were either working low-wage jobs or unemployed. The 256 primary caregivers identified a total of 685 children in their households. Fifty-three percent of the children were age 4 or younger; 47% of the children were elementary school age or adolescents. Twenty-five percent of the primary caregivers were responsible for one child, and 27%, 25%, and 23% for two, three, and four or more children, respectively. Fifty-six percent of primary caregivers were not married and did not have partners (e.g., boyfriends) living with them; another 17% were not married but were cohabiting with partners; 17% were married and living with their spouses; and 10% were married or separated and their spouses were not living in the home.

To gather ethnographic data on families, we employed a method of "structured discovery" in which in-depth interviews and observations focused on specific topics, but allowed flexibility to capture unexpected findings and relationships (Burton et al., 2001; Winston et al., 1999). Topics addressed in these interviews included health and health access experiences with TANF and other public assistance programs; education and work experiences and future plans; family economics; child development, parenting, intimate relationships; support networks; family routines; and home and neighborhood environments. In addition to these interviews, ethnographers engaged in participant observation with each family. This often involved accompanying a mother and her children to the welfare office, doctor, hospital, clinic, or workplace, and taking note of the interactions and contexts of those places.

Since an important goal of the ethnographic component was to describe the interaction of welfare policies, family behaviors, and child development, mothers with preschool children (whether partnered or not), rather than couples or fathers with preschool children, were chosen as the focal population for the study. This decision was made for several reasons. First, single mothers with children are the family constellation most likely to qualify for government cash assistance (Cherlin, 1995; Peterson, Song, & Jones-DeWeever, 2002). Therefore, they as a group would be most greatly affected by the work or educational requirements that were linked to assistance in the welfare reform legislation. Second, we assumed that decisions to work (or not to work) as part of compliance with welfare requirements would be complicated by the child care and developmental needs of children who were too young either to care for themselves or to attend some form of educational program. The ways in which mothers negotiated or resolved these issues would provide important information on the impact of welfare reform. Third, mothers overwhelmingly take on the responsibility and provide the majority of care for children, and the issues affecting their lives would invariably affect the lives of their children. Therefore, examining and describing interactions between the mothers in this study and the children to whom they provided the most care (i.e., preschool children) would provide valuable insight into potential impacts of welfare reform on child development. Even though families with resident fathers were not specifically recruited for the study, it is important to note that data were collected on all males relevant to the lives of the focal mothers and children.

Ethnographers met with each family once or twice each month, on average, for 12–18 months. In the follow-up stage, families were interviewed every 6 months to identify any changes in their lives, including welfare, work, health, and family status. Each interview was audiotape-recorded, and in addition, a written record for each interview was produced. These records took at least one (and sometimes more) of the following three formats: field notes, complete transcription, and targeted transcription (in which all information was recovered, and narrative accounts of significant events were transcribed word for word). The documents were then coded for entry into a qualitative data management (QDM) software application and summarized into a case profile for each family. The QDM program and case profiles enabled counts across the entire sample of ethnographic families, as well as detailed analyses of individual cases.

In the case of each family, a team of qualitative data analysts—using profiles developed on each family and the QDM software—assessed each family's typical-day status and the parenting histories.

Ethnographic Data for Parenting Analysis

As the first step in the analysis used for bridging research, we only examined data from the Chicago-based ethnographic component of the Three-City Study. The exploratory nature of the analysis, as well as the writers' actual field work at the site, were the primary rationales for using a subsample of the data. Moreover, the data set is voluminous, with over 45,000 pages of field notes. Therefore, we chose to engage in the bridging process in an incremental fashion (i.e., one city at a time).

Participants

Completed parenting interviews were available for 22 respondents at the time of the analysis (May 2002). Eight mothers (36%) in the sample were of Hispanic ethnicity, 10 (46%) were African American mothers, and four (18%) were non-Hispanic European American mothers—mirroring the diversity of Chicago's primary ethnic communities. Half of the sample was age 30 or younger (mean age = 31), and 59% of the mothers had received a high school diploma, a GED, or some form of postsecondary education. Thirty-six percent of mothers were not married and did not have partners (e.g., boyfriends) living with them; another 14% were not married but were cohabiting with partners; 41% were married and living with their spouses; and 9% were married or separated with the spouses not living in the home.

Data Collection

Multiple forms of the data—transcripts and field notes of the parenting interviews, family profiles, and general field notes—were analyzed in order to gain insight into the parenting practices of low-income mothers. However, the parenting interview data were foundational to our analysis of parenting practices and became the primary inclusion criteria. In this interview, mothers described their parenting perspectives and activities in reference to discipline, rewards, expectations, play, aspirations, safety, ethnicity, and child activity (Jarrett & Tubbs, 1999). Interviews were semistructured and took an average of 1 hour to complete.

BRIDGING RESEARCH: THE TRANSLATION PROCESS

In this section, we identify how findings from the ethnographic data and the SILM were used. Again, we use the term "bridging research" to describe the comparative analysis of findings from basic research with an applied model for the purpose of informing clinical interventions.

In the process of conducting our bridging research, we progressed through three phases, each building on the work of the prior phase. (As noted earlier in the chapter, we use roman numerals to refer to these phases, as opposed to arabic numerals for the phases of Frank et al.'s translation research model.) Phase I focused on an analysis of the informing research (i.e., the ethnographic data) in order to begin to understand the phenomenon of interest—parenting practices. Then Phase II compared the ethnographic findings with the constructs defining the two types of parenting practices outlined in the SILM. Finally, the third phase, Phase III, began the process of detailing strategies for incorporating the results of Phase II into creation or modification of interventions (see Figure 8.2). Figure 8.3 incorporates bridging research into the translation research model outlined by Frank and colleagues (2002).

Phase I. Informing Research: Parental Monitoring Analysis

The analysis in the first phase was undertaken as an initial effort toward utilizing ethnographic findings to inform parenting interventions for use with low-income, urban families of color (Tubbs, 2002a).

Methods

The primary research question guiding the analysis was "What are the parenting practices of low-income mothers?" Assumptions from systems theory and symbolic interaction theory provided the "sensitizing" concepts that guided the data analysis (Klein & White, 2002; Miles & Huberman, 1994). Relational and interactional interconnectedness and the holistic nature of systems were the systems theory assumptions employed; the symbolic nature of behavior and language, as well as the inherently interpretive nature of human cognition, were the assumptions based on symbolic interaction theory.

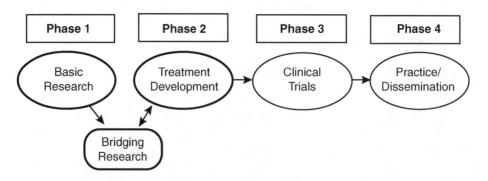

FIGURE 8.3. Translation research with bridging process. Data from Frank et al. (2002).

Content analysis of the data followed a generalized qualitative data analysis as outlined by Miles and Huberman (1994). Transcripts of interviews and field notes were the raw data that were coded, and coding progressed from descriptive coding to interpretive analyses (Patton, 2001). Although many parenting issues were identified (preventing behavioral problems, diminishing the effects of racism, teaching respect for others, promoting child physical health and emotional well-being, and disciplining children), ensuring children's physical safety was the most prevalent theme to emerge from the interviews (Tubbs, 2002a, 2002b).

Findings

Neighborhood safety was the concern most frequently cited by low-income, urban mothers, whether they were parenting preschool children or older, school-age children (ages 6–18). In addition, mothers reported that parenting behaviors to promote safety for children incorporated education and active intervention. In terms of intervention, mothers' attempts at direct intervention seemed to be more evident when children were more proximal in time and space, whereas attempts to intervene indirectly seemed to be more evident when children were more distal in time and space, and based on age. Direct interventions fell into two categories: checking on children and finding ways to contain children for their own safety. Indirect interventions were primarily verbal in nature and centered on various forms of safety advice transmitted from mother to child.

Phase II. Bridging Process: Comparative Analysis

A comparative analysis of the ethnographic findings and the SILM constituted Phase II. During this phase, salient themes from Phase I were compared to the constructs within the two types of parenting practices identified in the SILM. Since safety was the most prominent theme in the ethnographic data, it became the focal point of the comparative analysis.

When the SILM lens was used to view the safety construct and its constituent parts, there was a great deal of similarity between it and the SILM concept of monitoring. As we have noted earlier, monitoring refers to the ways parents keep track of their children's whereabouts and activities. Mothers' safety-enhancing behaviors (i.e., checking on and containing children) interfaced well with this construct. We interpreted mothers' emphasis on transmitting safety advice as an abstracted form of monitoring that incorporated temporal and spatial components.

However, there were aspects of the safety construct not articulated by the SILM, and therefore posing a challenge to outlining these unique aspects of safety.

Phase III. Treatment Development: Translation Process

Research on the SILM has found that monitoring is a positive parenting practice. The ethnographic data from the Three-City Study confirmed that most mothers in low-income neighborhoods engaged in this practice. However, mothers' reports indicated that their primary monitoring concerns were *not* born out of children's normative developmental issues, but rather out of distress about children's level of exposure to violence and violent victimization (Bureau of Justice Statistics, 2003; Finkelhor &

Ormrod, 2000). When the SILM template was overlaid on the ethnographic data, the unique area of difference was a form of monitoring that could be appropriately identified as "hypervigilance." Hypervigilance was manifested in mothers' pervasive concern with the safety of children's environments, as well as the potential violent intent of those who populated or traversed those environments—whether friend or foe, adult or child, at home or in the neighborhood. In most contexts, "hypervigilance" is understood as a pejorative term. However, in the context of adults' ensuring the safety of children in areas with high rates of violence, hypervigilance can be understood as an appropriate, and potentially necessary, parenting and personal strategy (Burton, 1991).

The translation of the ethnographic data to the realm of applied research included not only identifying the areas of uniqueness between the two, such as the notion of hypervigilance, but also determining how unique areas from the ethnography could inform the SILM and applied research using PMT, the psychoeducational intervention based on the SILM. (On the other side of the bridging research equation, though unaddressed in this chapter, the SILM's validity as an explanatory framework for parenting dimensions in low-income, urban families of color increased. Thereby it became an important model informing the interpretation of parenting in the Three-City Study data, as well as an important template for bridging the findings from these data to other quantitative and qualitative basic research. This process, called "iteration," increased the trustworthiness of the analysis [Strauss & Corbin, 1998].)

Using the hypervigilance finding as an example, we proposed that the SILM be modified in the following ways to increase its sensitivity to and accessibility by low-income, urban populations of color:

1. Although all the constructs in the two types of parenting practices are important, some may be more salient to certain populations because of their social location (i.e., ethnicity, income status, or geographical location). Therefore, in low-income, urban populations of color, additional emphasis should be given to the issue of monitoring.

2. Monitoring in high-crime areas should become part of the research on the SILM and of the curriculum in the PMT program. The information may or may not modify either as it is currently conceived. Nonetheless, both the model and the training can indicate that this unique aspect of parenting has been considered.

3. The salience of monitoring for safety is a noteworthy finding and should be used to explore how other parenting practices are ordered or viewed by the target population in terms of their ability to enhance or detract from safety. Findings on the relationship between these practices should be incorporated into the evaluation component of program delivery.

4. The PMT program should explore adding specific information on "safety proofing" the home, activities in the home, play areas outside the home, and family outings in public, in order to address mothers' concerns about safety. Whereas the intent of childproofing is to decrease children's access to dangerous situations, the intent of safetyproofing is to prevent dangerous activities from impinging on children's lives.

5. In addition, the PMT program should explore adding tip sheets on helpful advice that parents can rehearse with children to increase child safety when parents are not present.

6. Marketing of the PMT curriculum to the target population should emphasize

the safety component of the program as an incentive to enroll in and complete the program.

Iterative Process

The NIMH (Frank et al., 2002) workgroup asserts that the translation process should be an iterative process "that has a series of loops whereby at one point practice may stimulate the ideas for treatment development and at another time be the recipient of the change." Although we have outlined the process of bridging research in a linear fashion, we would be remiss if we left the reader with this impression of a lockstep agenda. Iteration is inherent in the process of bridging research, because of the bidirectional flow of information between informing research (whether basic or applied) and the intervention in order to ensure the emergence of best practices (see Figure 8.2). "Theoretical sampling," a term used in grounded theory approaches to data analysis to describe the process of finding and interpreting examples that both confirm and disconfirm an initial finding (in order to better understand the finding's nature and its relationship to other findings), is important to this process (Glaser, 1998; Glaser & Strauss, 1967; Strauss & Corbin, 1998).

DISCUSSION

Strengths and Limitations of Bridging Research

Strengths

The overarching strength of bridging research is its ability to bolster the link between research and practice, and to expedite movement of information from findings to concrete interventions. For our work, being rooted in ethnographic methodology reinforced this strength. As the basis for the bridging research described in this chapter, ethnographic data enhanced the translation process in four important ways. First, ethnography provided context-rich data that could be used to confirm or challenge existing clinical theory or models. Second, it moved our hunches about the data from the realm of anecdotes to the realm of "structured inquiries," or what Newman and Benz (1998) label "typicalities." Third, ethnography included observations in "real time" and in naturalistic contexts to accompany the narratives of participants. Finally, ethnography permitted us to assess whether a Type III error was being committed in the treatment development process. A Type III error is committed when a researcher begins his or her work asking the wrong question altogether (Newman & Benz, 1998).

Limitations

The dialectic of ethnography's characteristics would not be complete unless we also examined its limitations for the family therapy researcher. As the reader may already suspect, collecting interview, archival, and participant observation data (if applicable), transcribing interviews, and data analysis are extremely time-intensive processes (Miles & Huberman, 1994; Patton, 2001). Unless the clinical ethnographer employs strategies to reduce time drain, the use of traditional ethnographic research in the translation of family therapy research—and, in our opinion, bridging research—is limited. In addition, just as the translation process is segmented into distinct phases, the researchers who participate in each phase tend to specialize in that phase. Although some clinical researchers can equitably devote themselves to both research and practice, the probability of doing so is minimal. Therefore, the probability of bridging research's entering the phases of the translation research model is low. However, funding this type of effort will increase its practice.

Future Directions

Interest by funding agencies in identifying best practices has increased over the past decade (NIMH, 2003). The concept of "translation research" is becoming more familiar in all genres of research. Because of the greater emphasis placed on it by funding agencies and its growing visibility, translation research has entered the nomenclature of standard research practice (i.e., researchers acknowledge its import or incorporate a component of it into their research designs and proposals). Acknowledging the translation process is easily accomplished in policy recommendations and study implications. However, it is uncertain how translation research will be incorporated into proposed basic and applied research. To use the Frank and colleagues (2002) translation model as an example, it is not clear whether the bridging research we have proposed would be incorporated as a distinct phase in translation research or would be incorporated into the treatment development phase (Phase 2) of applied research.

Another potential direction for bridging research involves the role it plays in relaxing some of the disciplinary boundaries that seem to artificially segment the translation process. For family therapists, the outcome of diffusing these boundaries is the opportunity to be involved in more collaborative endeavors with family researchers in fields that have components emphasizing contextually based qualitative methodology, such as sociology and anthropology. Interfacing with researchers who are familiar with the nuanced and naturalistic aspects of family life should only serve to expedite the transition of basic research to effective practice.

CONCLUSION

Research has the ability not only to inform, but also to facilitate practical change and improvement in everyday life. For example, the introduction of aerospace and military technology into the daily life of the lay consumer has substantially increased communications, advanced medical care, and improved safety. The translation of research from specialized purposes to address the needs of broader groups of consumers has become a priority of funding agencies and a hallmark of exemplary research. In order for family therapy to continue increasing its legitimacy as a clinical field, it must increase its emphasis on translating basic family research to informed clinical interventions. This assertion does not imply that a family therapy clinical researcher should, or even ought to, engage in all phases of the translation research model. Good research is a time-intensive and sometimes highly specialized endeavor. However, the family therapy researcher should explore opportunities to maximize the strength of his or her area of expertise (whether basic, applied, or action research) by collaborating with other researchers (whether oriented toward basic, applied, or action research) to strengthen and expedite the translation process.

ACKNOWLEDGMENTS

We gratefully acknowledge the funders of the ethnographic component of Welfare, Children, and Families: A Three-City Study, including the National Institute of Child Health and Human Development; the Assistant Secretary for Planning and Evaluation, U.S. Department of Health and Human Services; the Social Security Administration; the Henry J. Kaiser Family Foundation; the Robert Wood Johnson Foundation; the W.K. Kellogg Foundation; and the John D. and Catherine T. MacArthur Foundation. We extend special thanks to our 210-member ethnographic team (see the project website, *http://www.jhu.edu/welfare*) and particularly the Penn State team, which provided the infrastructure, organization, and data management for the multisite ethnography. Most important, we thank the families that have graciously participated in the project and have given us access to their lives.

REFERENCES

Blau, S. (2003, September). *One chance only: Investigating the use of archaeology in search, location and recovery at disaster scenes.* Paper presented at the meeting of the Australian Disaster Conference, Canberra.

Brosseau, J. (2003). *The Center for Health Promotion and Translation Research applies medical research to clinical practice* (Health Care Discussions, Summer). Grand Forks, ND: Center for Rural Health. Retrieved from *http://www.bcbsnd.com/providers/discussions/summer2003/62_chptrapplies.pdf*

Bureau of Justice Statistics. (2003). *Victim characteristics: Violent crime victims—age.* Retrieved *http://www.ojp.usdoj.gov/bjs/ cvict_v.htm#age*

Burton, L. (1991). Drug trafficking schedules and childcare strategies in a high-risk neighborhood. *American Enterprise, 2*(3), 34–47.

Burton, L. M., Jarrett, R., Lein, L., Matthews, S., Quane, J., Skinner, D., et al. (2001). "*Structured discovery*": *Ethnography, welfare reform, and the assessment of neighborhoods, families, and children.* Paper presented at the biennial meeting of the Society for Research in Child Development, Minneapolis, MN.

Cabana, M. D., Rushton, J. A., & Rush, A. J. (2002). Implementing practice guidelines for depression: Applying a new framework to an old problem. *General Hospital Psychiatry, 24,* 35–42.

Center for Rural Health. (2001). *Center for Health Promotion and Translation Research.* Retrieved from *http://medicine.nodak.edu/crh*

Cherlin, A. J. (1995). Child care for poor children. In P. L. Chase-Lansdale & J. Brooks-Gunn (Eds.), *Escape from poverty: What makes a difference for poor children?* (pp. 121–137). Cambridge, UK: Cambridge University Press.

Childers, P., & Delany, P. (1994). Wired world, virtual campus: Universities and the political economy of cyberspace. *Works and Days, 23,* 61–78.

Donoghue J., & Hyla, T. R. (2001). Antidepressant use in clinical practice: Efficacy v. effectiveness. *British Journal of Psychiatry, 179,* 9–17.

Edelson, J. (2000, April 10). *Is childhood exposure to adult domestic violence a form of child maltreatment?* Paper presented at the conference on Children and Domestic Violence, Washington, DC.

Finkelhor, D., & Ormrod, R. (2000). Characteristics of crimes against juveniles. *Juvenile Justice Bulletin.* Retrieved from *http://www.ncjrs.org/html/ojjdp/2000_6_4*

Forgatch, M. S., & DeGarmo, D. S. (1999). Parenting through change: An effective prevention program for single mothers. *Journal of Consulting and Clinical Psychology, 67,* 711–724.

Forgatch, M. S., & DeGarmo, D. S. (2002). Extending and testing the social interaction learning model with divorce samples. In J. B. Reid, G. R. Patterson, & J. J. Snyder (Eds.), *Antisocial* behavior in children and adolescents: A developmental analysis and model for intervention (pp. 235–256). Washington, DC: American Psychological Association.

Forgatch, M. S., & Martinez, C. R., Jr. (1999). Parent management training: A program linking basic research and practical application. *Parent Management Training, 36,* 923–937.

Frank, E., Rush, A. J., Blehar, M., Essock, S., Hargreaves, W., Hogan, M., et al. (2002). Skating to where the puck is going to be: A plan for clinical trials and translation research in mood disorders. *Biological Psychiatry, 52,* 631–654.

Glaser, B. (1998). *Doing grounded theory: Issues and discussions.* Mill Valley, CA: Sociology Press.

Glaser, B., & Strauss, A. (1967). *The discovery of grounded theory: Strategies for qualitative research.* Chicago: Aldine.

Gudjonsson, G. H., & Haward, L. R. C. (1998). *Forensic psychology: A guide to practice.* New York: Routledge.

Jarrett, R., & Tubbs, C. Y. (1999). *Parenting interview guide. Welfare, Children, and Families: A Three-City Study.* State College: Population Research Institute, The Pennsylvania State University.

Klein, D., & White, J. (2002). *Family theories: An introduction.* Thousand Oaks, CA: Sage.

Kuczynski, L., & Hilderbrandt, N. (1997). Models of conformity and resistance in socialization theory. In J. Grusec & L. Kuczynski (Eds.), *Parenting and the socialization of values: A handbook of contemporary theory* (pp. 227–256). New York: Wiley.

Kuczynski, L., Marshall, S., & Schell, K. (1997). Value socialization in a bidirectional context. In J. Grusec & L. Kuczynski (Eds.), *Parenting and the socialization of values: A handbook of contemporary theory* (pp. 23–50). New York: Wiley.

Maccoby, E. A., & Martin, J. A. (1983). Socialization in the context of the family: Parent–child interaction. In P. H. Mussen (Series Ed.) & E. M. Hetherington (Vol. Ed.), *Handbook of child psychology* (4th ed.): *Vol. 4. Socialization, personality, and social development* (pp. 1–101). New York: Wiley.

McLaughlin, G. D. (1997). *The commercialization of the global positioning system.* Unpublished manuscript, Air Command and Staff College, U.S. Air Force.

Miles, M. B., & Huberman, A. M. (1994). *Qualitative data analysis: An expanded sourcebook* (2nd ed.). Thousand Oaks, CA: Sage.

Mrazek, P. J., & Haggerty, R. J. (Eds.). (1994). *Reducing risks for mental disorders: Frontiers for preventive intervention research.* Washington, DC: National Academy Press.

National Aeronautics and Space Administration. (n.d.). *Small business innovation research/small business technology transfer: Success stories.* Retrieved from *http://sbir.gsfc.nasa.gov/sbir/sbir.html*

National Institute of Mental Health (NIMH). (1999). *Bridging science and service: A report by the National Mental Health Council's clinical treatment and services research workgroup.* Bethesda, MD: Author.

National Institute of Mental Health (MINH). (2003). *Breaking ground, breaking through: The strategic plan for mood disorders research of the National Institute of Mental Health.* Retrieved from *http://www.nimh.nih.gov/strategic/mooddisorders.pdf*

Newman, I., & Benz, C. R. (1998). *Qualitative–quantitative research methodology: Exploring the interactive continuum.* Carbondale: Southern Illinois University Press.

O'Boyle, M. W., & Gill, H. S. (1998). On the relevance of research findings in cognitive neuroscience to educational practice. *Educational Psychology Review, 10,* 397–409.

Office of National Drug Control Policy (Producer). (2003a). *The enforcer* [Television public service announcement, National Youth Anti-Drug Media Campaign, Partnership for a Drug-Free America). Rockville, MD: Producer.

Office of National Drug Control Policy. (2003b). *Partnership attitude tracking study, national youth, 1999.* Rockville, MD: Author.

Parpal, M., & Maccoby, E. E. (1985). Maternal responsiveness and subsequent child compli-ance. *Child Development, 56,* 1326–1334.

Patton, M. Q. (2001). *Qualitative research and evaluation methods* (3rd ed.). Thousand Oaks, CA: Sage.

Patterson, G. R. (1986). Performance models for antisocial boys. *American Psychologist, 41,* 432–444.

Patterson, G. R. (1997). Performance models for parenting: A social interactional perspective. In J. Grusec & L. Kuczynski (Eds.), *Parenting and the socialization of values: A handbook of contemporary theory* (pp. 193–235). New York: Wiley.

Patterson, G. R., Reid, J. B., & Dishion, T. J. (1992). *A social learning approach to family inter-vention: Vol. 4. Antisocial boys.* Eugene, OR: Castalia.

Peterson, J., Song, X., & Jones-DeWeever, A. (2002). *Life after welfare reform: Low-income single parent families, pre- and post-TANF* (Research-in-Brief, IWPR Publication No. D446). Washington, DC: Institute for Women's Policy Research.

Reddy, P., Taylor, S. E., & Sifunda, S. (2002). Research capacity building and collaboration be-tween South African and American partners: The adaptation of intervention model for HIV/AIDS prevention in corrections research. *AIDS Education and Prevention, 14,* 92–102.

Rosier, K. B. (2000). *Mothering inner city children: The early school years.* New Brunswick, NJ: Rutgers University Press.

Satariano, W. A., & McAuley, E. (2003). Promoting physical activity among older adults: From ecology to the individual. *American Journal of Preventive Medicine, 25,* 184–192.

Schein, E. H. (1987). *The clinical perspective in fieldwork* (Qualitative Research Methods Series 5, A Sage University Paper). Newbury Park, CA: Sage.

Schwandt, T. A. (1994). Constructivist, interpretivist approaches to human inquiry. In N. K. Denzin & Y. S. Lincoln (Eds.), *Handbook of qualitative research* (pp. 118–137). Thousand Oaks, CA: Sage.

Sells, S. P., Smith, T. E., Coe, M. J., Yoshioka, M., & Robbins, J. (1994). An ethnography of couple and therapist experiences in reflecting team practice. *Journal of Marital and Family Therapy, 20,* 247–266.

Serradell, J., & Patwell, J. T. (1991). Unlabeled drug use patterns in a contemporary outpatient setting. *Journal of Pharmacoepidemiology, 2,* 19–43.

Shaw, D. S., Keenan, K., & Vondra, J. I. (1994). Developmental precursors of externalizing behavior: Ages 1 to 3. *Developmental Psychology, 30*(3), 355–364.

Snyder, J. J., & Huntley, D. (1990). Troubled families and troubled youth: The development of antisocial behavior and depression in children. In P. E. Leone (Ed.), *Understanding trou-bled and troubling youth* (pp. 194–225). Newbury Park, CA: Sage.

Strauss, A., & Corbin, J. (1998). *Basics of qualitative research: Techniques and procedures for developing grounded theory* (2nd ed.). Thousand Oaks, CA: Sage.

Tubbs, C. Y. (2002a). *Parental intent and monitoring behaviors in low-income families.* Poster session presented at the annual meeting of the American Family Therapy Academy, New York.

Tubbs, C. Y. (2002b). *The use of qualitative methods in informing clinical research and inter-ventions.* Paper presented at the annual meeting of the Family Research Consortium III, Charlotte, NC.

Ubelaker, D. H. (2000, July 24). *A history of Smithsonian–FBI collaboration in forensic anthro-pology, especially in regard to facial imagery.* Paper presented at the biennial meeting of the International Association for Craniofacial Identification, Federal Bureau of Investiga-tion, Washington, DC.

U.S. Department of Health and Human Services. (2002). Table 3.E8: Poverty guidelines for fam-ilies of specified size, 1965–2002 (dollars). *Federal Register 67*(31), 6931–6933.

U.S. Pharmacopeial Convention. (2003). *Off-label use: Frequently asked questions.* Retrieved from *http://www.usp.org/druginformation/offlabelsubmission/faq.html*

Van Maanen, J. (1995). An end to innocence. In J. Van Maanen (Ed.), *Representation in ethnography* (pp. 1–35). Thousand Oaks, CA: Sage.

Winston, P., Angel, R. J., Burton, L. M., Chase-Lansdale, P. L., Cherlin, A. J., Moffitt, R. A. et al. (1999). *Welfare, Children, and Families: A Three-City Study. Overview and design.* Baltimore: Johns Hopkins University.

Wolcott, H. F. (1995). Making a study "more ethnographic." In J. Van Maanen (Ed.), *Representation in ethnography* (pp. 79–111). Thousand Oaks, CA: Sage.

CHAPTER 9

Feminist Autoethnography

KATHERINE R. ALLEN
FRED P. PIERCY

> you fit into me
> like a hook into an eye
>
> a fish hook
> an open eye
>
> —ATWOOD (1971, p. 1)

Rarely do I go to the grave of my father. I find him, rather, in the photographs he took, in the letters he wrote, and in the person I try to be.

—QUINNEY (1996, p. 380)

For life is not lived realistically, in a linear manner. It is lived through the subject's eye, and that eye, like a camera's, is always reflexive, nonlinear, subjective, filled with flashbacks, after-images, dream sequences, faces merging into one another, masks dropping, and new masks being put on. In this world called reality, where we are forced to react, and life leaks in everywhere, we have nothing to hold on to but our own being.

—DENZIN (1992, p. 27)

In general, feminist researchers identify and address inequities in human relationships and the systems of domination that maintain them (Reinharz, 1992). Feminist family therapy researchers have employed quantitative methods and measures to do this (e.g., Avis, 1986; Black & Piercy, 1991; Chaney & Piercy, 1988; Haddock, MacPhee, & Zimmerman, 2001). More frequently, however, feminist scholars incorporate personal, reflexive dimensions into their research to shed light on how domination is reproduced in everyday life (Allen, 2000; Gailey, 1998; Laird, 2000). Similarly, researchers are increasingly using "ethnography"—a primary method to investigate other cultures, and in particular their family and kinship relations (Johnson, 2000)—to reflect on the layers of their own experience and culture (Gilgun, 1999; Tedlock, 2003). The epiphanous moments (Denzin, 1989) captured in this manner often have something to say to others. "Autoethnography" is the practice of going back and forth between inner vulnerable experience and outward social, historical, and cultural aspects of life, searching for deeper connections and understanding. As Ellis and Bochner (2003) explain, this particular genre of writing and research has been in circulation for at least two decades.

Many people enter the field of family therapy because of their needs to cure, rescue, or understand their own families (Framo, 1968). Similarly, family therapy educators' families of origin often peek out in their work (Fontes, Piercy, Thomas, & Sprenkle, 1998). This phenomenon also applies to those of us who research families (Allen, 2000). Autoethnography is a powerful way to "take back the night" from the potential violence of our unexamined projections and resist our own protestations that we are not biased. By telling a story *on* ourselves, we risk exposure to our peers, subject ourselves to scrutiny and ridicule, and relinquish some of our sense of control over our own narratives. Yet, as we will explain in this chapter, a paradoxical effect occurs: By giving up the power that comes from being disembodied and disinterested observers, we can claim a new sense of empowerment and add another dimension to our understanding of the human condition. Vulnerability is returned for strength.

In this chapter, we address how personal, reflective writing contributes to a richer feminism and how this reflective feminist inquiry intersects with a more personal ethnography. Feminist autoethnography is a method of being, knowing, and doing that combines two concerns: telling the stories of those who are marginalized, and making good use of our own experience. No longer must we insist on being dispassionate or positioned outside the hermeneutic circle in order to make valid contributions to knowledge. We propose that this connection between feminism and autoethnography offers a more fully human method of inquiry in the disciplines in which we teach, investigate, and practice—namely, family studies and family therapy.

BACKGROUND

Feminist Research and Knowledge

Feminist scholarship, in general, includes the experience of the researcher as part of the research process. Although there are infinite ways of applying feminist methodologies, epistemologies, ontologies, and ethics, feminists agree that "the observer and the observed are in the same causal scientific plane" (Harding, 1991, p. 11). As knowers, we are not invisible in the production of knowledge. Our experience counts and should be accounted for. In every respect, it matters just as much what we as researchers feel, know, and sense about the situation we are investigating as it does about the people, places, and artifacts we are trying to understand. All scientific knowledge is socially situated, and our role as ethical producers and consumers of knowledge is to demystify (i.e., make transparent) how we have generated our ideas (Haraway, 1988). Because society has historically devalued women, the currency of the day has included denial, distortion, silencing, misrepresentation, and repression of women's experiences. Those of us who are feminists have used reflection and conversation to unearth the social situatedness of knowledge and to define the standpoint of women (Smith, 1987). We use reflexivity to deconstruct "the way things are" and to reflect on how culture and socialization provide the specifications for what we know, how we know it, and how that knowledge changes over time, space, and circumstance (Bell, 1993).

Reflecting on one's experience in the world and thereby calling oneself a feminist constitute perhaps the one common definition of a feminist method. Reinharz (1992) demonstrated this in her exhaustive examination of 11 major types of feminist methods in the social sciences. Reinharz turns the typical question of "Is there a feminist research method?" into "What are feminists' actual ways of working?" To come to an understanding of this query that she could share with others, she applied the feminist method of talking and reflecting, stating that "My approach requires listening to the voices of feminist researchers at work and accepting their diversity" (p. 5). Feminists reflect on their experience and represent their experience in words or graphically (as in painting or film). This is a way women can validate and honor their own lives, particularly when the status quo reflects a version of reality that often excludes women's everyday experiences.

Change happens in the daily rhythms of life when courageous people break outside the circle of the status quo (Stanley & Wise, 1993). Inside the circle is the taken-for-granted reality of how and what to think, the actual vocabulary and the structures for thinking, and the ways of enacting personal and professional life. Feminist scholars and practitioners are critical of such unquestioned ways of being, doing, and knowing, because these ways dismiss women, people of color, and people who are lesbian, gay, bisexual, or transgendered as "the other." That is, the status quo disregards those who are not male, are not heterosexual, are not young, or fail in countless other ways to measure up to the ideal standard against which members of society judge what is more or less valued (Hare-Mustin & Marecek, 1990). This value system is irrational and outdated, based on an ideology that is not so useful in a postmodern world. (For lucid critiques of modernity, intimacy, family, and social science, see Cheal, 1991; Flyvbjerg, 2001; Giddens, 1992.)

The Social-Constructionist Turn in Family Therapy

Breaking outside the circle of the status quo is possible when we see so-called theoretical and scientific reality with the same multidimensionality that exists in our private lives, recognizing that "there is no center that can hold" (Gergen, 1999, p. 30). Social life is full of seams, "a collection of gaps and broken links, not iron-clad and inviolate at all" (Stanley & Wise, 1993, p. 183). Life, as Denzin (1992, p. 27) notes, is nonlinear and "leaks in everywhere." Reality is not fixed, but continuously under construction (Gergen, 1999).

Weingarten (1991) points out that therapists may be particularly well situated to confront the tensions and ambiguities in clients' private lives, and thus attentive to a social-constructionist way of seeing the world. The narrative turn in family therapy fits well with the power of language to shift meanings, definitions, and solutions to family problems, and therapists are adept at seeing life in alternative, fluid ways (Laird, 2000). Many clinical practices in the family therapy field are based on artistic and/or literary foundations, including narrative therapy (White & Epston, 1990), family sculpting (Satir, 1972), and experiential therapy (Whitaker & Keith, 1981).

Piercy and Benson (2005) observe that the richness that comes with this constructionist view—the irony, comedy, tragedy, drama, ambiguity, and tension of real life—can be flattened in the typical conventions of social science reporting, where statistics wipe away the nuances of emotional and behavioral complexities. Yet, on the other hand, researchers and therapists alike must be mindful to discuss the assumptions, rigor, and credibility of their methods, so that their reports will hold up under scrutiny (Denzin, 2003; Richardson, 2000a).

Feminist Consciousness in Family Therapy

In the field of family therapy, feminists (e.g., Goldner, 1985; Hare-Mustin, 1978; Luepnitz, 1988; McGoldrick, Anderson, & Walsh, 1989; Taggart, 1985) critiqued the theoretical underpinnings of the alleged neutrality of power and launched a period of "gendering" theories and practice models in the field (Laird, 2000). Scholars continue to address the politics of gender in family therapy and the passions that these issues stir among those who do not want the status quo to be challenged (Knudson-Martin, 1997; Silverstein & Goodrich, 2003).

Often blending reflexive narrative with feminist analyses of power in the "mirrored room" (Hare-Mustin, 1994), feminist therapists (e.g., Goodrich, Rampage, Ellman, & Halstead, 1988; Walters, Carter, Papp, & Silverstein, 1988) demonstrated early on how they experienced the vulnerabilities of transforming mainstream therapeutic practice into a more contested gender-sensitive therapy. They reshaped central concepts in the field by combining insights about power and domination with a social-constructivist perspective on meaning as co-constructed from dialogue and imbued with the power inherent in language. Weingarten (1991), for example, discusses previously untheorized dimensions of intimate and nonintimate encounters. Feminist family therapy scholars have generally demonstrated that gender, like race or class, is not an inherent property of individuals, but is "a socially prescribed relationship, a process, and a social construction" (Hare-Mustin & Marecek, 1990, p. 54) that cannot be renounced voluntarily.

Such groundbreaking work has transformed the field by insisting on a recognition of women's differential experiences in families and by challenging taken-for-granted assumptions about family systems theory, such as circularity, neutrality, and complementarity (Avis, 1996). Feminist scholars have recently introduced to family therapy the concept of "intersectionality" from critical race theory. Intersectionality sensitizes therapists and researchers to race, class, and sexual orientation, which largely have been erased from treatments addressing such issues as domestic violence (Bograd, 1999). Regarding practice, feminist family therapists have provided clinical tools, such as the "power equity guide," to train therapists to use and evaluate gender-informed family therapy (Haddock, Zimmerman, & MacPhee, 2000).

Defining Feminist Autoethnography

As we see it, to be feminist researchers is to be excruciatingly self-conscious (Stacey, 1988) about our location in a social system. As the word "excruciating" suggests, this is not a comfortable space, but it can be bittersweet. Reflexiveness helps keep researchers honest, especially with ourselves (Allen, 2000). When we strip away the layers of distortions imposed by our own limited perceptions, we allow ourselves to become edgy with the reminder that all knowledge is partial, and that there are flaws in the typical strategies we use to puff up our egos and distance ourselves from the "subjects" of our inquiry. When we tell and analyze our own stories, we begin to see how their content is derived from our culture. As we learn about ourselves and our own culture-bound constraints, we learn more about those binding our clients and the participants in our research. We become sensitized to their struggles as we reflect on those struggles in our own lives. This makes us better researchers and therapists. Likewise, it helps us in our efforts of social change, which is, after all, the ultimate goal of feminist practice—to change oppressive social conditions, regardless of our epistemological paradigm. (For a range of informative readings on this issue, see Bell & Klein, 1996; Freedman, 2002; Gergen, 1997a.)

Feminist autoethnography is a type of autobiographical method in the reflexive qualitative tradition where the researcher and the subject are one (Krieger, 1991; Richardson, 2000b). Feminist autoethnography is the explicit reflection on one's personal experience to break outside the circle of conventional social science and confront, court, and coax that aching pain or haunting memory that one does not understand about one's own experience. It is ideally suited for investigating hidden or sensitive topics, such as those dealing with sexuality or life course transitions about which little is known. Examples of such investigations include Philaretou and Allen's (2003) examination of male sexual anxiety, and Tenni, Smyth, and Boucher's (2003) critical analysis of dealing with the anxiety of self-produced data. Thus it can be adapted at any layer of the scholarly enterprise—research, teaching, or clinical practice—by providing a space to work through the fragments and missing pieces that echo in one's research project, classroom teaching, advising, supervision, or activities of daily living.

Richardson (2000b) calls the many forms of autoethnographic writing "creative analytic practices." This method requires variety and frequency in writing practices. Sher (1999) describes writing as a meditative practice that can precede, correspond with, or conclude any activity. Autobiographical writing takes discipline; it is not easy to confront the messiness of one's life and try to find meaning within it. Free writing is a good way to start the process, whether as a daily meditation on one's own feelings, or as a theoretical or methodological memo initiating a new research project. It is the process of moving back and forth between self and other, looking inside oneself and focusing outward on external institutions and structures, and making the connections that helps meaning take shape (Ellis & Bochner, 2003). Ideas are recorded and papers rewritten as one goes back and forth between rigor and imagination (Bateson, 1972), between the left brain and the right brain (Flemons, 1998), so that meaning emerges slowly and painstakingly. Consider the following examples from Katherine's autoethnographic writing in preparing this chapter.

FEMINIST AUTOETHNOGRAPHIC REFLECTIONS

Making Myself Vulnerable

When I (KRA) make myself so vulnerable by telling a story *on* myself, I confront the closest place to knowing myself that is possible in that moment. I enter and sustain a dialogue with myself and the characters in my own life. The benefit to my research is identification with the "subjects" (or "clients," or "students," or others in typically one-down positions from the one I occupy as the person with the power to name in my story). Using Goldberg's (1986) metaphor of "writing down the bones," writing raw, I work toward the smallest, most vulnerable part of myself. In that place of vulnerability, I am more open to hearing the voices of others, particularly those in marginalized positions. I am less ready to dismiss the experiences of others, or to superimpose theories that will distance myself from connecting with them.

Touchstones from the past also serve as powerful reminders of my vulnerability (Allen, 2000). "Touchstones" are memory fragments that help me negotiate the emotional terrain of the present. For me, touchstones are feelings of embarrassment, loss, shame, discomfort, anxiety, or pride—not what I would call "happy" emotions. It doesn't matter that I have a clinical label for a particular feeling, but rather that I am able to call upon the discomfort that can keep me grounded in this very moment. I want to let "this very moment be the perfect teacher," as Pema Chodron (1997, p. 12) describes, not by putting myself above the lives of those I'm inquiring about, teaching, or otherwise scrutinizing in my work as "scholar," but by feeling exactly what it feels to be nailed by life—no excuses, no bluffs, being right there in the moment, pierced through the heart.

As I write this chapter, one powerful touchstone from the past is the time I was a graduate student going for free therapy in the marriage and family therapy clinic at my university, seeing another student training to be a therapist. My boyfriend at the time went in for couple counseling with me. While I was in the waiting room and he was doing his intake with the therapist, he later told me that he had made a pass at her during their session. I felt horribly embarrassed. She was in the same classes with me. Feeling needy and trapped, but wanting someone to talk to anyway, I still went in for counseling with her. I really used to resent it when she would bum cigarettes off me.

This touchstone is a reminder about the ambivalent mix of emotions that has dogged me throughout my life and is returning once again as I prepare for my third marriage. No doubt there are countless other meanings to explore in this memory fragment, but what I find useful in this very moment is that it calls up my terror of being betrayed once again by a life partner and my resentment at the helper who is supposed to fix things. I believe that these memories have become a lens through which I too often see the world. Having written down my story (to the bone), something that actually occurred in 1978, and having examined it anew in the current context, I reexamine it with fresh insights, based on years of therapy, recent life events, and new friendships—one of which is my collaboration with my coauthor, Fred. For example, I can see in some new ways my own part in reproducing betrayal and resentment in personal and professional life. In dialogue with Fred over this memory fragment, he suggested that "many branches grow from this one root." This insight has led me to work on better ways to take responsibility for my actions and not be so quick to fight fire with fire. My reflections reminded Fred of the following story (from the film, *The Cup*; Norbu, 1999):

A Buddhist monk asks his followers, "Can we cover the earth in leather so it's soft wherever we go?"

"No," responds a student.

"So what can we do?"

"Cover our feet in leather," answers another.

Covering our feet in leather, the monk explains, is equal to covering the earth with leather.

"Likewise," he says, "enemies are as limitless as space. All enemies cannot possibly be overcome. Yet if one can just overcome hatred this will be equal to overcoming all enemies."

I am not there yet, but I like the story.

Not a Comfy Fit

> you fit into me
> like a hook into an eye
>
> a fish hook
> an open eye
>
> —ATWOOD (1971, p. 1)

Margaret Atwood's 1971 poem, which I first read as a 20-year-old college junior in 1974, caught hold of me, as a fish hook will. Wildly ambivalent with despair over yet another broken relationship with a man (boy) who wouldn't stay with me, but desperately wanting to find a person to love me (back), I felt the hook. It wasn't the comfortable fit in the eight stages of the family life cycle I read about in my marriage and family development textbook (Duvall, 1971). Teaching Sunday school, getting good grades, planning for my future, meeting the man who would become my first husband, but having an affair with my professor, I was also experimenting sexually with abusive men, living through the terror of undiagnosed depression and blackout drinking episodes, and fretting about my parents' troubled commuter marriage.

This hook and eye would be labeled "dysfunctional" by the founding fathers of the family therapy field, whose theories of instrumental and expressive roles in companionate marriages and isolated nuclear families would have little to say to me beyond its shame-based labeling. Clearly, I was dealing with the ambiguity of my WASP upbringing, and who I was and wanted to be in a world that didn't always affirm me. The relational interchanges I experienced as a young woman coming of age in the 1970s were biting, unsentimental, rough, and sometimes violent. In her 16-word poem, Margaret Atwood captured my experience perfectly. Nobody in my major of child development and family relations was talking about contested intimacy issues. This was a decade before the discourse on wife abuse had entered the mainstream of family studies and family therapy. In 1988, Yllo and Bograd's now classic text *Feminist Perspectives on Wife Abuse* was published, and as is true for many academic women, the text began to read me (Allen, 1994). My personal and professional lives bled together, and I never managed to compartmentalize work and love as the theories of adult development suggested (Levinson, 1980). As I read about and taught such topics as wife abuse, sexual assault, women's unpaid labor, and economic inequities at work, I came face to face with my own gendered legacy and personal history of abuse. Age, privilege, experience, humility, and learning to care (a little bit) less about what others think of me has allowed me to take greater risks in becoming more transparent in my research. Intimate life, to me, is a dangerous terrain. The personal is part of the professional, and I would be obscuring a primary source of ideas, motivation, and insight in my work if I pretended otherwise.

Through feminist reflexive work, I've learned the survival skill of taking care of "my side of the street" as a precaution to not projecting my own unresolved or untheorized motivations onto others. From a social-constructionist perspective, research is not a neutral endeavor, but a representation of one's own perception. It is in the stubbornly naïve not-knowing that we can truly do harm to others, as Avis (1996) so eloquently explains in her review of harm done in family therapy when practitioners are not educated about issues such as the battering of women or the tendency to blame mothers for child outcomes.

A feminist autoethnographic approach to research is grounded in humility—one of several paradoxes that seems apt for this type of method. As a new feminist scholar, I was most resistant to the notion of humility, but now, paradoxically, I push the goal of my work from dispassionate proof to more clear-sighted honesty. I want to tell the truth of my story (or your story, or our story; see Ellis & Berger, 2003) toward connecting body, spirit, head, and heart. Feminist autoethnography is being achingly honest with oneself in the service of finding a deeper understanding of self and society (Krieger, 1991). On the day before my father died, I wrote in my diary:

> My brother just called to say that my father has less than 2 weeks to live from the cancer that is ravaging his body. His death is coming at a strange time in my life. My mother is losing her husband of 51 years. Five days ago she lost her own mother, who died at 96. My father's death resurrects for me thoughts of my loss of a child I helped to bring into this world, a son by my former lesbian partner, who left me over 3 years ago and took him with her. I mourn the loss of the families in which I lived, including the family from my first marriage, in which I was a wife, had a husband, and a child. Tomorrow, for Thanksgiving, my ex-husband and his wife and their two children will come to my home to visit our son, my new fiancé, and me. My father's impending death reminds me of my loss of that first family, and my loss of my lesbian partnership and second son. Now I'm taking a chance on a third marriage, and my older son and I are living in a new family. And my father is dying and my grandmother is gone. There is this hole in my heart that I know I must go back and work through all over again.

My father's death reminds me in new ways of how the meaning of family changes as we live our lives. Autoethnography helps me delve deeply into my experience in a way that traditional social science methodologies have yet to tap—blending theoretical analysis with storytelling and the content of life. The particular self becomes subject and is used to inform broader issues of relevance to social science (Krieger, 1991). This method can provide first-person details of culture—details that help us understand and critique the social structures and processes constituting that culture. Not only do I find the reflexive writing a healing process for coping with the rush of emotions at a time of personal loss, but the discipline of daily writing practice helps me not rush to judgment over any idea, feeling, or sensation that emerges. If I do my job well, my experience connects with that of the reader, and the reader can reflect on the losses of his or her life and the issues it raises through my own sharing (Richardson, 2000b).

Where Is Fred in This Chapter?

Katherine asked me (FPP) to join her in writing this chapter because of my background in family therapy and because I am committed to research that liberates (Piercy & Thomas, 1998). However, as a male, I have had misgivings about coauthoring a chapter about feminism. Being an advocate for a group I am not part of has always been a balancing act for me. When do I step forward, and when should I take a back seat? I remember coleading HIV prevention workshops in Indonesia with my Indonesian colleagues. I wanted to support their success, so I generally stayed in the background in the workshops. I received feedback after one of the workshops that I should "maju depan" ("step forward") more.

In this chapter, as then, I want to contribute but not take up too much space. I worry about whether I should even have my name on this chapter as a white, privileged male. Shouldn't others be writing about feminism? That's my stay-in-the-background side speaking. My family of origin was big on support and encouragement, but not too good at coming into the light. I remember my mom singing "We Shall Overcome" in our kitchen as she made us dinner. She wanted to march for women's rights, but never did. Not many in her generation did. If my name ends up on this chapter, and if this section becomes part of the chapter (and as I write these words, that remains a big "if"), it will be, in a way, to rewrite my own family legacy. It will also be because of Katherine's encouragement. She doesn't want me to be invisible—a tribute to her life travels and open heart.

I appreciate the power of Katherine's reflections. A little secret in academia is that a lot of research is so removed from human experience that it is eviscerated—disemboweled of passion. Consequently, the typical research presentation is as exciting as stale bread. New graduate students sense this, and learn quickly to be polite and tolerant of the once-removed culture of dispassionate inquiry. They even learn to be dispassionate themselves. The authenticity and spirit of autoethnography attract me. I want to enliven the research process, and to be enlivened by it. Good autoethnography holds promise as a research method that can touch the soul and raise the dead.

A NOTE ON PARADIGMS

Feminist autoethnography is useful, regardless of the epistemological paradigm in which one works. In my (KRA) earlier work on the life histories of older never-married women (Allen, 1989), a reflexive analysis helped me reflect later on how the text promised new meanings 10 years after I completed the initial data collection and analysis. This occurred after several significant life changes, such as getting a divorce from my husband and coming out as a lesbian; I felt invited to reflect on my data in new ways (Allen, 1994). Years passed, and as that partnership ended, I found myself reflecting again on how changes in my private life entered my interpretations of data. I described in a narrative analysis some of the transformations the ending of my lesbian partnership created in my relationship with my teenage son (Allen, 2001). These examples show that whether employing empirical social science methods or postmodern strategies that blur the boundaries between science and humanities (Ellis & Flaherty, 1992), "self as subject" can be a fruitful, innovative, and insightful method to gain greater access to knowledge (Krieger, 1991). And just as feminist family therapy is being integrated with other therapy methods (e.g., Vatcher & Bogo, 2001), we see elements of feminist autoethnography potentially enriching other research methods. This is because feminist autoethnography is likely to connect with the heart as well as the head (Piercy & Benson, 2005). More social science research should do this.

To us as family scholars and practitioners, however, it is evident that our field is often divided between those who are concerned about taking a foundational approach versus a social-constructionist approach. Our view is that we need fewer empiricist versus constructionist "shootouts" and more conversations about how scholars can learn from each other (Acock, van Dulmen, Allen, & Piercy, 2005). As Gergen (1997b) reminds us, feminists are adept at blending categories. We do not have to be locked into a rigid adherence to relativism or foundationism. Gergen observes that a new breed of scholar has emerged on the scene: the "empiricist social constructionist," a scholar who has evolved by taking the best from both worlds. Gergen also reminds us of the necessity of improvising. Feminist researchers are adept at researching the situation at hand, perhaps because we have had to scramble for funding. Or perhaps it is because of our choice of understudied topics relevant to women (Fonow & Cook, 1991). Often our own lives are the most accessible—hence the rise of feminist autoethnography.

Gergen (1997b) lists seven challenges to take on this journey into the strange new land where categories are further mixed up, and empirical and constructionist paradigms are borrowed from and blended in ways that may seem bizarre or heretical to purists in either camp. Her insights bear repeating:

- Language is not a transparent representation of the world.
- Realities are cultural constructions.
- Polarities do not exist in nature, but in language.
- Facts are neither true nor false, except by the ordination of the social groups involved.
- We must apply values via a leap of faith alone.
- Political actions are deeds of faith.
- Identity and knowledge are critically dependent upon interaction to be created, and are partial, fragmented, and temporary.

APPLICATION: REFLECTIVE QUESTIONS FOR RESEARCHERS

In a human development research methods course, in which we train graduate students in areas such as family studies and family therapy, I (KRA) use feminist autoethnographic strategies to help students locate their own vulnerabilities and strengths and use them to benefit their research. For example, a warm-up exercise includes asking students on the first day of class the following questions, with the aim of immediately closing the distance between knower and known:

1. When was the last time you talked with anyone about research?
2. Have you ever been a subject in a research study? How did you feel?
3. Have the findings in a research study ever helped you?
4. What is the major obstacle you face in starting your own study?
5. If you were to follow a personal passion, what would you study?
6. If you could have the answer to any question, what would that question be?
7. What would you learn about yourself if you started a research project?
8. What is the latest insight you've had about your own behavior?
9. Give a definition of "analysis" that makes sense to you.
10. What kind of research might leave participants better off than when they began the study? In what ways, if any, is this important to you?

In this class, students write research proposals and critique the work of others. I ask them to reflect on their own experiences, and I give them time in class and in writing to process their responses. Students work individually, in dyads, in small groups, and in the class as a whole to treat research as a reflexive experience. A few questions that help to deemphasize the dispassionate nature of research training draw from principles and practices of feminist autoethnography:

1. How committed are you to your study and the way you constructed the proposal?
2. Having examined the feedback of your proposal, what is one issue you now understand about the study that was not clear to you previously?
3. What do you feel is the strength of your study? How was your perception supported by the feedback provided?
4. In what ways have your ideas not been understood or appreciated? What would you like to explain now that was unclear or misunderstood in your first draft?
5. What parts of your study, if any, are you ready to clarify and refine?
6. What parts of your study, if any, do you want to completely rethink?
7. What is the most helpful advice you have received about your study?
8. In what ways was the process of reviewing another student's proposal helpful to you?

Similarly, I (FPP) have an assignment option in my qualitative research class that allows students to experiment with autoethnography. Here is the assignment:

"Try your hand at writing an autoethnographic performance text, using poetry and/or prose. You will be engaging the reader with a deeply personal account of your lived experience. At the same time, your effort should work as cultural criticism—a tool to critique a cultural norm, or to write an alternative story, and to move the reader to greater awareness or action. You will have succeeded if you engage the reader and raise his or her consciousness about a particular issue. Some projects will take more thought and time than others (e.g., a script to be acted out vs. a one-page stream-of-consciousness poem). Thus the number of points you will receive will depend on both the degree to which you meet the criteria of engaging and raising consciousness, and the amount of work that you put into this option. Also, please include a short introduction to your work and a section that situates your work within the field of qualitative research. In this section, be sure to explain your intent and appropriate criteria for judging your work and interpretive/aesthetic pieces like it."

This assignment has encouraged students to focus on themselves and their own cultures as valid areas of study. A number of family therapy students have published their autoethnographies (e.g., McLaurin, 2003; Piercy & Benson, 2005; Ricci, 2003). All have learned to embrace their own experience as something from which to draw and learn.

CONCLUSION

Actually, there is no conclusion. Self-reflection is an ongoing endeavor. And feminist self-reflection that focuses on the violence done within the context of family, experienced and shared by us as researchers, has much to teach us all. Is it credible research? Yes, to the extent to which it touches readers and points them to learnings that they can apply to better understand and help families. In fact, the act of doing this research itself is intervention. And the evocative nature of this work has the promise of connecting with the reader in a manner that statistics usually do not. To paraphrase Stalin, one death is a tragedy, but a million deaths are just a statistic. Through our reflective work, we can bring to life truths that may otherwise be missed. But, then again, this isn't a conclusion. This work has just begun.

EXEMPLARS

Ellis, C. (1995). The other side of the fence: Seeing black and white in a small southern town. *Qualitative Inquiry, 1,* 147–167.

Krieger, S. (1996). *The family silver: Essays on relationships among women.* Berkeley: University of California Press.

Richardson, L. (1997). *Fields of play: Constructing an academic life.* New Brunswick, NJ: Rutgers University Press.

Tillmann-Healy, L. M. (1996). A secret life in a culture of thinness: Reflections on body, food, and bulimia. In C. Ellis & A. P. Bochner (Eds.), *Composing ethnography: Alternative forms of qualitative writing* (pp. 76–108). Walnut Creek, CA: AltaMira Press.

Wellman, D. (1996). Red and black in white America: Discovering cross-border identities and other subversive activities. In B. Thomson & S. Tyagi (Eds.), *Names we call home: Autobiography on racial identity* (pp. 29–41). New York: Routledge.

REFERENCES

Acock, A., van Dulmen, M., Allen, K., & Piercy, F. (2005). Contemporary and emerging research methods in studying families. In V. Bengtson, A. Acock, K. Allen, P. Dilworth-Anderson, & D. Klein (Eds.), *Sourcebook of family theory and research* (pp. 59–89). Thousand Oaks, CA: Sage.

Allen, K. R. (1989). *Single women/family ties: Life histories of older women.* Newbury Park, CA: Sage.

Allen, K. R. (1994). Feminist reflections on lifelong single women. In D. L. Sollie & L. A. Leslie (Eds.), *Gender, families, and close relationships: Feminist research journeys* (pp. 97–119). Thousand Oaks, CA: Sage.

Allen, K. R. (2000). A conscious and inclusive family studies. *Journal of Marriage and the Family, 62,* 4–17.

Allen, K. R. (2001). Feminist visions for transforming families: Desire and equality then and now. *Journal of Family Issues, 22,* 791–809.

Atwood, M. (1971). *Power politics.* New York: Harper & Row.

Avis, J. M. (1986). *Training and supervision in feminist-informed family therapy: A Delphi study.* Unpublished doctoral dissertation, Purdue University.

Avis, J. M. (1996). Deconstructing gender in family therapy. In F. P. Piercy, D. H. Sprenkle, J. L. Wetchler, & Associates, *Family therapy sourcebook* (2nd ed., pp. 220–255). New York: Guilford Press.

Bateson, G. (1972). *Steps to an ecology of mind.* New York: Ballantine Books.

Bell, D. (1993). Yes Virginia, there is a feminist ethnography: Reflections from three Australian fields. In D. Bell, P. Caplan, & W. J. Karim (Eds.), *Engendered fields: Women, men and ethnography* (pp. 28–43). London: Routledge.

Bell, D., & Klein, R. (Eds.). (1996). *Radically speaking: Feminism reclaimed.* North Melbourne, Victoria, Australia: Spinifex.

Black, L., & Piercy, F. P. (1991). A feminist family therapy scale. *Journal of Marital and Family Therapy, 17,* 111–120.

Bograd, M. (1999). Strengthening domestic violence theories: Intersections of race, class, sexual orientation and gender. *Journal of Marital and Family Therapy, 25,* 275–289.

Chaney, S. E., & Piercy, F. P. (1988). A feminist family therapy behavior checklist. *American Journal of Family Therapy, 16,* 305–318.

Cheal, D. (1991). *Family and the state of theory.* Toronto: University of Toronto Press.

Chodron, P. (1997). *When things fall apart: Heart advice for difficult times.* Boston: Shambhala.

Denzin, N. K. (1989). *Interpretive biography.* Newbury Park, CA: Sage.

Denzin, N. K. (1992). The many faces of emotionality: Reading *Persona.* In C. Ellis & M. G. Flaherty (Eds.), *Investigating subjectivity: Research on lived experience* (pp. 17–30). Newbury Park, CA: Sage.

Denzin, N. K. (2003). *Performance ethnography: Critical pedagogy and the politics of culture.* Thousand Oaks, CA: Sage.

Duvall, E. M. (1971). *Family development.* Philadelphia: Lippincott.

Ellis, C., & Berger, L. (2003). Their story/my story/our story: Including the researcher's experience in interview research. In J. A. Holstein & J. F. Gubrium (Eds.), *Inside interviewing: New lenses, new concerns* (pp. 467–493). Thousand Oaks, CA: Sage.

Ellis, C., & Bochner, A. P. (2003). Autoethnography, personal narrative, reflexivity: Researcher as subject. In N. K. Denzin & Y. S. Lincoln (Eds.), *Collecting and interpreting qualitative materials* (2nd ed., pp. 199–258). Thousand Oaks, CA: Sage.

Ellis, C., & Flaherty, M. G. (1992). An agenda for the interpretation of lived experience. In C. Ellis & M. G. Flaherty (Eds.), *Investigating subjectivity* (pp. 1–13). Newbury Park, CA: Sage.

Flemons, D. (1998). *Writing between the lines: How to compose riveting social science manuscripts.* New York: Norton.

Flyvbjerg, B. (2001). *Making social science matter: Why social inquiry fails and how it can succeed again.* Cambridge, UK: Cambridge University Press.

Fonow, M. M., & Cook, J. A. (1991). Back to the future: A look at the second wave of feminist epistemology and methodology. In M. M. Fonow & J. A. Cook (Eds.), *Beyond methodology: Feminist scholarship as lived research* (pp. 1–15). Bloomington: Indiana University Press.

Fontes, L., Piercy, F. P., Thomas, V., & Sprenkle, D. (1998). Self issues for family therapy educators. *Journal of Marital and Family Therapy, 24,* 305–320.

Framo, J. (1968). My families, my family. *Voices: The Art and Science of Psychotherapy, 4,* 18–27.

Freedman, E. B. (2002). *No turning back: The history of feminism and the future of women.* New York: Ballantine Books.

Gailey, C. W. (1998). Feminist methods. In H. R. Bernard (Ed.), *Handbook of methods in cultural anthropology* (pp. 203–233). Walnut Creek, CA: AltaMira Press.

Gergen, K. J. (1999). *An invitation to social construction.* London: Sage.

Gergen, M. M. (1997a). Life stories: Pieces of a dream. In M. M. Gergen & S. N. Davis (Eds.), *Toward a new psychology of gender* (pp. 203–221). New York: Routledge.

Gergen, M. M. (1997b). Skipping stone: Circles in the pond. In M. M. Gergen & S. N. Davis (Eds.), *Toward a new psychology of gender* (pp. 605–611). New York: Routledge.

Giddens, A. (1992). *The transformation of intimacy: Sexuality, love and eroticism in modern societies.* Stanford, CA: Stanford University Press.

Gilgun, J. F. (1999). Methodological pluralism and qualitative family research. In M. Sussman, S. K. Steinmetz, & G. W. Peterson (Eds.), *Handbook of marriage and the family* (2nd ed., pp. 219–261). New York: Plenum Press.

Goldberg, N. (1986). *Writing down the bones: Freeing the writer within.* Boston: Shambhala.

Goldner, V. (1985). Feminism and family therapy. *Family Process, 24,* 31–47.

Goodrich, T. J., Rampage, C., Ellman, B., & Halstead, K. (1988). *Feminist family therapy: A casebook.* New York: Norton.

Haddock, S. A., MacPhee, D., & Zimmerman, T. S. (2001). AAMFT master series tapes: An analysis of the inclusion of feminist principles into family therapy practice. *Journal of Marital and Family Therapy, 27,* 487–500.

Haddock, S. A., Zimmerman, T. S., & MacPhee, D. (2000). The power equity guide: Attending to gender in family therapy. *Journal of Marital and Family Therapy, 26,* 153–164.

Haraway, D. J. (1988). Situated knowledges: The science question in feminism as a site of discourse on the privilege of partial perspective. *Feminist Studies, 14,* 575–599.

Harding, S. (1991). *Whose science? Whose knowledge? Thinking from women's lives.* Ithaca, NY: Cornell University Press.

Hare-Mustin, R. T. (1978). A feminist approach to family therapy. *Family Process, 17,* 181–194.

Hare-Mustin, R. T. (1994). Discourse in the mirrored room: A postmodern analysis of therapy. *Family Process, 33,* 199–236.

Hare-Mustin, R. T., & Marecek, J. (1990). Gender and the meaning of difference: Postmodernism and psychology. In R. T. Hare-Mustin & J. Marecek (Eds.), *Making a difference: Psychology and the construction of gender* (pp. 22–64). New Haven, CT: Yale University Press.

Johnson, C. L. (2000). Kinship and gender. In D. H. Demo, K. R. Allen, & M. A. Fine (Eds.), *Handbook of family diversity* (pp. 128–148). New York: Oxford University Press.

Knudson-Martin, C. (1997). The politics of gender in family therapy. *Journal of Marital and Family Therapy, 23,* 421–437.

Krieger, S. (1991). *Social science and the self: Personal essays on an art form.* New Brunswick, NJ: Rutgers University Press.

Laird, J. (2000). Culture and narrative as metaphors for clinical practice with families. In D. H. Demo, K. R. Allen, & M. A. Fine (Eds.), *Handbook of family diversity* (pp. 338–358). New York: Oxford University Press.

Levinson, D. J. (1980). Toward a conception of the adult life course. In N. J. Smelser & E. H. Erikson (Eds.), *Themes of work and love in adulthood* (pp. 265–290). Cambridge, MA: Harvard University Press.

Luepnitz, D. (1988). *The family interpreted: Feminist theory in clinical practice.* New York: Basic Books.

McGoldrick, M., Anderson, C., & Walsh, F. (Eds.). (1989). *Women in families: A framework for family therapy.* New York: Norton.

McLaurin, S. L. (2003). Homophobia: An autoethnographic story. *The Qualitative Report, 8*(3), 481–486.

Norbu, K. (Director). *The cup* [Motion picture]. Bhutan/United States: FineLine Features.

Philaretou, A. G., & Allen, K. R. (2003). Macro and micro dynamics of male sexual anxiety: Theory and intervention. *International Journal of Men's Health, 2,* 201–220.

Piercy, F., & Benson, K. (2005). Aesthetic forms of data representation in qualitative family therapy research. *Journal of Marital and Family Therapy, 31,* 107–119.

Piercy, F., & Thomas, V. (1998). Participatory evaluation research: An introduction for family therapists. *Journal of Marital and Family Therapy, 24,* 165–176.

Quinney, R. (1996). Once my father traveled west to California. In C. Ellis & A. P. Bochner (Eds.), *Composing ethnography: Alternative forms of qualitative writing* (pp. 357–382). Walnut Creek, CA: AltaMira Press.

Reinharz, S. (1992). *Feminist methods in social research.* New York: Oxford University Press.

Ricci, R. (2003). Autoethnographic verse: Nicky's boy: A life in two worlds. *The Qualitative Report, 8*(4), 591–596.

Richardson, L. (2000a). Evaluating ethnography. *Qualitative Inquiry, 6,* 253–255.

Richardson, L. (2000b). Writing: A method of inquiry. In N. K. Denzin & Y. S. Lincoln (Eds.), *Collecting and interpreting qualitative materials* (pp. 499–551). Thousand Oaks, CA: Sage.

Satir, V. (1972). *Peoplemaking.* Palo Alto, CA: Science & Behavior Books.

Sher, G. (1999). *One continuous mistake: Four noble truths for writers.* New York: Compass.

Silverstein, L. B., & Goodrich, T. J. (Eds.). (2003). *Feminist family therapy: Empowerment in social context.* Washington, DC: American Psychological Association.

Smith, D. E. (1987). *The everyday world as problematic: A feminist sociology.* Boston: Northeastern University Press.

Stacey, J. (1988). Can there be a feminist ethnography? *Women's Studies International Forum, 11,* 21–27.

Stanley, L., & Wise, S. (1993). *Breaking out again: Feminist ontology and epistemology* (2nd ed.). London: Routledge.

Taggart, M. (1985). The feminist critique in epistemological perspective: Questions of context in family therapy. *Journal of Marital and Family Therapy, 11,* 113–126.

Tedlock, B. (2003). Ethnography and ethnographic representation. In N. K. Denzin & Y. S. Lincoln (Eds.), *Strategies of qualitative inquiry* (2nd ed., pp. 165–213). Thousand Oaks, CA: Sage.

Tenni, C., Smyth, A., & Boucher, C. (2003). The researcher as autobiographer: Analyzing data written about oneself. *The Qualitative Report, 8*(1), 1–12.

Vatcher, C., & Bogo, M. (2001). The feminist/emotionally focused therapy practice model: An integrated approach for couple therapy. *Journal of Marital and Family Therapy, 27,* 69–83.

Walters, M., Carter, B., Papp, P., & Silverstein, O. (1988). *The invisible web: Gender patterns in family relationships.* New York: Guilford Press.

Weingarten, K. (1991). The discourses of intimacy: Adding a social constructionist and feminist view. *Family Process, 30,* 285–305.

Whitaker, C., & Keith, D. (1981). Symbolic–experiential family therapy. In A. S. Gurman & D. P. Kniskern (Eds.), *Handbook of family therapy* (pp. 187–225). New York: Brunner/Mazel.

White, M., & Epston, D. (1990). *Narrative means to therapeutic ends.* New York: Norton.

Yllo, K., & Bograd, M. (Eds.). (1988). *Feminist perspectives on wife abuse.* Newbury Park, CA: Sage.

CHAPTER 10

Performance Methodology

CONSTRUCTING DISCOURSES AND DISCURSIVE PRACTICES IN FAMILY THERAPY RESEARCH

SALIHA BAVA

> Life can only be understood backwards, but it must be lived forwards.
> —KIERKEGAARD (quoted in Magee, 2001, p. 208)

Danish philosopher Søren Kierkegaard's words echo my experience of writing various research reports. I often find myself working backwards to construct what I have lived through. Even though I use a blueprint, I find myself at the "end" constructing a story to fit the acceptable frame in terms of using the "right" language, "right" format, and "right" presentation methods. There is a performative quality to the process, from proposal to research report. So when I had to work on my dissertation research, I chose to use an alternative research methodology that I call "performance." The form of performance methodology I used draws heavily from autoethnography (Ellis & Bochner, 1996; Reed-Danahay, 1997) and interpretive writing (Denzin, 2003; Richardson, 1997). Piercy and Benson (2005) describe my research project (which they call a "multimethod computer-assisted autoethnography") this way:

> Saliha Bava (2001) recently completed a virtual, completely-on-line dissertation at Virginia Tech. Her dissertation was an autoethnography of her research and personal experience during her family therapy internship at the Houston Galveston Institute. She immersed herself in and reflectively explored both the culture of the Institute, and her experience of it. She used many alternative forms of data representation—poetry, colors, animations, multiple conversations (with others, herself, and the literature), split dialogues, and other methods to bring her findings to life. Her styles of narration (words, graphics, prose, poetry, first person conversational texts, narratives, and collages) blurred the boundaries between academic writing, literature, and art. At the same time, she used hypertext to ground her own experience in relevant literature. She also had her committee reflect on their experiences of reading her dissertation (in a "reflections" section of her dissertation), and then responded to these reflections. In postmodern fashion, she built into her dissertation both recursion and reflection. (pp. 114–115)

In this chapter, I invite you to an overview of performance discourse and methodology, which I illustrate through discussing (and performing) selected parts of my dissertation research. I also provide a reflexive commentary on methodology as performance. Finally, in the discussion section, I address the questions raised by this book's editors in Chapter 1. This chapter itself represents a performance in discourse construction and discursive practices in research.

BACKGROUND

Constructing Performance Methodology

Setting: As the curtain rises, the audience walks into an ongoing conversation. Two researchers (R1 and R2) are seated in a coffee shop.

R1: I'm confused. Should I call it "performance methodology," or am I deconstructing methodology and reconstructing it is as performance?

R2: What does it matter, as long as your intent is to approach it as performance?

R1: It definitely matters, since the process is as important as the product. How I arrive at the end product is informed by what I assumed to be my beginning guides and by what and how I choose to include and exclude. My assumptions about performance are informing research and have implications for practice.

R2: All I care about is getting the research done and accepted as credible and useful.

R1: And how you go about doing it, and who sanction it as "research," are all parts of credibility building and utility. As Bentz and Shapiro (1998) point out, yesterday's frameworks, problems, and paradigms are replaced by new ones; so too are methodologies. We have adopted methodologies from other fields, and it's time to look and understand what performance studies discourses have to offer methodologically. Often I find that methodologies lag behind the epistemological assumptions that we adopt. Unfortunately, our assumptions of research practices are drawn from traditional schools of thought, even as our assumptions of what we know and how we know are changing. If we believe that we are living in postmodern times, then, in keeping with the performative turn, I ask you this: How are we performing methodologically?

R2: Wow! That's too heady for me! So is this a new research technique?

R1: I'm afraid that it will be received as a unitary method, rather than as something that is evolving. I think that in the search for the technique of performance methodology, we may risk losing sight of the idea that it is a way of framing the research process from a political–philosophical perspective.

R2: So is "performance" a qualifier of the type of methodology one chooses, or is it a philosophy that informs the research process—and thus one uses performance as a philosophical thread that ties together the techniques (drawn from other methods) to create the performance methodology?

R1: I fear that the editors, readers, consumers, and producers may be looking for a recipe for "performance methodology." I view it as a political–philosophical approach to research process that helps a researcher to construct a methodology in sync with his or her theory of knowledge construction (epistemology). However, due to the evolving constructions and the fluid nature of meaning making, especially in the realms of performative practices, I am hesitant to state what "performative practices" are or how they are enacted by researchers. I am afraid that if I do so, performance might get institutionalized. Rather than it being "received," I would prefer it to become part of an ongoing dialogue about our research practices and enhance our reflexivity about our methodological choices.

R2: So what is "performance"?

R1: One of the ideas is that performance is one of the cutting-edge practices of social constructionist theory, à la Kenneth and Mary Gergen and the East Side Institute (S. Levin, personal communication, 2003). The performative turn is related to the blurring of the boundaries between art and science, literary and scientific, real and virtual, and nature and nurture. Such turns are not only being heralded as innovative genres in clinical practices but also in research methodologies (Denzin, 2003; Piercy & Benson, 2005). Since both research and practice are imbued by theory, the performative "turn" does just that: It turns theory on itself and questions the boundaries among research, practice, and theory. It thus furthers the dialogue of blurring boundaries.

I entered the performance of writing this chapter with multiple voices, and reenacted the dialogue above as an ongoing internal and external dialogue that I continue to perform. My enactment is a postmodern dialogue I am performing as I write this chapter, complete with multiple voices and postmodern tensions that are informing this production. Hassan (quoted in Carlson, 1996) states:

> Postmodernism veers toward open, playful, optative, disjunctive, displaced, indeterminate forms, a discourse of fragments, an ideology of fracture, a will to unmaking, an invocation of silence—veers towards all these and yet implies their very opposition, their antithetical realities. (Carlson, 1996, p. 124)

At the risk of bringing forth a singularity—an antithesis from a postmodern perspective, yet very much in keeping with another postmodern notion of constructing diametrical opposites, herein the case of singularity–plurality—I introduce Kaye's (1994) notion of "performance." He states that "the condition of 'performance' may be read, in itself, as tending to foster or look towards postmodern contingencies or instabilities," and that performance "may be thought of as a *primary postmodern mode*" (quoted in Carlson, 1996, p. 123; emphasis added). Denzin (2003) elaborates on this: "Performance is an act of intervention, a method of resistance, a form of criticism, a way of revealing agency . . . performance is a form of agency, a way of bringing culture and the person into play" (p. 9). He distinguishes "performativity" and "performance" as "doing" and "done," as verb form and noun form. However, one of the pioneers of performance studies, Richard Schechner (2002), discusses performance in terms of "is" and "as":

> What is the difference between "is" performance and "as" performance? . . . There are limits to what "is" performance. But just about anything can be studied "as" performance. Something "is" a performance when historical and social context, conventions, usage, and tradition say it is. . . . One cannot determine what "is" performance without referring to specific cultural circumstances. There is nothing inherent in an action in itself that makes it

a performance. . . . Any behavior, event, action, or thing can be studied "as" performance, can be analysed in terms of doing, behaving, and showing. (pp. 30–31)

There is no consensus, then, about what performance is. All performances or actions that are culturally categorized as "performance" are socially constructed by the collective consensus of that sociocultural group within a particular time and space (historical period). Drawing on Schechner (2002), I assert that any methodology is performative and can be understood "as" performance. What makes it performance is when communities of academics and researchers or other authority-granting mechanisms agree to its performance construction. I view the notions of "performative," "as performance," and "performance" on a continuum. So a methodology act evolves from being a performative act to the act being understood as performance, to the act becoming performance. In other words, its construction evolves or is created from an adjective (qualifier function), to a metaphor (comparative notion), to a verb form (an action), or a noun (an object).

Schechner (2002) states that "a performance takes place only in action, interaction, and relation. Performance isn't 'in' anything, but 'between' " (p. 24). Turner (quoted in Schechner, 2002) states that the "liminal space" is "the betwixt and between spaces" where transformation occurs. Thus liminal spaces are where the discourses are constructed. One such space is among the research communities in universities.

Research Performances in Universities

City University of New York Distinguished Professor of English, poet, and essayist Charles Bernstein's (2000) critical commentary on dissertation styles captures the universities' research norms: "Let them be radical in what they say but not in how they say it." Bernstein asserts that "underneath the mask of career-minded concessions to normalcy is an often repressed epistemological positivism about the representation of ideas." Thus, from a "both–and" position, the research created by universities is guided by the discourses of political institutions (universities) and is not. The "not" consists of attempts by graduate students to experiment with alternative research methodologies (Bochner & Ellis, 2002; Denzin & Lincoln, 2003) such as autoethnography. Though some of these institutions offer students latitude with research methodologies, they are constrained by the larger discourse of acceptable and legitimate ways of researching and reporting or re-presenting.

In this chapter I illustrate performative methodologies, methodology as performance, and performance methodology as ways for researchers to situate their research and methodology. I present one way to construct, perform, and critically analyze methodology embedded in the performance discourse.

Philosophical Assumptions

The key assumptions that inform performance research methodology are these:

1. Research is a politically engaged activity. It is a transgressive performance that critically questions the status quo and is itself seeking legitimization or is legitimized by communal consensus of the authority-granting knowledge community.

2. Research is not a representation of an act or phenomenon that is studied; rather, it is a presentation of "exemplary and radical" alternatives and possibilities

(Carlson, 1996, p. 142) of the researched content. The substantive and the methodological aspects of research are critically scrutinized as part of the research process. Thus the methodology also becomes an integral part of the substantive material of the inquiry.

   3. The performative aspect of such a methodology is aimed at the destabilization of norms, the dissolution of certainties, and the presentation of critical questioning of what is constructed both as normative research and the researcher's product as research.

   4. Research is situated historically, socially, and culturally. It is written and read at particular times; with particular intents; under particular political conditions; and from particular cultural, economic, racial, class, gender, personal, and other perspectives. Research is a performance of contextualized multiple ideologies.

Historical Roots and Development

According to sociologist and social theorist Michal McCall (2003), "the term performance entered critical art and academic discourses in the 1970s, to name a new visual art form and to distinguish dramatic scripts from particular productions of them—that is, from performances on stage" (p. 112). Drawing on conventional histories, McCall locates the root of performance in the early 20th century.

   Denzin (2003) describes four groups of genealogical roots of performance text, each telling a different story. He traces performance through (1) language and narrative roots, beginning with Nietzsche and moving through critical pedagogy, feminist theory, and Marxist theory into ethnography; (2) "the dramaturgical turn," beginning with Erving Goffman and moving through anthropologists Bruke and Victor Turner to Mienczakowski's ethnodramas; (3) "performance art and performance studies" roots, as traced by McCall and concluding in the formation of performance ethnography, which draws on both social sciences and the arts and humanities; and (4) the "pedagogical turn," drawing on Paulo Freire's oppositional pedagogy, the discourses of critical pedagogy, and the works of McLaren and Giroux.

   Marvin Carlson (1996), professor of theatre and comparative literature at the City University of New York, provides a thorough critical review of the notion of performance from anthropological, sociological, psychological, linguistic, and artistic perspectives. In his book *Performance: A Critical Introduction*, he states that social performance theorists such as philosophers or psychologists tend to "emphasize the activities and operations of the performer" (1996, p. 38). However, sociologists (also identified as social performance theorists) and cultural performance theorists emphasize "the audience, or . . . the community in which performance occurs" (p. 38).

   Performance is a social constructionist (Anderson, 1997; Bava, 2003; K. Gergen, 1991, 1994a, 1994b, 1999; M. Gergen, 2001) notion of meaning making as a communal process, in that it occurs in language and dialogue. Performance metaphorically expands the symbolic meaning of dialogue. Such practice raises our reflexivity and heightens our sensitivity to the notion of shared inquiry as we ask one another, "What are we doing here?" (M. Gergen, 2001). The notion of performance as displayed via improvisational theater games[1] (Bava, 2003; Spolin, 1999) brings forth the notion of language games and of "discourse" as verb. It highlights the production of discursive cultural practices not unlike those we are involved in on a daily basis.

---

[1] A team of therapists at the Houston Galveston Institute has been experimenting with improvisational theater games as an evolving performance practice in therapy, consultation, and training.

Performance allows the unorthodox to occur. It has created space for the blurring of boundaries between science and fiction, academia and the arts (Bava, 2001; M. Gergen, 2001; Piercy & Benson, 2005). "Perform" becomes the verb form of discourse and brings forth the notion of "language games" (Wittgenstein, 1965). It is discourse in action. Consequently, performance is not limited to the postmodern discourse; rather, it expands the notion of discourse in action to include both modern and postmodern ideas and practices. The performance metaphor allows the traditional and the alternative to coexist, which is at the heart of the notion of postmodernism. This metaphor provides the researcher with expanding possibilities for what can be included in research practices. So, depending on one's theoretical frame and chosen discourses, if one wishes to locate oneself with the tradition of traditional academia and produce a report that is criticized by the alternative writing forums as being stale and dry, such a report can also be upheld as a performance. It can reflexively be identified as a *traditional academic performative act*, a "standard" way of writing that is itself a perfected art form.

METHODOLOGY: A PERFORMATIVE ACT

Performance can be viewed as a method of re-presentation or as a methodology. As a method for re-presentation (see Table 10.1), a performance script is created. According to McCall (2003), a script requires a cast and/or a performance and/or a staging. The parallels between research process and performance scripting are presented in Table 10.1, based on McCall's suggestions.

In performance as methodology, the philosophical assumptions are embodied and performed throughout the research process. So how these are performed in the plan-

TABLE 10.1. Parallels between Writing an Ethnographic Report and Writing a Performance Script

Research process	Ethnographic report	Performance script
Reading notes/data	Creating analytic themes	Creating characters that embody themes
	Orienting information	Is embodied in the script
Analysis and explanation	Analytical commentary	Done by the characters Characteristics of the actor
Research report	Writing up notes and reporting	Scripting
Data as quotations	Excerpts from field notes	Dialogue for the characters
Organizing the research report sections	Ordering of sections	Dividing script into acts
Chapter 1	Introduction	The stage setting
Chapter 2	Literature review	Scripts and characterization of the characters
Last chapter	Conclusion	The experience of the script

Note. Entries in the "Performance script" column are informed by or quoted from McCall (2003).

ning, research design, data collection, analysis, and presentation stages need to be reported.

We are consumers, producers, and products of discourses. As researchers, we are both situating ourselves in discourses and discursively producing them. By situating ourselves in selected discourses, we not only exhibit our consumption, but also illustrate how we are products of the discourses. For instance, in my research, by stating that I was drawing on phenomenology, heuristics, and ethnography, I positioned myself as a critical consumer. However, I was also a producer, as I drew critically from these approaches.

All research is performative. That is, an inquiry is a performative study of an activity that is presented as a performance. For instance, my dissertation was a threefold inquiry. First, I constructed the culture of internship in an institute of postmodern training, as experienced by me as a doctoral intern. Second, the work was my performance as a researcher of alternative methodology. Third, I employed hypertext (itself a performance) as a subversive activity to standard research presentations.

My dissertation, *Transforming Performances: An Intern-Researcher's Hypertextual Journey in a Postmodern Community* (Bava, 2001), was an intertextual script, a rendition, of my internship (1998–1999) and research (1998–2001) experiences. I performed the presentation as a dissertation web, a hypertext located within multiple discourses. In my research, I used this web as a performative medium to create a circular text rather then a linear text, where I challenged the canonical norms of how to present a research report. I constructed my dissertation as a website[2] with inter- and intralinked web pages. The reader is partially free to choose where he or she will go next by choosing from a variety of hyperlinks on any given page. Thus no two readers' experiences will be the same (except for statistical probabilities), due to the linked paths each reader chooses.

Research Questions

What family therapy research questions does this methodology answer? For me, it answered discursive questions subversive of the taken-for-granted ways of being. I raised and pondered research questions that were intertextual and critical, such that they questioned authority—my own, that of my peers, and that of institutionalized norms. Since research is constructed/enacted as political activity, research questions are intended to engage the researcher, the participants, and the readers in transgressive, resistant, reconstructive reflections of our everyday practices. Such questions emphasize relational and interactional understandings of the unit of inquiry (object). Thus the research questions are constructed as "what the object does, how it interacts with other objects or beings, and how it relates to other objects or beings" (Schechner, 2002, p. 24).

In my dissertation research, my main question was this: "What is the culture of internship in an institute of postmodern training, as experienced by me as a doctoral intern?" My goal was to perform this experience critically, as I self-consciously located

---

[2] Visit the website (*http://scholar.lib.vt.edu/theses/available/etd-01062002-234843*) and select either of two links (*11exclusive_diss_web.pdf* or *12intertextual_diss_web.pdf*).

   If the website is unavailable, go to Virginia Tech's Electronic Theses and Dissertations search page (*http://scholar.lib.vt.edu/theses/etd-search.html*) and enter the search word "Bava."

myself in the research process and subversively questioned more traditional research presentations via the performance of hypertext. In the ensuing section, drawing on my research, I illustrate how I constructed methodology as performance.

Methodology as Performance: An Illustration

As a producer and consumer of discourses, I drew on Kenneth Gergen's (1997) organization of textual traditions in human science writing. I chose to perform like an "autobiographer." On his web page, Gergen describes the autobiographer as one who

> typically strives to present the fullness of life as experienced. Similar to the mystical and the prophetic, autobiographical writing is replete with expressions of value. However, such expressions are not typically in the service of chastising the reader for his/her deficiencies, but for justifying actions taken. The reader is left, then, to draw object lessons from these accounts. The autobiography does share much with the myth, in terms of the commands of narrative coherence. However, these demands are often sacrificed for purposes of sharing the "lived experience" with the reader. . . . Perhaps the most significant characteristic of the genre is born of its attempt to share subjectivity, to enable the reader to stand in for the writer. This often means a high reliance on affectively charged language (for example, of the passions or the spirit, heavy usage of quotidian discourse (the reality shared by all), and a substantial reliance on metaphor (enabling the reader to sense the qualities of a unique experience).

The autobiographer draws the reader closer to the author, whose experience is rendered transparent and accessible. I further described my relationship with discourse as my reflexive understanding of my preferred position as a writer who is performing intertextually. My work was located within Gergen's scholarship (discourse), which provided me with a "language game" (Wittgenstein, 1965) as I created my performative dissertation web. I co-created the rules of the game along with members of the languaged community of performative scholarship, social construction, writing practices, academics, and other discourses. As I co-created the rules, I was scripting a performance discourse. I was defining how to be as an autoethnographer, an autobiographer—a researcher and an intern. And, recursively, the various discourses molded my performance as a researcher and an intern.

Performing Discourse

> The motivating spirit of experimentation is thus anti-genre, to avoid the reinstatement of a restricted canon like that of the recent past.
>
> —MARCUS AND FISCHER (1999, p. 42)

My dissertation web was thus located within multiple discourses—postmodernism, performance, hypertext, academic writing, crises of representation, textual practices, internships, training, and the Houston Galveston Institute's cultural and historical discourses, to name a few. I chose and located myself among the various discourses, depending on the context and the relationships. Harlene Anderson (personal communications, 1998–2001) states that relationships form, inform, and disform our conversations, and that our conversations form, inform, and disform our relationships. Thus at any given moment I was performing a number of discourses, depending on my relationships and conversations.

Performing Meaning

In my dissertation, I performed meaning primarily via intertextual presentations. These intertextual presentations took two primary forms: "narratives" and "hypertexts." Narratives are chunks of texts telling a story of my internship or research process experience. I identified the narratives as "swirling–fragmented narratives." Each story is part of the whole—the dissertation web of my experience. At any given moment, each swirling–fragmented narrative is detached and incomplete; simultaneously, it is also a whole—a story in itself. However, depending on the context of meaning construction, the reader may experience the text as fragmented or as a whole; and as a structured metaphor of my experience or a structuring element of my experience.

Hypertexts consist of chunks of text connected to each other electronically. According to Kolb (2000), hypertext is more of a technological utilization than a literary form, even though the hypertext writing style varies from print text. For some hypertext writers (Bernstein, 1999, 2001; Landow, 1997), hypertext is more about the patterns of link rather than the electronic linking of the text. The pattern of linking adds another level of complexity to the narratives, thus introducing the notion of polyvocality as a performance of the consensual community members co-constructing knowledge.

Another way of understanding performing meaning is to view my research writing as a threefold performance: (1) as an academic discourse acted out, (2) as a creation of the writer in dialogue with self and others/readers, and (3) as an art of re-presenting and re-(new)-creating of the research process.

Performing Writing

> In short, the poetic essay offers a more nuanced account in keeping with the spirit of the performative event itself. The performance scholar, then, might wish to articulate what he/she knows not through the mirroring positivistic logic but through a reliance on the poetic.
>
> —PELIAS (1999, p. xi)

I want to tell the story of my struggle with "how I should perform the text." I used three performative writing practices in an effort to draw the reader, as far as possible, into my world—unfamiliar and nonduplicable—to experience my story vicariously. First, I created an experience of circularity—no fixed beginning or end. Second, I (re)created fragmentation as experienced in my internship and the research process as an integral part of the backdrop of the text for the reader. Third, I practiced multiple interpretive positioning (Tillmann-Healy, 1996).

Writing, like an art, is a dynamic process (Richardson, 1997) and a construction among people (the writer and the intended readers—editor, committee chair and members, colleagues, friends and family, etc.). However, most students are not told about how the writing gets done because of the separation of scholarly work from teaching (Becker, 1986). The process of writing, editing, and rewriting is the process of knowledge construction for a consensual community. In this instance, the academic community constituted the consensual knowledge community as deemed by my research committee. However, before I even gave people a draft of my writing, I was engaged in numerous conversations about my writing. I wrote several beginning drafts before I decided upon a particular format. One of my beginning drafts was a description of the year as a play. On reviewing it, I thought it lacked the "oomph" I wanted and did not convey the story I wanted to share within a particular context. Even though it seemed to be innovative, it lacked certain postmodern dimensions—reflexivity, nonlinearity, multiple entries and exits, scholarly connections to multiple scholarly works—that I wanted to include. So I dropped the story line of a script for a play. However, the incomplete play provided me with a condensed version of my experience. I could see how the plot was built around a conflictual interpersonal relationship. Though that was part of the internship story I wanted to tell, I did not want it to be the only story. I also wanted to narrate the stories of how I grew as a therapist, of myself as a researcher studying myself, and of how I struggled within the challenges of what is doable as research. The initial drafts were ways I processed my intense feelings about the internship. I wrote these over a period of 4–5 months.

Writing-in-Inquiry

> The play with writing techniques brings to consciousness and the sense that continued innovation in the nature of ethnography can be a tool in the development of theory.
>
> —MARCUS AND FISCHER (1999, p. 42)

Though Marcus and Fischer (1999) are talking about innovation in ethnography, their statement captures for me the process of writing as a performance of and performing theory. The ensuing text is a reaccount of the process of writing as performing inquiry.

"Writing-in-inquiry" is the process of theory development (co-creating knowledge), innovation, and transformation via writing. It is a reflexive practice that generates creativity and innovation and is not limited by disciplinary boundaries or discourses. Traditional writing practices (third-person, authoritative genres that distance the reader) are limiting for a number of writers and readers (Richardson, 1997). Thus writing-in-inquiry is a practice that includes the traditional and new literary forms, which blur disciplinary boundaries.

Over the past 15 years, writing genres using the new literary forms have been growing in the fields of sociology, anthropology, women's studies, and critical cultural schools, thus closing the gap between scientific and literary discourses that has existed since the 17th century (Richardson, 1997). We have seen an evolution of plurality, polyphony, dialogue, reflexivity, and deconstruction as a critique and response to positivism, objectivism, and crises of representation. Other forms of postmodern praxis include the new writing genres in social sciences, such as performance scripts (McCall & Becker, 1990), second-voice device, decentering original texts (Schneider, 1991), poetry (Richardson, 1993, 1997), drama (Ellis & Bochner, 1996; Richardson, 1993, 1997; Richardson & Lockridge, 1991), polyvocal texts (Schneider, 1991), and web text (Pockley, 1999, 2000). However, such genres are relatively new to the disciplines of psychology in general and of marriage and family therapy (MFT) in particular. Both MFT and psychology could gain from these types of writing-in-inquiry. Feminist critique and postmodern approaches have added a critical edge to MFT. Such critique has introduced innovative therapeutic practice strategies; however, postmodern and critical ideas are not very prevalent in the field's research writing practices. There has been a proliferation of qualitative studies, but the push for quantitative methodologies that reflect standard scientific practice remains.

Writing-in-inquiry that uses alternative writing practices is not yet common in MFT, even though qualitative research has increased. The writing has moved to be more inclusive of the research participants' voices; however, an authoritative authorial presence generally continues. And as long as we continue moving in the direction of being diagnosticians of mental health, we continue to risk privileging a researcher's final word over a participant's word. Writing as being-in-inquiry, rather than as a way of presenting the results of a research, is consistent with our field's move in the direction of therapists as conversational partners who share expertise with individuals, couples, and families.

I describe below how I attempted to bring to life the practice of writing-in-inquiry with respect to data collection, re-presentation, analyses, and interpretation.

WRITING TO COLLECT DATA

Journal.

> The journal is a journey. . . . Its purpose, in part, is to give voice to the heart and sound of one's domestic and far-flung thoughts."
>
> —BRONER (quoted in Schiwy, 1996, back cover)

I felt that the process of journaling my experiences at the Institute, though private, could also touch universal experiences—hope, fears, confusions, and magical moments. Journaling has been widely used by writers in women's studies and other fields to make sense of their own experience, to find their own voices, and to heal themselves (Baldwin, 1977); it is a powerful tool of creative expression as well (Baldwin, 1977; Bell-Scott, 1994; Hogan, 1991; Schiwy, 1996; Simons, 1978).

Journaling from the feminist perspective has often been viewed as giving voice to the subjugated, to the other, to what a woman has denied to herself (Bell-Scott, 1994). The emphasis has been on a woman finding her inner self or owning what is rightfully hers. Though all this seemed to make sense to me, it did not fit for me or the purpose for which I wanted to use journaling in my research. My feminist readings did refer to the self in relation to others, but this was very different from the "relational self" (K. Gergen, 1991, 1994b), which refers to the self as constituted by language and dialogue (K. Gergen, 1991, 1994a, 1994b). According to the narrative metaphor, the self is storied and is ever changing (Polkinghorne, 1988). I took a social-constructionist position, which emphasizes the historicity and fluidity of gendering (Agger, 1998).

I used journaling as one of my predominant methods of data collection, for this reason:

> Any change in ourselves, any move toward greater self-awareness, authenticity, and openness, will affect those around us. Each step we take toward genuine creative expression sends ripples out into the world, and often, they may spread much further than we might imagine. The personal is universal. (Schiwy, 1996, p. 300)

"Self" means the relational self; self-awareness is a sociocultural product; and culture defines and constitutes the boundaries of the self, just as the self constitutes culture (Lock, 1981). Thus constituting myself as an *intern* in my journals was constructing the sociocultural practices of the Institute in that moment of journaling.

The journals I kept of my internship experience over a period of 10 months were intended to be daily entries. In the initial months of the internship, I kept daily entries of the activities I attended and reflections of my experience. However, as the daily conflictual interchanges increased, the entries became sketchy. There were days when I did not make entries because I found myself exhausted from interactions, and I did not want to write about negative exchanges since I did not want to relive those moments. When I had proposed the journal as the primary source of data collection, I had not anticipated the potential emotional impact of writing about "negative experiences." Even though I had expected that there might be certain surprises that I might not like, I had not expected the experiences to be so overwhelmingly depressing. In the initial months of my internship, I taped some conversational clusters that I was part of, but discontinued the process as the internship climate changed.

Autobiography.

> Autobiography adheres more closely to the true potential of the genre the more its real subject matter is character, personality, self-conception—all those difficult-to-define matters which ultimately determine the inner coherence and the meaning of a life.
>
> —WEINTRAUB (quoted by Broughton & Anderson, 1997, p. 182)

Another form of data collection method of personal experience is autobiography (Clandinin & Connelly, 1994). Autobiography is closely linked to journal writing. Indeed, a journal is a kind of autobiographical writing. Autobiographical writing attempts to capture the whole context of life, while journals include the small fragments of experience that lack this context (Clandinin & Connelly, 1994, p. 421).

In the book *Names We Call Home*, Thompson and Tyagi (1996) illustrate the power of autobiography via contributors' stories of how they "became raced" by recounting their childhood experiences of contradictions about race. Thompson and Tyagi used autobiography to illustrate "why racial identity formation occurs at the intersection of a person's subjective memory of trauma and collective remembrance of histories of domination" (p. xii).

Contributors to Thompson and Tyagi's (1996) book found that autobiography enabled them to explore their individual life histories as they tapped into communal memory and experience. Similarly, in the process of telling my story, I tapped into my memory and experience of how I became aware of the larger social process of discourse and emerging discourse formations. I also found autobiography to be a useful means of data collection, since personal narratives bring forth the politics of self-definition (Thompson & Tyagi, 1996). Self-definition is a process of social meaning making (Lemke, 1995) via conversations (Anderson, 1997) in the context of ever-present discourses and emerging discourses. One's own self-definition reflects one's values and belief system, which are recursively defined by one's culture (Lock, 1981). My story, then, re-presents a "politics of self-definition." Furthermore, my experiences of the research training I had in ethnography and my dissertation research experiences are captured in the words of Thompson and Tyagi: "Many of the contributors' most complex and startling insights were ones they didn't actually 'know' until they wrote them" (p. xiii). This was certainly true for me, and it is also one reason why journaling and writing are used in therapy as homework and used by therapists in letters to their clients (White & Epston, 1990).

(Re)telling methodology is performance in autobiographical storytelling. Or one may also view (re)telling methodology as performing a story. The former is a creation of a script, and the latter involves acting the script. However, both are performances; one is scripting a performance, and the other is performing a script.

Research Audit. As part of the research process, I kept a research audit from the time of writing the research proposal until the final submission of the dissertation to the graduate school. The audit included my comments on the process, my feelings, and my notes on how or what I was changing in the research. The audit also included my thoughts on different sections and plans for future writing.

Reviews. Viewing various texts as "data," I maintained an e-folder with notes from my readings of various texts. Flemons (1998), in his book *Writing between the Lines*, describes a method to manage one's literature review data. Adopting his method, I had an e-file for each reading—each book, article, dissertation, or website I consulted. I maintained quotes and my reflections for each reading in its e-file. Subsequently, I created a thematic e-file where I collated the notes from various authors by such themes as narrative, hypertext, content and form, collaborative learning communities, and so on.

WRITING TO RE-PRESENT

> We write in the moment and reflect our minds, emotions, environment in that moment. This does not mean that one is truer than the other—they are all true.
>
> —GOLDBERG (1986, p. 115)

Goldberg's words capture my experience with writing. I found myself writing and rewriting a number of times. And I knew everything I wrote was "true." The questions I kept asking myself were "Which of my experiences do I choose to include or exclude?", "What goes in or out?", "How do I decide what goes in or out?", and the like.

Writing to re-present involved mixing genres. I combined a number of new literary forms along with narrative prose in my (hyper)textual production. The intention was to convey the complexity of the research and internship experiences and to provide the reader with a window into my multiple selves. I used layered accounts, swirling–fragmented narratives, scripts, and poetry as forms of writing to re-present my lived experiences as an intern and a researcher.

Layered Accounts. Ronai (1992) defines a "layered account" as "shifting forward, backward, and sideways through time, space, and various attitudes in a narrative format" (p. 103). I used layered accounts in sections I called "The Story of Stormy Emotions" and "Poetic Re-presentation of Methodology" to invite the reader to my experiences of temporal and spatial shifts.

Swirling–Fragmented Narratives. I combined the notion of fragmentation (Bava, 2001; Bloom, 1998) with narrative to introduce the notion of a "swirling–fragmented narrative." Each story (a "lexia") is part of the whole—the dissertation web of my experience. Each lexia is detached and incomplete, and simultaneously a whole—a story in itself. However, depending on the context of meaning construction, the reader may experience the text as fragmented or as a whole, as a structured metaphor of my experience or a structuring of my experience. My intention was (and is) to invite the reader to construct the context jointly with me in virtual space and time, and thus together we will perform each "reading"—fragmented or defragmented.

Scripts. I used dialogues to perform the multiple voices I was bringing to life in my experience as a researcher and as an intern. Utilizing scripts also introduced polyvocality—that is, other interns' experiences. I did this not by describing any particular intern's experience in detail, but by tapping into my various intern conversations. Thus, by blurring the boundary between "fact" and "fiction," I created an interpreted description of interns' commentary on the Institute.

Poetry. I interspersed prose with poetry, which emerged as a form of presentation to "capture" my sense of the recreated experiences. Poetry has the power to create subjunctive texts that are fluid and inviting, while conveying a fluid "description" of the experience.

WRITING TO ANALYZE AND INTERPRET

> Meanings are made within communities and . . . the analysis of meaning should not be separated from the social, historical, cultural and political dimensions of these communities.
>
> —LEMKE (1995, p. 9)

Analyses and interpretations are cultural practices of the communities we belong to and are matters of opinion (Wolcott, 1994). Coffey and Atkinson's (1996) position that analysis is a reflexive activity informed my data collection, writing, and further data collection. I viewed analysis and interpretation as a dialogical conversation within a consensual community interwoven with "data collection," rather than a post-data-collection activity. The reflexive process of writing to re-present was inclusive of my interpretation, since while writing I felt the presence of my colleagues over my shoulders (Wolcott, 1994). According to Wolcott (1994), "our interpretations are our claims to the independent creation of new knowledge" (p. 258) that we do to be profound; however, they are always matters of consensus within the traditions in which we locate ourselves (Bruffee, 1999; Lemke, 1995; Wolcott, 1994).

Approaching analysis and interpretation as social practices of the academic community, and language as social semiotics or communal meaning making (Lemke, 1995), I utilized the following practices in the performances of the various stories of my internship and research.

Stories as Interpretations. I wrote stories about my internship experiences and research as interpretations about my experiences. The stories are not *the* experiences. The practices of making sense of my experiences and presenting them as narratives, poetry, script, or multimedia were all interpretive constructions of the experiences that I was writing about.

Stories about Stories. Related to the preceding was the practice of constructing texts, interpretive texts, as stories about stories. Every storytelling was an interpretive effort; thus the whole dissertation web was (and is) an illustration of stories about stories. The stories of textual production are another layer of interpretation of my efforts at meaning making.

Afterwords. An "afterwords" (Richardson, 1997) included words that I wrote from a reflective position after I completed a thematic lexia. The afterwords might be stories about stories, process reflections of my writing experience (and in turn of my research experience), and/or epilogues.

Interwoven Reflexive Narratives. Within the stories of my internship and research, I interspersed narratives as reflections of what I was doing textually. Drawing on the notion of reflexivity, I created narratives questioning the built-in interpretations of the texts. Thus I was (and am) suggesting that the reader read the text on a number of different levels and continually stay in a critically questioning dialogue with whichever interpretation he or she takes away from the text.

Decentering Text. Drawing on sociologist Joseph Schneider's (1991) critiques of textual authority, I boldfaced certain words as a practice of **reflexivity** and **analysis**, so that the focus of the reader might shift from the content of a lexia to the phrases and words in boldface. At times the hyperlinks served the same purpose. My intent was to draw attention to my reflexivity, as a further commentary on the textual production.

Reflexive Afterwords: Constructing Performance Methodology

I have written this chapter as a performance. At many points, the writing is itself a dissent from what should be written or how it should be written (i.e., the editors' guidelines for chapter authors). I have been constantly gripped by thoughts that maybe I should have just written the chapter strictly according to the suggested section subheadings. But to diverge is to create. Did I do what I did to create divergence or to create dissent? Did I do it because I had a hard time following an outline? Did I do it to illustrate performativity in action? Did I do it because this is more suited to my writing style? To answer any one or all of these questions in the affirmative is in itself a performance of meaning making. This goes exactly to my point about discourse construction. That is, as researchers we are constantly in the processes of constructing discourses. By choosing to be informed by a particular methodology and to "follow the steps" of that particular methodology, we are participating in the formation, building, and legitimizing of that research methodology's community or discourse community. To call it a performance is to recognize our (researcher selves') processes of participating in the political act of discourse or culture (re-)formation (Denzin, 2003). These processes are illustrated in both the reader's reflexivity and the researcher's reflection.

I have chosen to write this chapter in first person, as a way to personalize it and reach out to form a relationship with you, the reader. The writing is an illustrative performance of discourse construction as a performative act. It is the creation of what I call "performance methodology." The distinction between the performative act and methodology as performance should blur. But as a reader, you have to judge whether it is a performance. Thus, as the adjective "performative" and the metaphoric notions of "performance" blur, the act of being a performance is defined relationally and communally, thus bringing forth the process of legitimizing within the knowledge community.

Previously, when I would talk about my dissertation, I would describe my methodology as performance, autoethnography, and writing-in-inquiry. As I stand back in time and reflect on the dissertation processes in the context of the varied dialogues about performance and its application to my clinical, training, and research practices, I view performance today as an umbrella. Autoethnography and writing-in-inquiry are subsumed under performance.

My dissertation is a performance text. Its style and form make it a performance text. In addition to text, I used collages and multimedia to perform my experiences. All of it is a performance script, since I have continued to live it into my everyday life today as an administrator, therapist, researcher, and trainer. So, from McCall's (2003) perspective, I fulfill the criteria of script, character, and staging. The dissertation is a performance space and a liminal space of meaning making and transformation. It is the closest I have come thus far to illustrating how an experience is an experience of the process of making meaning, which is reflexive, contextual, and social. My dissertation is a performative space where meaning making can be acted out.

Though the emphasis of social construction is on communal construction and on a collective that grants this construction legitimacy, there is an inherent privileging of the local. The local can be pegged as the individual. Thus an inherent contradiction is set up between the collective and the individual. I was born and raised in New Delhi, India. I was thus raised in a culture that is labeled "collective," yet in a family that was much more "nuclear" and "individualistic." I became an active consumer of the notion of being a product of my "collective" culture, until I was working toward my PhD in an "individualistic" culture. In this culture, I initially constructed myself as being a critical observer and as becoming a receiver of the individualistic culture. Eventually, I redefined myself as co-constructing my identity and culture. In the process of doing this, I was in the process of privileging my voice, raising my voice. I experienced this as quite healthy and freeing. In this sense, my research project was autoethnographic. Since I was a woman from India headed to do my internship at one of the premium institutes for postmodern practices in the United States, I was entering into a legitimizing community or collective knowledge-making community that not only sanctioned my inquiry, but also legitimized it. The irony was in the process of constructing knowledge as a collective consensus, but through an intertextually individualized voice. Thus, if I had privileged only my voice (role of the performer) or the context (the performance context), I would be playing more of the same role as I did in India—that of a consumer, someone adapting to and legitimizing a particular culture. However, the difference lay in the fact that the performance was a critical performance. I was not aiming to privilege only the performer, as social performance theorist or the context of performance or the audience, as cultural performance theorists. I was focusing on the relationship of the discourses to the construction of the text, and on the relationship among my roles as the researcher, the reader, and the producer. Thus, as I was creating a localized multivocal narrative, I was also creating a transformational text of relational subversive performances. That is, no truth was swallowed whole or performed as *the* "truth."

As I have stated earlier, what is acceptable methodologically still lags behind our assertions that we are living in postmodern times. From a postmodern cultural perspective, there is a blurring of boundaries between avant-garde or high culture on the one hand and mass culture on the other. However, in academia and research, such blurring is slower to come. Often such blurring is questioned in the name of validity, replicability, or some other culture-bound concept of our current specifications for research. Yet I welcome such blurring and questioning in the name of theoretical consistency, and of the vitality that can be part of performance methodology. Schechner (2002) states:

One of the decisive qualities of postmodernism is the application of the "performance principle" to all aspects of social and artistic life. Performance is no longer confined to the stage, to the arts, and to ritual. Performativity is everywhere linked to the interdependence of power and knowledge. (p. 114)

So performativity already exists in our reports, whatever form we use. By accepting the cultural traditions of "academic writing," we are performing textually. However, varying forms of performativity are rising (Bava, 2001; Bochner & Ellis, 2002; Denzin, 2003; Ellis & Flaherty, 1992; Piercy & Benson, 2005) and are being legitimized as research.

DISCUSSION

Strengths and Weaknesses of the Methodology

As a researcher turns on an alternative research process to criticize it, he or she does so by using the very medium it was created to subvert. Thus, if the act of subversion is an action of resistance, it is inescapably wrapped in the remnants of the dominant discourses that it attempts to resist. So there is no escaping the dominant. Rather, the subversive act is a performance in reflexivity that questions "what has been" or "what can be." There will be others more committed to the dominant research specifications who will be all too happy to call performance methodology trivial, nonscientific, and more. Clearly, depending on where one stands, reflexivity, multivocality, and interpretive texts will be seen as possessing both strengths and weaknesses (F. P. Piercy, personal communication, 2003).

Reliability and Validity

Denzin (2003) states that some performances work and others don't. Every act of writing and research is assessed by the researcher and its community of evaluators for its structure of values, for its understanding of the phenomenon being studied, and consequently for its worldview—which is based on certain conceptual assumptions, such as what is assumed to be natural or constructed, genuine or fake, credible or incredible, research or fiction. When a research report is approached as a performance of constructing literature, then all aspects of the narrative may be viewed as signs that make claims, often implicitly, about the nature of the world as understood by the narrator. Furthermore, the reader assigns meaning to the research report as the researcher does—on the basis of his or her socially, politically, and culturally positioned discourses, which are informed by economy, race, gender, class, and other perspectives.

The postmodern turn challenges the standard assumptions about what valid knowledge is and how it is constituted (Bentz & Shapiro, 1998). The challenge lies in evaluating performances about how knowledge shapes people's lives and "how they enact cultural meanings in their daily lives" (Denzin, 2003). According to Denzin (2003), a "good performance text must be more than cathartic—it must be political, moving people to action, reflection, or both" (p. xi). He states that critical performance ethnographies are doubly reflexive—turning the theory on itself (i.e., reflecting on the researcher's location and the research process). Such performances "forfeit any claim to universal authority," and the final say rests in "its power to affect the world through praxis" (McLaren, quoted in Denzin, 2003, p. 33).

Not unlike literature or art, a performative inquiry calls forth certain types of responses, experiences, and values from the reader. The responses evoked in the reader are informed by the inquiry's style/form, language, narrative, and images. Thus the reader is the judge of the work. Consequently, not only does the substantive content inform the reader, but also the reader's response informs the substantive meaning of the inquiry. In my work, I invited various readers to experience the dissertation web, and I included our dialogue as another lexia of my dissertation. This added another reflexive layer that invited a multiplicity of experiences and experiences of experiences—generative conversations between and among researchers/readers.

Texts have evolved from being representational (reflecting "*the* truth") to presentational (interpreting and constructing "truths"). Performance texts are more than presentational; they are formative. Not only do they criticize the current performance, but they also perform alternative performances. For instance, in my dissertation I was not only resisting the traditional research discourses of presentation, but also co-creating the alternative forms. In creating the alternative forms, I was hesitant to view and discuss the work in terms of presentational forms, since it was more than such forms. The presentational forms were the contents through which I was constructing the embedded alternative discourse that was criticizing and rewriting what research is.

Skills

The art of doing such performative writing is to transpose oneself from being the writer to being the reader, and to write as if one were distanced from the original writing. This is easier said than done, since one is still the writer, yet one assumes the reader position. This is different from writing to an audience. One is writing as if one *is* the audience—a sort of participant observer. One observes through participation. One writes as the reader. This removes one from one's own experience, yet it is one's own experience that one is writing about. Perhaps, more importantly, the writing also invites the actual reader to be a coparticipant in meaning making.

If reading the preceding paragraph makes you dizzy, then that comes close to the experience of overanalyzing the accuracy of skillful application. Simply tell yourself, "I'm now going to read and respond [write] as a reader." Ask yourself, "Who is my reader?" Another approach is to ask, "What other historical and/or cultural distance from the research process and substantive area of research can I introduce?"

Bridging Research and Practice

This kind of writing creates evocative text that is more accessible to the reader. The work can be translated into performances that can be conducted in classrooms to explore the research experientially (Piercy & Benson, 2005). Clinicians can become involved in the research process by becoming performers of the discourse. They consume the performance and produce the performance of research as an activity in community meaning making, a shared inquiry. The inquiry does not stop with the product—that is, reports, scripts, or performance. The inquiry continues, furthered by dialogue among the readers, audience, and researchers who continue to make sense of the product, which thus becomes an experience in sense making. Such ideas transform the gap between research and practice.

Future Directions

This approach is relatively new to our field, though the notions of script writing and clinical performances are not. Reflexivity has also been a tool in the clinician's and researcher's toolbox. So it may come more easily to a clinician to be a performative methodologist if he or she is mindful of the role performance plays in clinical work. That is, clinicians co-construct performances with clients all the time. The postmodern clinician is also adept in the process of inquiry as a way to understand a client's story and problem. The performative inquiry thus requires approaching the research process with the tools that one already posseses as a clinician, but utilizing them with a slightly different intentionality.

A FOREWORD

For those who welcome the emerging wave of performance methodologies and alternative writings, I suggest that you review the works of Bochner and Ellis, (2002), Denzin (2003), Ellis and Bochner (1996), Ellis and Flaherty (1992), Patton (1999), and Piercy and Benson (2005), along with my research, to expand on performative ways of research design and implementation.

I now pause this performance with an invitation[3] to you, the reader, to communicate your ideas with others and me as an ongoing conversation. Let us critically question how and what we are doing methodologically and how we are constructing our consensual knowledge communities.

ACKNOWLEDGMENTS

I deeply appreciate Fred Piercy's skillful and pertinent edits and encouragement with the crafting of this performance. I also appreciate Carolyn Callahan's encouragement and feedback with the early chapter drafts. I am thankful to the HGI writing circle members who supported and helped me refine my manuscript. Finally, I am deeply appreciative of my dissertation committee, which sanctioned and gave me space to bring to fruition the ideas based on which this chapter is performed.

REFERENCES

Agger, B. (1998). *Critical social theories: An introduction.* Boulder, CO: Westview Press.
Anderson, H. (1997). *Conversation, language, and possibilities: A postmodern approach to therapy.* New York: Basic Books.
Bava, S. (2001). *Transforming performances: An intern-researcher's hypertextual journey in a postmodern community.* Doctoral dissertation, Virginia Polytechnic Institute and State University. Retrieved from *http://scholar.lib.vt.edu/theses/available/etd-01062002-234843*
Bava, S. (Ed.). (2003). *The show must go on: Families growing through divorce. Training guide for facilitators.* (Available from Houston Galveston Institute, 3316 Mt. Vernon, Houston, TX 77006)

---

[3] My email address is sbava@vt.edu.

Baldwin, C. (1977). *One to one: Self-understanding through journal writing.* New York: M. Evans.

Becker, H. S. (1986). *Writing for social sciences.* Chicago: University of Chicago Press.

Bell-Scott, P. (Ed.). (1994). *Life notes: Personal writings by contemporary black women.* New York: Norton.

Bentz, V. M., & Shapiro, J. J. (1998). *Mindful inquiry in social research.* Thousand Oaks, CA: Sage.

Bernstein, C. (2000). *Frame lock.* Retrieved from *http://epc.buffalo.edu/authors/bernstein/essays/frame-lock.html*

Bernstein, M. (1999, 2001). *Patterns of hypertext.* Retrieved from *http://www.eastgate.com/patterns/Print.html*

Bloom, L. R. (1998). *Under the sign of hope: Feminist methodology and narrative interpretation.* Albany: State University of New York Press.

Bochner, A. P., & Ellis, C. (2002). *Ethnographically speaking: Autoethnography, literature, and aesthetics.* Walnut Creek, CA: AltaMira Press.

Broughton, T. L., & Anderson, L. (Eds.). (1997). *Woman's lives/women's times: New essays on auto/biography.* Albany: State University of New York Press.

Bruffee, K. (1999). *Collaborative learning: Higher education, interdependence, and the authority of knowledge* (2nd ed.). Baltimore: Johns Hopkins University Press.

Carlson, M. (1996). *Performance: A critical introduction.* New York: Routledge.

Clandinin, D. J., & Connelly, F. M. (1994). Personal experience methods. In N. K. Denzin & Y. S. Lincoln (Eds.), *Handbook of qualitative research* (pp. 413–427). Thousand Oaks, CA: Sage.

Coffey, A., & Atkinson, P. (1996). *Making sense of qualitative data.* Thousand Oaks, CA: Sage.

Denzin, N. K. (2003). *Performance ethnography: Critical pedagogy and the politics of culture.* Thousand Oaks, CA: Sage.

Denzin, N. K., & Lincoln, Y. S. (Eds.). (2003). *Strategies of qualitative inquiry.* Thousand Oaks, CA: Sage.

Ellis, C., & Bochner, A. (Eds.). (1996). *Composing ethnography: Alternative forms of qualitative writing.* Walnut Creek, CA: AltaMira Press.

Ellis, C., & Flaherty, M. (Eds.). (1992). *Investigating subjectivity: Research on lived experience.* Newbury Park, CA: Sage.

Flemons, D. (1998). *Writing between the lines: Composition in the social sciences.* New York: Norton.

Gergen, K. (1991). *The saturated self.* New York: Basic Books.

Gergen, K. (1994a). Exploring the postmodern. *American Psychologist, 49*(5), 412–416.

Gergen, K. (1994b). *Realities and relationships: Soundings in social construction.* Cambridge, MA: Harvard University Press.

Gergen, K. (1997). *Who speaks and who replies in human science scholarship?* Retrieved from *http://www.swarthmore.edu/SocSci/kgergen1/whospeak.html*

Gergen, K. (1999). *An invitation to social construction.* Thousand Oaks, CA: Sage.

Gergen, M. (2001). *Feminist reconstructions in psychology: Narrative, gender, and performance.* Thousand Oaks, CA: Sage.

Goldberg, N. (1986). *Writing down the bones.* Boston: Shambhala.

Hogan, R. (1991). Engendered autobiographies: The diary as a feminine form. *Prose Studies, 14*(2), 95–107.

Kaye, N. (1994). *Postmodernism and performance.* New York: St. Martin's Press.

Kolb, D. (2000). *Hypertext as subversive?* [e-journal]. Retrieved from *http://culturemachine.tees.ac.uk/frm_f1.htm*

Landow, G. (1997). *Hypertext: The convergence of contemporary critical theory and technology* (2nd ed.). Baltimore: Johns Hopkins University Press.

Lemke, J. L. (1995). *Textual politics: Discourse and social dynamics.* Bristol, PA: Taylor & Francis.

Lock, A. (1981). Universals in human conception. In P. L. F. Heelas & A. J. Lock (Eds.), *Indigenous psychologies: The anthropology of the self* (pp. 19–36). London: Academic Press.

Magee, B. (2001). *The story of philosophy*. New York: DK.

Marcus, G. E., & Fischer, M. M. (1999). *Anthropology as cultural critique: An experimental moment in the human sciences* (2nd ed.). Chicago: University of Chicago Press.

McCall, M. M. (2003). Performance ethnography: A brief history and some advice. In N. K. Denzin & Y. S. Lincoln (Eds.), *Strategies of qualitative inquiry* (2nd ed., pp. 112–133). Thousand Oaks, CA: Sage.

McCall, M. M., & Becker, H. S. (1990). Performance science. *Social Problems, 37*(1), 117–132.

Patton, M. (1999). *Grand Canyon celebration: A father–son journey of discovery*. Amherst, NY: Prometheus Books.

Pelias, R. J. (1999). *Writing performance: Poeticizing the researcher's body*. Carbondale: Southern Illinois University Press.

Piercy, F., & Benson, K. (2005). Aesthetic forms of data presentation in qualitative family therapy research. *Journal of Marital and Family Therapy, 31*, 107–119.

Pockley, S. (1999/2000). *The flight of ducks: Duck song*. Retrieved from *http://www.duckdigital.net/FOD/FOD0004.html*

Polkinghorne, D. (1988). *Narrative knowing and the human sciences*. Albany: State University of New York Press.

Reed-Danahay, D. E. (Ed.). (1997). *Auto/ethnography: Rewriting the self and the social*. New York: Berg.

Richardson, L. (1993). Poetics, dramatics, and transgressive validity: The case of the skipped line. *Sociological Quarterly, 35*, 695–710.

Richardson, L. (1997). *Fields of play: Constructing an academic life*. New Brunswick, NJ: Rutgers University Press.

Richardson, L., & Lockridge, E. (1991). The sea monster: An ethnographic drama and comment on ethnographic fiction. *Symbolic Interaction*, 335–341.

Ronai, C. R. (1992). The reflexive self through narrative: A night in the life of an erotic dancer/researcher. In C. Ellis & M. G. Flaherty (Eds.), *Investigating subjectivity: Research on lived experience* (pp. 102–124). Newbury Park, CA: Sage.

Schechner, R. (2002). *Performance studies: An introduction*. New York: Routledge.

Schiwy, M. A. (1996). *A voice of her own*. New York: Fireside Books.

Schneider, J. W. (1991). Troubles with textual authority in sociology. *Symbolic Interaction, 14*(3), 295–319.

Simons, G. (1978). *Keeping your personal journal*. New York: Ballantine.

Spolin, V. (1999). *Improvisation for the theater* (3rd ed.). Evanston, IL: Northwestern University Press.

Thompson, B., & Tyagi, S. (Eds.). (1996). *Names we call home*. New York: Routledge.

Tillmann-Healy, L. (1996). A secret life in a culture of thinness: Reflections on body, food, and bulimia. In C. Ellis & A. P. Bochner (Eds.), *Composing ethnography: Alternative forms of qualitative writing* (pp. 76–108). Walnut Creek, CA: AltaMira Press.

White, M., & Epston, D. (1990). *Narrative means to therapeutic ends*. New York: Norton.

Wittgenstein, L. (1965). *Philosophical investigations* (G. E. M. Anscombe, Trans.). New York: Macmillan.

Wolcott, H. F. (1994). *Transforming qualitative data: Description, analysis and interpretation*. Thousand Oaks, CA: Sage.

CHAPTER 11

Future Directions for Qualitative Methods

RONALD J. CHENAIL

The only certain thing about the future is that it will surprise even those who have seen furthest into it.

—E. J. HOBSBAWM

INTRODUCTION

Prediction is very difficult, especially about the future.

—NIELS BOHR

Most writings about the future of qualitative methods (e.g., Gergen & Gergen, 2000; Lincoln & Denzin, 1994, 2000; McLeod, 2001; Page, 2000) seem to include the same cautionary disclaimer: Neither the past nor the present may be the best guide for predicting the future, but the present and the past are all we have to work with at this time. Given this conundrum, I have taken a similar path in researching and writing this chapter, knowing full well the potential folly in such an endeavor. Having said that, I still have enjoyed the opportunity to reflect on what has transpired in the marriage and family therapy (MFT) field over the last few decades, to observe the growth of qualitative research as a viable research method, to scan the contemporary qualitative inquiry landscape for emerging trends and informing contexts, and to squint carefully at the horizon that lies ahead. This exercise to me suggests a hopeful future for qualitative research in our field.

CURRENT STYLES OF QUALITATIVE RESEARCH

The future is here. It's just not widely distributed yet.

—WILLIAM GIBSON

In attempting to make sense of the world of qualitative methods, some authors have approached the subject in terms of developmental moments over time (e.g., Denzin & Lincoln, 1994b, 2000b), while others have come to understand the phenomenon in

191

terms of its contrasting styles: scientific, artistic, critical, and participatory (Eisner, 1981). For discussing future directions of qualitative research in MFT, I favor the contrasting-styles conceptualization to assess the trends of today and to suggest the patterns of tomorrow. It is a useful way to show what forms of qualitative research predominate in the MFT literature, and it can also give some clues to the directions in which researchers may take these methods.

Scientifically Styled Qualitative Research

Qualitative researchers who operate from the scientific perspective have a tendency to organize their work in relationship to the social and natural sciences. Their work resembles the products of their experimental, quantitative colleagues, in that they emphasize epistemologies that favor postpositivist or realist views of the world; their methods are rich in descriptions of their sampling procedures, data selection, preparation, and analysis; and they carefully describe their efforts at building validity and reliability into their studies (see King, Keohane, & Verba, 1994). The results of their studies are published in reporting formats that resemble those used by their quantitative colleagues. They also tend to situate their qualitative work in relation to quantitative projects (e.g., qualitative research as prestudy preparation, qualitative data analysis as a means for triangulation with quantitative data analysis, and qualitative inquiry as post hoc analysis of a completed quantitative study) (Patton, 2002).

Within this science-dominated inquiry, many qualitative researchers have successfully created qualitative research approaches that offer complementary naturalist alternatives to the quantitative studies. Grounded theory is a good example of how qualitative researchers have established a rigorous method for exploring a wide range of phenomena (see Glaser & Strauss, 1967; Strauss & Corbin, 1998). Qualitative researchers operating within the scientific worldview have also been influential in introducing phenomenological, constructivist, constructionist, and postmodern perspectives into the mix (see Lincoln & Guba, 2000, for a fuller discussion). In the MFT world, scientifically oriented qualitative research is the predominant form (see Faulkner, Klock, & Gale, 2002; Gehart, Ratliff, & Lyle, 2001).

Artistically Styled Qualitative Research

Qualitative researchers who favor the artistic approaches emphasize the roots of qualitative research in the arts and humanities. Their projects have a tendency to celebrate interpretation, story, performance, evocation, the audience, and improvisation (see Bochner & Ellis, 2002; Denzin, 2003; Ellis, 2004; Ellis & Bochner, 1996; and Bava, Chapter 10, this volume). Their studies are presented in the forms of stories, plays, poems, and other vehicles that emphasize aesthetics, poetics, characters, themes, plots, and moods. They are concerned with how their work makes readers sensitive to voices and events previously unheard or unappreciated; how it generates "aesthetic quality" and "interpretive vitality"; and how it stimulates, provokes, and moves their audience (Patton, 2002, pp. 544–545; Piercy & Benson, 2005). Although it is difficult to find a large number of contemporary examples of this approach in MFT literature (see Karl, Cynthia, Andrew, & Vanessa, 1992; McAdams, Josselson, & Lieblich, 2001), at one time our field was rich with this kind of research report—as exemplified in the work of its leaders, such as Augustus Napier and Carl Whitaker's (1978) *The Family Crucible*,

Salvador Minuchin's (1984) *Family Kaleidoscope*, and Murray Bowen's (1967/1972/ 1978) anonymous account.

Critically Styled Qualitative Research

The critical branch of the qualitative research family tree organizes its inquiries around a particular orienting theory, such as feminist theory (e.g., Visweswaran, 1994), Marxist theory (e.g., Carspecken, 1996), or queer theory (Gamson, 2000). In this kind of qualitative approach, data are collected along lines similar to those found in scientific or artistic approaches; at a certain point in the process, however, the data are subjected to a dialogical or critical stage during which the orienting theory is juxtaposed with the data to produce a dialectical relationship through which an interpreted result is produced (see Carspecken, 1996). The products produced from this line of inquiry can be in the form typical of the scientific style, or can take an alternative form as seen with the artistic projects. The researchers working in this style seek to increase consciousness about injustices, focus on sources of inequalities, and inspire those involved to take action (Patton, 2002, p. 545). Some recent examples of this style of qualitative research in MFT can be found in the papers by Schindler Zimmerman, Holm, and Starrels (2001) and Sparks (2002), as well as the work of the Just Therapy team (Waldegrave, Tamasese, Tuhaka, & Campbell, 2003).

Collaborative or Action Approaches to Qualitative Research

The participatory or action approaches to qualitative research emphasize the collaborative relationship between researchers and participants as they work together to assess, to innovate, and to change some aspect of the participants' world (e.g., an organization, a family, or a community) (see Jason, Keys, Suarez-Balcazar, Taylor, & Davis, 2004; Kemmis & McTaggart, 2000). These applied modes of inquiry are usually organized in terms of ongoing circular processes in which the researcher–participant (or stakeholder) team identifies a problem or focus of change, collects information about the problem, reflects on possible solutions, implements a potential remedy, measures the results of the intervention, and begins the cycle anew based upon the feedback received during the assessment phase. Researchers working within the participatory or action style emphasize cooperation, the generation of practical meaning, and the production of change (Piercy & Thomas, 1998). Recent exemplars of this approach in MFT can be found in the work of Deacon and Piercy (2000) and McDowell and colleagues (2003). (See also Mendenhall & Doherty, Chapter 6, this volume.)

Current Tensions and Future Directions

Even though the scientific style of qualitative inquiry dominates the current research landscape, the influence of the artistic, critical, and participatory approaches on scientifically minded researchers is considerable today and will continue to be a factor tomorrow. In important works such as the two editions of the *Handbook of Qualitative Research* (Denzin & Lincoln, 1994a, 2000a), in some leading journals (e.g., *Qualitative Inquiry*), and even in some research guides for psychologists (e.g., Camic, Rhodes, & Yardley, 2003; Kopala & Suzuki, 1999), the sheer volume of prescriptive writings on such issues as the self of the researcher, the importance of research participants and readers (i.e., the "others"), and notions of voice and representation strongly suggests that the scientifically styled research of the future will continue to be informed by the other styles. This may be seen in a greater use of excerpts from research diaries in published accounts, to create a greater degree of openness and reflexivity in reports of how categories were created (Constas, 1992; Smith, 1999); an expanded role of research participants in the member checking, so that they become almost like consultants to the research process (Asher & Asher, 1999); and a utilization of literary styles to represent findings (Flemons & Green, 2002; Ricci, 2003).

The presence of all these major styles of qualitative research suggests a healthy and diverse methodological environment within the contemporary MFT world and a solid foundation for further development. So, if qualitative research is here for the foreseeable future, then what other factors or tensions may help to shape how this family of methods develops and evolves over the next decade or so?

GENERIC OR DESIGNER METHODS

The future is made of the same stuff as the present.
—SIMONE WEIL

Currently, qualitative researchers are divided along the lines of either practicing from a generic perspective or organizing their work along specific designer guidelines (Caelli, Ray, & Mill, 2003). Such a split can also be seen in the MFT world (Gehart et al., 2001).

In the designer approach, qualitative researchers adhere to a well-established model or school of inquiry, such as phenomenology, ethnography, conversation analysis, case study, or grounded theory. They conduct their studies according to well-known practices and produce products that are easily recognizable by others of their school. The strength of this approach is that the methods offer clearly defined practices for researchers to conduct the projects and to produce the results, and for reviewers to evaluate the submitted reports. Weaknesses of the designer approach include a possible misfit between the method and the research question, or possibly method underutilization (e.g., someone may use grounded theory but may not produce theory in the finished project).

In the generic approach, the method is usually described in such terms as "qualitative research" or "qualitative inquiry," and its method choice points are not restricted to any particular school or model or theory (e.g., ethnography, phenomenology, grounded theory, etc.). These researchers—or, as Denzin and Lincoln (2000b, pp. 4–6) call them, "bricoleurs" or "quilt makers"—must master a variety of the skills inherent in many of the designer approaches, and mix and match these applications to fit the needs of their studies at hand. The strength of this approach lies in its flexibility, although this is also a potential weakness. If the challenge for designer-informed researchers is to stay true to their school, the real challenge for generic-minded researchers is to create a project that is internally coherent (Chenail, 1997) or externally recognizable to reviewers.

Future Trends

Both generic and designer methods will persist in the MFT world, and the quality of each will also improve through the abundance of literature on "quality in qualitative research" (e.g., Seale, 1999). These highly prescriptive writings make it easier for qualitative researchers to decide how to conduct a particular part of a study (Ayres, Kavanaugh, & Knafl, 2003), how to evaluate the outcome of the act (Bailey, 1996), how to present the report of the act in a published account of the research (Anfara, Brown, & Mangione, 2002), and how to assess the representation of the act in written form (Byrne, 2001).

Although there is a certain amount of criticism of these guides (e.g., Barbour, 2001), the apparent reality is that these prescriptive lists of suggestions can make the daunting processes of conducting research studies (Patton, 1999), producing publishable results (Drisko, 1997; Rowan & Huston, 1997), and reviewing and judging reports (Russell & Gregory, 2003) clearer. Interestingly enough, this trend can also be seen with the more artistically minded researchers (e.g., Angen, 2000; Denzin, 2003; Piercy & Benson, 2005). As such, I think that we will see a continued proliferation of these guides, and that their influence will become greater with qualitative researchers and reviewers—especially if movements such as evidence-based practice continue to grow.

PRACTICE-BASED EVIDENCE AND EVIDENCE-BASED PRACTICE

Our imagination is the only limit to what we can hope to have in the future.

—CHARLES F. KETTERING

According to Scott Miller and Barry Duncan's website, TalkingCure.com (*http:// www.talkingcure.com/latest.htm*), MFT today is dominated by two schools of thought and practice when it comes to the delivery and evaluation of clinical work: the "practice-based evidence" and the "evidence-based practice" groups. The gold standard of evidence for therapists and researchers operating from the practice-based evidence perspective is to judge the effectiveness of their work by carefully speaking with clients to learn what works for them and why (e.g., Duncan & Miller, 2000; Hubble, Duncan, & Miller, 1999). Clinicians and researchers working from the evidence-based practice point of view rely heavily on the use of systematic reviews of multiple randomized controlled trials as their gold standard for determining the effectiveness of treatments (Liddle, Santisteban, Levant, & Bray, 2002; Sprenkle, 2002). If the future of MFT continues to be organized around both of these two worldviews, the prospects for qualitative research appear bright.

Because qualitative research methods work well when practice-based evidence researchers want to discover and explore phenomena in depth, they will continue to be used widely to study clients' perspectives on therapy (e.g., Gehart & Lyle, 1999; Kuehl, Newfield, & Joanning, 1990; Sells, Smith, & Moon, 1996), as well as to examine other clinical processes and outcomes (Maione & Chenail, 1999; McLeod, 2001). Even though the scientific styles of qualitative research have dominated so far, the strengths of the artistic approaches in their abilities to feature stories and emotions should also prove to be informative to researchers and therapists working within the practice-based evidence approach.

Although many in the MFT field worry about the rise of the evidence-based practice approaches, for qualitative researchers there is much to be gained. For example, the stage model employed in the development of evidence-based approaches presents a series of challenges for researchers working in this style (Rounsaville, Carroll, & Onken, 2001). When these researchers work to develop and refine manuals to guide the delivery of the therapy, they need research methods that help them to systematically observe what works in the therapy room in a case-by-case process. For this task, qualitative methods have already shown their worth (see Pote, Stratton, Cottrell, Shapiro, & Boston, 2003). Qualitative research can also bring value to the evidence-based approach because of the methods' strength at exploring a subject in great depth, studying a phenomenon where theory is lacking, assisting in the study of social interaction, appreciating cultural differences, focusing on nonclinical factors, and addressing instances when there are contradictory results (Barbour, 2000, pp. 157–158, 161).

A major hurdle confronting the evidence-based practice approach to qualitative research will be how well the evidence produced by qualitative studies will be accepted by those who construct systematic reviews of effectiveness reports, such as the Cochrane Review Methodology Database (*http://www.cochrane.org*). The biggest challenges in this area, according to Dixon-Woods, Fitzpatrick, and Roberts (2001, pp. 129–130), are the need to overcome methodological prejudice and methodological difficulties, the challenges of searching for qualitative evidence in databases, and the appraisal of quality in qualitative research. Luckily, measures to improve the future of qualitative research in systematic reviews are already underway. These can be seen in the efforts of such groups as the Cochrane Collaboration Qualitative Methods Network (*http://www.iphrp.salford.ac.uk/cochrane*), which is a worldwide community dedicated to exploring the scope for incorporating qualitative research into the Cochrane Reviews; and Economic and Social Data Service's Qualidata (*http://www.esds.ac.uk/qualidata*), which provides access and support for a range of social science qualitative data sets. The "quality in qualitative research" movement mentioned earlier in this chapter (e.g., Seale, 1999) is also proving to be invaluable to creators and critics of qualitative research, in that they present clear guidelines for the production and review of the work.

Future Trends

For researchers operating within both the practice-based evidence and evidence-based practice worlds, the future will be about making connections. For McLeod (2001, pp. 205–208), "making connections" means inviting and facilitating replication and developing knowledge communities by weaving the findings of previous studies into these projects; comparing this work to that of others working in the area; conducting qualitative meta-analysis and metasynthesis; thinking of future researchers who will be exploring the topic by reporting findings explicitly; embracing networks of people who collectively share in the knowledge of how to do something; developing a review literature that will enable others to learn, explore, and critique qualitative methods; learning from those outside the MFT field; and publishing articles on the Internet in order to encourage ongoing discussion (see the new journal *Discourse Analysis Online*, *http://www.shu.ac.uk/daol*, for an exciting look into the future of this last type of interaction).

Lastly, in any discussion of the many relationships between therapy and qualitative research, the possibility of qualitative methods' actually being used as therapeutic approaches is another intriguing option. Over the last few years, several writers have examined the apparent therapeutic quality of qualitative research when it is used with clinical populations (Berger & Malkinson, 2000; Boudah & Lenz, 2000; Gale, 1992; Murray, 2003). The work of these authors suggests that one future direction for qualitative research in the clinical arena is for it to become a clinical approach itself.

FUNDING

The future, according to some scientists, will be exactly like the past, only far more expensive.

—JOHN SLADEK

Funding for qualitative research is another important factor when we are contemplating the future (Gilgun, 2002). For many academia-based researchers, this is a crucial challenge that must be successfully met in order to ensure job security, raises, and promotions. Although the challenge is daunting, the door is certainly open for funding of scientifically styled qualitative research. For example, on the federal level, the National Institutes of Health (NIH) Office of Behavioral and Social Sciences Research has shown strong support for funding qualitative research (Heurtin-Roberts, 2002). In 1999, the NIH Culture and Qualitative Research Interest Group (CQRIG), with support from the National Institute of Mental Health and the National Institute on Alcohol Abuse and Alcoholism, organized a workshop entitled "Qualitative Methods in Health Research: Opportunities and Considerations in Applications and Review"; the proceedings of this workshop were later published as an online monograph (National Institute of Mental Health, 2001).

The CQRIG (*http://tango01.cit.nih.gov/sig/home.taf?_function=main&SIGInfo_SIGID=101*) is another promising sign itself. The CQRIG works to promote awareness of the impact of culture, ethnicity, racial categories, and class on public health research for members of NIH and for those seeking funding through NIH. Its goals include encouraging the use of theory-based conceptualization of these terms and their inclusion as variables in NIH and NIH-sponsored qualitative and quantitative research.

There is also a growing body of papers providing "tips of the trade" for those qualitative researchers seeking extramural funding (e.g., Carey & Swanson, 2003; Sandelowski & Barroso, 2003). In these works, authors not only share the insights from their successful awards, but also walk readers through the "nuts and bolts" entailed in writing each section of the proposal. These lessons will be invaluable to MFT researchers looking to enter the world of federally funded research.

Future Trends

Education of reviewers and review panels, as well as of institutional review boards for the protection of human subjects, remains a challenge for qualitative researchers seeking funding, especially for those who wish to use less traditional qualitative approaches (Morse, 2003a). Just as some authors have presented suggestions to these reviewers and peers when it comes to the more scientifically styled qualitative research (e.g., Morse, 2003b), qualitative researchers in the future will need to write similar guides to educate the next generation of boards to the strengths and utilities of artistic, critical, and collaborative approaches as well.

TECHNOLOGY

Any sufficiently advanced technology is indistinguishable from magic.
—ARTHUR C. CLARKE

As it will be in many aspects of our everyday lives, technology will have a greater and greater influence on the future direction of qualitative research, especially as the children of today begin to enter graduate school and learn these modes of inquiry. Through playing computer games, future qualitative researchers are developing skills that allow them to navigate online with ease; to grasp information coming from text, images, symbols, and sounds; and to collaborate with others from around the world (Gee, 2003). These students of tomorrow will want to work with multimedia, hypertextuality, and hypermedia (Barrett, 1992) and will have the skills and mindsets to do so.

For qualitative researchers, this means that we will see more image-based research (Prosser, 1998) and other multimedia works (e.g., Bauer & Gaskell, 2000). In an ironic turn, this development actually harks back to earlier studies in family therapy and psychotherapy, when researchers used images and innovative data displays to represent their results. For example, Pittenger, Hockett, and Danehy (1960) used "Dutch door" pages to present transcripts and commentary, and Scheflen's (1973) classic study incorporated drawings and transcripts on pull-out, "accordion" pages to represent in-session process. Whereas the costs of production today have limited such creativity, the advent of the Internet as a publication source, along with inexpensive software on the desktop, will lead us to see more and more qualitative research that incorporates multimedia.

The most commonly recognized usage of technology in qualitative research today is computer-aided qualitative data analysis software (CAQDAS) (Ryan & Bernard, 2000; Weitzman, 2000). At the same time, these programs are also some of the most misunderstood ingredients in the qualitative research mix (see Matheson, Chapter 7, this volume). For some researchers, CAQDAS programs represent the false hope that the software will do the analysis for them; for others, they present the false fear that the programs cannot help with the analysis process (Weitzman, 2000, pp. 806–808). Neither of these statements is quite true, but the usage of these packages is challenging for many, to say the least. Thankfully, there is now more information available via the World Wide Web to provide help and support for researchers trying out these packages (e.g., the CAQDAS Networking Project at *http://caqdas.soc.surrey.ac.uk*). This availability of help and the overall improvement of the programs mean that we will see more researchers using these packages, especially as we see a rise in the use of teams in qualitative research.

Future Trends

Speaking of teams, the communication and collaborative strengths of the Internet and the next generation of communication networks will make the use of groups in qualitative research projects more commonplace in the future (Mann & Stewart, 2000). The availability of high-speed, large-capacity networks such as Internet 2 (*http://www.internet2.edu*) and the National LambdaRail (*http://www.nationallambdarail.org*) will make teleconferencing ubiquitous. These large conduits will also make it easier for researchers to exchange large data sets or for multiple researchers to work on one data set simultaneously. These speedy fiber optic networks will also make it much more convenient to work with multimedia and other image-rich data sources, such as videotaped therapy sessions. These sources could be a boon for artistic approaches in particular.

NEW AND EMERGING RESEARCH METHODOLOGIES

> The future belongs to those who believe in the beauty of their dreams.
> —ELEANOR ROOSEVELT

As discussed above, the contemporary world of qualitative research methodologies is populated by both generic and designer approaches. Among the designer methods, current researchers favor such long-standing approaches as content analysis, ethnography, case study, phenomenology, grounded theory, and conversational analysis (Faulkner et al., 2002). Even though these methods, along with the generic approaches, may dominate the qualitative research used in MFT for the time being, a number of newer and as yet little-used approaches may become the next wave of methods in the field. The following is just a sample of these useful but not well-known methods that are available for MFT researchers to explore.

Autoethnography

Ellis and Bochner (2000) state, "Autoethnography is an autobiographical genre of writing and research that displays multiple layers of consciousness, connecting the personal to the cultural" (p. 739). The key feature of the approach is the interplay of a wide-angle lens (i.e., the ethnographic approach, which exposes cultural, social, and other meaningful contexts) and a narrow-focus perspective through which an individual researcher peers inwardly to expose a "vulnerable self" (Ellis & Bochner, 2000, p. 739). Autoethnographers employ a variety of literary styles to present their accounts and explore their lives in context (Ellis, 2004). In their collections of works, Bochner and Ellis (2002; Ellis & Bochner, 1996) present numerous examples of this method's highly effective use in studies of life transitions, chronic illness, and death. (See also Allen & Piercy, Chapter 9, this volume.)

Portraiture

As the portrait artist who paints a likeness of a subject on canvas does, the portraiture researcher attempts to balance elements of context, thematic structure, relationship, and voice into an aesthetic whole. In creating this portraiture of a person, setting, organization, or family, such a researcher endeavors to create a sense of coherence among all of these elements (Davis, 2003, p. 199). Portraiture is a challenging qualitative research method and demands a style of writing that is both rigorous and artistic (Lawrence Lightfoot & Davis, 1997). Mary Catherine Bateson's (1989) work represents an outstanding example of this approach to the study of narrative in context.

Recursive Frame Analysis

Recursive frame analysis (RFA) was developed by Bradford Keeney (see Chenail, 1990–1991) to serve as a means for therapists to observe and chart their conversations in therapy sessions. In this process, clinicians note topics in the flow of conversation (marking semantic differences that make clinical differences as "frames") and then chart semantic turns in the sessions as they occur. Therapists can then track their clinical discourse, so that they can pinpoint how talk in the sessions moves from problem-focused discussions to solution-focused or resourceful conversations (Ray & Keeney, 1993). From this useful notation system, my colleagues and I have helped to develop RFA into a tool used by qualitative researchers to study conversations, to render figures of speech, and to present "understandings of understandings." With RFA, qualitative researchers can perform semantic, sequential, pragmatic, and contextual analyses in recursive relationships to study all types of spoken and written texts (Chenail, 1991, 1995; Rambo, Heath, & Chenail, 1993; Rudes, Shilts, & Berg, 1997).

Zaltman Metaphor Elicitation Technique

Zaltman Metaphor Elicitation Technique (ZMET; see *http://www.olsonzaltman.com*) was developed by a Harvard Business School professor, Gerald Zaltman (2003). It is a patented qualitative research tool that enables participants to understand their own thinking more fully and to share this thinking with others (Duffy & Chenail, 2004). It allows researchers to elicit basic constructs or ideas in the form of images, pictures, or drawings made and/or collected by participants, and to explore the connections among images as ideas (i.e., metaphors) in order to make participants' mental models or constructs overt (Christensen & Olson, 2002, p. 478). The individual constructs are then grouped together to form a consensus map that represents the relationships between the various constructs (Zaltman, 1996, pp. 16–19). ZMET presents an alternative to the basic open-ended interview, and it is also unique in its reliance on visual images contributed by the participants to explore their metaphors.

Metasynthesis

Although the number of qualitative studies has increased greatly in recent years, there have been few attempts to examine the collective works on one topic to see what patterns, if any, are emerging from different studies on the same phenomenon. This disjointed nature of qualitative research can be seen as a hindrance when it comes to demonstrating the collective worth of its inquiries. One solution to the challenge of examining qualitative research results collectively is to develop a unique, qualitative approach to synthesize the studies while maintaining the integrity of individual studies (Sandelowski, Docherty, & Emden, 1997). One approach to this quandary is "metasynthesis," a qualitative method used to make the results of qualitative studies more accessible to clinicians, other researchers, laypersons, and policymakers. To this end, these researchers "synthesize" findings from related studies to create a meta-analysis of the various studies. The method is relatively new; it was first developed in 1994, and since that time several variations of metasynthesis have emerged. The results of these metasyntheses have been theory building, theory explication, and substantive descriptions of various phenomena (Finfgeld, 2003). Although at present metasynthesis is primarily used in nursing (e.g., Barroso & Powell-Cope, 2000; Clemmens, 2003), it has great promise for MFT researchers looking to bring the contributions of qualitative researchers into the systematic review movement.

Appreciative Inquiry

If action research can be understood as a problem-focused approach to change, then "appreciative inquiry" can be conceptualized as a solution-focused alternative. Whereas action research begins its cycle of change by studying what's wrong in an organization or family, appreciative inquirers start their "4-D cycle" with a "discovery" phase, in which participants are asked what they appreciate about the company, the organization, or the family. From this point, the process goes to the other three phases: "dream" (i.e., envisioning impact), "design" (i.e., co-constructing), and "destiny" (i.e., sustaining) (Cooperrider & Whitney, 1999, p. 11). Appreciative inquiry uses a variety of qualitative research approaches to gather information about what is appreciated, to learn (along with the participants) what is best about their lives, and to measure the effectiveness of the changes brought about by the 4-D cycle (Cooperrider, Sorensen, Whitney, & Yaeger, 2000). Another aspect of appreciative inquiry that makes it an interesting approach is its practitioners' sense of community, both in how they conduct their inquiries and in how they relate to one another (e.g., the Appreciative Inquiry Commons—see *http://connection.cwru.edu/ai*).

Narrative Inquiry

"Narrative inquiry" is the process of interacting with others in order to gather data and information for the purpose of representing life experiences through storytelling. The recursive quality of narrative inquiry means that the research process is focused on both participants' stories and their stories about their stories, along with an emphasis on including the stories of the researchers as well. In this fashion, researchers engaging in narrative inquiry write accounts of their experiences that include stories of the others they encountered in the field (Clandinin & Connelly, 2000). The sheer variety of narrative inquiry and narrative analysis is partially derived from the multiple fields that understand and study life in terms of story. These include psychology, literature, linguistics, art, history, and the sciences (e.g., Daiute & Lightfoot, 2004; Josselson, Lieblich, & McAdams, 2003). This wealth of options presents MFT researchers with a breadth of approaches for studying clients and themselves.

EDUCATING THE NEXT GENERATION

> We cannot always build the future for our youth, but we can build our youth for the future.
>
> —FRANKLIN D. ROOSEVELT

One of the greatest challenges facing qualitative researchers today is how best to educate the next generation of researchers in the time allotted in most graduate programs. For many MFT programs, the whole work of understanding and practicing qualitative methods is contained in one, or possibly two, semester-length classes. This means that students usually receive a solid introduction to the well-known scientifically styled methods, such as ethnography, phenomenology, and grounded theory, but there may be scant time for learning about the artistic, critical, and participatory approaches. Another factor in this time crunch is that many students may learn pieces of the skills needed to conduct a study, but do not have the opportunity to participate in a study from beginning to end within their standard curriculum (Webb & Glesne, 1992).

Some educators (e.g., Hoshmand, 1989) have proposed lengthier tracks for learning qualitative approaches, and some institutions, such as the University of Georgia, now offer graduate certificate programs in qualitative inquiries (*http://www.coe.uga.edu/edpsych/qualinquiry.html*). However, the fact remains that most qualitative researchers do not receive the training and supervision they really need in order to bring the overall caliber of the field to a new level. It also means that the diversity of methods will remain limited, thus making it difficult for researchers to locate methods to fit their questions. Sadly, the result is that the well-known methods will drive the questions explored.

Future Trends

Despite the gloomy picture painted above of contemporary graduate education in qualitative methods, some exciting developments occurring today do inspire hope for tomorrow. The literature on how best to teach qualitative research is growing, and these authors suggest that an activity-driven style of learning may be the best way to develop expertise in these challenging methods (e.g., Cobb & Hoffart, 1999; Fontes & Piercy, 2000). There is also a new trend of teaching qualitative research to undergraduates (e.g., Clark & Lang, 2002; Reising, 2003), which will help those teaching these methods to students at the graduate level. The Internet and other communication networks of the future also raise hopes. There is an ever-growing abundance of websites and web pages dedicated to all aspects of qualitative research, including teaching (e.g., see *http://www.wcer.wisc.edu/tqm* for the University of Wisconsin's Teaching Qualitative Methods site). This should help faculty and students alike.

Someday, we may see a more collaborative approach to educating our next generation, so that the burden of helping students learn the best methods available will not fall solely on the faculty of the students' department. In the future, we will move from static websites of qualitative research links and papers to dynamic, active online communities that will be something like a combination of Disney World's Epcot and North Carolina's Research Triangle Park. In such a community, students and faculty from around the world can visit the Qualitative Research Pavilion; have access to human and virtual park guides who can help parkgoers explore new methods and work with actual data; join research teams and work on cutting-edge projects, regardless of where they are living in the world; learn how to use the latest CAQDAS packages from the packages' creators themselves; and even earn credit by demonstrating through outcomes that they have mastered skills and have acquired knowledge. With luck, these online research parks of tomorrow will be here before we know it (see Chenail, 2004).

CONCLUSION

The best way to predict the future is to invent it.
—ALAN KAY

Therapists, clients, researchers, educators, and policymakers will all have a hand in shaping the future directions qualitative methods will take in the world of MFT. I remain hopeful that qualitative researchers will continue to demonstrate the value of their work to all MFT stakeholders. The diversity of the qualitative approaches represents these methods' greatest strength and is the crucial source of their long-term success. Because qualitative researchers can communicate their findings in forms that clinicians, clients, faculty, the public, and other investigators can all understand, their work will continue to inform knowledge, practice, and wisdom for years to come.

REFERENCES

Anfara, V. A., Jr., Brown, K. M., & Mangione, T. L. (2002). Qualitative analysis on stage: Making the research process more public. *Educational Researcher, 31*(7), 28–38.

Angen, M. J. (2000). Evaluating interpretive inquiry: Reviewing the validity debate and opening the dialogue. *Qualitative Health Research, 10*(3), 378–395.

Asher, N. S., & Asher, K. C. (1999). Qualitative methods for an outsider looking in. In M. Kopala & L. A. Suzuki (Eds.), *Using qualitative methods in psychology* (pp. 135–144). Thousand Oaks, CA: Sage.

Ayres, L., Kavanaugh, K., & Knafl, K. A. (2003). Within-case and across-case approaches to qualitative data analysis. *Qualitative Health Research, 13*(6), 871–883.

Bailey, P. H. (1996). Assuring quality in narrative analysis. *Western Journal of Nursing Research, 18*(2), 186–194.

Barbour, R. S. (2000). The role of qualitative research in broadening the 'evidence base' for clinical practice. *Journal of Evaluation in Clinical Practice, 6*(2), 155–163.

Barbour, R. S. (2001). Checklists for improving rigour in qualitative research: A case of the tail wagging the dog? *British Medical Journal, 322,* 1115–1117.

Barrett, E. (Ed.). (1992). *Sociomedia: Multimedia, hypermedia, and the social construction of knowledge.* Cambridge, MA: MIT Press.

Barroso, J., & Powell-Cope, G. M. (2000). Metasynthesis of qualitative research on living with HIV infection. *Qualitative Health Research, 10*(3), 340–353.

Bateson, M. C. (1989). *Composing a life.* Boston: Atlantic Monthly Press.

Bauer, M. W., & Gaskell, G. (2000). *Qualitative researching with text, image and sound: A practical handbook.* London: Sage.

Berger, R., & Malkinson, R. (2000). "Therapeutizing" research: The positive impact of family-focused research on participants. *Smith College Studies in Social Work, 70*(2), 307–314.

Bochner, A. P., & Ellis, C. (Eds.). (2002). *Ethnographically speaking: Autoethnography, literature, and aesthetics.* Walnut Creek, CA: AltaMira Press.

Boudah, D. J., & Lenz, B. K. (2000). And now the rest of the story: The research process as intervention in experimental and qualitative studies. *Learning Disabilities Research and Practice, 15*(3), 149–159.

Bowen, M. (1978). On the differentiation of self. In M. Bowen, *Family therapy in clinical practice* (pp. 467–528). New York: Aronson. (Original work presented 1967, published anonymously 1972)

Byrne, M. M. (2001). Evaluating the findings of qualitative research. *Association of periOperative Registered Nurses Journal, 73*(3), 703–706.

Caelli, K., Ray, L., & Mill, J. (2003). 'Clear as mud': Toward greater clarity in generic qualitative research. *International Journal of Qualitative Methods, 2*(2). Article 1. Retrieved from *http://www.ualberta.ca/~iiqm/backissues/2_2/html/caellietal.htm*

Camic, P. M., Rhodes, J., E., & Yardley, L. (Eds.). (2003). *Qualitative research in psychology: Expanding perspectives in methodology and design.* Washington, DC: American Psychological Association.

Carey, M. A., & Swanson, J. (2003). Funding for qualitative research. *Qualitative Health Research, 13*(6), 852–856.

Carspecken, P. F. (1996). *Critical ethnography in educational research: A theoretical and practical guide.* New York: Routledge.

Chenail, R. J. (1990–1991). Bradford Keeney's cybernetic project and the creation of recursive frame analysis. *The Qualitative Report, 1*(2–3). Retrieved from *http://www.nova.edu/ssss/QR/QR1-23/keeney.html*

Chenail, R. J. (1991). *Medical discourse and systemic frames of comprehension.* Norwood, NJ: Ablex.

Chenail, R. J. (1995). Recursive frame analysis. *The Qualitative Report, 2*(2). Retrieved from *http://www.nova.edu/ssss/QR/QR1-2/rfa.html*

Chenail, R. J. (1997). Keeping things plumb in qualitative research. *The Qualitative Report, 3*(3). Retrieved from *http://www.nova.edu/ssss/QR/QR3-3/plumb.html*

Chenail, R. J. (2004). When Disney meets the research park: Metaphors and models for engineering an online learning community of tomorrow. *Internet and Higher Education, 7,* 107–121.

Christensen, G. L., & Olson, J. C. (2002). Mapping consumers' mental models with ZMET. *Psychology and Marketing, 19*(6), 477–501.

Clandinin, D. J., & Connelly, F. M. (2000). *Narrative inquiry: Experience and story in qualitative research.* San Francisco: Jossey-Bass.

Clark, R., & Lang, A. (2002). Balancing yin and yang: Teaching and learning qualitative data analysis within an undergraduate quantitative data analysis course. *Teaching Sociology, 30*(3), 348–360.

Clemmens, D. (2003). Adolescent motherhood: A meta-synthesis of qualitative studies. *American Journal of Maternal/Child Nursing, 28*(2), 93–99.

Cobb, A. K., & Hoffart, N. (1999). Teaching qualitative research through participatory coursework and mentorship. *Journal of Professional Nursing, 15*(6), 331–339.

Constas, M. A. (1992). Qualitative analysis as a public event: The documentation of category development procedures. *American Educational Research Journal, 29*(2), 253–266.

Cooperrider, D. L., Sorensen, P. F., Whitney, D., & Yaeger, T. F. (Eds.). (2000). *Appreciative inquiry: Rethinking human organization toward a positive theory of change.* Champaign, IL: Stipes.

Cooperrider, D. L., & Whitney, D. K. (1999). *Appreciative inquiry.* Williston, VT: Berrett Koehler Communications.

Daiute, C., & Lightfoot, C. (2004). *Narrative analysis: Studying the development of individuals in society.* Thousand Oaks, CA: Sage.

Davis, J. H. (2003). Balancing the whole: Portraiture as methodology. In P. M. Camic, J. E. Rhodes, & L. Yardley (Eds.), *Qualitative research in psychology: Expanding perspectives in methodology and design* (pp. 199–217) Washington, DC: American Psychological Association.

Deacon, S. A., & Piercy, F. P. (2000). Qualitative evaluation of family therapy programs: A participatory approach. *Journal of Marital and Family Therapy, 26*(1), 39–45.

Denzin, H. K. (2003). *Performing ethnography: The politics of culture.* London: Sage.

Denzin, H. K., & Lincoln, Y. S. (Eds.). (1994a). *Handbook of qualitative research.* Thousand Oaks, CA: Sage.

Denzin, H. K., & Lincoln, Y. S. (1994b). Introduction: Entering the field of qualitative research. In N. K. Denzin & Y. S. Lincoln (Eds.), *Handbook of qualitative research* (pp. 1–17). Thousand Oaks, CA: Sage.

Denzin, H. K., & Lincoln, Y. S. (Eds.). (2000a). *Handbook of qualitative research* (2nd. ed.). Thousand Oaks, CA: Sage.

Denzin, H. K., & Lincoln, Y. S. (2000b). Introduction: The discipline and practice of qualitative research. In N. K. Denzin & Y. S. Lincoln (Eds.), *Handbook of qualitative research* (2nd ed., pp. 1–28). Thousand Oaks, CA: Sage.

Dixon-Woods, M., Fitzpatrick, R., & Roberts. K. (2001). Including qualitative research in systematic reviews: Opportunities and problems. *Journal of Evaluation in Clinical Practice, 7*(2), 125–133.

Drisko, J. W. (1997). Strengthening qualitative studies and reports: Standards to promote academic integrity. *Journal of Social Work Education, 33*(1), 185–198.

Duffy, M., & Chenail, R. (2004). Qualitative strategies in couple and family assessment. In L. Sperry (Ed.), *Assessment of couples and families: Contemporary and cutting-edge strategies* (pp. 33–63). New York: Brunner-Routledge.

Duncan, B. L., & Miller, S. D. (2000). *The heroic client: Doing client-directed, outcome-informed therapy.* San Francisco: Jossey-Bass.

Eisner, E. W. (1981). On the differences between scientific and artistic approaches to qualitative research. *Educational Research, 10*(4), 5–9.

Ellis, C. (2004). *The ethnographic I: A methodological novel about autoethnography.* Walnut Creek, CA: AltaMira Press.

Ellis, C., & Bochner, A. P. (Eds.). (1996). *Composing ethnography: Alternative forms of qualitative writing.* Walnut Creek, CA: AltaMira Press.

Ellis, C., & Bochner, A. P. (2000). Authoethnography, personal narrative, reflexivity: Researcher as subject. In N. K. Denzin & Y. S. Lincoln (Eds.), *Handbook of qualitative research* (2nd ed., pp. 733–768). Thousand Oaks, CA: Sage.

Faulkner, R. A., Klock, K., & Gale, J. E. (2002). Qualitative research in family therapy: Publication trends from 1980 to 1999. *Journal of Marital and Family Therapy, 28*(1), 69–74.

Finfgeld, D. L (2003). Metasynthesis: The state of the art—so far. *Qualitative Health Research, 13*(7), 893–904.

Flemons, F., & Green, S. (2002). Stories that conform/stories that transform: A conversation in four parts. In A. P. Bochner & C. Ellis (Eds.), *Ethnographically speaking: Autoethnography, literature, and aesthetics* (pp. 87–94, 115–121, 167–171, 189–192). Walnut Creek, CA: AltaMira Press.

Fontes, L. A., & Piercy, F. P. (2000). Engaging students in qualitative research through experiential class activities. *Teaching of Psychology, 27*(3), 174–179.

Gale, J. (1992). When research interviews are more therapeutic than therapy interviews. *The Qualitative Report, 1*(4). Retrieved from *http://www.nova.edu/ssss/QR/QR1-4/gale.html*

Gamson, J. (2000). Sexualities, queer theory, and qualitative research. In N. K. Denzin & Y. S. Lincoln (Eds.), *Handbook of qualitative research* (2nd ed., pp. 347–365). Thousand Oaks, CA: Sage.

Gee, J. P. (2003). *What video games have to teach us about learning and literacy.* New York: Palgrave Macmillan.

Gehart, D. R., & Lyle, R. R. (1999). Client and therapist perspectives of change in collaborative language systems: An interpretive ethnography. *Journal of Systemic Therapies, 18*(4), 78–97.

Gehart, D. R., Ratliff, D. A., & Lyle, R. R. (2001). Qualitative research in family therapy: A substantive and methodological review. *Journal of Marital and Family Therapy, 27*(2), 261–274.

Gergen, M. M., & Gergen, K. J. (2000). Qualitative inquiry: Tensions and transformations. In N. K. Denzin & Y. S. Lincoln (Eds.), *Handbook of qualitative research* (2nd ed., pp. 1025–1046). Thousand Oaks, CA: Sage.

Gilgun, J. (2002). Conjectures and refutations: Governmental funding and qualitative research. *Qualitative Social Work, 1*(3), 359–375.

Glaser, B. G., & Strauss, A. L. (1967). *The discovery of grounded theories: Strategies for qualitative research.* Chicago: Aldine.

Heurtin-Roberts, S. (2002). Thoughts on qualitative research methods at NIH. *Qualitative Social Work, 1*(3), 376–379.

Hoshmand, L. T. (1989). Alternate research paradigms: A review and teaching proposal. *Counseling Psychologist, 17*(1), 3–79.

Hubble, M. A., Duncan, B. L., & Miller, S. D. (Eds.). (1999). *The heart and soul of change: What works in therapy.* Washington, DC: American Psychological Association.

Jason, L. A., Keys, C. B., Suarez-Balcazar, Y., Taylor, R. R., & Davis, M. I. (Eds.). (2004). *Participatory community research: Theories and methods in action*. Washington, DC: American Psychological Association.

Josselson, R., Lieblich, A., & McAdams, D. P. (Eds.). (2003). *Up close and personal: The teaching and learning of narrative research*. Washington, DC: American Psychological Association.

Karl [Tomm], Cynthia, Andrew, & Vanessa. (1992). Therapeutic distinctions in an on-going therapy. In S. McNamee & K. J. Gergen (Eds.), *Therapy as social construction* (pp. 116–135). London: Sage

Kemmis, S., & McTaggart, R. (2000). Participatory action research. In N. K. Denzin & Y. S. Lincoln (Eds.), *Handbook of qualitative research* (2nd ed., pp. 567–605). Thousand Oaks, CA: Sage.

King, G., Keohane, R. O., & Verba, S. (1994). *Designing social inquiry: Scientific inference in qualitative research*. Princeton, NJ: Princeton University Press.

Kopala, M., & Suzuki, L. A. (Eds.). (1999). *Using qualitative methods in psychology* (pp. 135–144). Thousand Oaks, CA: Sage.

Kuehl, B. P., Newfield, N. A., & Joanning, H. (1990). A client-based description of family therapy. *Journal of Family Psychology*, *3*(3), 310–321.

Lawrence Lightfoot, S., & Davis, J. H. (1997). *The art and science of portraiture*. San Francisco: Jossey-Bass.

Liddle, H. A., Santisteban, D. A., Levant, R. F., & Bray, J. H. (Eds.). (2002). *Family psychology: Science-based interventions*. Washington, DC: American Psychological Association.

Lincoln, Y. S., & Denzin, N. K. (1994). The fifth moment. In N. K. Denzin & Y. S. Lincoln (Eds.), *Handbook of qualitative research* (pp. 575–586). Thousand Oaks, CA: Sage.

Lincoln, Y. S., & Denzin, N. K. (2000). The seventh moment: Out of the past. In N. K. Denzin & Y. S. Lincoln (Eds.), *Handbook of qualitative research* (2nd ed., pp. 1047–1065). Thousand Oaks, CA: Sage.

Lincoln, Y. S., & Guba, E. G. (2000). Paradigmatic controversies, contradictions, and emerging confluences. In N. K. Denzin & Y. S. Lincoln (Eds.), *Handbook of qualitative research* (2nd ed., pp. 163–188). Thousand Oaks, CA: Sage.

Maione, P. V., & Chenail, R. J. (1999). Qualitative inquiry in psychotherapy: Research on the common factors. In M. A. Hubble, B. L. Duncan, & S. D. Miller (Eds.), *The heart and soul of change: What works in therapy* (pp. 57–88). Washington, DC: American Psychological Association.

Mann, C., & Stewart, F. (2000). *Internet communication and qualitative research: A handbook for researching online*. Thousand Oaks, CA: Sage.

McAdams, D. P., Josselson, R., & Lieblich, A. (Eds.). (2001). *Turns in the road: Narrative studies of lives in transition*. Washington, DC: American Psychological Association.

McDowell, T., Fang, S.-R., Gomez Young, C., Khanna, A., Sherman, B., & Brownlee, K. (2003). Making space for racial dialogue: Our experience in a marriage and family therapy training program. *Journal of Marital and Family Therapy*, *29*(2), 179–194.

McLeod, J. (2001). *Qualitative research in counseling and psychotherapy*. London: Sage.

Minuchin, S. (1984). *Family kaleidoscope*. Cambridge, MA: Harvard University Press.

Morse, J. M. (2003a). The adjudication of qualitative proposals. *Qualitative Health Research*, *13*(6), 739–742.

Morse, J. M. (2003b). A review committee's guide for evaluating qualitative proposals. *Qualitative Health Research*, *13*(6), 833–851.

Murray, B. L. (2003). Qualitative research interviews: Therapeutic benefits for the participants. *Journal of Psychiatric and Mental Health Nursing*, *10*(2), 231–238.

Napier, A. Y., & Whitaker, C. A. (1978). *The family crucible*. New York: Harper & Row.

National Institute of Mental Health. (2001, December). *Qualitative methods in health research:*

Opportunities and considerations in applications and review (NIH Publication No. 02-5046). Retrieved from *http://obssr.od.nih.gov/publications/qualitative.pdf*

Page, R. (2000). Future directions in qualitative research. *Harvard Educational Review, 70*(1), 100–108.

Patton, M. Q. (1999). Enhancing the quality and credibility of qualitative analysis. *Health Services Research, 34*(5), 1189–1209.

Patton, M. Q. (2002). *Qualitative research and evaluation methods* (3rd ed.). Thousand Oaks, CA: Sage.

Piercy, F. P., & Benson, K. (2005). Aesthetic forms of data representation in qualitative family therapy research. *Journal of Martial and Family Therapy, 31*(1), 107–119.

Piercy, F. P., & Thomas, V. (1998). Participatory evaluation research: An introduction for family therapists. *Journal of Marital and Family Therapy, 24*(2), 165–176.

Pittinger, R. E., Hockett, C. F., & Danehy, J. J. (1960). *The first five minutes: A sample of microscopic interview analysis.* Ithaca, NY: Paul Martineau.

Pote, H., Stratton, P., Cottrell, D., Shapiro, D., & Boston, P. (2003). Systemic family therapy can be manualized: Research process and findings. *Journal of Family Therapy, 25,* 236–262.

Prosser, J. (1998). *Image-based research: A sourcebook for qualitative researchers.* London: Falmer Press.

Rambo, A. H., Heath, A. W., & Chenail, R. J. (1993). *Practicing therapy: Exercises for growing therapists.* New York: Norton.

Ray, W. A., & Keeney, B. (1993). *Resource focused therapy.* London: Karnac Books.

Reising, D. L. (2003). Establishing student competency in qualitative research: Can undergraduate nursing students perform qualitative data analysis? *Journal of Nursing Education, 42*(5), 216–219.

Ricci, R. J. (2003). Autoethnographic verse: Nicky's boy: A life in two worlds. *The Qualitative Report, 8*(4), 591–596. Retrieved from *http://www.nova.edu/ssss/QR/QR8-4/ricci.pdf*

Rounsaville, B. J., Carroll, K. M., & Onken, L. S. (2001). A stage model of behavioral therapies research: Getting started and moving on from Stage I. Clinical. *Psychology: Science and Practice, 8*(2), 133–142.

Rowan, M., & Huston, P. (1997). Qualitative research articles: Information for authors and peer reviewers. *Canadian Medical Association Journal, 157*(10), 1442–1447.

Rudes, J., Shilts, L., & Berg, I. K. (1997). Focused supervision seen through a recursive frame analysis. *Journal of Marital and Family Therapy, 23*(2), 203–215.

Russell, C. K., & Gregory, D. M. (2003). Evaluation of qualitative research studies. *Evidence-Based Nursing, 6*(2), 36–40.

Ryan, G. W., & Bernard, H. R. (2000). Data management and analysis methods. In N. K. Denzin & Y. S. Lincoln (Eds.), *Handbook of qualitative research* (2nd ed., pp. 769–802). Thousand Oaks, CA: Sage.

Sandelowski, M., & Barroso, J. (2003). Writing the proposal for a qualitative research methodology project. *Qualitative Health Research, 13*(6), 781–820.

Sandelowski, M., Docherty, S., & Emden, C. (1997). Focus on qualitative methods. Qualitative metasynthesis: Issues and techniques. *Research in Nursing and Health, 20*(4), 365–371.

Scheflen, A. E. (1973). *Communicational structure: Analysis of a psychotherapy transaction.* Bloomington: Indiana University Press.

Schindler Zimmerman, T., Holm, K. E., & Starrels, M. E. (2001). A feminist analysis of self-help bestsellers for improving relationships: A decade review. *Journal of Marital and Family Therapy, 27*(2), 165–175.

Seale, C. (1999). *The quality of qualitative research.* Thousand Oaks, CA: Sage.

Sells, S. P., Smith, T. E., & Moon, S. (1996). An ethnographic study of client and therapist perceptions of therapy effectiveness in a university-based training clinic. *Journal of Marital and Family Therapy*, 22(3), 321–342.

Smith, B. A. (1999). Ethical and methodologic benefits of using a reflexive journal in hermeneutic–phenomenologic research. *Image: Journal of Nursing Scholarship*, 31(4), 359–363.

Sparks, J. A. (2002). Taking a stand: An adolescent girl's resistance to medication. *Journal of Marital and Family Therapy*, 28(1), 27–38.

Sprenkle, D. H. (Ed.). (2002). *Effectiveness research in marriage and family therapy*. Alexandria, VA: American Association for Marriage and Family Therapy.

Strauss, A., & Corbin, J. (1998). *Basics of qualitative research: Techniques and procedures for developing grounded theory*. Thousand Oaks, CA: Sage.

Visweswaran, K. (1994). *Fictions of feminist ethnography*. Minneapolis: University of Minnesota Press.

Waldegrave, C., Tamasese, K., Tuhaka, F., & Campbell, W. (2003). *Just therapy: A journey*. Adelaide, South Australia: Dulwich Centre.

Webb, R. B., & Glesne, C. (1992). Teaching qualitative research. In M. D. LeCompte, W. L. Millroy, & J. Preissle (Eds.), *The handbook of qualitative research in education* (pp. 771–814). San Diego, CA: Academic Press.

Weitzman, E. A. (2000). Software and qualitative research. In N. K. Denzin & Y. S. Lincoln (Eds.), *Handbook of qualitative research* (2nd ed., pp. 803–820). Thousand Oaks, CA: Sage.

Zaltman, G. (1996). Metaphorically speaking. *Marketing Research*, 8(2), 13–21.

Zaltman, G. (2003). *How customers think: Essential insights into the mind of the market*. Boston: Harvard Business School Press.

PART III
MIXED METHODS

CHAPTER 12

Survey Research in Marr2iage and Family Therapy

THORANA S. NELSON
DAVID D. ALLRED

BACKGROUND

"Survey," as a verb, means "to examine, inspect or consider carefully" (Guralnik, 1966, p. 749). As a noun, a survey is a "general study: as a *survey* of public opinion" (Guralnik, 1966, p. 749). McGraw and Watson (1976) define "survey research" as "a method of collecting standardized information by interviewing a sample representative of some population" (p. 343). Survey research "studies large and small populations by selecting and studying samples chosen from the population to discover the relative incidence, distribution, and interrelations of sociological and psychological variables" (Kerlinger, 1986, p. 378). Warwick and Lininger (1975) describe survey research as a "method of collecting information about a human population in which direct contact is made with the units of the study (individuals, organizations, communities, etc.) through such systematic means as questionnaires and interview schedules" (p. 2). Common terms that emerge in definitions of survey research are "sample," "information," "questionnaire" or "interview schedule," and (for our purposes) "sociological variables" and "psychological variables." The sample is the *who* of the study, the variables are the *what*, and the questionnaire is the *how*. Survey research, then, is a method of collecting data from or about a group of people and asking questions in some fashion about things of interest to the researcher for the purpose of generalizing to a population represented by the group or sample.

Broadly, a sample is a part selected to represent a larger whole (Warwick & Lininger, 1975). The "sampling frame" is the set of people who have a chance of being selected (Fowler, 2002). The variables are the concepts or information in which the researcher is interested. A questionnaire or interview schedule is a series of questions presented to the sample in person by an interviewer, over the telephone, through a self-administered mailed paper-and-pencil instrument, through the Internet, or in some other way. The data analyses and reports are then used to describe the group or to draw inferences about the variables, their relation to each other, and their relation to the population of interest.

Surveys usually focus on people—facts about them or their opinions, attitudes, motivations, behaviors, and so on—and the relationships among variables under study related to these people. For example, survey research might be used to compare demographic characteristics of a sample of people in a particular location, their access to mental health services, and their perceptions about the efficacy of those services. This information could be used to make recommendations about improving the services for that population or the methods for delivering them. In marriage and family therapy (MFT) research, Wetchler (1989; Wetchler, Piercy, & Sprenkle, 1989) surveyed both supervisors and supervisees about their impressions of their supervision experiences, and made suggestions about MFT training based on responses to his survey.

For the purposes of this chapter, survey research methods do not include those that involve experiments, as in therapy outcome research; discussions related to family therapy process research; or discussions of single-case studies, small samples, or observational methods of collecting data. This chapter *does* include discussions of methods related to gathering information from samples of volunteers for the purpose of describing, explaining, and/or exploring (1) particular aspects of the participants' experience, (2) ways these data relate to each other and to other data, and (3) ways the results of data analyses can be used to draw generalizations about larger populations. *Qualitative* research, designed to provide rich descriptions or to develop new theory based on in-depth personal interviews or content analysis of responses to open-ended questions, is described elsewhere in this volume. Readers interested in detailed discussions of instrument or questionnaire development are referred elsewhere (e.g., Dillman, 2000; Fowler, 2002) and to texts dedicated to instrument and questionnaire development).

The remainder of this chapter describes the history of survey research, various methods related to different stages of designing and conducting survey research, strengths and weaknesses of the method, issues of reliability and validity, researcher skills, and ways that survey research can be used to form bridges between clinicians and researchers. Because of space limitations, much of this chapter may seem sketchy to some readers. Readers are referred to appropriate texts for more in-depth discussions. Examples from the Basic Family Therapy Skills (BFTS) Project (e.g., Figley & Nelson, 1989) are used extensively to illustrate various points. Following is a brief description of the BFTS Project to provide context for the illustrations. Throughout the chapter, we will refer to this series of publications as the "BFTS Project," rather than repeating the citations. Readers may want to return to the description after reading this chapter and use the chapter for critiquing the study.

Basic Family Therapy Skills Project

One of us (TSN) and her colleagues (Figley & Nelson, 1989, 1990; Nelson & Benson, 2004; Nelson & Boxley, 2000; Nelson & Figley, 1990; Nelson, Heilbrun, & Figley, 1993; Nelson & Webb, 2001) embarked on an ambitious survey of family therapy supervisors, trainers, students, and trainees to determine their opinions about the essential skills for beginning and intermediate family therapists. The studies were designed to provide comprehensive lists of skills rather than consensus reports. The studies were carried out in several phases. In the first phase, we contacted all American Association for Marriage and Family Therapy (AAMFT)–approved supervisors and all members of the American Family Therapy Academy (AFTA)—describing our purposes and the scope of the study, outlining the criteria for participating, and inviting people to participate in a several-phase study. Invitations were personalized by using the merge capabilities of a word processor to enhance response rate (Dillman, 1978; Dillman & Frey, 1974). As much as possible, personal touches were used throughout the study. Dillman (2000) has since updated his survey method, which will be described later in this chapter.

Questionnaires were sent to those who responded and were eligible ($n = 688$). These asked for demographic information and experience as family therapists/trainers/ educators, and solicited nominations for essential, basic skills for beginning family therapists. Participants were asked to nominate skills from their theoretical preferences as well as generic basic skills. After the nominations were sorted and consolidated, lists of generic skills were sent to the participants in Phase II. Each questionnaire listed the nominated skills and asked the participants to rate each in terms of its importance for beginning-level family therapy trainees. Participants were also invited to provide comments.

To enhance the response rate of Phase II, participants received only one-quarter of the nominated items, making the questionnaires more manageable in length for each person. Multiple questionnaires of the model-specific items were sent to those requesting them in Phase III of the project. The model-specific questionnaires included the same Likert-type response choices as the generic survey plus several categorical response choices based on feedback from the participants in Phase II. That is, in each phase of the survey, we used information from earlier phases to enhance the quality of the data. In each phase, follow-up postcards were sent to the sample to enhance response rates.

Data from the generic survey were analyzed by computing means, sorting the items accordingly, and producing a ranked list; these data were reported by Figley and Nelson (1990). Data from the model-specific phase (Phase III) were analyzed by first comparing the responses of participants who were self-expressed users of a particular model with those of participants who reported that they used a different model. In no case were the groups judged different (according to chi-square tests) in their responses to the items. Items were then ranked by means and standard deviations. Several of the model-specific results have been published (Figley & Nelson, 1989, 1990; Nelson & Figley, 1990; Nelson et al., 1993).

Data from these phases were combined with information from the literature, as well as from graduate programs accredited by the Commission on Accreditation for Marriage and Family Therapy Education (COAMFTE) about their evaluation procedures. This resulted in an instrument to evaluate students on their skills development (Nelson & Johnson, 1999). Additional phases of the project have surveyed students on their ideas about what they need to learn (Nelson & Webb, 2001), supervisors of intermediate trainees (those who have graduated and are working toward MFT licensure or clinical membership in AAMFT; Nelson & Boxley, 2000), and the trainees themselves (Nelson & Benson, 2004).

History of Survey Research

Surveys have been used for nearly as long as recorded history. Egyptians and Romans used census surveys to gather information about their citizenry for purposes of developing tax rates, conducting military conscription, and meeting other administrative needs (Warwick & Lininger, 1975). John Howard, an 18th-century British reformer, surveyed prison conditions in England and their effects on inmates' health. An economist, Frederic LePlay, surveyed income and expenses of households in 19th-century France to aid in social planning. He also checked his information against independent sources: observations and reports of others. In the late 19th century, Charles Book, a statistician, studied poverty in England, asserting that effective change required accurate data on a problem (Warwick & Lininger, 1975).

The 1930s and 1940s saw an alliance between the developments of probability sampling techniques from agriculture (developed to estimate crop yields) and controlled interviewing methods (Warwick & Lininger, 1975). Prior to this time, social science considered sampling methods too difficult to gather an accurate picture of a population. Rensis Likert, creator of the famous Likert (1932) scale used so much in social science research today, pioneered the study of people's attitudes, beliefs, and behaviors. Paul Lazersfeld moved beyond even this sort of descriptive survey to causal explanations and hypothesis testing using survey sampling techniques.

In family therapy research, many surveys have been designed to determine what clinicians think or do. Survey research has been used to ask clinicians about their use of assessment instruments (Boughner, Hayes, Bubenzer, & West, 1994), their actions when faced with ethical dilemmas (Green & Hansen, 1986, 1989), their practice patterns (Doherty & Simmons, 1996; Nelson & Palmer, 2001; Northey, 2002), barriers to their participating in research (Sandberg, Johnson, Robila, & Miller, 2002), their uses or views of their clinical training (Carter, 1989; Coleman, Avis, & Turin, 1990; Keller, Huber, & Hardy, 1988; Wilson & Stith, 1993), and their attitudes toward aging (Ivey, Wieling, & Harris, 2000).

Survey research has also been used to query directors of training programs about their views of accreditation standards (Keller et al., 1988), theory-of-change projects (Nelson & Prior, 2003), ways of dealing with the situations of impaired students (Russell & Peterson, 2003), uses of clinical research in their programs (McWey et al., 2002), views of admission and program requirements (O'Sullivan & Gilbert, 1989), and issues related to ethnicity and gender in their curricula (Coleman et al., 1990; Wilson & Stith, 1993). Students have been surveyed about their ethnic minority status and related experience in training (Wilson & Stith, 1993) and about their experiences as therapists in training (Anderson, Rigazio-DiGilio, & Kunkler, 1995; Anderson, Schlossberg, & Rigazio-DiGilio, 2000; Wetchler, 1989; Wetchler et al., 1989). Supervisors have been asked about their training practices (Lewis & Rohrbaugh, 1989; Nichols, Nichols, & Hardy, 1990), about their views of essential basic family therapy skills (BFTS Project), and about the essential elements of MFT and MFT supervision (White, Edwards, & Russell, 1997; White & Russell, 1995). Individuals also have been surveyed for their opinions about their experiences as clients in therapy, including which components of therapy were most influential for them. Nylund and Thomas (1994) conducted this sort of survey to determine whether or not letters Nylund had written (a narrative approach) had been helpful to his clients and, if so, to what extent. The responses to his survey yielded information about his approach not only for his own enlightenment, but also as a way of informing his clinical practice in the context of managed care and brief therapy.

Delphi models, a particular form of survey research, are often used to query a panel of experts on a topic through several phases of inquiry and feedback; these models are discussed more extensively by Stone Fish and Busby (Chapter 13, this volume).

Experts have been surveyed in other ways, however, to obtain their views on a number of topics—including family therapy skills (BFTS Project) and, interestingly, family therapy workshops (Heath, McKenna, & Atkinson, 1988).

On occasion, members of the general population or a class of clients have been surveyed to determine their experiences of a particular issue. Examples include wives' experience of their husbands' posttraumatic stress disorder (PTSD) symptoms or combat stress reactions (Solomon, Ott, & Roach, 1986), PTSD in Holocaust child survivors (Lev-Wiesel & Amir, 2000), depression and marital adjustment in infertile couples (Peterson, Newton, & Rosen, 2003), divorce and coparenting (Baum, 2003), love (Riehl-Emde, Thomas, & Willi, 2003), and the effects of differing wake–sleep patterns on marital relationships (Larson, Crane, & Smith, 1991). Halik, Rosenthal, and Pattison (1990) measured personal authority (Bray, Williamson, & Malone, 1984) of daughters of Jewish Holocaust survivors or immigrants. Finally, although this was not strictly survey research using *people*, medical records have been surveyed to determine the cost offset of mental health care utilization (Crane & Law, 2002; Law, Crane, & Burge, 2003). These examples of survey research pertain to family therapy by virtue of the constructs measured and are often easily extrapolated into family therapy interventions.

METHODOLOGY

Planning Survey Research

Fowler (1988, 2002) suggested a "total design" concept for planning survey research. In this concept, each stage of the project—from determining the goals and purposes of the study through reporting the results—operates recursively with every other stage, each one informing the others until a clear plan emerges. This kind of careful planning helps prevent both sampling error (described below) and nonsampling error, which includes errors related to the questions asked of the participants, their responses, coding and processing the data, analyzing the data, and reporting the results of the study. As much as possible, error should be limited in each area so that the researcher has confidence in the results of the study. Researchers should consult books and articles (e.g., de Vaus, 1986; Dillman, 2000; Fink & Kosecoff, 1985; Fowler, 2002; Hackett, 1981; Jolliffe, 1986; Miller, 1986; Warwick & Lininger, 1975) and statistical consultants, and should conduct pilot studies to refine their projects.

Goals and Purposes

The first step in the planning stage of survey research is determining the purpose of the project and setting goals. At this time, investigators should think about the later stages of the project: the analyses and report writing. By working back and forth through each stage of the project, an investigator ensures that each stage is strong in the context of the others, limits error as much as possible, and ensures that the project can be appropriately executed.

For example, in the BFTS Project, our original end goal was to produce a textbook for master's-level family therapy students and instructors, based on empirically derived basic family therapy skills. As we thought about this goal, we began to realize that other goals were desirable, including developing instruments that could be used to evaluate family therapy trainees (Nelson & Johnson, 1999) and to determine which aspects of family therapy are predictive of successful therapy outcomes. These new goals required us to rethink the methods of the project, adding procedures that would help develop an instrument.

Research Questions in Survey Investigations

Survey research is often used to determine characteristics or descriptions of samples (and thus of populations). For example, a researcher might want to know typical characteristics of families who enter therapy. Information could be gathered about variables such as age, income, education, ethnicity or race, types of presenting problems, family structures, and/or other factors. In addition to demographic descriptions, the researcher could gather information related to who does what, why, how, how well, and with what effect. The researcher could correlate the elicited information with demographic descriptions of the sample.

Researchers can investigate questions related to behavior, influences on behaviors, attitudes, beliefs, values, and the relationship between beliefs and behaviors. For example, clinicians may believe that they are quite sensitive to and aware of the cultural contexts of their clients. These beliefs can be explored through attitude questionnaires or probing interviews. Data can then be correlated with responses to questions posed after each clinician has read a case study vignette designed to elicit clinical choices. At the same time, clients can be surveyed regarding their experiences in therapy related to contextual issues. All the information can then be analyzed together to provide a picture of how well therapists do what they believe they do.

Ivey and colleagues (2000) wanted to compare attitudes of nonclinicians, therapists in training, and marriage and family therapists related to issues of aging. They presented respondents with a vignette about a couple in therapy. Two versions were randomly assigned; in one version the partners were in their 30s and in the other they were in their 60s. Respondents were then asked a series of questions designed to elicit attitudes toward older couples.

In the BFTS Project, we were interested in the kinds of skills that supervisors from specific theoretical perspectives thought were most important for therapy trainees. We compared groups on the variable "preferred theoretical perspective" and noted that, for the most part, the groups were similar in the way they rated different skills for particular theories. That is, those who used a particular family therapy theory in their own practices tended to rate the skills in a fashion similar to that of supervisors who preferred other theories. This suggested to us that the skills nominated by our sample were indeed derived from generic constructs rather than from preferred personal practice.

Survey methods use information gathered *directly* from the participants themselves. However, this information can be compared to other information to answer complex questions. For example, an administrator of a family therapy clinic may want to evaluate the effectiveness and efficiency of therapy performed to enhance an effort to secure a certain kind of therapy contract (e.g., a health maintenance organization panel or a state domestic violence contract). Administrators can survey a sample of the clinic's former clients using a variety of instruments that assess family dynamics (e.g., the Family Assessment Device; Epstein, Baldwin, & Bishop, 1983); they also can ask questions about the clients' satisfaction with the clinic's services, using their own instrument and/or other questions. Furthermore, administrators can ask the therapists about their opinions of the clients' therapy, and then compare all the data with clinic records: scores on assessment instruments, number of sessions, presenting problems, economic levels, race/ethnicity, and so on. In the BFTS Project, after surveying supervisors regarding their ideas about essential beginning skills, we surveyed the literature, compared the skills reported there to our supervisors' ideas, and generated a new, more comprehensive list of skills.

It is critical for researchers to develop their research questions carefully so that the variables are appropriate and are clearly defined and operationalized. A thorough discussion of types of variables and measurements can be found in many standard measurement textbooks. In general, however, investigators must determine the independent and dependent variables and their levels of measurement; they also must decide whether they want to *describe* a population or *draw inferences* about it, in terms of either how the variables are associated with each other or how groups compare. There are many excellent texts that can help students and researchers learn the art of formulating research questions. Some of these include Creswell (2003) and Patten (2002). Both the Pyrczak and Sage publishing houses have books on nearly every aspect of research, survey and otherwise.

The variables of interest and their measurement level (nominal, ordinal, interval, or ratio) determine the way the data will be obtained (forms of questions and collecting strategy) and the analysis strategies. Thus the research questions must be formulated in the context of other stages of the project. Statistical consultation can be very helpful at this stage to ensure that the form of the data is adequate for the kinds of analyses required to answer the research questions.

Sampling

Although each element of the survey method is critical to the overall design of a good research project, the ability to generalize the results will be only as good as the sampling techniques used (Fowler, 2002). Sampling error is one of the most common and poorly described problems in survey research. "Sampling error" is that error associated with how well or how poorly the sample represents the population of interest. All samples result in some error. That is, no sample is perfectly representative of the population from which it is drawn; by chance, some error will occur. However, sampling error can result from poorly designed sampling strategies or from strategies that are not followed carefully; this is the type of error that should be avoided.

Sample Size

Although the size of the sample is important, a large sample will not make up for poor selection methods or lack of adherence to the method chosen. Fowler (2002) points out that determining a sample size is a complex process. The aim is to select a quality and quantity of units that will provide sufficient data to answer the research questions with an adequate level of confidence. The sample size also is determined by the sampling method (smaller size when one is using simple random methods than when one is using convenience samples), levels of variance in the variables (smaller n for more homogeneous samples), and expected response rate (higher n when expected response rate is low), in addition to the level of precision required or power desired.

As the sample size increases, the size of the margin of error increments decreases, and power increases. At a certain point, the costs associated with a larger sample size do not justify the slightly higher level of precision and confidence obtained. For a simple random sample with a fairly high expected response rate (60–75%), sample sizes of 150–200 are sufficient for confidence that the sampled mean is in fact similar to the population mean, within an acceptable margin of error (Fowler, 2002). (See Kraemer & Thiemann, 1987, for a more detailed discussion of power and sample sizes.)

Representativeness

A critical issue in sampling is representativeness. That is, the sample chosen must represent the population of interest sufficiently that the analyzed data can be generalized to the population. In general, the researcher must be sufficiently confident in the sampling procedures and the results of the study to say that the outcome is probably true for the sampled population. For example, it would not be helpful in an evaluation study to state that clients are generally satisfied with a service if the sampled group did not include those who were least satisfied. In such a case, the researcher must be certain to sample all segments of a population that might give diverse responses to the study's questions.

In family therapy research, we are sometimes less interested in the precision of generalization to larger populations than in feeling rather certain that the information gathered is sufficiently comprehensive to be useful for informing recommendations or opinions about a topic. That is, does the information represent all or most opinions rather than the "average" opinion? In the BFTS Project, we were less interested in the precision of the information than in its comprehensiveness—and therefore its usefulness to a broader population of family therapy supervisors and their trainees and to the field of family therapy in general.

Sampling Techniques

Sampling begins with a decision about the size of the sample desired and the method for selecting the sample. As noted at the beginning of this chapter, "sampling frame" is the group or list used for selecting potential respondents. This may be a complete list of the population or some subgroup. Two types of selection may be used: probability and nonprobability techniques. Probability sampling techniques are less prone to sampling error and thus are more representative of the population of interest. Nonprobability techniques may be used if generalizing to a population is not a critical issue but the information itself is needed and probability techniques are not possible or are too costly. In either case, the limitations of the method must be noted in reports. (See Jolliffe, 1986, for a more thorough discussion of error-estimating techniques associated with different kinds of sampling methods; see Fowler, 2002, and Warwick & Lininger, 1975, for detailed discussions of sampling methods.)

PROBABILITY SAMPLING

Probability sampling techniques (simple, systematic, stratified, and cluster) yield participants from the population of interest, each of whom has a known chance of being selected for the sample. Simple random sampling is considered the best method and the one with the least error (Hackett, 1981; Jolliffe, 1986; Kerlinger, 1986; Kerlinger & Lee, 1999). In this method, a complete list of the targeted population is used and participants are chosen through random selection procedures. This may mean assigning a number to each potential subject and using a computer- or table-generated list of random numbers to select the sample. Such a method might be useful if one needed a sample of clinical members of the AAMFT.

Systematic sampling involves determining the proportion of the population needed in the sample and choosing each nth subject in a list. Instead of using a table of random numbers to determine each member of the sample, the researcher could choose one number from the table and then count out each nth person after that. For example, if there were 5,000 people in the population and 200 were needed for the sample, the researcher would use a table of random numbers to pick a starting point and then select each 25th person.

Stratified sampling involves random selection of participants from essential subgroups of a population (Miller, 1986). This ensures adequate representation from each group for description or comparison. For example, it may be important to describe or compare a population based on race. By chance, too few participants from some racial groups could be chosen if simple random sampling techniques were used. In this case, a proportionate number (based on known proportions of each group in the population) could be randomly chosen from each group. If the number of cases chosen in this way is too small for some groups, disproportionate numbers can be chosen from each group (Miller, 1986). Although the results of the study might not generalize well to the entire population, it is more likely that the data will be comprehensive and representative of the diversity of the population.

Finally, cluster (or "multistage") sampling may be used to assist in selecting respondents when the population is very large or there is no available listing of the total population. In this method, participants are selected in stages, beginning by randomly choosing sections of the population and then randomly choosing participants from within these sections. For example, if a researcher wanted to survey licensed or certified marriage and family therapists in the United States, obtaining a complete list would be very difficult. However, a researcher could randomly choose several states that certify or license marriage and family therapists, and then obtain lists of certified or licensed therapists from those states. Participants would then be selected from those lists.

NONPROBABILITY SAMPLING

Nonprobability sampling techniques may be used when representativeness of a whole population is not as important as the information itself or when probability sampling is not feasible. Nonprobability sampling significantly increases sampling error and introduces bias into the sample (Miller, 1986). Sometimes this bias can be accounted for and taken into consideration when one is reporting the results of the project. At other times it will compromise the results so badly that they are not useful. This is most obvious when the bias is related to the purpose of the project. For example, a health survey that could not question hospitalized participants could yield extremely skewed and therefore useless data. In any case, the limitations and strengths of the method should be explained in reports so that readers may draw their own conclusions about potential sample bias.

"Judgmental," "purposive," or "expert" sampling may be appropriate when data from a particular group are required and the researcher uses some rational method for selecting participants. In the BFTS Project, we were interested in opinions from those who were most expert at training family therapists. Therefore, we used lists of AAMFT approved supervisors and members of AFTA as our expert panel. Because we did not have access to a list of *all* supervisors or trainers in family therapy (whether members of organizations or not), ours was not a probability sample and thus contained both known and unknown bias.

"Quota" sampling involves determining how many people from particular groups or subgroups are needed and then selecting participants nonrandomly until the determined number for each group is reached. Although this method ensures adequate numbers from each group to represent the population, it does not satisfy the criterion that each subject in the population has a known chance of being selected; persons in the smaller groups have a greater chance of being selected than those in the larger groups. However, economy of time and other resources may make this method expeditious, particularly when there are unequal numbers in groups.

A third nonprobability method of selecting participants uses "haphazard" or "convenience" techniques. These methods often entail using participants who are "handy," but the sample will probably not be representative of a population. For example, family therapy researchers may be interested in certain characteristics of therapists. It would be very difficult to obtain a list of all therapists, but relatively easy to determine the names of therapists at local agencies. The researchers may draw some tentative conclusions from this sample about therapists, but the data actually describe only local volunteer therapists.

"Snowball" or word-of-mouth samples also are convenience samples (Miller, 1986). In this strategy, participants are solicited who then suggest other potential participants. The danger is that the bias of the sample becomes compounded (e.g., students tend to suggest other students). This is a reasonable method, however, when a nonclinical sample is needed that matches a clinical sample in terms of age, education, and socioeconomic status. The participants in the clinical sample are likely to suggest people similar to themselves for the matched sample.

All sampling techniques have limitations as well as advantages. It is important for researchers to understand and comment on the limitations of the sampling techniques they use. It also is important to state any deviance from standard techniques. For example, a mail survey may yield an unacceptably low response rate. The researcher may telephone or e-mail those participants he or she believes will respond with a little encouragement. This method was used to survey COAMFTE-accredited programs about their theory-of-change projects (Nelson & Prior, 2003) and increased the response rate to an acceptable level. Although this technique may increase the response rate, it also biases the sample. The tradeoff may be worth the bias introduced, but it is important that the researcher include the potential for this bias in the research reports. Suggestions for increasing response rates are included in a later section of this chapter.

Decisions regarding sampling techniques should take into account many factors, including the resources of the researcher, as well as the questions being investigated. When precision is required, random sampling techniques that may cost more in terms of time and money are essential. However, when the research is exploratory, the potential population quite large, lists difficult to obtain, the potential biases of a sample well known, precision or ability to generalize to a population not essential, and/or the resources of the researcher low, convenience samples may be more appropriate or acceptable. On occasion, a mixed method of sampling will be adequate, with multiple stages and mixes of probability and nonprobability methods. Researchers should be aware, however, that sampling techniques are critical when articles are being judged for publication.

Nonrespondents

It often is as important in survey research to know the biases of the nonrespondent portion of the sample as to know those of the participants. Because, to some extent, most survey research involves self-selected nonrespondents (those who choose not to respond), the reasons for not participating are often quite important. In the BFTS Project, for example, our response rate for Phase IV was lower than in other phases. We surmised that this had as much to do with fatigue from our barrage of questionnaires, waning interest, and competing demands for time as with any other reason. Ideally, we would have found some way to sample nonrespondents to ascertain potential bias. However, this process would have required that these people *respond*—something we did not think they were likely to do. Therefore, we examined demographic variables to determine differences between this group of participants and groups from earlier phases of the project. We noted that the participant group in this phase, compared with other phases, contained a higher percentage of supervisors who had doctoral degrees and who listed university settings as primary places of employment and "researcher" as a secondary professional identity. We then surmised that these people were more likely to participate in the project because the results of our survey might apply to their work or they felt an obligation to help fellow researchers. We also hypothesized that this group included a higher proportion of supervisors working with master's-level graduate students—an ideal situation for our research, because we needed those who supervised *beginners* (who were working with their first families in therapy, and therefore who were in graduate school). If we had been looking for a broader array of items generalizable to all trainees, our results would have been much less useful.

Generating hypotheses about the characteristics of the nonrespondent portion of a sample can be quite challenging. Researchers can attempt to compare the demographic distribution of the responding sample (e.g., education, sex, age, etc.) to the population. For example, characteristics of a sample of AAMFT clinical members can be compared to the latest statistics about the demographic characteristics as generated by the AAMFT.

Data-Gathering Techniques

In survey research, the investigator gathers data by asking people questions. Strictly speaking, an "interview" is the format that the investigator uses to ask questions; it can be conducted in person, over the telephone, through mailed questionnaires, or in some other way. Internet technology (e-mail and web-based questionnaires) and interactive voice response (IVR; Mundt, Bohn, King, & Hartley, 2002) are newer methods of gathering interview data and are discussed in a later section of this chapter. A "questionnaire" is the list of questions or items used in any of the interview methods. Each method has its own advantages and disadvantages.

The format for gathering data should follow from the research questions asked. Researchers also must consider issues related to costs in terms of money, personnel, training time, and so on, and choose the method that best suits their research questions and available resources. Sometimes it is better to reframe a research question so that an appropriate method can be afforded than to choose a design that cannot yield adequate data. For example, the first phase of the BFTS Project yielded many hundreds of nominated skill items. Many of these were worded rather vaguely or in ambiguous terms. It might have been better at that point to abandon (or modify) the mailed questionnaire interview format and phone a sample of respondents so that we could ask probing questions. We might have had fewer participants (with different limitations) but better data to work with. A researcher can rarely have a high-quality, inexpensive project that takes a minimal amount of time. One of these three characteristics nearly always must be sacrificed and the researcher must find the best balance for the project.

Personal and Telephone Interviews

Personal interviews can be used for asking questions from a structured or semistructured questionnaire and are the most effective means for gathering in-depth information from people about their opinions, beliefs, or attitudes (Kerlinger, 1999). Personal interviews are the best means for gathering data that will be analyzed via qualitative methods. Personal interviews also are useful when the researcher is generalizing to *theory* rather than to *populations* (Moon, Dillon, & Sprenkle, 1990). That is, such interviews yield qualitative data that inform the evolving nature of theory (e.g., how people decide to get divorced), rather than some characteristic of a population. The chief disadvantage of personal interviews for survey research is their cost in terms of time and money relative to the number of participants surveyed.

Telephone interviews offer many of the advantages of personal interviews with different disadvantages. They are more effective when larger numbers of people must be interviewed (Warwick & Lininger, 1975), or when the respondents are known to have a stake in the research and have previously agreed to participate. They may not be as effective, however, if personal or sensitive questions are asked (Fowler, 2002). A great disadvantage is the increasing tendency of people to refuse to respond. Response rates may be increased by sending advance letters explaining the purpose and usefulness of the survey, or by combining phone questions with in-person or mailed questions.

The format for the interviews in either in-person or telephone questionnaires can be structured, semistructured, or unstructured. Structured interviews are those in which the interviewer must follow a set list of questions, using verbatim phrases and clarifying statements that are consistent across all participants. Semistructured interviews ask closed questions, which may then be followed by open questions for clarification or depth. They also may ask predetermined open questions followed by probing or clarifying questions. This method often provides both quantitative and qualitative data. Unstructured interviews are those informed by the purpose of the study; the researcher, in these cases, may become the "instrument." (See Downs, Smeyak, & Martin, 1980, and Tanur, 1992, for excellent texts on interviewing techniques and cognitive aspects of surveys.)

Self-Administered Questionnaires

The most common method for gathering survey data in MFT to date is through mailed, self-administered questionnaires (SAQs). Typically, a population is identified, lists of potential participants are gathered and sampled, and questionnaires are mailed to the selected sample. This method has advantages over personal or telephone interviews when the information needed is easily obtained from written, self-administered questionnaires; when the sample is likely to be interested in the subject matter; when larger numbers of participants are needed; and when the researcher wishes to keep the data-gathering time to a minimum.

The disadvantages of SAQ formats are not inconsequential. Often, it is difficult or impossible to determine the response bias of the sample. More important, however, is the inability to know the "response set" of the respondents because follow-up or probing questions are uncommon. In the BFTS Project, for example, many of the skill items were rather vaguely worded (we used the exact words of the nominated items whenever possible) and so were vulnerable to interpretation. We do not know how differently the members of our sample interpreted the items, or whether they gave them Likert scores rather than admit a lack of familiarity with the items. That is, some respondents may have had a "set" (i.e., been predisposed) to use the Likert responses. Some may even have had a "set" to answer "very important" more frequently, reducing the variance in their responses.

In addition to deciding how to obtain the information required for the research project, the researcher also must decide how to format the questionnaires. A good SAQ is designed with two issues in mind: (1) motivating participants to complete the questionnaire, and (2) providing reliable, valid data for the research analyses. Questions are typically classified as either "closed" or "open." Closed questions are those that ask for "yes–no" or fixed-choice responses. Questions about demographic information usually fall into this category, as do checklists, ratings, rankings, or any question that requires simply marking or otherwise indicating a specific response from two or more choices. Closed questions are easier to code for analysis and are easily quantifiable. Open questions are those that allow respondents to respond in their own words. Although open questions require more from the investigator in terms of coding and analyzing the data, these responses are less restrictive and often contain less researcher bias. For example, the researcher may ask, "What kind of supervision do you prefer: live or case consultation?" The information obtained from this closed question will be very different from that obtained through the open question, "What kind of supervision best facilitates your learning?"

Closed or fixed-choice questions can be followed with probing, open ones. They also can be followed with invitations to add to a list or comment on the question. The researcher needs to think carefully about potential bias in the questions, in their presentation, and in the format allowed for responses. Pretesting or pilot testing is invaluable at this stage. Pretesting also helps determine how long an interview or SAQ may take a participant to complete.

Questions can be asked through an investigator's own, personally developed questionnaire or through one that has been standardized with known utility, validity, and reliability. Much research uses a combination of standardized and self-developed questionnaires. Many standardized instruments have themselves been developed via survey methods. Whole books have been dedicated to the listing of instruments related to individuals, couples, and families, as well as instruments that are designed to measure clinical variables and change (e.g., Corcoran & Fischer, 2000a, 2000b; Filsinger, 1983; Fredman & Sherman, 1987; Grotevant & Carlson, 1989; L'Abate & Bagarozzi, 1993; Lopez & Snyder, 2003; Touliatos, Perlmutter, & Straus, 2001). Lopez and Snyder's (2003) volume looks at positive measures and constructs that underlie them.

Often, researchers must develop their own questionnaires. There are many excellent resources available to help MFT researchers with this task, including Snyder and Rice (1996), Tinkelman (1971), and Wiersma and Jurs (1990). Snyder and Rice wrote an excellent chapter on scale development for the first edition of this book.

A researcher must take great care to construct questions that yield usable responses. In the BFTS Project, we solicited Likert-type ratings of many different nominated basic skill items. After the first phase, we needed to add several categorical response choices for further phases because members of our sample told us that they did not understand the meaning of some items and needed, for example, "don't understand this item" as a response choice.

Good questions are short and simple, ask for only one answer, are unambiguous, are not leading, are positive (do not use "not"), tap knowledge the respondent has (rather than asking for information about something unfamiliar), will be understood similarly across participants, and are not unnecessarily detailed or objectionable (de Vaus, 1986). In the BFTS Project, we did not define "skills" for our sample, resulting in responses that included what some might call "personality characteristics." This was serendipitous for us, but investigators should be careful to anticipate their participants and make sure that they will get usable information by not asking ambiguous questions. Pilot testing is invaluable for this purpose. Other factors must be balanced in terms of the time it takes participants to answer the questions, the face validity of the instrument, and the comprehensiveness of the questions.

In addition to thinking about the particular questions asked, the investigator should pay careful attention to the ordering, formatting, and aesthetics of the questionnaire. Questions in different forms can be asked in different orders to reduce fatigue or boredom. Mailed SAQs should be easy to read, with sufficient white space that participants are not daunted. Type style and size should be plain and clear and instructions should be repeated frequently so that respondents do not need to page back and forth to find response choices. Response rates can be increased by making sure that the questionnaires are appropriate for the average reading level of the sample. They also should be free of typographical and spelling errors. These ideas may seem obvious, but more than one poorly proofread questionnaire has been tossed into the round file. Pilot studies can reduce this particular cause of nonresponse. See Dillman (2000) and Fowler (2002) for more discussion. Dillman also describes Internet survey design.

The Internet and Other Newer Technologies

The use of the Internet for e-mail and World Wide Web survey methods has changed many aspects of conducting survey research. For the most part, the advantages of using these technologies include ability to reach larger audiences, ease of use for participants, attractiveness of surveys, and ease of use in entering and storing data, thus reducing data error and reducing dollar costs for conducting the research. Disadvantages include lower response rates in some cases, unknown response rates in other cases, and the need to limit samples to those who are computer-literate and who tend to use the Internet (Fowler, 2002). Although more and more people are using the Internet, survey research is in its infancy in this medium. Some factors that need to be kept in mind include the need for accurate addresses or salient groups to which one advertises the survey, ways of maintaining security of the site and the data, and ways to track participants so that each person can complete the survey only once. Decisions need to be made about formatting; it is very easy to get excessive in the use of fancy fonts and colors, which may deter responses. Researchers need to keep in mind that not all participants use the same browsers or operating systems, may have slow modem access to the Internet, and may not have screens as large as the researchers'. Decisions also need to be made whether to use e-mail notices with attached surveys that can be returned via e-mail (with less confidentiality) or printed and either faxed or mailed; web-based surveys using commercial sites that maintain good security and return data stripped of identifiers; web-based methods that download the data to researchers' secure servers; or other methods that are not yet developed. We suggest that readers consult the latest literature on the use of the Internet for survey research.

DVD, CD, and web-based interactive methods are increasing the possibilities for participants to watch video clips and respond to questions based on the clip. Subsequent questions can be automated so that respondents automatically skip unnecessary questions or are given follow-up, probing, or other open questions about their responses. In this way, technology can reduce costs of using interviewers in some situations and still allow for gathering in-depth information.

Finally, IVR (Mundt et al., 2002) technologies are allowing researchers to gather data from respondents about sensitive topics that may otherwise reduce response rates or reliability of data. In these technologies, participants use researcher-provided or respondent-selected identification codes to access telephone-automated response systems. By using voice or touch-tone technology, participants respond to questions in many formats (e.g., multiple-choice or open questions), are automatically advanced to appropriate questions based on their responses, and can do all of this at their own convenience. For example, a researcher might want to know about the sex habits of HIV-positive individuals. Interviewing such individuals might not yield reliable data. However, allowing the participants to call an IVR line and respond to questions such as "How often did you have protected sex this week?" might make the participants feel more comfortable about responding to sensitive questions. Simply saying, for example, "Two times" would allow the system to record the response. Alternatively, the participant might push the key with the number 2 on it. Mundt and colleagues (2002) have reported high response rates for these technologies, which are particularly useful and cost-effective when data must be gathered from the same participant many times.

Increasing Response Rates

Methods for carrying out mail survey research and increasing response rates have been suggested by Dillman (1978, 2000) and Dillman and Frey (1974). When followed, Dillman's methods yield acceptable response rates (60–80%) for generalizing at least some information to the population of interest and for reporting both aggregate and comparative data analyses.

In the second edition of his book, Dillman calls his data-gathering process the "tailored design" method rather than the "total design" method. This method emphasizes tailoring data-gathering procedures to each situation and often using multiple methods to increase response rates. New technologies allow for multiple methods (regular mail, telephone, e-mail) for contacting people and for tailoring protocols through computer-enhanced procedures. Dillman and others (Cook, Heath, & Thompson, 2000) now recommend prenotification through e-mail or regular mail, alerting each potential participant to the purpose and procedures for the study; sending a copy of the questionnaire through regular mail or e-mail; sending a thank-you/reminder postcard about 2 weeks later; sending a replacement questionnaire about 2 weeks after that; and making a final contact through phone or email. For especially important studies, researchers can send replacement questionnaires or reminders through overnight delivery or priority mail to enhance salience for the participants. Dillman also suggests that researchers personalize the study as much as possible by using participants' real names, using real letterhead (rather than photocopying), and using real signatures. He also has found that using real stamps on the return envelopes increases response rates. Finally, he suggests that researchers use prepaid financial incentives of $1–$5.

To enhance confidentiality and anonymity, Dillman (2000) suggests enclosing postcards with questionnaires that participants can return at the same time they mail the survey to the researcher. Names can be checked off from lists and data are thus never linked to individual participants through codes on surveys. Similarly, codes on surveys can be checked against lists by a third person who is not involved in data entry or analysis. In this way, participants are not sent reminder postcards and this reduces dollar costs for the study. Links and lists are always destroyed after data are collected.

Cook and colleagues (2000) also suggest prior notices when researchers are using Internet technologies. Their research suggests that Internet technologies (e-mail and web-based) work best with specialized populations (e.g., university professors) who are computer- and Internet-savvy; when representativeness of the population is less likely to depend upon response rates (when populations are more homogeneous or when information rather than representativeness is required); and when there is no need for random sampling. These methods are fast, flexible, and much cheaper than personal interviews, telephone interviews, or mailed SAQ studies. In Cook and colleagues' meta-analysis of 49 studies that reported on 68 surveys, the most important variables for increasing response rates included university sponsorship, prenotification, salience, and follow-up. Survey length did not seem to affect response rates. However, there seemed to be a point of diminishing returns with additional follow-up reminders. Cook and colleagues found that the second contact almost doubled response rates in Internet research. Curiously, incentives actually seemed to decrease response rates, perhaps because these were associated with very long surveys.

Mundt and colleagues (2002) found that IVR methods yielded significantly greater response rates when used in projects that required multiple uses of the method per participant, when the topic was particularly sensitive (e.g., recent alcohol use), and when accessibility and staff time were issues. The method was compared to traditional ways of using a particular instrument and seemed actually to serve as an intervention. That is, participants were more likely to report alcohol use and their scores tended to decrease from Time 1 to Time 2.

Finally, Dillman (2000) suggests using multiple methods for informing potential participants of the survey (e.g., e-mail), providing the questionnaire (e.g., e-mail, regular mail, websites); reminding and thanking respondents; and following up with both replacement surveys and personal reminders. He suggests that response rates can remain reasonable, although with large ranges (30–80%) because of the nature of the variables involved: the type of sample, the availability of lists of persons most likely to be interested, the type of questionnaire, and the salience of the study to the participants.

Data Coding and Storing

After the data are collected, they must be analyzed. To do this, they must be transformed into usable data units for either quantitative or qualitative analysis. Many researchers do not put enough thought into this phase early enough in the project and begin coding and entering data into a database without carefully considering how the data will be analyzed. Consultations with data managers or statisticians can be very helpful at this time.

Data from survey research are usually converted to numbers of some kind with each number representing either a category of information (e.g., race) or a numerical value placed on an item by a participant (as with Likert-type ratings). In either case, and however the researcher wishes to code and store data, a codebook is essential. This book should list all methods in the study, including research variables, their positions in database records, and the meanings of different values. It is useful to know the details of how the statistical software manages data while setting up the codebook and database structures. The data codebook should also include a narrative developed over the life of the project, describing decisions, procedures, and so forth. Although this may seem cumbersome and time-consuming, it can be invaluable later when a manuscript reviewer asks, "What about . . . ?", or when a researcher wants to recall why a particular decision was made.

As with all research, it is extremely important to "proof" or "clean" data that have been entered into a database. Each record in the database should be compared to its corresponding raw data and corrected in the master database. Once the master database has been "cleaned," it should be stored in some form that cannot be changed and a written copy should be kept in a safe place. Optical scanning has made data entry and assurance of accuracy much easier and should be used whenever possible. It is also useful to include descriptions of the data in the database in the form of "comments." Too many data have been scrapped because no one knew the meaning of numbers in a database.

Data Analysis

Data from survey research are analyzed according to the kinds of research questions asked and the kinds of data gathered. That is, are the research questions asking for descriptive, associative (correlational or comparative), or predictive results? Are the data qualitative or quantitative? Are they nominal, ordinal, interval, or ratio? Other chapters of this book, other texts, and statistical consultants can help determine the best analytical methods for the project. A thorough discussion is beyond the scope of this chapter, and the following material is introductory only.

Statistical analyses can be grouped as univariate, bivariate, or multivariate, depending on the number of variables being considered. Univariate statistics provide descriptions of single variables: frequencies and distributions of values (how this sample responded in an overall picture), statistics of central tendency (the average or most frequent response), and dispersion (how much variability there is in the responses; the range of responses; Miller, 1986). These analyses yield results that describe the sample on the variables of interest, both independent and dependent. Reports usually include descriptions of demographics or independent variables. Analyses of dependent variables usually require adhering to assumptions about randomly selected samples and normal distributions of responses or scores; therefore, it is important to report sampling methods and descriptive statistics so that readers can judge the appropriateness of the inferential analyses or compare other samples to the one reported.

Bivariate and multivariate analyses are usually considered "inferential" because they infer characteristics or comparisons of random samples rather than directly observing them. Bivariate analyses consider two variables simultaneously. Crosstabulations are frequency tables that group nominal variables against each other in distributions. For example, a researcher may want to know how variables are distributed across sex and educational level. Researchers may want to know how variables are associated (correlated or compared) and how strong the association is. This requires analyses such as correlations, chi-squares, t-tests, or analyses of variance.

Multivariate analyses involve more than two variables, either independent or dependent. They include canonical correlations, multiple analysis of variance (MANOVA), and analyses that take into account variables that *covary* in some way (analysis of covariance, or ANCOVA). Multiple variables can be collapsed into new variables with underlying common dimensions by using factor analyses. Factor analysis is especially useful in developing new instruments. Participants can be formed into groups according to shared patterns of responses by using cluster analyses. Finally, dependent variables can be predicted from multiple independent variables through analyses such as regression, discriminant-function analysis, and path analysis. Path analysis and other structural modeling tools can be used to test hypotheses of how variables should relate according to theoretical principles. Andrews and colleagues (1998) lead the researcher through a decision tree to appropriate statistical tests that can be used for data analyses, depending on levels and number of variables and on how the researcher wants these variables treated.

Reporting

A very important and little-discussed issue relates to how and where research is reported. Survey research has many uses and can be reported in many legitimate forums, including newspapers; refereed journals (both paper and online); and state, regional, national, and international conferences. At least as important as where the research is reported is *how* it is reported. Researchers should think carefully about their audiences and tailor their writing to the needs of those audiences. For readers to gain as much as possible from the report, researchers must include clear descriptions of the research questions, as well as of the methods used for sampling the population and gathering the data. Specific topics covered should include methods used to increase response rates, incentives, the characteristics of the sample, interview strategies, the types of questions on the questionnaires, analysis methods, and analysis results. Researchers should take particular care in describing the limitations of the research, including sample bias and any information that may be known about those who did not respond to the survey, as well as limitations related to the questionnaire or methods for collecting data. Conclusions and recommendations should clearly relate to the data with logical connections that will make sense to the audience. Results and speculations that do not relate clearly to the research questions or data can be confusing and misleading.

DISCUSSION

Strengths and Weaknesses

The greatest strength of survey research lies in its ability to gather large amounts of data from a number of participants in a relatively short amount of time. It is the method of choice when a researcher wants opinions from a number of readily identified people who are willing and able to answer the questions and when they are the *only* ones who can answer the questions (e.g., about beliefs, opinion, attitudes, or values; Miller, 1986). For appropriately conducted, large-sample research, researchers are able to make inferences about a population with reasonable certainty. It certainly is the method of choice when general descriptions about "normal" distributions of variables in a population are required. It is an extremely flexible method, allowing much latitude in the variables studied and the strategies for studying them. Surveys that question clinicians and report the results in forums and formats that are useful to them add to the credibility of family therapy research.

The greatest weakness of survey research is the ease with which each step can be done carelessly, adding considerably to both sampling and nonsampling error, and thus producing biased or nonvalid results. Each step assumes certain things, and to the extent that these assumptions are violated, the method will produce results that are not valid. Survey research also is not useful when respondents may be unwilling or unable to provide accurate, reliable information.

It often is difficult to replicate survey research, even when each step has been clearly described in the research report. There are many unknown aspects of the process that cannot be described, replicated, or controlled: the response sets, recall ability, cohort effects, or unique reactions of the participants, for example. In this sense, meta-analytical methods may be more appropriate for discerning "true" distributions of variables.

A final concern about survey research relates to its meaning. Scientific inquiry is usually interested in the statistical significance of research results. In the field of family therapy, we are also interested in the practical or clinical significance of results. This means that analyses may produce results suggesting that two or more groups are indeed statistically different, but this difference may not make a practical or clinical difference; that is, it may not have meaning to either the researcher or the readers of a report. Is a difference of 2 points between groups when the maximum possible score is 150 points practically meaningful, even though it most likely did not occur by chance? In discussion sections, this is the "so what" of the research: What difference does this finding make, beyond its veracity, to further research or to clinical practice?

Survey research is usually carried out from a perspective of attempting to discover some "truth" or fact about a population or sample, without taking into account perspectives that might suggest alternative ways of viewing the problem (is it indeed a problem? for whom?), the constructs behind the questions, and the multiplicity of ways that participants make meaning out of what is presented to them. That is, survey research may produce accurate numbers about a variable, its distribution in a sample, and its relationship to other variables. What the descriptions and relationships *mean*, however, is a subjective issue of interpretation. Researchers should be careful to distinguish the difference.

Reliability

Research is useful only if the information received is reliable and valid. In survey research, the reliability (accuracy and dependability) of responses is greatly affected by many factors in the participants' contexts, many of which cannot be controlled by the researcher or are unknown. Fortunately, the reliability of averages is greater than the reliability of individual responses (Kerlinger & Lee, 1999). That is, although a single participant may respond differently to a questionnaire, depending on mood, current issues, or misunderstanding, many participants as a whole are less subject to the same variations. Outliers do not affect results as much.

Researchers should use statistical tools to determine the reliability of their surveys. Participants may be asked to respond to the instrument a second time some weeks after the first administration of the instrument. This method has obvious drawbacks in terms of the bias introduced with such a self-selected sample. Wetchler (1989; Wetchler et al., 1989) asked participants in the first survey whether they would be willing to participate in a reliability test–retest study. He then randomly sampled from this list of participants. Because survey research by definition entails the use of self-selected samples in many ways, this method may compound the bias. A second method is to resurvey a randomly selected subsample. Self-selection is a factor in this method also, but less so than in the first. The responses can be compared by using agreement correlations, frequently Cohen's kappa (Cohen, 1960, 1968). Other statistics (e.g., Cronbach's [1951] alpha) may be used with some instruments to determine the consistency of the participants in responding to questions that are part of a composite or global measure.

The easiest method to increase reliability in survey research is to make sure that the questions are clear and unambiguous so that the responses are not as likely to change from participant to participant. Reliability can also be increased by having a sufficient number of items for all subscales and by making the length of the survey reasonable so that fatigue does not hinder the participants' ability to be thoughtful. Finally, there are occasions when reliability in the form of consistency (alpha) is preferable to test–retest reliability, so that changes in scores over time reflect true change in a variable (e.g., distress level) rather than vagaries of responses (e.g., ambiguous questions or response sets that lead to uncertain responses).

Validity

Data are useful only to the extent that they correspond to the research questions and measure what they are intended to measure. There are three basic kinds of validity: criterion, content, and construct. For criterion validity, the data are compared to existing measures of the same concept or phenomenon. This is often difficult in MFT research. For example, attempts to measure Bowen's (1978) concept of differentiation of self are notoriously difficult. In contrast, however, outcome measures (e.g., marital satisfaction) can be validated during the instrument development stages by comparing results of the new instrument to those of existing instruments with established validity that have been reported in the literature. For content validity, different aspects of the content of the question are tied to definitions of the concept. For example, in the BFTS Project, we asked our respondents to consider basic skills for beginning family therapists and sampled only those supervisors who had recent experience with beginning trainees; we defined these trainees as "ones with fewer than 100 clinical contact hours," rather than using the participants' personal definitions of "beginners." This enhanced validity for beginning-level skills. Finally, construct validity is established by noting a questionnaire's performance compared to theoretical notions. Less experienced therapists, for example, might theoretically have experience with fewer ethical dilemmas than more experienced therapists, and therefore might list few dilemmas in a survey. This may not mean that they are not aware of ethical issues in family therapy, but simply that they are less experienced with them. "In the end," however, "there is no ideal way of determining the validity of a measure" (de Vaus, 1986, p. 49). If there were, direct observations of the phenomena would suffice.

In family therapy survey research, validity is often established through careful examination of the items used in the inquiry. Independent judges, knowledgeable in the topic of interest, can make recommendations about how well the items address the researcher's questions. Because most surveys are unique and the questionnaires may not have already established reliability and validity, comparing whatever information is possible can help establish the validity of the data. For example, if a researcher claims that a sample is representative of the population on many demographic variables, evidence of this in terms of known demographic statistics would enhance the researcher's claims to validity.

One difficulty in establishing validity relates to the response set of the participants when they respond to the questionnaire. Not only does mood affect the reliability of the information given; it also can affect the validity, especially when the questions are ambiguous or worded in ways that require a particular response set. For example, asking which items are most important from a list is very different from asking which items are important; the first response set may assume that all items are important to some degree, whereas the second suggests that some items are important and others are not. The researcher must be very careful in interpreting data from such questions because claiming that items with low scores are "not important" rather than "less important" may not be a valid conclusion of the study. Again, using opinions from independent judges who have expertise in the subject matter and who might be similar to the surveyed sample can increase the strength of the data.

Skills

To a great extent, a survey researcher must possess the skills of both an experimental researcher and a case study researcher. As in all research, the project is only as strong as its total design—from formulation of research questions or hypotheses through design of the procedures and sample selection, careful choices or design of instruments, and good knowledge of research analysis and reporting procedures. The survey researcher must also be a skilled consumer of research. That is, in order to obtain good results and report them in a meaningful way, the researcher must be familiar with the field of study, issues of sampling and potential bias, and the meaning of the data in the context from which they are drawn and in which they are reported. It does little good to survey family therapy educators about the strengths and weaknesses of their programs if the researcher is not familiar with the external standards or institutional constraints on programs, but recommends sweeping and impossible reforms.

An essential skill for the survey researcher is in consulting with others. Good researchers use experts to help formulate questions for interviews or questionnaires; run pilot tests on knowledgeable participants to refine the questionnaires' content and appearance, as well as the data-gathering procedures; and consult early with statisticians about the design of the study, before needing help with analyses of data. It is interesting that some of the best reported research was accomplished by doctoral candidates for their dissertations under the watchful eye of committees. Although students perennially complain about the rigor of research done in this context, the results are often more meaningful and less wasteful of resources. Proposals written for grant funding are often reviewed by experts in the field, which helps researchers with rigorous design. In some ways, editors and journal reviewers serve a similar function, but at the end rather than at the beginning of a project. Researchers can keep this in mind, however, as they design their studies, and use colleagues as peer reviewers at early stages.

The survey researcher must have patience and an ability to plan with great detail. This same patience can make analyzing the data more fruitful when the researcher is skilled at seeing patterns in data that may not be apparent in the numerical statistics generated from the data. That is, in looking over the questionnaires or listening to recorded interviews, the researcher may begin to see patterns that suggest further interesting analysis, refinement of the research, or future studies.

Bridging Research and Practice

Survey research is a good way to bridge the gap between researchers and clinicians because it can easily use clinicians and their clients as participants. Other survey research in family therapy has asked questions of training programs and supervisors; these data are of interest to clinicians because we all have opinions about the strengths and weaknesses of our training and about what should be included in family therapy education. In other ways, survey research responds to questions that clinicians ask: What are people doing, how are they doing it, and what do they think about it? Clinicians should be able to use the results of research to keep themselves current in their practices. Researchers should survey clinicians about what kinds of research they pay attention to, what kinds of research they would like to see conducted, how they would use this research, and how they might be willing to participate.

A most useful way that researchers help bridge the gap between their work and that of their colleagues is how they report the results. Publishing articles in refereed professional journals is useful for tenure and promotion, but may not be the best way to capture the interest and attention of clinician nonresearchers. Venues such as *The Psychotherapy Networker* or conference presentations and workshops may be better suited for this purpose. In these instances, the report language and formatting must be geared toward application, with many examples of clinical usefulness.

Future Directions

Future survey research through electronic media will be greatly enhanced with advances in technology. E-mail and web-based research will become easier and more attractive to both researchers and participants, although programming costs may keep it from being cheaper. Automated data entry will continue to increase the reliability of data and to decrease response error. Increased security technology will make sensitive topics easier to investigate. PC cameras, DVD technology, interactive programming possibilities, and enhanced Internet voice technologies also have possibilities. As the web becomes faster and more people have fast broadband access to the Internet in their homes, surveys will be more private and will be easier and faster to complete, transmit, code, store, and analyze.

EXEMPLARS

This section briefly describes what we consider the exemplary use of survey methods in several studies. That is, the sampling methods and follow-up procedures were appropriate for the research questions and population; the methods yielded acceptable response rates for the particular study; and the articles report details related to sampling, those who were sampled but not included in the analyses for various reasons, and the follow-up attempts to increase response rates. These methods seemed to yield the representation required for each study's purposes and reported the method in such a way that it could easily be replicated.

Chadi, Rafferty, and Pickard (2003) studied stressors for African American wives who provided caregiving for their elderly husbands. This was a specialized sample that required stratified random sampling, using zip code, age, and gender to assure representation in those demographic categories. Reverse sampling was used: Medicare recipients were contacted by telephone, screened, and provided with letters of explanation. These respondents then asked their caregivers to participate. The article reports clear criteria used for all phases of selection and sampling. African American interviewers contacted the participants in their homes for the structured, computerized questionnaires; participants were compensated with a $15 grocery coupon. These procedures resulted in an 88% response rate.

Ivey and colleagues (2000) looked at ageism in marriage and family therapists. Three samples were recruited in order to make valid comparisons: university students as nontherapists; therapists in training (associate members of AAMFT); and therapists (clinical members of AAMFT). Therapists in training and therapists were randomly sampled from the AAMFT lists. A notable feature was that four reminder letters were used, resulting in response rates of approximately 59%.

Northey (2002) published a study of AAMFT clinical members, sponsored by the Center for Substance Abuse Treatment (CSAT), which required a response rate of at least 70%. Members were sent prenotice letters from the AAMFT's executive director that explained the purpose of the study and informed members of an upcoming phone call by an outside agency. A copy of the questionnaire was included for the members to review before the interview. Northey's article provides a clear report of procedures and descriptions of subsamples that were not included for various reasons (e.g., refused, quit interview in middle, could not be reached by phone). Follow-up was conducted through two letters and numerous phone calls. This procedure yielded a response rate of 86%.

Results of these studies are not reported here because the results are not what made them exemplary for present purposes. Rather, the researchers could be confident in the validity of their results because of the careful methods that they followed. They also provided sufficient information for readers to judge the adequacy of the data and replicate the study if they desired.

The potential for survey research is in its breadth and depth: It can be used to ask many kinds of questions, from many kinds of populations and samples, and reported in a wide variety of ways. Its heuristic value for pointing the field in useful directions is well established because its results often pose more questions than they answer. It is precisely this stance of curiosity and openness that makes survey research in family therapy useful and informative, as researchers and clinicians apply its results to their practices, to their theory, and to further research.

REFERENCES

Anderson, S. A., Rigazio-DiGilio, S., & Kunkler, K. P. (1995). Training and supervision in family therapy: Current issues and future directions, *Family Relations, 44,* 489–500.

Anderson, S. A., Schlossberg, M. & Rigazio-DiGilio, S. (2000). Family therapy trainees' evaluations of their best and worst supervision experiences. *Journal of Marital and Family Therapy, 29,* 79–91.

Andrews, F. M., Klem, L., O'Malley, P. M., Rodgers, W. L., Welsh, K. B., & Davidson, T. N. (1998). *Selecting statistical techniques for social science data: A guide for SAS users.* Cary, NC: SAS Institute.

Baum, N. (2003). Divorce process variables and the co-parental relationship and parental role fulfillment of divorced parents. *Family Process, 42,* 117–131.

Boughner, S. R., Hayes, S. F., Bubenzer, D. L., & West, J. D. (1994). Use of standardized assessment instruments by marital and family therapists: A survey. *Journal of Marital and Family Therapy, 20,* 69–75.

Bowen, M. (1978). *Family therapy in clinical practice.* New York: Aronson.

Bray, J. H., Williamson, D. S., & Malone, P. E. (1984). Personal authority in the family system: Development of a questionnaire to measure personal authority in intergenerational processes. *Journal of Marital and Family Therapy, 10,* 167–178.

Carter, R. E. (1989). Residency training and the later use of marital and family therapy in psychiatric practice. *Journal of Marital and Family Therapy, 15,* 411–418.

Chadi, L. A., Rafferty, J., & Pickard, J. (2003). The influence of caregiving stressors, social support, and caregiving appraisal on marital functioning among African American wife caregivers. *Journal of Marital and Family Therapy, 29,* 479–490.

Cohen, J. A. (1960). A coefficient of agreement for nominal scales. *Educational and Psychological Measurement, 20,* 37–46.

Cohen, J. (1968). Weighted kappa: Nominal scale agreement with provision for scaled disagreement or partial credit. *Psychological Bulletin, 70,* 213–220.

Coleman, S. B., Avis, J. M., & Turin, M. (1990). A study of the role of gender in family therapy training. *Family Process, 29,* 365–374.

Cook, C., Heath, F., & Thompson, R. (2000). A meta-analysis of response rates in Web- or Internet-based surveys. *Educational and Psychological Measurement, 60*(6), 821–836.

Corcoran, K., & Fischer, J. (2000a). *Measures for clinical practice: A sourcebook* (Vol. 1). New York: Free Press.

Corcoran, K., & Fischer, J. (2000b). *Measures for clinical practice: A sourcebook* (Vol. 2). New York: Free Press.

Crane, R. D., & Law, D. D. (2002). Conducting medical offset research in a health maintenance organization: Challenges, opportunities, and insights. *Journal of Marital and Family Therapy, 28*(1), 5–19.

Creswell, J. W. (2003). *Research design: Qualitative, quantitative, and mixed methods approaches* (2nd ed.). Thousand Oaks, CA: Sage.

Cronbach, L. J. (1951). Coefficient alpha and the internal structure of tests. *Psychiatrika, 16,* 297–334.

de Vaus, D. A. (1986). *Surveys in social research.* Boston: George Allen & Unwin.

Dillman, D. A. (1978). *Mail and telephone surveys: The total design method.* New York: Wiley.

Dillman, D. A. (2000). *Mail and Internet surveys: The tailored design method* (2nd ed.). New York: Wiley.

Dillman, D. A., & Frey, J. H. (1974). Contribution of personalization to mail questionnaire response as an element of a previously tested method. *Journal of Applied Psychology, 59,* 297–301.

Doherty, W. J., & Simmons, D. S. (1996). Clinical practice patterns of marriage and family therapists: A national survey. *Journal of Marital and Family Therapy, 22,* 9–25.

Downs, C. W., Smeyak, O. P., & Martin, E. (1980). *Professional interviewing.* New York: Harper & Row.

Epstein, N. B., Baldwin, L. M., & Bishop, D. S. (1983). The McMaster Family Assessment Device. *Journal of Marital and Family Therapy, 11,* 171–180.

Figley, C. R., & Nelson, T. S. (1989). Basic family therapy skills, I: Conceptualization and initial findings. *Journal of Marital and Family Therapy, 15,* 349–365.

Figley, C. R., & Nelson, T. S. (1990). Basic family therapy skills, III: Brief and strategic schools of family therapy. *Journal of Family Psychotherapy, 4,* 49–62.

Filsinger, E. E. (Ed.). (1983). *Marriage and family assessment: A sourcebook for family therapy.* Newbury Park, CA: Sage.

Fink, A., & Kosecoff, J. (1985). *How to conduct surveys: A step-by-step guide.* Newbury Park, CA: Sage.

Fowler, F. J., Jr. (1988). *Survey research methods.* Newbury Park, CA: Sage.

Fowler, F. J., Jr. (2002). *Survey research methods* (3rd ed.). Thousand Oaks, CA: Sage.

Fredman, N., & Sherman, R. (1987). *Handbook of measurements for marriage and family therapy.* New York: Brunner/Mazel.

Green, S. L., & Hansen, J. C. (1986). Ethical dilemmas in family therapy. *Journal of Marital and Family Therapy, 12,* 225–230.

Green, S. L., & Hansen, J. C. (1989). Ethical dilemmas faced by family therapists. *Journal of Marital and Family Therapy, 15,* 149–158.

Grotevant, H. D., & Carlson, C. I. (1989). *Family assessment: A guide to methods and measures.* New York: Guilford Press.

Guralnik, D. B. (Ed.). (1966). *Webster's new world dictionary of the American language.* Nashville, TN: Southwestern.

Hackett, O. (1981). Survey research methods. *Personnel and Guidance Journal, 59,* 599–604.

Halik, V., Rosenthal, D. A., & Pattison, P. E. (1990). Intergenerational effects of the Holocaust: Patterns of engagement in the mother–daughter relationship. *Family Process, 29,* 325–339.

Heath, A. W., McKenna, B. C., & Atkinson, B. J. (1988). Toward the identification of variables for evaluating family therapy workshops. *Journal of Marital and Family Therapy, 14,* 267–276.

Ivey, D. C., Wieling, E., & Harris, S. M. (2000). Save the young—the elderly have lived their lives: Ageism in marriage and family therapy. *Family Process, 39,* 163–175.

Jolliffe, F. B. (1986). *Survey design and analysis.* New York: Halstead Press.

Keller, J. F., Huber, J. R., & Hardy, K. V. (1988). Accreditation: What constitutes appropriate marriage and family therapy education? *Journal of Marital and Family Therapy, 14,* 297–305.

Kerlinger, F. N. (1986). *Foundations of behavioral research.* New York: Holt, Rinehart & Winston.

Kerlinger, F. N., & Lee, H. B. (1999). *Foundations of behavioral research* (4th ed.). New York: Harcourt College.

Kraemer, H. C., & Thiemann, S. (1987). *How many subjects?: Statistical power analysis in research.* Newbury Park, CA: Sage.

L'Abate, L., & Bagarozzi, D. A. (1993). *Sourcebook of marriage and family evaluation.* New York: Brunner/Mazel.

Larson, J. H., Crane, D. R., & Smith, C. W. (1991). Morning and night couples: The effect of wake and sleep patterns on marital adjustment. *Journal of Marital and Family Therapy, 17,* 53–65.

Law, D., Crane, D. R., & Berge, J. (2003). The influence of individual, marital, and family therapy on high utilizers of health care. *Journal of Marital and Family Therapy, 29,* 353–363.

Lev-Wiesel, R., & Amir, M. (2000). Posttraumatic stress disorder symptoms, psychological distress, personal resources, and quality of life in four groups of Holocaust child survivors. *Family Process, 39,* 445–459.

Lewis, W., & Rohrbaugh, M. (1989). Live supervision by family therapists: A Virginia survey. *Journal of Marital and Family Therapy, 15*, 323–326.

Likert, R. (1932). A technique for measurement of attitudes. *Archives of Psychology, 140,* 52.

Lopez, S. J., & Snyder, C. R. (Eds.). (2003). *Positive psychological assessment: A handbook of models and measures.* Washington, DC: American Psychological Association.

McGraw, D. L., & Watson, G. L. (1976). *Political and social inquiry.* New York: Wiley.

McWey, L. M., West, S. W., Ruble, N. M., Handy, A. K., Handy, D. G., Koshy, M., et al. (2002). The practice of clinical research in accredited marriage and family therapy programs. *Journal of Marital and Family Therapy, 28*, 85–92.

Miller, B. C. (1986). *Family research methods.* Beverly Hills, CA: Sage.

Moon, S. M., Dillon, D. R., & Sprenkle, D. H. (1990). Family therapy and qualitative research. *Journal of Marital and Family Therapy, 16*, 357–373.

Mundt, J. C., Bohn, M. J., King, M., & Hartley, M. T. (2002). Automatic standard alcohol use assessment via interactive voice response technology. *Alcohol: Clinical and Experimental Research, 26*(2), 207–211.

Nelson, T. S., & Benson, M. (2004). *Intermediate family therapy skills: Trainee perspectives.* Unpublished manuscript, Utah State University.

Nelson, T. S., & Boxley, S. (2000). *Intermediate family therapy skills: Supervisor perspectives.* Unpublished manuscript, Utah State University.

Nelson, T. S., & Figley, C. B. (1990). Basic family therapy skills, II: Structural family therapy. *Journal of Marital and Family Therapy, 16*, 225–239.

Nelson, T. S., Heilbrun, G., & Figley, C. R. (1993). Basic skills in family therapy, IV: Transgenerational theories of family therapy. *Journal of Marital and Family Therapy, 19*, 253–266.

Nelson, T. S., & Johnson, L. N. (1999). The Basic Skills Evaluation Device. *Journal of Marital and Family Therapy, 25*, 15–30.

Nelson, T. S., & Palmer, T. R. (2001). Practitioner profiles and practice patterns for marriage and family therapists in Utah. *Journal of Marital and Family Therapy, 27*, 403–407.

Nelson, T. S., & Prior, D. (2003). Theory of change projects in marriage and family therapy programs. *Contemporary Family Therapy, 25*, 133–151.

Nelson, T. S., & Webb, N. (2001). *Basic family therapy skills: Student perspectives.* Unpublished manuscript, Utah State University.

Nichols, W. C., Nichols, D. P., & Hardy, K. V. (1990). Supervision in family therapy: A decade restudy. *Journal of Marital and Family Therapy, 16*, 275–285.

Northey, W. F., Jr. (2002). Characteristics and clinical practices of marriage and family therapists: A national survey. *Journal of Marital and Family Therapy, 28*, 487–494.

Nylund, D., & Thomas, J. (1994, November–December). The economics of narrative. *Family Therapy Networker, 18*(6), 38–39.

O'Sullivan, M. J., & Gilbert, R. K. (1989). Master's degree programs in marital and family therapy: An evaluation of admission and program requirements. *Journal of Marital and Family Therapy, 15*, 337–347.

Patten, M. L. (2002). *Proposing empirical research: A guide to the fundamentals* (2nd ed.). Los Angeles: Pyrczak.

Peterson, B. D., Newton, C. R., & Rosen, K. H. (2003). Examining congruence between partners' perceived infertility-related stress and its relationship to marital adjustment and depression in infertile couples. *Family Process, 42*, 59–70.

Riehl-Emde, A., Thomas, V., & Willi, J. (2003). Love: An important dimension in marital research and therapy. *Family Process, 42*, 253–267.

Russell, C. S., & Peterson, C. M. (2003). Student impairment and remediation in accredited marriage and family therapy programs. *Journal of Marital and Family Therapy, 29*, 329–338.

Sandberg, J. G., Johnson, L N., Robila, M., & Miller, R. B. (2002). Clinician identified barriers to clinical research. *Journal of Marital and Family Therapy, 28*, 61–67.

Snyder, D. K., & Rice, J. L. (1996). Methodological issues and strategies in scale development. In D. H. Sprenkle & S. M. Moon (Eds.), *Research methods in family therapy* (pp. 216–237). New York: Guilford Press.

Solomon, J., Ott, J., & Roach, A. (1986). A survey of training opportunities for predoctoral psychology interns in marriage and family therapy. *Journal of Marital and Family Therapy, 12*, 269–280.

Tanur, J. M. (Ed.). (1992). *Questions about questions: Inquiries into the cognitive bases of surveys*. New York: Russell Sage Foundation.

Tinkelman, S. N. (1971). Planning the objective test. In R. L. Thorndike (Ed.), *Educational measurement* (pp. 46–80). Washington, DC: American Council on Education.

Touliatos, J., Perlmutter, B. F., & Straus, M. A. (Eds.). (2001). *Handbook of family measurement techniques*. Thousand Oaks, CA: Sage.

Warwick, D. P., & Lininger, C. A. (1975). *The sample survey: Theory and practice*. New York: McGraw-Hill.

Wetchler, J. L. (1989). Supervisors' and supervisees' perceptions of the effectiveness of family therapy supervisor interpersonal skills. *American Journal of Family Therapy, 17*, 244–256.

Wetchler, J. L., Piercy, F. P., & Sprenkle, D. H. (1989). Supervisors' and supervisees' perceptions of the effectiveness of family therapy supervisory techniques. *American Journal of Family Therapy, 17*, 35–47.

White, M. B., Edwards, S. A., & Russell, C. S. (1997). The essential elements of successful marriage and family therapy: A Delphi study. *American Journal of Family Therapy, 25*, 213–231.

White, M. B., & Russell, C. S. (1995). The essential elements of supervisory systems: A modified Delphi study. *Journal of Marital and Family Therapy, 31*, 33–53.

Wiersma, W., & Jurs, S. G. (1990). *Educational testing and measurement* (2nd ed.). Boston: Allyn & Bacon.

Wilson, L. L., & Stith, S. M. (1993). The voices of African-American MFT students: Suggestions for improving recruitment and retention. *Journal of Marital and Family Therapy, 19*, 17–30.

CHAPTER 13

The Delphi Method

LINDA STONE FISH
DEAN M. BUSBY

BACKGROUND

Dear Reader,

   We would like to ask your help in a research study of considerable significance for family therapy researchers and clinicians. The present study is designed to compare and contrast the various research methodologies in the field by examining the opinions of prominent family therapists. The completion of the three questionnaires that will make up this study will require a total of no more than 1½ hours of your time. In appreciation of your participation, a complete summary of the findings and a list of the other panelists will be sent to you.

   This study will employ the Delphi technique, a widely used method of gathering group consensus from a panel of knowledgeable persons. The Delphi technique assures anonymity of responses, reduces group pressure for conformity, and takes less time for panelists than traditional methods of pooling opinion. As an expert in the field of family therapy, your participation in the present research will be greatly appreciated.

   With your help, this research will help clarify various research methodologies and their role in the family therapy field. We look forward to working with you in the weeks to come.

   Respectfully,
   Linda Stone Fish, PhD   *Dean M. Busby, PhD*

Sound interesting? This is the way Delphi research often begins. Researchers are curious about a particular topic in the field. They may perceive the seeds of an idea germinating in the soil of family therapy (e.g., feminist-informed family therapy in the 1980s), or they may perceive discrepancies in ideas that are fueling theory and practice (e.g., how structural and strategic therapies are similar vs. different). Or they may have an opinion about a particular topic relevant to the field and want to know how expert colleagues around the country think about the same things (e.g., the strengths and weaknesses of families at the present time). Regardless of the idea, the researchers want to pool experts on the subject. The researchers want to structure communication about the idea so that consensus can be reached. They do not have the financial resources to pay all the experts to meet in one place. The Delphi method provides researchers with a way to gather consensus without face-to-face interaction. They do not want to do traditional surveying, because then they would just gather everyone's opinions without the benefit of participants' receiving feedback from other survey participants. They want more of a dialogue about ideas, and the Delphi method allows this type of dialogue to take place.

Philosophical Assumptions

The Delphi method is based on the philosophical assumption that "n heads are better than one" (Dalkey, 1972). It is a procedure designed to sample a group of knowledgeable persons in order to gain a consensus of opinion on a particular topic. The Delphi method structures the communication of individuals in a way that allows a group of individuals to deal with complex problems (Linstone & Turoff, 1975).

The Delphi structures the communication by providing a forum in which participants are able to express their opinions anonymously, gather feedback from the group about their views, access other views of the same ideas, and have an opportunity to revise their views. How a researcher designs and implements the Delphi technique is not as important as the philosophical assumption underlying its usage. The Delphi method rests on the idea that it is possible and often quite valuable to reach consensus through a collective human intelligence process (Linstone & Turoff, 1975). The view that truth is relative underlies the attempt to gather myriad opinions on a particular topic. Mitroff and Turoff (1975) explain the underpinnings of the Delphi by utilizing different components of the philosophies of Locke, Leibniz, Kant, Hegel, and Singer. They are quick to suggest, however, that we must be careful not to rigidly define the philosophical assumptions underlying the Delphi:

> We certainly no longer seem able to afford the faulty assumption that there is only one philosophical base upon which a technique can rest if it is to be "scientific." Indeed if our conception of inquiry is "fruitful" (notice, not "true" or "false" but "productive") then to be "scientific" would demand that we study something (model it, collect data on it, argue it, etc.) from as many diverse points of view as possible. (Mitroff & Turoff, 1975, p. 36)

Scheele (1975), another Delphi method specialist, utilizes the ideas of Merleau-Ponty to define the assumptions underlying the philosophical base of the Delphi method. According to Scheele,

> the Merleau-Pontyean is concerned with the particular reality created by the "bracketing" of an event or idea out of the great din of experience, rather than explicating a pragmatic reality that can be used to define possible actions. Truth to the Merleau-Pontyean is agreement that enables action by confining or altering "what is normal" or to be expected. (p. 43)

The Delphi method attempts to negotiate a reality that can then be useful in moving a particular field forward, planning for the future, or even changing the future by forecasting its events. The philosophical underpinnings of the Delphi are thus more concerned with the application of useful knowledge than with the attempt to define the truth.

Historical Roots and Development

The Delphi method was named after the Greek town of Delphi. The ancient Greeks believed that Apollo—son of Zeus and god of light, purity, the sun, and prophecy—killed the dragon Python in Delphi. The temple in Delphi then contained the famous oracle, Pythia, whom Apollo chose to speak through to predict the future. She would turn around in frenzy and utter strange sounds, which would then be used for prediction. The Delphi method that is used today, based in a more rational, scientific paradigm, had its first usage in attempting to predict the future.

Although Quade (1967) reports the Delphi method's earliest use in the prediction of horse race outcomes, other leading Delphi specialists argue that the method originated at the Rand Corporation and had its first application in defense and military matters (Dalkey & Helmer, 1963). The first Rand Corporation utilization of the Delphi, "Project Delphi," was an attempt to forecast the probability of a particular event. The Air Force was interested in what U.S. experts believed the Soviet Union thought was the optimal U.S. industrial target and how many A-bombs it would take to reduce the munitions output (Linstone & Turoff, 1975). Had the research team attempted to study this idea with extant research practices, they would have had to use extremely difficult computer programs for the 1950s and would have had to estimate much of the input subjectively. Instead, they decided to gather a consensus of opinion as a means to identify the "truth."

Although defense practices were the first subject for the Delphi technique, it did not receive much publicity until Gordon and Helmer (1964) utilized it to forecast long-range trends in science and technology and their impact on society. This study—coupled with a monograph by Helmer and Rescher (1960) entitled *On the Epistemology of the Inexact Sciences*, both done through the Rand Corporation—were used as catalysts for many other researchers to utilize the Delphi technique (Linstone & Turoff, 1975). The methodology proliferated in the 1960s and 1970s and continues to find applications in fields dealing with other complex problems that face society, such as the environment, health, education, and transportation. The Delphi technique is also commonly used in psychology, sociology, and political science.

The Delphi technique found its way into family therapy through Sam Cochran of East Texas State University. Cochran utilized his experience as part of the Rand Corporation to bring the Delphi to the psychology department. He became a committee member for Wayne Winkle's family therapy dissertation. Under the advisorship of Fred Piercy, Winkle used the Delphi to reach a consensus of opinion about a model family therapy curriculum in the late 1970s (Winkle, Piercy, & Hovestadt, 1981). Family therapy researchers have been using the Delphi since the early 1980s, although most of the research utilizing this approach has been archived in dissertation abstracts. Whereas the general field of psychotherapy has seen a number of studies utilizing the approach (e.g., Goplerud, Walfish, & Broskowski, 1985; Kaufman, Holden, & Walker, 1989; Norcross, Alford, & DeMichele, 1992; Thomson, 1990), the family therapy field has only seen a limited number of published articles using this technique.

The traditional Delphi technique has been used in five family therapy research articles since the publication of Winkle and colleagues' article in 1981. First, Stone Fish and Piercy (1987) used the Delphi to examine the similarities and differences between structural and strategic family therapies. In the second article, Stone Fish (1989) compared the results of the Stone Fish and Piercy (1987) study with those of an unpublished Delphi poll conducted by Wheeler (1985), which explored the differences between extant family therapy practices and feminist-informed family therapy. In the third study, Rago and Childers (1990) used the Delphi to survey family therapists about revisions in family therapy theories that might better accommodate the changing U.S. family. Stone Fish and Osborn (1992) also used the Delphi to survey family therapy experts about the current strengths and weaknesses of family life in the United States. The final traditional Delphi study published in the family therapy literature to date surveyed panelists on their conceptual and practical ideas of the reflecting team approach to family therapy (Jenkins, 1996).

A more recent trend in the family therapy literature is to use a modified version of the Delphi technique. There have been five studies using modified versions of the technique in the family therapy literature since Winkle and colleagues' (1981) study. In the first such study, Nelson and colleagues (Nelson & Figley, 1990; Nelson, Heilbrun, & Figley, 1993) surveyed a large group of family therapists about basic family therapy skills. In the second, White, Edwards, and Russell (1997) modified the traditional Delphi to identify the principal components necessary for successful outcomes in marriage and family therapy. Blow and Sprenkle (2001) also used a modification of the Delphi to identify common factors across marriage and family therapy theories. Hovestadt, Fenell, and Canfield (2002) modified the Delphi technique to survey rural mental health service providers about effective marriage and family therapy in rural settings. Lastly, Nelson, Piercy, and Sprenkle (in press-a) modified the Delphi to survey family therapy experts about Internet infidelity.

METHODOLOGY

Research Questions

As a field undergoing continual transformation and encountering constant theoretical and practical challenges, family therapy is well positioned to find the Delphi method useful. The family therapy research questions that are best answered by this methodology are those in which researchers are trying to reach some consensus of opinion about a particular area. An additional use of this method is to develop policy issues for a field or profession regarding a relatively new phenomenon (e.g., AIDS in the early 1990s). Often what occurs is that particular ideas or series of thoughts are germinating in the literature. The Delphi technique is available to help researchers reach a consensus about such ideas or to predict the future of these ideas in the field.

A good example of the utility of the Delphi method occurred in the early 1980s. Structural and strategic family therapies, two of the most popular approaches at the time, lacked both conceptual and practical clarity. There was much confusion in the field about whether to integrate the two approaches. It was often difficult to differentiate them because of overlap in both theory and practice. Clinicians throughout the country were calling themselves "structural/strategic family therapists," and outcome research combined the two schools into the same category (Stanton, Todd, & Associates, 1982). On the other hand, many leading theoreticians in the field (de Shazer, 1984; Fraser, 1982; MacKinnon, 1983; Rohrbaugh, 1984) believed that it would be a grave mistake to integrate the two approaches. A need existed to define both the structural and strategic approaches to family therapy, as well as their similarities and differences.

Although family therapy theorists (e.g., Beavers, 1981; Liddle, 1980; Sprenkle, 1976) were suggesting that the best family therapy practices are linked to some research base, it was proving difficult to research a therapy approach that lacked theoretical clarity. A consensus of opinion from a panel of expert structural and strategic therapists as to the similarities and differences inherent in these two approaches would help clarify the therapies and move the field forward. The Delphi method proved to be an excellent vehicle for researching this dilemma.

Sampling and Selection Procedures

Panel selection is a critical element in the Delphi method. Dalkey (1969) reports that panelists' knowledge of the subject matter at hand is the most significant assurance of a high-quality outcome when the Delphi method is used. Therefore, Delphi panelists are chosen for their expertise rather than through a random process. The researcher selects the panelists based on their knowledge of the subject matter of interest. It is also possible to contrast opinions from an expert panel with those from a panel of nonexperts.

In the Delphi research comparing structural and strategic therapists, panelists were selected who met three of the following criteria: They (1) had published at least two articles or books on structural or strategic family therapy, (2) had at least 5 years of clinical experience in structural or strategic family therapy, (3) had at least 5 years of experience teaching structural or strategic family therapy, (4) had made at least two national convention presentations on structural or strategic family therapy, and (5) possessed a qualifying degree in a mental health discipline. A list of panelists was generated by perusing family therapy journals and books, and selecting authors who wrote about structural and strategic therapies. Those panelists from this first list who were asked to participate were also asked to provide the names of other family therapists who met the criteria listed above. These latter therapists were then sent letters asking them to participate. A short demographic questionnaire was sent with the Delphi to confirm the panelists' expertise in the subject matter. Of the panelists who were selected for the structural/strategic study, the 32 panelists who agreed to participate and completed the three rounds of the Delphi were quite expert in the field. Twenty-six were educators in the field. The average panelist had more than 8 publications and 10 national presentations

Data Collection Procedures

Data collection utilizing the traditional Delphi technique involves a three-part questionnaire. Delphi experts agree "that a point of diminishing returns is reached after a few rounds. Most commonly, three rounds proved sufficient to attain stability in the responses; further rounds tended to show little change and excessive repetition was unacceptable to the participants" (Linstone & Turoff, 1975, p. 229). According to Linstone and Turoff (1975), data collection undergoes four distinct phases. First, the subject is explored by the participants, and each panelist gives as much input as he or she would like about the topic under study. The second phase is characterized by pulling together the individual information and understanding how the group views the subject. The third phase deals with the disagreements encountered among panelists with differing views. The final phase occurs after the initial information has been fed back to the individuals for their analysis. How these phases are accomplished is left up to the research team. Most important is the opportunity for panelists to express their opinions about the subject matter and for the research team not to prematurely close off disagreements among members. Usually the team designs a questionnaire that is sent out to a large group of expert panelists. The research team then pools the responses and sends them out again (at least once) to the panelists, so that they can re-evaluate their answers based on group responses. The research team attempts to reach a consensus of opinion about the initial responses during the last phase of the Delphi.

The Delphi technique, according to Dalkey (1972), has overcome the following drawbacks of the traditional methods of pooling opinion: (1) the influence of dominant individuals, (2) irrelevant and biasing communication, and (3) group pressure for conformity. Anonymity in the Delphi technique reduces the effect of dominant individuals; controlled feedback reduces irrelevant communication; and the use of statistical procedures reduces group pressure for conformity (Dalkey, 1972). It allows greater participation from panel members with economy of time and expense, avoids the pressures of face-to-face contacts, and aids the formation of opinion consensus.

The Delphi technique that was employed in the structural/strategic study involved three questionnaires designed by the research team (Stone Fish, Piercy, Sprenkle, and Constantine) and sent to each participant. Delphi Questionnaire I (DQI) was an open-ended form with major category headings supplied by the team to stimulate and guide participants' thinking (see Figure 13.1). The major headings asked the panelists to associate authors with structural therapy or strategic therapy; to identify major theoretical assumptions and techniques, how change occurs, and the major goals of therapy; and to discuss the differences and similarities inherent in the two approaches.

The completed DQI was returned to the primary researcher, who compiled every panelist's responses, creating Delphi Questionnaire II (DQII) (see Figure 13.2). DQII was sent to panelists with a 7-point scale next to each item. The structural DQII had 213 items, and the strategic DQII contained 271 items. Every panelist was asked to rate each item in regard to its importance in defining either strategic or structural family therapy, and to return these ratings to the primary researcher. A rating of 1 indicated complete disagreement with the item's being important in defining the different approaches, whereas a rating of 7 indicated complete agreement (see Figure 13.2). The ratings from DQII were analyzed by computing the median, quartiles one and three, and the interquartile range for each item. This statistical information, a new 7-point scale, and each respondents' ratings of DQII items were combined to form Delphi Questionnaire III (DQIII; see Figure 13.3). In light of this new information, DQIII asked the respondents once again to rate the items on a 7-point scale indicating disagreement–agreement and return them to the primary researcher.

For the final profile of the strategic and structural questionnaires, medians and interquartile ranges were computed in the fashion of previous Delphi studies in family therapy (e.g., Redenour, 1982; Winkle et al., 1981). A high level of consensus and agreement was set in accordance with Binning, Cochran, and Donatelli (1972), to ensure that those items that became part of the final profile were those considered most important by the panelists. Those items that received a median of 6.00 or above and an interquartile range of 1.50 or less were selected as items on the final profile of strategic and structural family therapies (see Table 13.1).

Please complete this questionnaire. It is designed to compile a composite profile of structural family therapy. Please answer all the questions, using the reverse side of the paper if necessary. Feel free to make any other major categories or statements you feel would add to an understanding of structural family therapy.

Name: _____

What authors do you associate with structural family therapy?

_____

_____

_____

What are five major theoretical assumptions underlying structural family therapy?

1. _____
2. _____
3. _____
4. _____
5. _____

What are the differences between structural and strategic family therapies?

_____

_____

_____

_____

_____

_____

FIGURE 13.1. A sample Delphi Questionnaire I (excerpts).

Data Analysis Procedures

Delphi data are analyzed by calculating medians and interquartile ranges, to identify the rates of group agreement and consensus for each item that a panelist makes as a statement. Medians provide information on the central tendency of responses, indicating where most items fall on the disagreement–agreement scale. A "median" is a measure that divides the distribution into two equal parts if the distribution is a normal bell curve. Another term for the median is the "50th percentile," or the point below which 50% of the cases fall. However, when the distribution of responses is skewed toward the high of low ends of a scale—as it is in many of the questions from a Delphi study, where an attempt is made to obtain consensus—the median will often be close to the highest or lowest possible score. An example of a frequency distribution for an item from a Delphi study is presented in Table 13.2. The results in Table 13.2 are com-

Please circle one number for each item, indicating the degree of importance it assumes in the final profiles of structural family therapy.

What authors do you associate with structural family therapy?

Disagree–Agree

1 2 3 4 5 6 7   1. Harry Aponte

1 2 3 4 5 6 7   2. Lynn Hoffman

1 2 3 4 5 6 7   3. Salvador Minuchin

1 2 3 4 5 6 7   4. Ron Liebman

1 2 3 4 5 6 7   5. Braulio Montalvo . . .

What are the major theoretical assumptions underlying structural family therapy?

Disagree–Agree

1 2 3 4 5 6 7   6. Families are hierarchically organized with rules for interacting across subsystems.

1 2 3 4 5 6 7   7. Family structure is defined by family transactional patterns (rules).

1 2 3 4 5 6 7   8. Family structure determines the effectiveness of family functioning.

1 2 3 4 5 6 7   9. Family members relate to each other in patterned ways that are observable.

1 2 3 4 5 6 7   10. Conflict is not to be avoided but used for change . . .

What are the differences between structural and strategic family therapies?

Disagree–Agree

1 2 3 4 5 6 7   11. The goals and techniques are the same. The degree that each is emphasized is different.

1 2 3 4 5 6 7   12. Strategic therapy focuses more on the presenting problem.

1 2 3 4 5 6 7   13. Strategic therapy focuses more on the rules that maintain the problem.

1 2 3 4 5 6 7   14. The strategic therapist utilizes more direct reliance on paradox.

1 2 3 4 5 6 7   15. Strategic therapists do not use family maps . . .

FIGURE 13.2. A sample Delphi Questionnaire II (excerpts).

Please reconsider your responses to each item on Delphi Questionnaire III in light of the new information presented.

The new information summarizes the responses of all other panelists to each item. The information is reported in terms of the median (MDN) and the interquartile range (IQR). The median is the point below which 50 percent of the responses fell. The interquartile range contains the middle 50 percent of the responses. Its size gives an indication of how widely the responses differed from one another. Your previous answers to each item on Delphi Questionnaire II are given for you to compare. The following is an example.

What authors do you associate with structural family therapy?

Delphi Questionnaire			III Delphi Questionnaire II (Your previous response)

Disagree–Agree	MDN	IQR	Disagree–Agree
1 2 3 4 5 6 7	6.83	0.92	1 2 3 4 5 6 7 1. Harry Aponte
1 2 3 4 5 6 7	3.00	3.50	1 2 3 4 5 6 7 2. Lynn Hoffman

In the example above, the median for Item 1 is 6.83, indicating strong agreement. The interquartile range is 0.92, which is narrow and indicates a high degree of consensus among panelists. Your response on DQII to Item 1 was 7.

The median of Item 2 is 3.00, indicating moderate disagreement. The large interquartile range of 3.50 indicates that there is not strong consensus on this item. Your response on DQII to Item 2 was 4.

Please reconsider each item carefully and present new ratings in the scale under Delphi Questionnaire III. Remember to rate each item and to circle only one number for each item.

FIGURE 13.3. A sample Delphi Questionnaire III (excerpts).

TABLE 13.1. A Sample of the Final Results of a Delphi Study

Median	Interquartile range	
		Authors associated with structural family therapy
7.00	0.50	Salvador Minuchin
6.96	0.54	H. Charles Fishman
6.87	0.64	Harry Aponte . . .
		Major theoretical assumptions of structural therapy
6.80	0.82	Families are hierarchically organized with rules for interacting across and between subsystems.
6.73	0.85	Insight is not sufficient for change.
6.60	0.90	Normal developmental crises can create problems within a family.
6.67	0.99	Inadequate hierarchy and boundaries maintain symptomatic behavior . . .
		Differences between structural and strategic therapies
6.33	1.17	Different approaches to resistance.
6.30	1.32	Strategic therapists focus more on between session change.
6.07	1.05	The strategic therapist utilizes more direct reliance on paradox . . .

TABLE 13.2. A Sample Frequency Distribution of a Delphi Item

What authors do you associate with structural family therapy?

Disagree–Agree
1 2 3 4 5 6 7   Harry Aponte

Response	Frequency	Cumulated frequency
1	0	0
2	0	0
3	1	1
4	3	4
5	5	9
6	13	22
7	18	40

Note. Mean = 6.1; median (50th percentile) = 6.85; 25th percentile = 6.08; 75th percentile = 7; interquartile range = 0.92.

mon for many items obtained in Delphi studies. The median is 6.83, which is almost equal to the highest possible score of 7. This indicates that the distribution is skewed toward the high end of the scale.

The degree to which panelists have reached a consensus of agreement on a particular response is determined by the "interquartile range." Interquartile ranges provide information about the variability in the data without being affected by extreme scores. Interquartile ranges are calculated by taking half the difference between the "upper quartile," or the point in the distribution below which 75% of the cases lie (the 75th percentile), and the "lower quartile," the point below which 25% of the cases lie (the 25th percentile). This type of statistic provides information about the range of scores that lie in the middle 50% of the cases, and in doing so provides information about the consensus of response on a particular item.

Table 13.2 contains results that are common for the interquartile range of high-consensus items. The upper quartile (75th percentile) is 7, and the lower quartile (25th percentile) is 6.08. The interquartile range is calculated by subtracting the upper quartile from the lower quartile (7 – 6.08), which equals 0.92. This is a small interquartile range, indicating high consensus from the panelists.

An attractive aspect of the Delphi method is that most researchers can calculate all of the necessary statistics by hand, using simple formulas. The formulas for calculating the 25th, 50th, and 75th percentiles are as follows (Nachmias & Nachmias, 1981):

$$25\text{th percentile} = Li + \frac{(n/4 - \text{CumF})Wi}{Fi} \quad \text{or the minimum score}$$

$$50\text{th percentile} = Li + \frac{(n/2 - \text{CumF})Wi}{Fi}$$

$$75\text{th percentile} = Li + \frac{(3n/4 - \text{CumF})Wi}{Fi} \quad \text{or the maximum score}$$

where Li is the lower real limit of the interval containing the desired percentile; n is the number of cases; CumF is the accumulated sum of the frequencies of all intervals preceding the interval containing the desired percentile; Fi is the frequency of the interval containing the desired percentile; and Wi is the width of the interval containing the desired percentile.

An example using the data from Table 13.2 follows. To obtain the median, the numbers from Table 13.2 can be inserted into the formula for the 50th percentile. It is necessary to know how many people are in the sample; in Table 13.1, there are 40. The researcher then knows that the median will fall in the interval containing the 20th case—in this instance, the response choice of 6. The 25th percentile will fall in the interval containing the 10th case—in this instance, the response choice of 6. The 75th percentile will fall in the interval containing the 30th case—in this instance, the response choice of 7.

$$50\text{th percentile} = 6 + \frac{(40/2 - 9)1}{13} = 6 + \frac{20 - 9}{13} = 6.84$$

$$25\text{th percentile} = 6 + \frac{(40/4 - 9)1}{13} = 6 + \frac{(10 - 9)}{13} = 6.07$$

$$75\text{th percentile} = 7 + \frac{(3 \cdot 40/4 - 22)1}{18} = 7 + \frac{(30 - 22)}{18} = 7.44 \text{ or } 7$$

The 75th percentile cannot be any higher than the maximum score, so although the formula produces a score of 7.44, the answer is 7.

Reporting

Delphi studies are typically reported in the literature as research articles, and are commonly published in refereed journals. A review of the literature about the content of the report is followed by a methodology section, which describes both the Delphi method in general and the particular application of the method in the research study. Findings are reported both in narrative form and in tables. Conclusions are usually drawn about the results in a discussion section following the results. The discussion section also includes the idiosyncratic and interesting challenges that have occurred throughout the research process. For example, in one Delphi study, Stone Fish and Osborn (1992) asked family therapists to express their views about family life in the United States. In the discussion section, they reported:

> There is a final profile of the U.S. family with which family therapy panelists from diverse backgrounds are able to reach consensus. There were, however, great misgivings by many, when asked to reach a consensus about U.S. family life. Panelists wrote on the edges of their surveys and on additional pieces of paper. The content of these misgivings had to do with the panelists' reluctance to make general statements about all families today when families are so diverse, depending both on the culture they are embedded in and their own shape and size. (p. 414)

DISCUSSION

Strengths and Weaknesses

The Delphi approach is particularly well suited for examining emerging areas of inquiry and for building consensus among a group of experts. When it is used for these purposes, few weaknesses exist. Still, there are several pitfalls that researchers should be aware of when conducting a Delphi study.

Regression to the Mean

It is common for respondents to change their answers to become more similar to the group mean if too many iterations are conducted. In other words, after three questionnaires are administered, the only significant change that occurs in the responses is that they begin to cluster closer to the mean. This problem is most easily avoided by only sending out one questionnaire in which respondents are aware of the group means. This is usually the last questionnaire.

Minimization of Diversity

In most instances, the researchers are searching for consensus from a sample of very diverse people. Because the final items that are selected are often dependent on small interquartile ranges, diversity is sacrificed for consensus. It is possible to report the outlying responses or to allow bimodal distributions in which groups of experts split into different camps if the researchers are flexible enough to relax the standard of tight interquartile ranges. A scatterplot is particularly useful for determining whether bimodal or other types of unusual distributions exist in the data.

Time Commitment

The respondents, if they take the time to think carefully about their answers. can often expend several hours on completing the questionnaires. Because panels of experts are typically surveyed and experts are usually very busy people, there is an immediate difficulty in obtaining an adequate sample. However, some people respond to being called "experts" and will complete the surveys just to be included in the expert group. In other instances, financial incentives can be used, or shorter questionnaires can be constructed.

Narrow Perspectives

With increasing time in the field, experts can become more and more specialized. This can produce a perspective that is too narrow to be useful or one that is impossible to mesh with others' views. If researchers are interested in opinions about issues that are likely to involve complex systems, it is questionable whether specialized experts are the best persons to provide useful opinions.

The "So What" Factor

Finding out that most experts think that families are important has little practical value, even though high consensus can be reached. If the questionnaire is not constructed creatively, or if responses are grouped together into categories that are too broad, significance can be sacrificed for consensus. One of the first indicators that the questionnaires are not useful is a low response rate. Additional indicators of poorly constructed questionnaires are small numbers of unique responses on the first questionnaire and uncharacteristically high levels of consensus on the second questionnaire.

Reliability and Validity

Traditional types of reliability and validity are not easily obtained or applicable to the Delphi approach. Because the questionnaires are open-ended and general in nature, it is probably not useful to conduct typical reliability estimates. The issue of test–retest reliability could be explored by having the same group of experts complete the same questionnaire twice. However, experts are likely to be less tolerant of this repetition than are freshmen students in an introductory psychology class. An estimation of reliability between the first and second questionnaires can be estimated by exploring the consensus rates of the respondents. If a reasonable level of consensus is produced on many items on the second questionnaire, it is likely that a researcher has adequately summarized the meaning behind the responses of the first questionnaire.

The issue of validity is directly related to the selection of the panel of experts. Consensus of opinion is easily obtained with most samples; the important question is whether the experts fit the area of inquiry. If the criteria for selection of the experts are evaluated for content validity by several professionals in the field, this can go a long way toward ensuring some level of validity. Whenever an open-ended approach is used, a researcher takes a bigger risk in the area of validity. Validity asks the question "Am I really measuring what I set out to measure?" Because the panel of experts is only given general topics to follow, it is possible that many of the experts may diverge from the topic of interest into their own pet issues. As with qualitative studies, it is possible that the end product will reflect a different topic from that of the beginning research question. The only solution to wandering is to tightly define the area of interest. This may improve validity, but most experts will show a surprising ability to break free from restrictions on their freedom of expression. An example of this was evidenced in Stone Fish and Osborn's (1992) study, where the experts simply used the margins and other pieces of paper to freely express their opinions that did not fit into the predefined categories.

Skills

The Delphi method does not demand special statistical skills or clinical expertise. Medians and interquartile ranges can be computed by hand or with a calculator. Some creativity is necessary to capture the interest of the experts and to sell the idea of the research project. One study has demonstrated that the number of words needed to describe a topic area or event is related to the amount of information and the consensus rates that are obtained (Linstone & Turoff, 1975). This finding suggests that authors need to avoid using too few or too many words when constructing Delphi questionnaires if they hope to elicit accurate responses and build consensus.

Bridging Research and Practice

The characteristics of the Delphi make it particularly well suited for bridging the gap between research and practice. This approach does not demand large samples, statistical expertise, or a great amount of financial resources. As a result, clinicians can use the Delphi method to survey "expert" clients, expert referral sources, or any other group of individuals whose opinions are important. It is especially useful for developing policies about new problems that can crop up in agency work. When offered the choice of completing a few short questionnaires or attending several committee meetings that are likely to produce endless dialogue, most practitioners would elect to complete the questionnaires.

The results from the Delphi questionnaires are presented in the language of the respondents, rather than shrouded in excessive theory or statistical jargon. This attribute alone can help bridge the gap between research and practice, in that the interest level is usually higher when readers can speak the same language as the authors.

Future Directions

As the helping professions continue to struggle with populations that are increasingly diverse and a delivery system that is experiencing dramatic changes, opinions of leaders in the field will be helpful for developing new programs and policies. It is likely that the Delphi approach will become as common in all fields of psychotherapy as it is in education and political science. It is surprising how few studies there are in marriage and family therapy that use this technique. In order for this approach to become more commonplace in the field, students must be exposed to it in the early stages of their training. It is a method of inquiry that could easily fit the skills and interests of graduate students who are attempting to complete dissertations and theses.

Since the publication of the first edition of this book, a new trend in Delphi research has gained popularity in the marriage and family therapy field: Using a modified version of the Delphi technique is now more popular than using the traditional version. The modification has been either to use fewer rounds and/or different analysis (Hovestadt et al., 2002; Nelson & Figley, 1990; Nelson et al., 1993; White et al., 1997), or to add a qualitative and/or an Internet component to the survey data (Blow & Sprenkle, 2001; Nelson et al., in press-a). In place of the third round of questionnaires traditionally used by Delphi researchers, Blow and Sprenkle (2001) qualitatively interviewed six panelists about discrepancies in the data. Nelson, Piercy, and Sprenkle (in press-b), modified the Delphi and surveyed panelists in seven phases. They surveyed panelists, then created vignettes to comment on, and also gave panelists the option to respond directly to a website (providing a qualitative iteration to the Delphi). The use of qualitative interviews and access to the Internet as adjuncts to or substitutes for the traditional questionnaires may change the face of the Delphi method in the field of family therapy. Researchers who want to use multiple methodology for study into unexplored phenomena, and/or who want to experiment with using the Internet in survey research, may find the modified Delphi a useful tool.

REFERENCES

Beavers, W. R. (1981). A systems model of family for family therapy. *Journal of Marital and Family Therapy*, 7, 299–307.

Binning, D., Cochran, S., & Donatelli, B. (1972). *Delphi panel to explore post-secondary needs in the state of New Hampshire*. Manchester, NH: Decision Research.

Blow, A., & Sprenkle, D. (2001). Common factors across theories of marriage and family therapy: A modified Delphi study. *Journal of Marital and Family Therapy*, 27, 385–402.

Dalkey, N. (1969). Experimental study of group opinion. *Futures*, 1, 408–426.

Dalkey, N. (1972). *Studies in the quality of life*. Lexington, MA: Lexington Books.

Dalkey, N., & Helmer, O. (1963). An experimental application of the Delphi method to the use of experts. *Management Science*, 9, 458–467.

de Shazer, S. (1984). Fit. *Journal of Strategic and Systemic Therapies*, 3, 34–37.

Fraser, J. S. (1982). Structural and strategic family therapy: A basis for marriage or grounds for divorce? *Journal of Marital and Family Therapy*, 8, 13–22.

Goplerud, E. N., Walfish, S., & Broskowski, A. (1985). Weathering the cuts: A Delphi survey on surviving cutbacks in community mental health. *Community Mental Health Journal*, 21, 14–27.

Gordon, J., & Helmer, O. (1964). *Report on a long-range forecasting study*. Santa Monica, CA: Rand Corporation.

Helmer, O., & Rescher, N. (1960). *On the epistemology of the inexact sciences*. Santa Monica, CA: Rand Corporation.

Hovestadt, A., Fennell, D., & Canfield, D. (2002). Characteristics of effective providers of marital and family therapy in rural mental health settings. *Journal of Marital and Family Therapy*, 28, 225–231.

Jenkins, D. (1996). A reflecting team approach to family therapy: A Delphi study. *Journal of Marital and Family Therapy*, 22, 219–238.

Kaufman, K. L., Holden, E. W., & Walker, C. E. (1989). Future directions in pediatric and clinical child psychology. *Professional Psychology: Research and Practice*, 20, 148–152.

Liddle, H. A. (1980). On teaching a contextual or systemic therapy: Training content, goals, and methods. *American Journal of Family Therapy*, 8, 58–69.

Linstone, H. A., & Turoff, M. (Eds.). (1975). *The Delphi method: Techniques and applications*. Reading, MA: Addison-Wesley.

MacKinnon, L. (1983). Contrasting strategic and Milan therapies. *Family Process*, 22, 425–437.

Mitroff, I. I., & Turoff, M. (1975). Philosophical and methodological foundations of Delphi. In H. A. Linstone & M. Turoff (Eds.), *The Delphi method: Techniques and applications* (pp. 17–36). Reading, MA: Addison-Wesley.

Nachmias, D., & Nachmias, C. (1981). *Research methods in the; social sciences* (2nd ed.). New York: St. Martin's Press.

Nelson, T., & Figley, C. (1990). Basic family therapy skills: III. Brief and strategic schools of family therapy. *Journal of Family Psychology*, 4, 49–62.

Nelson, T., Heilbrun, G., & Figley, C. (1993). Basic family therapy skills: IV. Transgenerational theories of family therapy. *Journal of Marital and FamilyTherapy*, 19, 253–266.

Nelson, T., Piercy, F., & Sprenkle, D. (in press-a). Internet infidelity: A multi-wave Delphi study. *Journal of Couple and Relationship Therapy*.

Nelson, T., Piercy, F., & Sprenkle, D. (in press-b). Internet infidelity: A multi-wave Delphi study. In F. Piercy, K. Hertlein, & J. Wetchler (Eds.), *Handbook of infidelity treatment*. New York: Haworth Press.

Norcross, J. C., Alford, B. A., & DeMichele, J. T. (1992). The future of psychotherapy: Delphi data and concluding observations. *Psychotherapy*, 29, 150–158.

Quade, E. S. (1967). *Cost-effectiveness: Some trends in analysis*. Santa Monica, CA: Rand Corporation.

Rago, A. M., & Childers, J. H. (1990). Perceived changes in theories of family therapy in response to the changing American family. *TACD Journal*, *18*, 23–45.

Redenour, C. (1982). *A Delphi investigation of alternative futures for Texas marriage and family therapists*. Unpublished doctoral dissertation, East Texas State University.

Rohrbaugh, M. (1984). The strategic systems therapies: Misgivings about mixing models. *Journal of Strategic and Systemic Therapies*, *3*, 28–32.

Scheele, D. S. (1975). Reality construction as a product of Delphi interaction. In H. A. Linstone & M. Turoff (Eds.), *The Delphi method: Techniques and applications* (pp. 37–71). Reading, MA: Addison-Wesley.

Sprenkle, D. H. (1976). The need for integration among theory, research, and practice in the family field. *The Family Coodinator*, *25*, 124–127.

Stanton, M. D., Todd, T. C., & Associates. (1982). *The family therapy of drug abuse and addiction*. New York: Guilford Press.

Stone Fish, L. (1989). Comparing structural, strategic, and feminist-informed family therapies: Two Delphi studies. *American Journal of Family Therapy*, *17*, 303–314.

Stone Fish, L., & Osborn, J. (1992). Therapists' views of family life: A Delphi study. *Family Relations*, *41*, 409–416.

Stone Fish, L., & Piercy, F. P. (1987). The theory and practice of structural and strategic family therapies: A Delphi study. *Journal of Marital and Family Therapy*, *13*, 113–125.

Thomson, B. R. (1990). Appropriate and inappropriate uses of humor in psychotherapy as perceived by certified reality therapists: A Delphi study. *Journal of Reality Therapy*, *10*, 59–65.

Wheeler, D. (1985). *The theory and practice of feminist-informed family therapy: A Delphi study*. Unpublished doctoral dissertation, Purdue University.

White, M., Edwards, S., & Russell, C. (1997). The essential elements of successful marriage and family therapy: A modified Delphi study. *American Journal of Family Therapy*, *25*, 213–231.

Winkle, W. C., Piercy, F. P., & Hovestadt, A. J. (1981). A curriculum for graduate-level marriage and family therapy education. *Journal of Marital and Family Therapy*, *7*, 201–210.

CHAPTER 14

Task Analysis of Couple and Family Change Events

BRENT BRADLEY
SUSAN M. JOHNSON

BACKGROUND

The air in the room weighed heavy as the couple and therapist once again hit an impasse. "If I could only talk about my fear," confided the husband as he gazed down at the floor. The atmosphere was tense as the couple therapist aided the more blaming spouse in "softening" toward his partner—a pivotal change event in the emotionally focused approach.

A chance for Change was knocking on the office door.

Panic coursed through the therapist's veins. His tensing body screamed, "What do I do now? I can feel that this is big. I've never seen him this vulnerable. This is really important. I've got to help him, and both of them. But I don't know what to do when he talks so deeply of his 'fear.'"

"My fear is just so big," the husband continued.

Change rapped even more loudly on the door, now demanding to be let in.

The husband took a deep breath and sighed.

The therapist had read the theories and the research studies many times, but though these gave an overview, he desperately needed a more detailed map. The therapist was stuck, paralyzed.

"But I just can't talk about it," the husband declared in defeat. "It's just too much."

The room fell awkwardly silent. The opportunity for Change was missed.

Therapists face similar situations on a daily basis. After learning about a new theory or intervention, or reading a research study, a therapist may think, "This makes sense. I am going to start doing this." But in sessions with clients, things often don't go as smoothly as they are presented in the abstract pages of a manual or lists of interventions in a research study.

Mountains of research support and charismatic presenters matter little when clinicians are unable to translate application into the moment-to-moment process of a key session. As the therapist in the scenario discovered above, the abstract "map" given in clinical handbooks and described and tested in research studies is often not detailed enough to guide a therapist through the actual in-session terrain. Beutler, Williams, and Wakefield (1993) report a strongly consistent criticism of the research literature among clinicians—namely, that there is a startling lack of research focusing on therapist and/or client behaviors that lead to important moments of change in therapy sessions. As Pinsof and Wynne (2000) astutely point out, our research thus far too often offers little to guide the clinician in his or her in-session decision making. In fact, the process of couple and family therapy (CFT) is described and debated, but little is really known about how interpersonal change actually occurs (Friedlander, Wildman, Heatherington, & Skowron, 1994). CFT researchers have understandably emphasized outcome research to provide efficacy support for these modes of intervention (Jacobson & Addis, 1993; Pinsof & Wynne, 1995, 2000). A shortcoming of outcome research, however, is that it fails to target what is specifically helpful or unhelpful in the ongoing process of therapy (Johnson & Lebow, 2000; Pinsof & Wynne, 2000). Outcome research is often primarily interested in emphasizing the evaluation of whether a general model of CFT works, rather than building a framework that focuses on *how* it works. Process research is needed to build minitheories focused on specified change events occurring throughout the process of therapy (Diamond & Diamond, 2002; Greenberg, Heatherington, & Friedlander, 1996; Johnson, 2003; Pinsof & Wynne, 2000). Too often, family therapists conceptually understand theory and or general intervention models, but are uncertain about how to translate these into moments of change in the therapy session.

The opening vignette reflects a larger concern in the CFT field referred to as the "research–practice gap" (Sprenkle, 2002). Emotionally focused therapy (EFT; Greenberg & Johnson, 1988; Johnson, 1996), for example, is one of a few empirically validated and empirically supported approaches. And although the EFT practitioner described in the vignette was well versed in the approach, the breakdown occurred at a more micro level that has not yet been sufficiently addressed in the literature. Therapists need more than outcome research; they need studies that answer relevant process questions and help them in their daily work to create moments of change with real families in diverse communities. These kinds of concerns led the therapist in the vignette (who was actually one of us, BB) to conduct a task analysis (Greenberg, 1984) study addressing relevant therapist questions such as these: "What am I supposed to do when someone keeps talking about his or her immense fear? What specific interventions are used? What themes are focused on? What does the typical successful EFT softening change process *really* look and sound like?"

Task analysis is a process research methodology that seeks to discover how change occurs in various "events" throughout the course of psychotherapy. It is a kind of "bottom-up" rather than "top-down" research methodology that focuses on key tasks and steps in the therapeutic change process. Task analysis has proven useful for both researchers and clinicians, because it builds theory and clarifies successful change interventions. It is the kind of methodology recommended to narrow the research–practice gap in CFT (Johnson, 2003; Pinsof & Wynne, 2000; Sprenkle, 2002).

In this chapter, we present an adaptation of task analysis that clearly demonstrates clinical relevance for practicing therapists struggling "in the trenches" on a daily basis. Task analysis is often presented in the context of a research program (Greenberg, 1999), and although we allude to these possibilities, we want to present it as accessible to students or clinicians interested in studies focusing on the process of change. Clinician-researchers may or may not have access to assistants or other professionals seasoned in research. In our presentation, we focus mainly on the discovery-oriented aspect of task analysis, which is the heart of the approach. We believe that task analysis can be utilized by students, experienced therapists, and researchers alike to uncover the pivotal change processes so needed in CFT research.

Philosophical Assumptions

Historically, the areas of process research and outcome research have been seen as separate domains (Greenberg & Pinsof, 1986). Process research often dealt with what happened in the session, while outcome research was mainly concerned with whether clients improved significantly from the beginning to the end of therapy. Process research, which was initiated more than 50 years ago, previously emphasized naturalistic designs where frequency counts of variables across sessions were correlated with outcomes or other processes (Diamond & Diamond, 2002). In this manner, both process and traditional psychotherapy research methods operated under a "uniformity myth"—that is, the assumption that process is uniform throughout the course of treatment (Greenberg et al., 1996).

Contemporary process researchers have answered such criticism by emphasizing a discovery-oriented paradigm (Elliot, 1984; Greenberg & Pinsof, 1986; Johnson, 2003; Mahrer, 1988; Rice & Greenberg, 1984). Task analysis lends itself to this new direction for process research. It is an intensive, discovery-oriented process research method for conducting structured, clinically relevant investigations of specific change processes. The primary goal of research within this paradigm is to examine actual change processes in therapy. Although we have to be clear when inferences are made, we can examine and denote patterns of behavior.

A core assumption of task analysis is that therapist and client behaviors occur in events that differ at various stages of the therapeutic process. Researchers study key events to gain a better understanding of how change happens at a smaller, more micro level. For example, knowing the frequency count of interventions used in an initial stage of therapy as compared to an ending stage is of limited value to the clinician. Such findings do not aid in tracking key client change processes, or in recognizing when to utilize specific interventions. They also do not take into account the very different client and therapist tasks involved at different stages in the overall therapy process. Establishing an initial therapeutic alliance in EFT, for example, is a very different process from the later task of exploring and expanding primary attachment-related emotion associated with a withdrawn spouse's position in the relationship. Even if similar interventions are utilized, they occur in different contexts and for different purposes. The specific "whys," "whens," and "hows" that task analysis taps into are immensely helpful for clinicians, theoreticians, and researchers alike, because they create a map of change terrain.

Historical Roots and Development

Task analysis discerns the nature of change by drawing on the tradition of critical-incident research, where key events are examined (Flanagan, 1954), and protocol analysis or process research, in which verbal interactions are studied (Greenberg & Pinsof,

1986). Rice and Greenberg (1984) recognized that traditional research methods failed to capture multidimensional tasks or events occurring in smaller numbers of sessions. This weakness is multiplied over the course of therapy, where multiple events occur at multiple stages. These researchers noted that in traditional research, the dynamic interaction among therapist, client, model, intervention, and environment is ignored. They introduced a new research paradigm called "task analysis," which emphasizes the examination of therapy "events." Initially it was most often applied to the study of change processes in individual psychotherapy (e.g., Clarke, 1990; Greenberg, 1983).

Increasingly, CFT scholars are advocating the use of task analysis for discovering mechanisms of change with couples and families (Johnson & Lebow, 2000; Nichols with Schwartz, 2004; Sprenkle, 2002). These scholars believe that its application would spur differentiated treatment development; aid in the training of clinicians; and enhance treatment potency, cost-effectiveness, and transportability (Diamond & Diamond, 2002). CFT researchers have applied task analysis to examine change within a variety of theoretical approaches, such as structural family therapy (Heatherington & Friedlander, 1990), constructivist family therapy (Coulehan, Friedlander, & Heatherington, 1998), multidimensional family therapy (Diamond & Liddle, 1996; Diamond, Liddle, Hogue, & Dakof, 1999), and EFT (Bradley & Furrow, 2004; Johnson & Greenberg, 1988; Johnson, Makinen, & Millikin, 2001). It is the most developed and widely used discovery-oriented methodology, repeatedly demonstrating effectiveness in uncovering in-session change in CFT.

METHODOLOGY

Task analysis serves the clinician well, because it supplies a stringent methodology for discovery-oriented investigation. It answers normal, everyday, and relevant practitioner questions such as these: "That session was powerful; what just happened?" "How did we accomplish that?" "Everything was going well, and then it just went in the other direction. What is this family trying to tell me that I am missing?" Therapy is seen as a set of meaningful and change-producing events occurring throughout the course of treatment. These events vary in context and content, and can be examined to capture pivotal change elements involving both therapist and client behavior (Friedlander et al., 1994).

In the opening vignette, the therapist was working from within the EFT approach (Johnson, 1996). EFT is an empirically validated short-term approach to modifying distressed couples' constricted interaction patterns and emotional responses, and fostering the development of a secure bond. EFT is consonant with empirical research on the nature of marital distress (Gottman, 1994), and the EFT conceptualization of adult love ties into the now abundant research on adult attachment (Cassidy & Shaver, 1999; Johnson, 2003). Secure attachment bonds are associated with physical and mental health, resilience in the face of stress, couple satisfaction, a strong sense of self, and positive communication behaviors such as empathy and assertiveness (Johnson & Whiffen, 1999). EFT has been found to obtain excellent posttherapy results (Johnson, Hunsley, Greenberg, & Schindler, 1999), and evidence shows that these results are stable, even in high-risk populations (Clothier, Manion, Gordon Walker, & Johnson, 2002). This collaborative approach integrates a Rogerian focus on the construction of emotional experience with a systemic focus on changing interaction patterns.

The three stages of EFT are "deescalation," "restructuring of interactions," and "consolidation." Throughout this chapter, two task analyses exemplify application of the methodology. The two change events examined in these task analyses are the "blamer-softening event" and the "resolution of attachment injuries." Both occur in Stage 2 of EFT, restructuring of interactions. The softening task analysis examines pivotal *therapist intervention*, whereas the attachment injuries task analysis captures *client process* en route to change.

Successful completion of the blamer-softening event is predictive of positive outcome in EFT (Johnson & Greenberg, 1988). In the culmination of this event, the more blaming partner softens toward the other partner, creating the beginning of mutual accessibility and responsiveness between the partners. The softening event is often the most difficult element of the approach for both therapist and couple (Greenberg & Johnson, 1988). The therapist in the opening illustration (again, BB) had read the literature and been trained by the originators of EFT, but remained uncertain when attempting to process softening events. To address this clinical need, a task analysis was performed to uncover what therapists actually do when facilitating successful softening events (Bradley & Furrow, 2004). Key therapist themes and interventions employed by an expert therapist were consistently found across successful softening events. This task analysis illustrates effectiveness in tracking crucial therapist behaviors that facilitate change.

Other recent process research has begun examining attachment injuries, which are key impasses in the restructuring of interactions (Stage 2 of EFT). This task analysis outlines client steps in the process of resolving in these impasses. The resolution of an attachment injury involves the creation of both forgiveness and reconciliation (Johnson et al., 2001). The task analysis methodology is explained and illustrated here according to these two task analysis research studies.

Task Analysis of Couple and Family Change Events

Our adaptation of the steps of a task analysis is summarized in Table 14.1 and discussed in detail below.

Formulating an Initial Map of Tasks

The initial conceptualization of key tasks within change events should be framed within a specific theoretical conceptualization (e.g., EFT, structural therapy). This allows expert clinicians to provide a beginning framework (Greenberg & Newman, 1996).

TABLE 14.1. Task Analysis of Change Events

1. Formulating an initial map of tasks
2. Identifying components of the change event
3. The rational analysis: Mapping the process
   a. Client process
   b. Therapist process
4. The empirical analysis: Building the minitheory
5. Verification

The degree to which a type of event is reflected in the current literature can vary greatly. This need not stifle the inquisitive clinician-researcher. The recent softening task analysis, for example, built upon an earlier study of client processes in successful softenings (Johnson & Greenberg, 1988). The attachment injuries task analysis, however, actually began by recognizing a *new* event that for the most part was not previously recognized in the literature. Examining such a new event requires more time and effort in the early steps of task analysis. The key here is to begin outlining a general understanding of key tasks involved in a change event.

It is vital that either the lead researcher or someone on the research team be well versed in the chosen theoretical approach. This clinician-researcher has to draw on his or her tacit understanding of change to help formulate key tasks and change events, and then to capture and articulate an often intricately nuanced change process.

APPLICATION EXAMPLE

The study of client processes in the attachment injuries task analysis began with a question: What happened when couples improved but did not recover from relationship distress in EFT? The conjecture was that Stage 2 change events (withdrawer reengagement and blamer softening) were not properly completed in the therapy session, and that the mutual emotional responsiveness necessary for a more secure bond was not then set in place. Tapes of sessions containing attempted softening events were then examined to begin tracking this specific process of therapy. A pattern became apparent: In an improved but not recovered couple, the therapist was unable to support the more blaming partner in reaching for the other partner from a position of vulnerability and pulling the other toward him or her. In fact, this partner, when asked to risk being vulnerable to the other partner, reacted with a "Never again" response and retreated to a defensive position. This appeared to predict improvement rather than recovery from relationship distress. The blaming partner then articulated a traumatic incident of abandonment and betrayal at a crucial moment of need, and refused to move to a position of trust. Only when the therapist shifted to resolve this injury did the couple progress to complete a softening and move into recovery. Intensive observation then allowed for the formulation of a specific impasse in a key change event and the tentative delineation of the path through such an impasse.

Identifying Components of the Change Event

Once this pattern emerged from intensive observation, more video session examples of the attachment injuries change event were collected, so that clients' processing steps in successful resolution events leading to forgiveness and reconciliation might be tentatively outlined. We often find it helpful to separate client from therapist activities to be examined; this is evidenced in the two task analyses reviewed in this chapter. In reality, these two types of processes always overlap, and both *can* be examined within a single task analysis. A change event consists of the following four components: (1) a problem marker, followed by (2) therapist interventions and (3) a sequence of client responses, which if successful (4) result in the family or couple achieving an effective resolution to the problem. Defining the marker and resolution components are key aspects of this step.

APPLICATION EXAMPLE

Client Process: The Attachment Injuries Task Analysis. In the attachment injuries task analysis, when we examined a small number of tapes, the marker for the emergence of the injury became clearer and clearer. As a therapist worked to assist a couple in disclosing attachment needs and taking the risk of a new level of emotional engagement, the more blaming partner would balk and evoke a past event when he or she had been vulnerable and the other partner had not responded to them. The more blaming partner would speak of this event in the present tense and become exceedingly distressed. This person would then refuse to risk further, and the softening event was therefore not completed. The resolution component was defined as effective and observable resolution to the problem in the therapy session.

Therapist Process: The Blamer-Softening Task Analysis. In the softening task analysis, the literature was reviewed to locate descriptions, actual transcripts, and professional videos of softening events. Based on subjective and theoretical conceptualizing, the event marker was identified as therapist initiation or direction of the softening enactment. This would occur when the therapist asked the blaming partner to turn toward his or her partner from a position of vulnerability, expressing his or her attachment-related needs and wants. The intervention directing this enactment would be restructuring and reshaping interactions by turning new emotional experience into a new response to the partner. We described this intervention during the softening event as a "softening reach," where the softened blamer would reach for the other partner. The resolution of the event was hypothesized to occur when there was mutual acceptance from each partner of the softening blamer's emerging position.

The Rational Analysis: Mapping the Process

It is during the rational analysis that the clinician creatively wrestles with and begins diagramming maps of the steps in the unfolding change process. He or she (and the team, if applicable) scrutinizes a number of recorded sessions and begins diagramming the process of the change event. Researchers should categorize the process in terms of the concepts and language that make the most sense to them. If there is a team, its members work together as a consensus group. The goal of this step is to create a detailed map that represents the best estimate of the process of change, based on a literature review, clinical experience, intuition, and intense examination of recorded events. Types of questions used to help form a rational map of the event may include the following (Greenberg, 1999):

1. What therapist interventions are utilized?
2. What is/are the intentional theme(s) of the therapist throughout the event/ task? What are the patterns in partner or family member responses? Describe and detail how themes unfold.
3. Describe how this task/event ends unsuccessfully or resolves. What impact does this seem to have on the couple or family?

The investigator continues to observe recorded performances from a previously collected data set of a couple or family involved in the designated change event. The clinician-researcher identifies, diagrams, and refines the articulation of the interactional steps taken by family members as they proceed through the marker and components of a change event. This process involves successive repetitions of comparing, contrasting, and elaborating between the evolving rational model and each newly examined event. This allows the clinician-researcher to corroborate, refine, or successively reformulate the steps in the evolving model of a change event. This process continues as long as the comparing, contrasting, and elaborating continue to produce new findings that further discriminate the emerging model. This structured repetition produces a conceptual minitheory of the change event.

Creation of a rational model allows the researcher to consider how family and/or therapist responses in the selected event would be best measured. This occurs in the next step of task analysis—the empirical analysis. Instruments need to be sensitive enough to detect and help expand on the client and therapist processes that have been identified. Therapist interventions were a key focus of the recent softening task analysis, for example. At this stage in the study, we realized that we were going to need an instrument sensitive enough to code and distinguish among specific EFT interventions. Thus we created a coding scheme based on the EFT interventions noted in the literature.

APPLICATION EXAMPLE

Client Process: The Attachment Injuries Task Analysis. In the study of attachment injuries, a small number of examples were thoroughly examined, and the beginning marker for each event was confirmed. The themes arising in the client process were then outlined, together with typical therapist interventions and completion or lack of process through the attachment injury impasse, progressing to the completion of a softening event.

As attachment injuries were examined, the patterns in the drama of the event emerged as follows (Johnson et al., 2001):

1. The therapist heightened attachment longings and needs, and asked the blaming partner to emotionally engage with these and articulate them to the other partner.
2. This partner refused and described a vivid example of hurt at the hands of the other partner.
3. The theme of this hurtful incident was abandonment or betrayal at a moment of intense need, such as at the time of a miscarriage or death of a parent.
4. The hurt partner became intensely upset and expressed the desire to protect him- or herself from risking such pain again.
5. The other partner sometimes tried to remain responsive, but at other times retreated to a defensive position, often saying, "Not this again."
6. The hurt partner spoke of his or her perception of a lack of remorse and responsibility on the part of the injuring partner.
7. The therapist attempted to validate both partners and get them to access and reveal emotional responses.
8. When this was successful, the hurt partner was able to articulate the injury clearly.

9. The other partner was then able to respond by admitting responsibility and apologizing in an emotionally engaged and remorseful way.
10. When this apology was accepted, the injured partner asked for comfort, and the other responded.
11. The partners were then able to talk generally about attachment needs and fears and soothe each other as the blamer moved into a softening.
12. If this did not occur, the partners stayed deescalated, but ended the session on a less engaged and more distant note. Softenings and the subsequent bonding events did not occur. The therapist was unable to structure an enactment where the blamer risked and became soothed by the previously withdrawn partner.

Therapist Process: The Blamer-Softening Task Analysis. At this step in the softening task analysis, the clinician-researchers asked process questions such as these: "What are the themes the therapist is focusing on in these softening segments? What seems important for the expert EFT practitioner to keep 'front and center' with the softening blamer and the other partner throughout the softening event? What words are used by therapists and clients when talking about attachment bonds?" Each therapist and client talk turn was analyzed for thematic content. This analysis yielded an initial performance diagram, which was then compared and contrasted with each collected softening event. Sequentially, the remaining softening event transcripts were compared, and the thematic sequence was modified. Results of this analysis were continually integrated into the evolving rational model.

The newly created minitheory yielded six distinct therapist process themes across blamer-softening events: (1) processing possible blamer reaching, (2) processing fears of reaching, (3) promoting actual blamer reaching, (4) supporting the softening blamer, (5) processing with the engaged withdrawer, and (6) promoting the engaged withdrawer's reaching back with support (Bradley & Furrow, 2004). In processing fears of reaching, the therapist expands the more blaming partner's fears of reaching to the other partner contextually from within internal working views of other and self (Bowlby, 1988). This finding highlights the importance of attachment theory to EFT at a crucial point in the approach's change process. The rational analysis provided a map of key expert therapist themes and interventions in successful softening events (see Figure 14.1).

The Empirical Analysis

Formal observational instruments can now be applied to check the newly created map empirically (see also "Data Analysis," below). The Structural Analysis of Social Behavior (SASB; Benjamin, Foster, Roberto, & Estroff, 1986), for example, allows raters to code responses from therapy tapes or transcripts into clear descriptive categories, such as "closeness" and "control." So, for example, "nurture" and "comfort" can be tracked. The investigator can follow the in-session process of what happens as one partner gently soothes the other without asking for anything in return, or when one partner puts the other one down by telling him or her, "Your ways are wrong." The themes outlined in the rational model are now refined or revised as specific responses emerge. The patterned sequence of responses that occur in the events can also be checked.

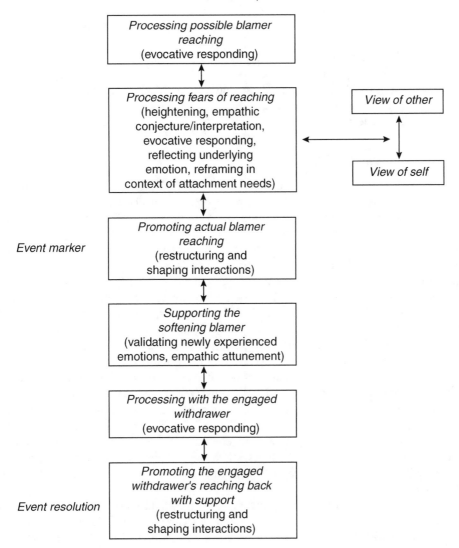

FIGURE 14.1. A map of therapist process themes and related interventions in blamer-softening events. From Bradley and Furrow (2004). Copyright 2004 by the American Association for Marriage and Family Therapy. Adapted by permission.

A useful component that to date has not been applied often in task analysis involves determining clients' responses to selected events. Clients can be asked to review and discuss selected moments on tapes. Interpersonal process recall (IPR; Elliot, 1986), in which a couple or family reviews a tape of an event and is asked questions concerning what each person was thinking and feeling during the session, is a helpful method for gaining an understanding of clients' processing. Typical questions in IPR may include the following:

1. "What happened for you in this segment that led to change or was significant?"
   a. "What happened inside of you [intrapersonally]?"
   b. "What happened between you [interpersonally]?"
   c. "What did your therapist do that was helpful? Not helpful?"
2. "What change possibly occurred?"
3. Specific questions relating to various particular studies can now be asked.

APPLICATION EXAMPLE

Therapist Process: The Blamer-Softening Task Analysis. The work leading up
to this point in the softening task analysis of therapist process proved very helpful in
discriminating exactly what we wanted our instruments to measure. Tracking and
coding the specific therapist interventions used in successful softening events were
important. The review of the EFT literature (completed in the first step of the task
analysis) had not yielded desired specificity. After searching the literature for couple
and family therapy process instruments, we determined that no current instrument
was sensitive enough to distinguish among EFT interventions. Based on this finding,
we created the EFT Coding Scheme (EFT-CS; Bradley, 2001), which included all of
the current EFT interventions. Second, an existing process coding instrument, the
Classification System for Counseling Responses (CSCR; Highlen, Lonborg, Hampl,
& Lassiter, 1984; Lonborg, Daniels, Hammond, Houghton-Wenger, & Brace, 1991),
was chosen to capture the softening process from a more atheoretical perspective.
The CSCR enables the coding of 19 therapist verbal behaviors, using moment-by-
moment intervals. The CSCR would also provide an opportunity to establish construct validity with the newly created EFT-CS. It is important to establish interrater
reliability on all measures used. Kappa coefficients for the three raters using the
EFT-CS ranged from .83 to .92, suggesting strong intercoder reliability. The percentage of agreement among the three CSCR raters ranged from 81% to 92% for the
four transcripts.

Session transcripts of softening events were analyzed by using the EFT-CS and the
CSCR to code therapist behaviors. This analysis categorized therapist behaviors according to both EFT interventions and a list of common therapist behaviors (CSCR).
Results indicated that frequent EFT interventions used in softening events involve in-
tensifying emotional experience and promoting intrapsychic awareness and interpersonal shifts in attachment-related interactions that define the relationship. Evocative
responding, heightening present and changing positions, and validation are often used
to facilitate a softening event.

The resulting empirical model provides a clinical map illustrating the development
of specific themes and related interventions leading to blamer softening (see Figure
14.1). In the opening vignette of this chapter, for example, the more blaming partner
confided, "If I could only talk about my fear." During that actual session, before the
softening task analysis, the therapist got stuck there, unsure of how to specifically address this "fear." The ensuing softening task analysis spotlighted that processing this
fear at this specific point in the EFT process is a vital part of a successful softening
event. The results of the task analysis provided a detailed map of how an expert therapist successfully navigates a softening.

Let us now creatively "reenter" this session. Based on the results of the softening task analysis, an expert EFT practitioner typically processes such fear in the following manner:

"If I could only talk about my fear," confided the husband as he gazed down at the floor. The atmosphere was tense as the EFT practitioner aided the more blaming spouse in "softening" toward his partner—a pivotal change event in the approach.

Change began knocking on the office door. The therapist recognized this "knock" as a client marker for a change event in EFT—a softening. The therapist warmly welcomed Change into the session as a trusted partner:

THERAPIST: There's this fear that grips you, right? Would you please help me understand this fear?

SPOUSE: My fear is just so big.

THERAPIST: It's big. It's like it is enveloping you right now. You're kind of gazing down at the floor and slowly shaking your head. What's happening inside?

SPOUSE: My shoulders are heavy. I carry this fear around all the time. I want to tell her things, but I am so afraid that these things are not acceptable to her—that she will see them as childish or wimpy, and she'll laugh at me.

THERAPIST: (*Softly*) A part of you wants to share some very important things with her. You want to confide in her, to risk with her. But another part of you is afraid of doing this. Maybe you'll get put down. Maybe you'll get ridiculed. Is that close?

SPOUSE: That's it. I am so afraid of being rejected by her. That word "rejected" sounds so adolescent-like. It's not like that. This is big, really heavy. It's like I walk around concealing these things about me, because I don't know if I could handle her seeing this about me and not being okay with it. It would just kill me.

THERAPIST: I hear you. You're saying, "Carolyn, I want you to see this part of me. I long to show it to you. But I am so afraid that you will find it not good enough. And that would be so hurtful. It'd . . . kill me."

SPOUSE: (*Nods head.*)

THERAPIST: Help me out here—but it's like this fear paralyzes you. It keeps you walled off from really being . . . known by Carolyn? Is that too strong?

SPOUSE: No. It's not too strong. That's it. That's where I am. No one knows this fear. (*His toes flex up and down rapidly as he stares at the floor.*)

THERAPIST: Right. So no one knows this fear. This fear is just too big, or too disgusting, I am not sure, but no one knows it. You hold this deep inside.

SPOUSE: I always have. It was the same with my parents. I wouldn't show my dad I was afraid. No way. If I did, he'd say I was a "sissy" or a "girly boy."

THERAPIST: You learned early on that it was not safe to show this fear. It sounds like if you did, you would be seen as somehow not good enough, or not worthy, or less than normal.

SPOUSE: I wouldn't be a real man. I'd be a loser. A failure.

THERAPIST: Um-hmm. Right. So, when this fear comes up with Carolyn, there's a *lot* going on inside for you, right? All of this history, all of these signals and messages you got from your parents—or your dad, as you said. My sense is that all of this is there chiming in as part of a loud chorus telling you, "Don't share that with her! She'll confirm the worst if you do! She'll laugh, or she'll see the real you, and . . . she won't like that a bit!" Yeah?

SPOUSE: Yeah. It's all there. It's just so powerful.

THERAPIST: It's like you're saying, "Carolyn probably won't be there for me if I share this. Nobody has else has been." [View of other] And on top of that, you're saying, "Why would anyone really want to be there and accept me, anyway?" Right? It's not just about Carolyn; this fear also grips you and says "You, you, Jeff, you're not worthy." Something like this? [View of self]

SPOUSE: A part of this is about Carolyn, yes. But another part of this is about me. I am afraid that no one will really accept me. Sometimes I wonder, "Who would? Why would they?"

THERAPIST: Right. Could you begin, just now, to start to tell Carolyn about this fear? You see, I think she rarely sees this part of you. This scared part. This vulnerable part. She sees this big man who has it all together, and gets angry and critical. But this is really different. Could you, in your own words, begin right now to share this fear with her?

Verification

The newly constructed minitheory can now be subjected to more traditional research methods, such as hypothesis testing. Typically, a group of specific resolution and nonresolution events from a newly collected set of data are compared to determine whether the model discriminates between successful and unsuccessful performances at a statistically significant level. If statistical analysis shows that the minitheory's components do indeed discriminate between resolution and nonresolution performances, the minitheory is seen as credible. Detailed explanations of the verification process, with appropriate measures, are available in the literature (see Diamond et al., 1999; Greenberg & Foerster, 1999).

    Relating process to outcome is a vital part of a task analysis research program. The clinician-researcher now seeks to answer the crucial question of whether couples and families who successfully engage in the process captured by the minitheory have better outcomes than those who do not. The minitheory allows increased control and explanation of the variability in couple and family change events. Subsequent studies benefit from larger sample sizes and better-matched samples at baseline.

Data Collection

Most event-based research methods require actual session recordings (video or audio). Researchers may, for example, collect data from their own work, from the practices of colleagues, or perhaps from a cooperating clinic. Researchers can also team with other colleagues or clinics to videotape sessions. Tapes may be obtained from an archive of previously collected data, from various commercially available videotapes, or from "expert" therapists themselves and their trained colleagues. The key is finding competently trained therapists working in a theoretically consistent manner that captures the event to be studied. In the softening task analysis, for example, one of us (SMJ) Dr. Johnson supplied nine taped sessions identified by EFT practitioners as possibly containing softenings. Gaining access to recorded sessions in which events of interest might have occurred is one of the challenges of this type of research. Within research programs, research projects can help generate such tapes. The tapes can be collected and stored over time, creating a library of possible events for examination. It is useful for researchers to collect as many sessions as possible, and not only the ones that appear to capture the "successful" families. Data may prove useful in later steps of a subsequent task analysis (e.g., comparing successful and unsuccessful resolution events).

Data Analysis

The field of psychology has a history of emphasizing experimental design in establishing cause, to the detriment of observing and measuring actual performance (Greenberg, 1995). Theorizing, observing, and measuring in-session change events are critical empirical steps that foster later investigations of explanation and prediction. Alexander, Newell, Robbins, and Turner (1995) provide a helpful two-dimensional scheme for observational coding, based on degree of content meaning and inference. As these authors note, when someone is coding behavior, inference always occurs. Meaning is dependent on some form of interpretation, whether that occurs at the level of the code creator, the coder, or the clinician-researcher who interprets that data. What is important is to be explicit about when the inference is being made. This then allows the researcher to utilize more interpretive concepts in coding, so long as reliability between coders can be demonstrated.

Measuring therapy process is currently an underdeveloped area of family research (Pinsof & Hambright, 2002). The choice of coding instruments must be guided by the particular research questions at hand. In the empirical analysis and verification steps of task analysis, a reliable coding instrument sensitive to distinct variables of particular interest is vital. As previously mentioned, for the recent softening task analysis, an existing instrument sensitive enough to identify and distinguish among specific EFT interventions could not be found. Thus we created our own instrument, the EFT-CS (Bradley, 2001). The EFT-CS was combined with the CSCR, a more general process coding scheme of therapist behaviors. Analysis of the EFT-CS provided initial support for reliability and construct validity (Bradley & Furrow, 2004).

Several different observational coding instruments are used in CFT process research. Johnson and Greenberg (1988) examined the process of change in best sessions of EFT by rating clients' performance, specifying the depth of experiencing and the quality of interpersonal interactions using the SASB (Benjamin et al., 1986) and the Experiencing Scales (Klein, Mathieu-Coughlin, & Kiesler, 1986). Heatherington and Friedlander (1990) used the Family Relational Communication Control Coding System (Friedlander & Heatherington, 1989) to observe changes in parent–child interactions in structural family therapy. Diamond and Liddle (1996) used the Beavers Timberlawn Family Evaluation Scale (Lewis, Beavers, Gossett, & Phillips, 1976) to verify the presence of a shift intervention, in their study exploring the process of re-solving an in-session impasse between a parent and an adolescent in family therapy. Pinsof and Wynne (2000) recommend ethnographic methods such as IPR (Elliot, 1986) to enrich quantitative analyses. Greenberg (1995) applied the SASB and IPR in a task analysis study to better understand couples' internal processing and perceptions in episodes of conflict resolution. Many resources provide guidance in the selection and application of observational coding (see Greenberg & Pinsof, 1986; Heppner, Kivlighan, & Wampold, 1999; Hill, 1991).

Reporting

Examples of journals that have published task analysis studies include the *Journal of Marital and Family Therapy, Journal of Family Psychology, Journal of Clinical Psychology, Journal of Consulting and Clinical Psychology, Journal of Counseling Psychology*, and *Psychotherapy Research*. This list is by no means exhaustive. Task analyses are published at various steps within the overall methodology. Johnson and colleagues (2001), for example, reported on the completion of a rational analysis of attachment injuries in couple relationships. Bradley and Furrow (2004) completed an empirical analysis that yielded a minitheory of expert therapist behaviors involved in EFT softening events.

DISCUSSION

The great potential of this kind of research is that it offers the clinician a map of the change process—a map that can be put on every therapy room wall. This research translates the abstract language of means and medians into an "if this, then that" document. The field of CFT has to move away from abstract models of therapy, even when these models can demonstrate that they lead to positive change at the end of therapy. Clinicians are demanding to know exactly how change can occur in a specific context and what specific interventions offer them the best chance of positive outcome. This research can also feed back into theory and into refinement of clinical models.

In the attachment injuries study of client process, we have learned, for example, that apology is not enough. This alone does not have an impact on the hurt partner. This partner has to see remorse, and has to see that his or her pain affects and reso-nates within the other. This project has taught us about forgiveness and reconciliation, and confirmed the usefulness of an attachment model of adult love. The hurts incurred are most easily understood within an attachment model. The softening task analysis of therapist process has proven effective in uncovering key therapeutic themes and interventions at a level of detail previously unavailable. The therapist processes through six distinct attachment-related themes en route to blamer softening. Each of these themes involves a different set of EFT interventions. The softening event involves both intra-psychic (inner) and interpsychic (between-partner) processing, highlighting the experiential and systemic roots of EFT. The resulting map of the softening event has been implemented into the training of EFT practitioners and supervisors, and is being incorporated into the EFT literature (Johnson, 2003). A follow-up study of softenings with a larger sample size that builds on this initial rational–empirical examination is being planned.

Task analysis of change events in CFT holds great potential for building and testing theory based on actual in-session processes. It is extremely useful for refining intervention strategies at different stages across the therapy process. The results are helpful in the training of therapists and relevant to practicing clinicians, because they provide a map of change detailed enough to specify how to intervene and when. Task analysis of CFT change events adds to our theoretical understanding of change, combines qualitative and quantitative methods in a rigorous manner, and helps bridge the gap between clinicians and researchers by utilizing the strengths of each to investigate how change happens.

EXEMPLARS

Bradley, B., & Furrow, J. L. (2004). Toward a mini-theory of the blamer softening event: Tracking the moment-by-moment process. *Journal of Marital and Family Therapy, 30*(2), 233–246.

Diamond, G. S., & Liddle, H. A. (1996). Resolving a therapeutic impasse between parents and adolescents in multidimensional family therapy. *Journal of Consulting and Clinical Psychology, 64*, 481–488.

Greenberg, L. S., & Foerster, F. S. (1996). Task analysis exemplified: The process of resolving unfinished business. *Journal of Consulting and Clinical Psychology, 64*, 439–446.

Heatherington, L., & Friedlander, M. L. (1990). Applying task analysis to structural family therapy. *Journal of Family Psychology, 4*, 36–48.

Johnson, S. M., Makinen, J. A., & Millikin, J. W. (2001). Attachment injuries in couple relationships: A new perspective on impasses in couples therapy. *Journal of Marital and Family Therapy, 27*, 145–155.

REFERENCES

Alexander, J. F., Newell, R. M., Robbins, M. S., & Turner, C. W. (1995). Observational coding in family therapy process research. *Journal of Family Psychology, 9*, 355–365.

Benjamin, L. S., Foster, S. W., Roberto, L. G., & Estrof, S. E. (1986). Breaking the family code: Analysis of videotapes of family interactions by Structural Analysis of Social Behavior (SASB). In L. S. Greenberg & W. Pinsof (Eds.), *The psychotherapeutic process: A research handbook* (pp. 391–438). New York: Guilford Press.

Beutler, L. E., Williams, R. E., & Wakefield, P. J. (1993). Obstacles to disseminating applied psychological science. *Applied and Preventive Psychology, 2*, 53–58.

Bradley, B. (2001). *The process of blamer softening in emotionally focused therapy.* Unpublished doctoral dissertation, Fuller Theological Seminary, Pasadena, CA.

Bradley, B., & Furrow, J. L. (2004). Toward a mini-theory of the blamer softening event: Tracking the moment-by-moment process. *Journal of Marital and Family Therapy, 30*, 233–246.

Bowlby, J. (1988). *A secure base: Parent–child attachment and healthy human development.* New York: Basic Books.

Cassidy, J., & Shaver, P. R. (Eds.). (1999). *Handbook of attachment: Theory, research, and clinical applications.* New York: Guilford Press.

Clarke, K. M. (1990). Creation of meaning: An emotional processing task in psychotherapy. *Psychotherapy: Theory, Research, and Practice, 26*, 139–148.

Clothier, P. F., Manion, I., Gordon Walker, J., & Johnson, S. M. (2002). Emotionally focused interventions for couples with chronically ill children: A two year follow-up. *Journal of Marital and Family Therapy, 28*, 391–398.

Coulehan, R., Friedlander, M. L., & Heatherington, L. (1998). Transforming narratives: A change event in constructivist family therapy. *Family Process, 37,* 17–33.

Diamond, G. S., & Diamond, G. M. (2002). Studying a matrix of change mechanisms: An agenda for family-based process research. In H. A. Liddle, D. A. Santisteban, R. F. Levant, J. H. Bray, V. E. Holt, & R. F. Levant (Eds.), *Family psychology: Science-based interventions* (pp. 41–66). Washington, DC: American Psychological Association.

Diamond, G. S., & Liddle, H. A. (1996). Resolving a therapeutic impasse between parents and adolescents in multidimensional family therapy. *Journal of Consulting and Clinical Psychology, 64,* 481–488.

Diamond, G. M., Liddle, H. A., Hogue, A., & Dakof, G. A. (1999). Alliance-building interventions with adolescents in family therapy: A process study. *Psychotherapy, 36,* 355–367.

Elliot, R. (1984). A discovery-oriented approach to significant change events in psychotherapy: Interpersonal recall and comprehensive process analysis. In L. Rice & L. S. Greenberg (Eds.), *Patterns of change: Intensive analysis of psychotherapy process* (pp. 249–286). New York: Guilford Press.

Elliot, R. (1986). Interpersonal process recall (IPR) as a psychotherapy process research method. In L. S. Greenberg & W. M. Pinsof (Eds.), *The psychotherapeutic process: A research handbook* (pp. 503–527). New York: Guilford Press.

Flanagan, J. C. (1954). The critical incident technique. *Psychological Bulletin, 51,* 327–358.

Friedlander, M. L., & Heatherington, L. (1989). Analyzing relational control in family therapy interviews. *Journal of Counseling Psychology, 36,* 139–148.

Friedlander, M. L., Wildman, J., Heatherington, L., & Skowron, E. A. (1994). What we do and don't know about the process of family therapy. *Journal of Family Psychology, 8,* 390–416.

Gottman, J. (1994). *What predicts divorce?* Hillsdale, NJ: Erlbaum.

Greenberg, L. S. (1983). Toward a task analysis of conflict resolution in Gestalt therapy. *Psychotherapy: Theory, Research, and Practice, 20,* 190–201.

Greenberg, L. S. (1984). A task analysis of intrapersonal conflict resolution. In L. N. Rice & L. S. Greenberg (Eds.), *Patterns of change* (pp. 66–123). New York: Guilford Press.

Greenberg, L. S. (1995). The use of observational coding in family therapy research: Comment on Alexander et al. (1995). *Journal of Family Psychology, 9,* 366–370.

Greenberg, L. S. (1999). Ideal psychotherapy research: A study of significant change processes. *Journal of Clinical Psychology, 55,* 1467–1480.

Greenberg, L. S., & Foerster, F. S. (1996). Task analysis exemplified: The process of resolving unfinished business. *Journal of Consulting and Clinical Psychology, 64,* 439–446.

Greenberg, L. S., Heatherington, L., & Friedlander, M. L. (1996). The events-based approach to couple and family therapy research. In D. H. Sprenkle & S. M. Moon (Eds.), *Research methods in family therapy* (pp. 411–428). New York: Guilford Press.

Greenberg, L. S., & Johnson, S. M. (1988). *Emotionally focused therapy for couples.* New York: Guilford Press.

Greenberg, L. S., & Newman, F. L. (1996). An approach to psychotherapy change process research: Introduction to the special section. *Journal of Consulting and Clinical Psychology, 64,* 435–438.

Greenberg, L. S., & Pinsof, W. M. (Eds.). (1986). *The psychotherapeutic process: A research handbook.* New York: Guilford Press.

Heatherington, L., & Friedlander, M. L. (1990). Applying task analysis to structural family therapy. *Journal of Family Psychology, 4,* 36–48.

Heppner, P. P., Kivlighan, D. M., & Wampold, B. E. (1999). *Research design in counseling* (2nd ed.). Belmont, CA: Brooks/Cole Wadsworth.

Highlen, P. S., Lonborg, S. D., Hampl, S. P., & Lassiter, W. L. (1984). *Classification System for Counseling Responses (CSCR) manual.* Unpublished manuscript, Ohio State University.

Hill, C. E. (1991). Almost everything you ever wanted to know about how to do process research on counseling and psychotherapy but didn't know who to ask. In C. E. Watkins, Jr., & L. J. Schneider (Eds.), *Research in counseling* (pp. 85–118). Hillsdale, NJ: Erlbaum.

Jacobson, N. S., & Addis, M. E. (1993). Research on couples and couple therapy: What do we know? Where are we going? *Journal of Consulting and Clinical Psychology, 61,* 85–93.

Johnson, S. M. (1996). *The practice of emotionally focused marital therapy: Creating connection.* New York: Brunner/Mazel.

Johnson, S. M. (2003). The revolution in couple therapy: A practitioner-scientist perspective. *Journal of Marital and Family Therapy, 29,* 365–384.

Johnson, S. M., & Greenberg, L. S. (1988). Relating process to outcome in marital therapy. *Journal of Marital and Family Therapy, 14,* 175–183.

Johnson, S. M., Hunsley, J., Greenberg, L., & Schindler, D. (1999). Emotionally focused couples therapy: Status and challenges. *Clinical Psychology: Science and Practice, 6,* 67–79.

Johnson, S. M., & Lebow, J. (2000). The "coming of age" of couple therapy: A decade review. *Journal of Marital and Family Therapy, 26,* 23–38.

Johnson, S. M., Makinen, J. A., & Millikin, J. W. (2001). Attachment injuries in couple relationships: A new perspective on impasses in couples therapy. *Journal of Marital and Family Therapy, 27,* 145–155.

Johnson, S. M., & Whiffen, V. (1999). Made to measure: Adapting emotionally focused couples therapy to partners' attachment styles. *Clinical Psychology: Science and Practice, 6,* 366–381.

Klein, M. H., Mathieu-Coughlin, P., & Kiesler, D. J. (1987). The Experiencing Scales. In L. S. Greenberg & W. M. Pinsof (Eds.), *The psychotherapeutic process: A research handbook* (pp. 21–71). New York: Guilford Press.

Lewis, J. M., Beavers, W. R., Gossett, J. T., & Phillips, V. A. (1976). *No single thread: Psychological health in family systems.* New York: Brunner/Mazel.

Lonborg, S. D., Daniels, J. A., Hammond, S. G., Houghton-Wenger, B., & Brace, L. J. (1991). Counselor and client verbal response mode changes during initial counseling sessions. *Journal of Counseling Psychology, 38,* 394–400.

Mahrer, A. R. (1988). Discovery-oriented psychotherapy research: Rationale, aims, and methods. *American Psychologist, 43,* 694–702.

Nichols, M. P., with Schwartz, R. C. (2004). *Family therapy: Concepts and methods* (6th ed.). Boston: Allyn & Bacon.

Pinsof, W. M., & Hambright, A. B. (2002). Toward prevention and clinical relevance: A preventive intervention model for family therapy research and practice. In H. A. Liddle, D. A. Santisteban, R. F. Levant, J. H. Bray, V. E. Holt, & R. F. Levant (Eds.), *Family psychology: Science-based interventions* (pp. 177–194). Washington, DC: American Psychological Association.

Pinsof, W. M., & Wynne, L. C. (1995). The efficacy of marital and family therapy: An empirical overview, conclusions, and recommendations. *Journal of Marital and Family Therapy, 21,* 585–613.

Pinsof, W. M., & Wynne, L. C. (2000). Toward progress research: Closing the gap between family therapy practice and research. *Journal of Marital and Family Therapy, 26,* 1–8.

Rice, L. N., & Greenberg, L. S. (Eds.). (1984). *Patterns of change.* New York: Guilford Press.

Sprenkle, D. H. (2002). *Effectiveness research in marriage and family therapy.* Alexandria, VA: American Association for Marriage and Family Therapy.

CHAPTER 15

Program Evaluation Science and Family Therapy

JAY A. MANCINI
ANGELA J. HUEBNER
ERIC E. McCOLLUM
LYDIA I. MAREK

In addition to clinical practice, family therapists are often involved in the development and implementation of prevention and intervention programs. These programs are designed either to lessen the chances of problem behaviors occurring in the future, or to ameliorate problem behaviors once they have occurred. Evaluation science focuses on the interrelated areas of program development and evaluation research, and seeks to examine the logic of prevention and intervention programs, as well as to determine the progress and success of those programs. Evaluation science offers an array of powerful analytical tools to family therapists that increase their understanding of prevention and intervention activities, and enable them to assess and systematically address a program's results and the processes leading to those results. This chapter covers five main topics: (1) presentation of two hypothetical case studies that illustrate evaluation science principles and methods; (2) theory as it applies to evaluation science; (3) logic model approaches to link theory and methods; (4) particular evaluation science issues and methods that fit with theory and with logic modeling; and (5) implications for family therapists, including issues of ethics, model development, and education and training.

BACKGROUND

Program and Community Case Studies

In this chapter, evaluation science is applied to two hypothetical cases of interventions that are common in communities. One is a workshop for children in divorcing families, and the other is a community intervention in youth development. Although there are commonalities across these scenarios, they also illuminate distinctive elements of programs and evaluation science. The seminar for children in divorcing families is sponsored by a single community agency and is not considered a community-wide initiative. The intervention addressing youth development issues involves multiple agencies and organizations and is a community-wide effort.

Case Study 1: Children and Divorce Seminar

As a new employee at the local mental health center, you have inherited the "Children and Divorce Seminar," a 6-hour education program for divorced parents and their children. The seminar has been enormously popular in the community for 12 years. Judges order all divorcing couples with children to attend the seminar before granting them a final divorce. Community agencies refer a constant stream of participants. Parents who have completed the seminar have formed an ongoing support group that provides volunteers to help conduct the sessions. The program has found such wide acceptance in the community that a local foundation provides financial support. But does it work? This is the question that the mental health center director tells you needs to be answered as part of the center's reaccreditation. The accrediting body wants all programs it accredits to measure results and benefits for families. How do you answer such a question?

Case Study 2: Community Intervention in Youth Development

The newspaper headline read: "Five Local Students Attempt Suicide as Part of Pact." These students combined their parents' prescription drugs and vodka in an attempt to end their lives. Community leaders were alarmed, school officials were perplexed, and parents were frantic. Everyone was demanding action. Local mental health agency personnel were called in to address the problem. You have been asked to discover why these students attempted suicide, and to participate on a team that will develop an intervention to prevent such incidents from happening again. It seems that everyone in the community has a different view about the problem and what should be done. Parents think that a few "bad seeds" in the school are leading other teens down the wrong path. Teachers think that students are responding to the combined pressures of being adolescents and succeeding in school. Mental health workers are convinced that the increasing depression rate among youth is the problem. Still others think that the community is a poor environment in which to raise children and youth.

Though evaluation research is a process that begins with program design, in reality most evaluators face situations not unlike that of the Children and Divorce Seminar. They are asked to conduct an evaluation of a program that has been in place for some time; has a variety of stakeholders with different views of what constitutes a good outcome; and has goals that were never clearly articulated, have been lost in the agency's memory, or have radically changed over time. The scenario on community intervention in youth development has a different focus, in that it demonstrates a problematic issue said to affect the entire community. The county mental health services agency has been charged with leading the intervention, and the evaluator is part of the process from the outset. A community problem has surfaced because of risky and alarming behavior among some youth. There is no program in place that is targeted toward suicide prevention. It is unclear exactly what the community issues are that require professional attention. Multiple stakeholder groups are willing to get involved in solving the problem.

Evaluation Theory: Articulating Process and Results

Whether we are attempting to discover the effects of parent education or to build better communities for youth, we are faced with harnessing the ideas and efforts of community members and program professionals. Theory has an important part in systematically clarifying an issue, planning action to address it, and knowing how that action makes a difference. There is, in other words, "nothing as practical as good theory" (Weiss, 1995, p. 65). An evaluation theory of change makes explicit the assumptions about why something will make a difference, charts the course of how that change will occur, provides a road map for program developers and evaluators, and provides insight into a program's process and results. A key element is "articulation," which takes what is hidden, assumed, and presumed, and makes it stated, visible, and subject to examination. Assumptions that are not expressed well keep a program's professionals guessing about the reasons for the program's success or failure. Theory sharpens the focus on key aspects of the program, facilitates cumulating evaluation results into a richer understanding of program impacts, forces program professionals and evaluators to make their assumptions explicit, and can influence how policymakers view important issues because of this focused and cumulative knowledge base (Weiss, 1995). The professionals who have been tasked to develop a community intervention in youth development, for instance, have to decide exactly what the precursors are in their community that adversely affect youth. As their ideas are articulated, a framework for action emerges that includes intervention at multiple levels.

In evaluation science, theory is dynamic and emergent. Theory that informs program developers and evaluators about why a prevention or intervention activity should work is derived in part from the literature, but is usually expressed in far greater detail. Program professionals and evaluation researchers must also introduce their own theory into the process by contributing their beliefs to articulating why something should work. Sources of information for developing theory include science-based knowledge, experience with programs, and other sources (such as participants' insights) (Reneger & Titcomb, 2002). A good theory of change is plausible, doable, and testable, and occurs at community, organizational or institutional, person network/family, and individual levels (Connell & Kubisch, 1998). A solid program theory is clear about the level of change that it can effect. For instance, the leaders of the Children and Divorce Seminar realized that their program was best suited to influence dynamics inside families, and structured their program activities accordingly to focus on parental communication and conflict management.

Program theory articulates a program's impact and process. "Impact theory" focuses on causes and effects that link program activities with desired results (Rossi, Lipsey, & Freeman, 2004). An impact theory usually contains an "action hypothesis" (the most immediate effects that a program is expected to have) and a "conceptual hypothesis" (the effects of immediate results on longer-term results). The leaders of the Children and Divorce Seminar hypothesized that improved parental communication and conflict management would lead to better child adjustment, and ultimately that more positive interaction between divorcing parents would lead to decreased custody and visitation disputes. "Process theory" describes how the program is supposed to operate. It includes a "service utilization plan" (assumptions about how people will engage with the program, including how they will initially become connected and how they will stay connected) and an "organizational plan" (assumptions about what must happen in the program to facilitate transactions between the target population and the program that will produce the intended results) (Rossi et al., 2004). The community mental health professionals involved in the youth development program may assume that the schools will serve as an important portal for getting youth in need involved in programs, and decide that involving other youth in providing emotional support will keep needy youth engaged in the program.

When an intervention does not lead to expected changes in people's lives, it may be due to either theory failure or implementation failure. "Implementation failure" means that the program has not followed through with either its organizational plan or its utilization plan. The participants in the Children and Divorce Seminar may attend four sessions rather than six, with the result that important educational modules are not delivered to them. The role of teachers in the youth development community intervention may not be clearly explained to them, and consequently the involvement of teachers may be uneven. Thus there are deviations from the plans that have been designed to produce important outcomes. "Theory failure," on the other hand, suggests flawed thinking from the beginning of the program-planning process; that is, the program is implemented as planned, but the expected results have not occurred. Theory failure can occur with regard to anticipated short-term, immediate, and longer-term expected results. For example, parents may attend all sessions of the Children and Divorce Seminar and still not gain a significant amount of knowledge. This may also be true regarding expectations about gaining knowledge about symptoms of youth depression by attending classes. Or the Children and Divorce Seminar may lead to divorced parents' having more knowledge about good parenting, but it may not lead to their becoming better parents. In these instances, there is a flaw in the part of the articulated theory suggesting that information produces either better parenting or improved ability to detect youth depression.

METHODOLOGY

Logic Model Elements: Expressing Theory and Process

The practicality of program theory is demonstrated by the use of "logic models"—flow charts of the relationship among program results, resources/inputs, and activities targeted toward a specific issue (Julian, Jones, & Deyo, 1995; McLaughlin & Jordan, 1999). Logic models provide a visual picture of program theory in action. Of primary importance in developing a logic model is establishing and maintaining a focus on results (Orthner & Bowen, 2004). This is important because too often activities rather than results become the focus. When this happens, it is difficult to know whether positive changes are being made, much less to know exactly what is leading to such changes. Program professionals should be managing "results" rather than managing "activities."

Logic models help program professionals, evaluators, and stakeholders reach consensus about which elements are essential to a program (Millar, Simeone, & Carnevale, 2001; Orthner & Bowen, 2004). Consequently, program professionals and researchers are more able to identity faulty or implausible links at early stages. Our logic model examples include six elements: (1) need identification and analysis, (2) desired results, (3) measurable indicators, (4) activities, (5) monitoring, and (6) resources. Figures 15.1 and 15.2 depict how the two case studies in this chapter translate into usable logic model frameworks.

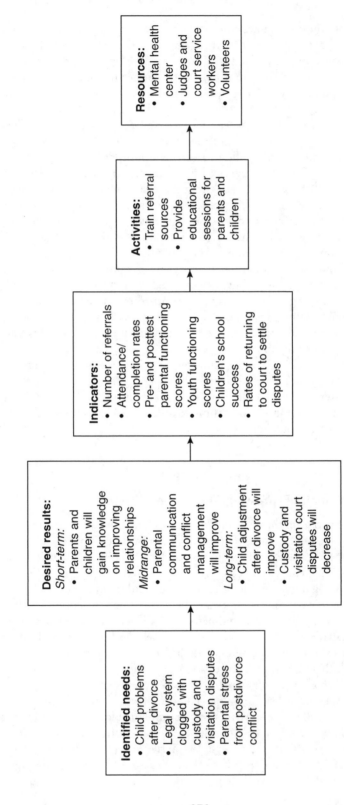

Identified needs:
- Child problems after divorce
- Legal system clogged with custody and visitation disputes
- Parental stress from postdivorce conflict

Desired results:
Short-term:
- Parents and children will gain knowledge on improving relationships

Midrange:
- Parental communication and conflict management will improve

Long-term:
- Child adjustment after divorce will improve
- Custody and visitation court disputes will decrease

Indicators:
- Number of referrals
- Attendance/completion rates
- Pre- and posttest parental functioning scores
- Youth functioning scores
- Children's school success
- Rates of returning to court to settle disputes

Activities:
- Train referral sources
- Provide educational sessions for parents and children

Resources:
- Mental health center
- Judges and court service workers
- Volunteers

FIGURE 15.1. Logic model of the Children and Divorce Seminar. *Note:* Monitoring and evaluation activities permeate all aspects of the logic model.

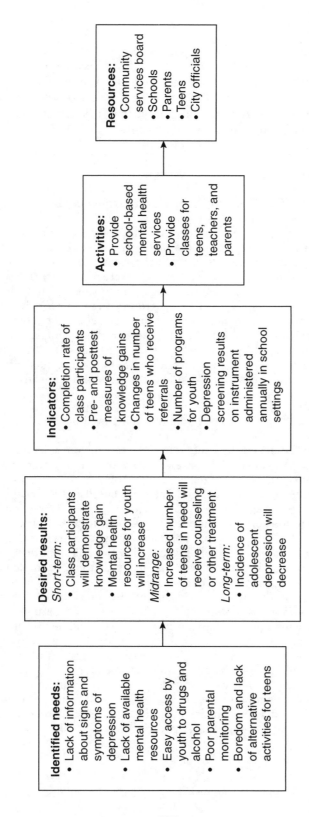

FIGURE 15.2. Logic model of a community intervention in youth development. *Note:* Monitoring and evaluation activities permeate all aspects of the logic model.

Need Identification and Analysis

Programs are developed because there is an identified need among families or within communities. A first step in creating a logic model is to ensure that stakeholders have clearly defined the issue (i.e., have identified the problem statement). Because this is the basis for the entire program, it is important that it be defined with accurate and valid information rather than uninformed hunches.

Case Study 1: Children and Divorce Seminar

In evaluating the Children and Divorce Seminar, the needs assessment that led to the program's development has to be reconstructed. The mental health center director tells you that in the beginning, two local family court judges approached him with their concerns: So many parents were coming back to court to deal with minor custody and visitation issues that the court calendar was overbooked. Local school counselors also reported that they were seeing increasing academic and behavioral indicators of problems among children whose parents had recently divorced. They wanted to begin offering group counseling for those children, but had no time or funds to do so. Finally, staff members at the mental health center reported an increase in referrals for adults whose major complaints were the stress and emotional turmoil involved in trying to coparent children after contentious divorces. "We were having an epidemic of children and adults suffering from divorces," the director tells you. "We felt like we had to do something."

Case Study 2: Community Intervention in Youth Development

To get a better handle on the issue of teen depression and suicide, you lead a team of professionals to isolate the causes of problems among teens. What does the community know about teen suicide attempts? You decide to work with the medical profession to get a sense of this. The team checks all the hospital admissions records for the past year. They are surprised to see that depression is the leading cause of hospitalization for youth ages 10–14 and the second leading cause for those ages 15–19. The agency also conducts a review of the research literature and makes a list of all the risk factors associated with adolescent depression. You decide to use this information to develop a survey that will be implemented with all the middle and high school students in the school.

Findings from the survey reveal that at least one out of every three students demonstrates symptoms of depression; that the symptoms are higher among girls and those students making the transition between middle and high school; and that many of the students have easy access to alcohol and prescription drugs. You decide to supplement the survey with interviews of groups of students. In focus group interviews, students readily admit that alcohol is a big part of their daily lives and that they do not have any clear plans for their future. When you and your team begin to plan how to get support for these youth, you discover that the school does not offer any on-site mental health services or related educational programs, and that the closest services are in a town 30 miles away.

Results

The second step in the logic model process is articulating the desired results or change in the problem. This is arguably the most important aspect of a logic model because it provides the focus that all successful programs need. At the completion of the program/intervention, how will the problem be different? Results should be defined as measurable objectives. Specifying short-term, midrange, and long-term objectives is useful because it gives program professionals a more realistic sense of how parts of the program theory fit, and what can reasonably be expected to change over a specific time period. In order to specify results effectively, a theory of change must be delineated. This involves understanding the chain of causal factors that influence the issue and that the intervention must affect.

Case Study 1: Children and Divorce Seminar

Desired results have to be inferred from various participants' memories of the beginnings of the program. As you listen to the various people who have been involved with the program over the years, you decide that there were several goals for the Children and Divorce Seminar. The short-term goal was to increase what program participants knew about how to improve family relationships. The intermediate goal was to improve parental communication and conflict management after divorce. The long-term goals were to decrease court appearances for postdivorce custody and visitation disputes, and to improve children's postdivorce adjustment.

Case Study 2: Community Intervention in Youth Development

The community mental health agency identifies several levels of desired results. The first desired result is that students, parents, and teachers will increase their knowledge about youth risk factors and about depression. The intermediate goal is that more depressed teens who need support will receive counseling or other treatment. The long-term goal is to decrease the incidence of adolescent depression by 50% by the end of the program's fourth year.

Measurable Indicators

Effective evaluation science incorporates measurable indicators across the evaluation process, from need assessments through periodic program monitoring. When programs are planned, there must be discussions among program professionals and evaluators about program activities and results that can be measured and tracked (Mancini, Marek, Byrne, & Huebner, 2004). Consequently, notions, hunches, hearsay, and anecdotes are not good indicator candidates. Indicators can be far-ranging, including results from surveys and focus groups, agency administrative data, and population data, as well as psychological tests (DeVellis, 2003; McKillip, 1998).

Case Study 1: Children and Divorce Seminar

Finding measurable indicators of success for the Children and Divorce Seminar proves challenging. The next question you try to answer is what data might be available to you to assess various outcomes. The records of the seminar itself contain only a satisfaction questionnaire comprising three questions: "What was most helpful?", "What was least helpful?", and "Any other comments about the seminar you would like to share with us?" This form was apparently developed for the first seminar session and was never revised. Also in the records are copies of some of the artwork that children did during seminar sessions, and copies of the "Parental Conflict Form" (a self-report instrument to be filled out by divorced parents concerning their levels of conflict and cooperation).

Your next stop is the county clerk of court's office, where you find that it is possible to access the court records of all divorced couples to see how often they return to court following the final decree, and what the issues and outcomes are. You also have access to a roster of participants in the seminar for the past 5 years. You could conceivably track and compare those who participated with those who did not, to see whether there is a difference in the number of couples that have returned to court.

School district personnel say that with parental consent, they can provide records of school achievement and behavioral problems for any child. There appear to be no existing data that will let you assess changes in parental adjustment as a result of participating in the seminar. And up until now, there has not been a control or comparison group of parents and children, therefore making it very difficult to know the seminar outcomes. Overall, you discover that there are a number of indicators connected with the program results. However, for some of these indicators, you cannot rely on available data and must implement some type of impact assessment.

Case Study 2: Community Intervention in Youth Development

Several measurable indicators seem reasonable. These include hospital admissions records; youth reports of depression; the provision of mental health services and educational classes in school; the number of youth, parents, and teachers attending educational sessions; reported changes in students' leisure behavior and parental monitoring; and the number of youth clients receiving counseling or referrals. There is thus a wide array of indicators that you can use to monitor this community initiative to help youth.

Activities

After the need is identified, the desired results are specified and informed by the program theory of change, and indicators are determined, specific activities or program interventions can be determined. These activities should logically fit the program theory and lead to the desired results. Program professionals should be able to conclude that there is a logical fit between activities—whether they are classes, home visitation, or public service announcements—and desired results.

Case Study 1: Children and Divorce Seminar

To understand the activities involved in the seminar, you sit in on a typical session. The day begins with children and adults being split into separate groups. In addition, two groups of adults are formed, so that ex-spouses are not in the same group if they are attending together. The adult group is psychoeducational in nature. The leaders lecture about the importance of cooperative parenting, and show videos of good and bad examples of postdivorce parenting. Group discussion is encouraged as a way for participants to apply the principles taught in the lectures to their own situations.

The children's group is activity-oriented. The younger children write and produce a puppet show about what divorce feels like for a child. The teens do "teen-on-the-street" interviews with each other, in which they describe their experiences of divorce in their families and give advice to parents on how to make life better for children after a divorce. They tape-record the interviews. At the end of the day, the younger children put on their puppet show, and the teens play portions of their tapes for the assembled adult group. As you watch the adults' reactions, you see a number of teary eyes and looks of recognition as the children describe parental actions that make postdivorce life difficult for them.

Case Study 2: Community Intervention in Youth Development

To achieve these results, agency personnel implement school-based mental health services. They conduct depression screening with adolescents entering the ninth grade (a particularly vulnerable period of development). They provide educational sessions to students, parents, and teachers about the signs and symptoms of depression. Several sessions about healthy lifestyles are included in the teen sessions, in an effort to give adolescents alternatives to drinking and using drugs to alleviate boredom. Parents receive information about parental monitoring and the importance of securing prescription drugs. When adolescents with depression are identified, counselors work with them and their families to provide mental health services. They also coordinate with the adolescents' family physicians to examine the necessity of medication.

Resources

As the members of an evaluation team identify its desired results and the associated activities, they also need to know whether there are adequate resources to field and monitor the initiative. How much of an investment is required with regard to money, people, and time? Partnerships are important in initiatives that have multiple components. The issue of time is particularly important, because the personnel of an agency must be clear about how much time they are willing to commit to training staffers; collecting and analyzing survey, focus group, or observational data; and tracking participants— all activities that must occur in addition to actual program implementation.

Case Study 1: Children and Divorce Seminar

Three staff members at the mental health center are assigned part-time to staff and coordinate the seminar. In addition to providing services themselves, they recruit and train a group of volunteers who help with the sessions, and they serve as liaisons with the schools and with the local family court judges and court service workers to identify families that might benefit from participation.

Case Study 2: Community Intervention in Youth Development

The community mental health agency will provide two full-time staff persons to work at the school. School personnel will allow class time to be used for educational programming. School administrators will provide office space for the on-site mental health agency personnel. The local parent–teacher association has sent out information to parents about the educational classes, and intends to provide transportation and on-site child care to enhance participation.

Monitoring and Evaluation

An important part of the logic model is how the intervention will be monitored and evaluated, including program implementation and its intended results. Monitoring and evaluation permeate all parts of a logic model. There are multiple objectives for monitoring and evaluation: to identify the initial extent of need or a problem; to track how the need or problem may change over time; to document how well program implementation protocols are being followed; to mark progress toward achieving results; to know when results have been met; and to discern how resource use has supported particular program efforts and subsequent results.

Case Study 1: Children and Divorce Seminar

As you retrospectively reconstruct the logic model for the Children and Divorce Seminar, it becomes clear that monitoring and evaluation were not part of the initial planning for the seminar. Staff members made changes to the seminar curriculum based on their informal assessments that changes were needed, and data for evaluation purposes were never consistently collected. One outcome of the current evaluation will be to develop and implement an ongoing monitoring and evaluation component for the seminar.

Case Study 2: Community Intervention in Youth Development

The mental health agency personnel develop a plan for monitoring that cuts across all program dimensions as represented in the logic model. For each of the desired results and indicators, they include a timeline for when information will be collected, how it will be analyzed, and how it will be used to restructure educational programs. The team decides that monitoring information will be used to modify the intervention on an ongoing basis. It is your responsibility to oversee this monitoring process, including interpreting the data and reporting back to the individuals and agencies sponsoring this initiative.

Evaluation Science Research: Particular Methods and Strategies

Evaluation theory provides the basic conceptual framework for thinking about problems and how change should occur. Logic models provide valuable ways to organize that thinking around evaluation research. This section focuses on specific issues family therapists must address and methods they can use as they plan and implement effective evaluations. Each of these relates to one or more aspects of the logic model. These include (1) developing program evaluation research questions; (2) needs analysis; (3) program monitoring and formative evaluation; (4) research design and summative evaluation; (5) indicators and measurement; (6) triangulation of qualitative and quantitative data; (7) data analysis; and (8) evaluation feedback and reporting results.

Developing Program Evaluation Research Questions

Developing clear, concise, and answerable research and evaluation questions that flow from program theory has a major impact on what is ultimately known about program success. A poor research question is often grandiose (e.g., "Does this program improve the quality of life for families?"), whereas focusing on specific results leads to questions that can be answered (Mancini et al., 2004; Rossi et al., 2004). Examples of answerable questions include "Does this program provide improved parenting skills to divorcing parents?" and "Does working through the schools improve early identification of depressed youth?" Guidelines for developing questions include the following:

1. Involve key stakeholders in discussions. This is likely to increase the relevancy of questions, due to the diversity of perspectives.
2. Ask whether the program has a little or a lot to say about the research question and the desired program result. For example, any one program has very little control on overall quality of life for families, whereas a program may have relatively more influence on a particular aspect of family interaction.
3. Determine whether the intervention is strong enough to influence families. It is critical to understand the power of the intervention and whether it can reasonably address the research question.
4. Develop research questions that are informed by the therapy, social science, and behavioral science literature. Research-based or evidence-based evaluation benefits from the related work accomplished by other family therapists or researchers.
5. Develop concrete questions that evaluation research methods can address.
6. Match general research questions with particular elements of the program, including its activities, participants, and staff. For example, there may be insufficient staff members to conduct intensive activities that are expected to produce the desired results.

Needs Analysis

"Needs analysis" is a systematic way of gathering information that examines needs (need identification) and helps set priorities (need assessment) for action (Gaber, 2000; McKillip, 1998). In the logic model process, the information that evaluators are gathering in order to understand the severity of a problem also assists them in determining program priorities, as well as the results that accrue from program activities. Census data, observations, existing records and databases, and literature reviews are sources of existing information to identify needs (Witkin & Altshuld, 1995). Witkin and Altshuld (1999) suggest three phases of needs assessment: (1) preassessment exploration (surveying what data already exist, and deciding what additional data are needed to understand needs and problems); (2) assessment data gathering (the process of accumulating and integrating information that can be used to support the program); and (3) postassessment utilization (the process of taking action on what is learned, including planning dimensions of a logic model from needs to desired results, etc.). In the community intervention case study, the following data sources are used: hospital records showing that 30% of teenage admissions are due to depression-related illnesses; an examination of mental health service offerings, revealing few programs available to youth; and the adolescent development literature describing predictors of depression among youth and effective intervention approaches (e.g., Juszczak, Melinkovich, & Kaplan, 2003; Simmons & Blyth, 1987). In the absence of extant records, need analysis information is gathered through questionnaires, interviews, or focus groups (Gaber, 2000). In the community intervention case study, a focus group with teens reveals reasons for their engaging in substance use.

Program Monitoring and Formative Evaluation

"Formative evaluations" are conducted with the purpose of improving program processes (Scriven, 1997) and are particularly valuable in the early stages of program development, since they provide feedback about program implementation quality. Valuable information about unanticipated consequences of program implementation can be discovered. Monitoring supports formative evaluation because it provides information that can be directly applied to program processes.

Program monitoring is a primary method for ensuring implementation integrity. Monitoring allows program professionals and evaluators to gauge how well program plans are being followed, how well the intervention activities are refined and explained, and whether or not activities are consonant with desired program results; it also provides insight into how programs can be fine-tuned (Owen & Rogers, 1999). Questions that program monitoring is designed to answer include the following:

1. Are the appropriate people receiving services or involved in the program?
2. Are the program activities clearly explained to staff members, so that they can be implemented as intended?
3. Are there enough staff members to implement the activities?
4. Are resources used effectively and efficiently?
5. Are program participants satisfied with their experiences?

Program monitoring is centered on the systematic documentation of program-related activities and situations that indicate whether or not implementation is proceeding as planned. "Business information technology systems" (also called "management information systems") are excellent tools to guide the collection, management, and analysis of program monitoring data. For example, Savaya (1998) used such a system in a family counseling agency, and used these data to check on the status of clients, to monitor treatment progress, to develop profiles of the people using clinic services, and to conduct research on treatment success.

Research Design and Summative Evaluation

How theory is used and how the research is designed are major influences on the success of evaluation research. "Summative evaluations" provide information about whether a particular program is achieving its intended results (Fitz-Gibbon & Morris, 1987) and are facilitated by use of rigorous research designs, so that alternative explanations of observed changes can be controlled. More sensitive designs detect smaller meaningful changes that result from an intervention; that is, they enable the family therapist to conclude that the intervention has had an effect, even when the difference between participants who receive it and those who do not is relatively slight (Leber, St.

Peters, & Markman, 1996; Mohr, 1995). Since a primary goal of evaluation is to determine the effects of a prevention or intervention effort, there must be a focus on determining whether anything would have improved had there been no program. This condition in the absence of the program is called the "counterfactual" (Hollister & Hill, 1995). To know program effects, the evaluator must know what would have happened if there was no program initiative. Expansive discussions of research design are provided by Mohr (1995), Rossi and colleagues (2004), Leber and colleagues (1996), and Tebes, Kaufman, and Connell (2003).

Certain factors can lead to false conclusions about program effects. A primary consideration in evaluating a program intervention is deciding how to minimize threats to internal and external validity. "Internal validity" refers to whether differences between the program (treatment) and control (comparison) groups can be genuinely attributed to the intervention (Campbell & Stanley, 1966; Cook & Campbell, 1979). The research design must be rigorous enough to account for the variety of influences that will interfere with drawing a valid conclusion of a cause–effect relationship between the program intervention and observed changes in program participants. History, selection, and contamination are primary threats to internal validity. Internal validity can be threatened if (1) there is an outside influence that affects the results of the intervention, such as a natural catastrophe or even involvement in another intervention program at the same time; (2) too many participants drop out of the program prior to its conclusion; (3) a pretest is taken that may influence performance on the posttest, thus artificially inflating scores; (4) there are extreme responses on a measure, because there is a tendency for scores to be naturally less extreme over time; (5) certain situations change with age and experience, without requiring an intervention program to do so; (6) there are initial, preprogram differences between the program (treatment) group and the control group; (7) the intervention program is delivered inconsistently (i.e., not according to established protocols); and/or (8) program and control groups are subject to influence by different environmental factors, such as changes in neighborhoods, schools, or the weather.

"External validity" refers to how well evaluation findings can be generalized to other samples, groups, or populations. Socioeconomic status, culture, and region can vary dramatically and therefore make generalizability suspect. Societal change may also affect the generalizability of findings. The setting in which a program is delivered may affect program outcomes as well: The more laboratory-like the setting, the greater the threat to external validity because of the disparity between this controlled setting and a naturalistic setting. Although parenting skills may be learned in a class, for example, parenting practices occur in the home. Does classroom learning translate into changed behavior at home? A major complicating factor establishing external validity involves how well the intervention was understood in the first place; consequently, how the program is operationalized in other settings is subject to interpretation. Another source of external invalidity is the pretest, because in some respect it is part of the intervention and may increase intervention effects (McCollum et al., 1996).

The "experimental design" maximizes internal validity because it utilizes participants from a common pool and then employs random assignment. If the number of eligible participants is large, random selection can be used prior to random assignment. A control group is of paramount importance because it gives the family therapist a better sense that differences are due more to the program than to extraneous influences. History-related threats to internal validity, such as external events and normal aging or development, are not a danger in experimental studies because of the control group feature. Initial group differences threats also pose no problem in experiments, unless there is flawed randomization when the program and control groups are formed. Experiments and their randomization and control group features are not immune to inconsistency in program delivery. Experimental design fares better with regard to internal validity than to external validity, because by definition this type of design creates a laboratory-like, less naturalistic setting.

"Quasi-experimental designs" form comparison groups through methods other than random assignment (one method is called the "constructed control groups" approach, whereas another equates groups through statistical procedures). Care must be used in all of these designs in establishing group equivalence. The "regression–discontinuity" quasi-experimental design is very similar to the experimental design in giving the researcher a clearer indication of true intervention effects. This design employs a sharp cutting point that separates the program and control groups, and then statistically controls for the original selection variable. This design works best when the researcher has valid and reliable quantitative criteria for forming the program and control groups. The matched constructed control group quasi-experimental design is commonly used in evaluation research and forms its control group by matching as closely as possible key characteristics of the program group. A third quasi-experimental design equalizes program and control groups by instituting statistical controls on key known differences between the groups.

Indicators and Measurement

When clinician-researchers are developing indicators and data collection instruments, validity and reliability are important measurement issues. Whether a family therapist is examining how well items within a measure interrelate ("internal consistency"), whether different combinations of items in a measure yield similar findings ("split-half reliability"), or whether repeated testing produces similar findings ("test–retest reliability"), the primary concern is whether a measure performs in expected and consistent ways (DeVellis, 2003). "Content validity" and "criterion-related validity" are also important considerations for therapists, especially when assessing a program's results (including behavior, attitudes, and knowledge). Content validity focuses on how well a set of items (questions) represents the content area (e.g., adolescent depression or parenting skills). For criterion-related validity to be established, the set of items must empirically relate to one or more criteria in predicted ways (e.g., a couple communication score relates to more positive interaction concerning custody issues). Measurement issues do not only apply to psychological tests, but apply equally to any indicator that family therapists may use in evaluation. Any qualitative or quantitative observation, recording, or counting of what people do, say, or believe is subject to measurement problems.

Triangulation of Qualitative and Quantitative Data

As family therapists choose measures and indicators, they will often need to make choices between two very different types of approaches. Qualitative research strategies are particularly useful when therapists are conducting process evaluations (understanding the dynamics of program operations), individualized outcome evaluations (matching program services to individual needs), case studies (documenting individual client outcomes), implementation evaluations (examining program fidelity), and formative evaluations (improving program quality) (Patton, 1987). Qualitative methods are beneficial in that they can facilitate understanding meaning and context, identifying unanticipated phenomena, identifying processes that influence actions, and developing causal explanations (Maxwell, 1998). In contrast, because quantitative approaches use standardized measures across a potentially large response pool, quantitative methods facilitate comparison and statistical aggregation of data and subsequent generalization (Patton, 1987). Quantitative research strategies are particularly useful in summative evaluations (Fitz-Gibbon & Morris, 1987).

The choice of whether to mainly use a qualitative or a quantitative design depends on the research question. Ideally, methods of both types should be applied to an evaluation. In our case studies, methods of either type can be readily employed. Qualitative approaches include individual interviews or focus groups (with open-ended questions) and surveys (with open-ended questions), whereas quantitative approaches include surveys and standardized interviews (with determined response categories).

"Triangulation" refers to using more than one data-gathering strategy to examine a particular process or result (Jick, 1979). An evaluation study of the Children and Divorce Seminar, for instance, should triangulate findings by gathering data from more than one stakeholder group (e.g., seminar participants and leaders, attorneys who refer clients, and local judges), and by using both quantitative and qualitative data to measure processes and results (a validated measure of child functioning, as well as interviews with children and their parents). Triangulation serves a variety of purposes (Goetz & LeCompte, 1984; Marshall & Rossman, 1989). It lends credibility to findings when there is consensus between the various data sources being used. If parents participating in the seminar report that they are more able to cooperate with their ex-spouses as a result of participation, and referring attorneys report that contentious couples go back to court much less often following the seminar, the assertion that the seminar helps to reduce postdivorce conflict is more believable (though not definitive in the absence of a control or comparison group). Triangulation can also produce a more complete and complex picture of the results being measured.

Triangulation also illuminates unexpected or contradictory findings. At an early version of the Children and Divorce Seminar, the staff gave pre- and posttest parental conflict surveys to participating parents. Analysis of the data showed an increase in parental conflict over the course of the seminar. Through interviews with parents, researchers discovered that at the beginning of the seminar they were very suspicious about how the information gathered would be used and tried to present themselves in the best possible light as parents. However, as they came to trust that the information would not be used to hurt them in court, they were able to answer more honestly and reflectively. What looked like a decline in effective parenting could actually be understood as an indication of increased trust.

Data Analysis

Data analysis provides the opportunity to test the underlying program theory and the hypothesized relationship among the logic model activities and outcomes. Since other chapters in this book focus on the particulars of data analysis, we briefly mention two issues integral to evaluation research: Type I/Type II errors and practical significance.

Evaluators who are trying to determine the impact of prevention and intervention programs attempt to avoid Type I and Type II errors. A Type I error is a "false positive," or a conclusion that a program makes a difference when it does not. A Type II error is a "false negative," or a conclusion that a program does not make a difference when in fact it does. Using a stricter significance level in a statistical test minimizes the chances of a false-positive error, but at the same time increases the chances of a false-negative error. Both types of errors can be minimized by increasing the sample size in an evaluation or by statistically controlling other factors that can cloud a program result (Lipsey, 1990). A decision must be made about the balance between the possibilities of false-positive and false-negative errors, and the family therapist must decide which type of error can be better tolerated (Lipsey, 1990; Thye, 2000). Considerations in making this judgment include cost of the intervention, risk to participants, and alternatives to the intervention.

Evaluation researchers must also consider the practical significance of findings. Findings that are statistically significant are not necessarily practically or clinically significant (Deal & Anderson, 1995; Rosnow & Rosenthal, 1988; Tebes et al., 2003). For example, though it is statistically significant, is a 2-point decrease in a depression score among youth enough to warrant program continuation? Is a 5-point increase in knowledge about the effects of divorce on children enough to justify the Children and Divorce Seminar? One way to determine practical significance is through examination of "effect sizes." Effect sizes provide an estimate of the magnitude or importance of effects, rather than just their statistical significance (Cohen, 1988; Deal & Anderson, 1995). However, care must be exercised to avoid committing Type I errors by accepting low effect sizes as indications that a program is making a difference.

Providing Evaluation Feedback and Reporting Results

We discuss two aspects of presenting evaluation results: providing feedback to program professionals and evaluators connected with the intervention, and reporting results to other professionals and stakeholder groups. Our logic model is predicated on the generation of information to address program process and program results. There are several questions to ask when one is developing a summary of evaluation results: Who will be the consumers of the information? How will they use the information? Will the information be useful to them? A family therapist who is evaluating a program may be providing short-term result data to others connected with the program. If the goal is to improve the program while it is in progress, then the evaluator will place those findings in the context depicted by the logic model (e.g., discussing how intervention activities are contributing or not contributing to the result).

A comprehensive evaluation report includes these major sections: an executive summary; background information on the program (including program origin, goals, clients, program activities, and staff involvement); particulars of the evaluation research (including purposes, research design, and result measures); results; discussion of results (including confidence in attributing change to the intervention); costs and benefits of the program (both economic and noneconomic); and recommendations and implications (Morris, Fitz-Gibbon, & Freeman, 1987). In choosing an effective method of communication, it is important to know the audience and to have a specific goal as a presenter (Mancini & Shea, 1987). Presenting information to a group of parents of youth is best done via oral presentation, whereas providing information to other professionals on effects of improved parental monitoring on youth risk behavior is best accomplished by a written report accompanied by an oral presentation. The key in making a difference with regard to communicating effectively is shaping the communication to the particular audience, presentation goals, and presentation method.

DISCUSSION: IMPLICATIONS FOR FAMILY THERAPISTS

Education and Training

As family therapists and other mental health professionals are increasingly called upon to demonstrate not only the efficacy of their treatment models but the effectiveness of those models in actual practice, education in evaluation methods is vital. Such education should have two outcomes as its target. First, marriage and family therapy (MFT) practitioners need to have a clear understanding of how to apply the systemic learning that grounds the practice of MFT to evaluation research. For instance, a logic model that does not take into account the contextual nature of an intervention like the Children and Divorce Seminar may miss the theoretical connections between various interventions and the interactional view of postdivorce conflict. MFT students who plan primarily on clinical practice will probably be called upon to participate in, and understand the findings of, evaluation studies. They will find themselves in the position of needing to choose programs and models to implement for both prevention and intervention services. This decision process will be informed if MFT students are trained to critically assess programs or models (Stufflebeam, 2001). More importantly, however, MFT practitioners need to know the effectiveness of their own services, in order to demonstrate to managed care companies and other providers that these services are credible and do produce meaningful, positive outcomes. This demonstration of credibility will depend both on controlled outcome trials and on evaluations of how treatments are delivered in the community (Andrews, 1999; Beutler & Howard, 1998; Pinsof & Wynne, 1995).

Education in evaluation science can sensitize MFT students to the necessity of linking practice with results, and to the iterative process by which treatment programs and models are developed and then refined. No longer will therapists' position and persuasive abilities suffice as the basis for credibility, even in the realm of clinical practice. Learning what evaluation science is and how to apply it to clinical models and programs will provide MFT students with the ability to choose appropriate programs and models and to demonstrate clear and measurable outcomes. At the master's level, MFT students should be exposed to evaluation research, along with clinical trial research and process research, as part of their coursework in research methods. Doctoral preparation in MFT should include coursework in program evaluation methodology as well as program development, since these two tasks are duties most MFT practitioners will be called on to perform during their careers. It is imperative that program evaluation and development be taught as related activities, and that the recursive process between them be emphasized.

Ethical Practice in Evaluation Science

Evaluation studies are located in political contexts, where findings lead to actions with real-world consequences. Evaluation study findings are used to justify discontinuing ineffective programs, making major modifications in programs, and awarding contracts for services to competing agencies. Under these conditions, family therapists must serve a variety of masters, including policymakers, program sponsors, evaluation sponsors, program participants, program management, program staff, program competitors, and those groups and individuals in the immediate community who will be indirectly affected by changes in the program being evaluated. Each of these groups will probably bring a different vision of success and different needs to the table as the results of the evaluation are judged. Evaluators have an ethical obligation to make sure that findings are presented accurately and disseminated to as many stakeholder groups as possible for inclusion in the political realm of policy and decision making (American Evaluation Association, 2003; Fitzpatrick, 1999; Joint Committee on Standards for Educational Evaluation, 1994).

Quality of the research design must be considered as family therapists balance potential costs and benefits of a study. A poorly designed project that is not likely to yield meaningful findings is not worth even minimal risk to participants. Similarly, there is little rationale for doing a study whose findings have a low likelihood of use, thereby exposing participants to risk with little promise of any meaningful outcome. Thus family therapists must be able to demonstrate that a program will be able to provide credible responses to the needs and problems that have been identified. This is an especially important consideration for those who tend to overestimate the benefits of their work and to underestimate its risks to participants (Mark, Eyssell, & Campbell, 1999).

Contribution of Evaluation Results to Model Development

Although evaluation is most often used to examine existing intervention programs, the findings from such studies (particularly process studies) may lead to changes in the intervention model, thus promising to make it more effective. For example, an evaluation may suggest that certain model components do not add to overall results and can be dropped from the model. Conversely, the findings may suggest that the model can be improved by adding components to it. Such a decision should only be made when there are empirical and theoretical reasons to believe that the change will improve effectiveness. The modified model can then be subjected to subsequent evaluation to determine whether the modification has had an impact. In the case of dropping components from the model, a finding of no difference may still have significance, since dropping the component in question may result in a more streamlined and cost-effective intervention.

To illustrate the way in which evaluation findings can contribute to model development, let us return to the Children and Divorce Seminar. Interviews with a number of parents who were participants in an earlier version of the program revealed that many of them had found using the skills taught in the program relatively easy for the first few weeks after the seminar ended. However, as time went on, they reported that the level of conflict with their ex-spouses rose, and that they found themselves again embroiled in an ongoing cycle of argument followed by withdrawal and no communication about the children. Several suggested that "booster sessions" be provided, available to any former participant who wanted to attend, to reinforce the skills taught during the seminar. The Children and Divorce Seminar staff felt that this was an important suggestion for the intervention and implemented it.

EVALUATION SCIENCE AND FAMILY THERAPY: CONCLUSIONS

We have focused on some essential elements of evaluation science that we believe are relevant for program development and implementation activities of family therapists. Evaluation science provides a knowledge base that can facilitate how MFT practitioners think about program initiatives and how they determine their effectiveness. Much of evaluation science is practiced in the field rather than in the laboratory; therefore, it is a field that has dealt with the challenges of applied research. Evaluation science has a great deal to offer family therapy research in this regard. Evaluation science and family therapy share the characteristics of being located in community settings, focusing on complex issues, instigating and examining change, and helping families and communities to improve their conditions. The evaluation science framework we have presented focuses on how to think about prevention and intervention programs, articulate program processes and results, and apply evaluation methods.

EXEMPLARS

Green, B. L., Mulvey, L., Fisher, H. A., & Woratschek, F. (1996). Integrating program and evaluation values: A family support approach to program evaluation. *Evaluation Practice*, *17*, 261–272.

Irvine, A. B., Biglan, A., Smolkowski, K., Metzler, C. W., & Ary, D. (1999). The effectiveness of a parenting skills program for parents of middle school students in small communities. *Journal of Consulting and Clinical Psychology*, *67*, 811–825.

Kirby, R. H., & Kirby, J. J. (2000). Strengthening evaluation strategies for divorcing family support services: Perspectives of parent educators, mediators, attorneys, and judges. *Family Relations*, *49*, 53–61.

Kumpfer, K. L., & Alvarado, R. (2003). Family strengthening approaches for the prevention of youth problem behaviors. *American Psychologist*, *58*, 457–465.

Matthews, J. M., & Hudson, A. M. (2001). Guidelines for evaluating parent training programs. *Family Relations*, *50*, 77–86.

RECOMMENDED RESOURCES ON EVALUATION SCIENCE

Rossi, P. H., Lipsey, M. W., & Freeman, H. E. (2004). *Evaluation: A systematic approach* (7th ed.). Thousand Oaks, CA: Sage.

Weiss, C. H. (1998). *Evaluation: Methods for studying programs and policies* (2nd ed.). Upper Saddle River, NJ: Prentice Hall.

ACKNOWLEDGMENT

The comments of Deborah L. Mancini on an earlier version of this chapter are appreciated.

REFERENCES

American Evaluation Association. (2003). *Guiding principles for evaluators*. Retrieved from *http://www.evalorg/EvaluationDocuments/aeaprin6.html*

Andrews, G. (1999). Efficacy, effectiveness and efficiency in mental health service delivery. *Australian and New Zealand Journal of Psychiatry, 33*, 316–322.

Beutler, L. E., & Howard, K. I. (1998). Clinical utility research: An introduction. *Journal of Clinical Psychology, 54*, 297–301.

Campbell, D. T., & Stanley, J. C. (1966). *Experimental and quasi-experimental designs for research.* Chicago: Rand McNally.

Cohen, J. (1988). *Statistical power analysis for the behavioral sciences* (2nd ed.). Hillsdale, NJ: Erlbaum.

Connell, J. P., & Kubisch, A. C. (1998). Applying a theory of change approach to the evaluation of comprehensive community initiatives: Progress, prospects, and problems. In K. Fulbright-Anderson, A. C. Kubisch, & J. P. Connell (Eds.), *New approaches to evaluating community initiatives: Vol. 2. Theory, measurement, and analysis* (pp. 15–44). Washington, DC: Aspen Institute.

Cook, T. D., & Campbell, D. T. (1979). *Quasi-experimentation: Design and analysis issues for field settings.* Boston: Houghton Mifflin.

Deal, J., & Anderson, E. (1995). Reporting and interpreting results in family research. *Journal of Marriage and the Family, 57*, 1040–1048.

DeVellis, R. F. (2003). *Scale development: Theory and applications* (2nd ed.). Thousand Oaks, CA: Sage.

Fitz-Gibbon, C. & Morris, L. L. (1987). *How to design a program evaluation.* Newbury Park, CA: Sage.

Fitzpatrick, J. L. (1999). Ethics in disciplines related to evaluation. *New Directions in Evaluation, 82*, 5–14.

Gaber, J. (2000). Meta-needs assessment. *Evaluation and Program Planning, 23*, 139–147.

Goetz, J. P., & LeCompte, M. D. (1984). *Ethnography and qualitative design in educational research.* Orlando, FL: Academic Press.

Hollister, R. G., & Hill, J. (1995). Problems in the evaluation of community-wide initiatives. In J. P. Connell, A. C. Kubisch, L. B. Schorr, & C. H. Weiss (Eds.), *New approaches to evaluating community initiatives: Vol. 1. Concepts, methods, and contexts* (pp. 127–172). Washington, DC: Aspen Institute.

Jick, T. (1979). Mixing qualitative and quantitative methods: Triangulation in action. *Administrative Science Quarterly, 24*, 602–611.

Joint Committee on Standards for Educational Evaluation. (1994). *The program evaluation standards.* Thousand Oaks, CA: Sage.

Julian, D., Jones, A., & Deyo, D. (1995). Open systems evaluation and the logic model: Program planning and evaluation tools. *Evaluation and Program Planning, 18*, 333–341.

Juszczak, L., Melinkovich, P., & Kaplan, D. (2003). Use of health and mental health services by adolescents across multiple delivery sites. *Journal of Adolescent Health, 32*, 108–118.

Leber, D., St. Peters, M., & Markman, H. J. (1996). Program evaluation research: Applications to marital and family therapy. In D. H. Sprenkle & S. M. Moon (Eds.), *Research methods in family therapy* (pp. 485–506). New York: Guilford Press.

Lipsey, M. W. (1990). *Design sensitivity: Statistical power for experimental research.* Newbury Park, CA: Sage.

Mancini, J. A., Marek, L. I., Byrne, R., & Huebner, A. J. (2004). Community-based program research: Context, program readiness, and evaluation usefulness. *Journal of Community Practice, 12*, 7–21.

Mancini, J. A., & Shea, L. (1987). Presenting information to others. In W. J. McAuley (Ed.), *Introduction to applied research and problem-solving in gerontology* (pp. 214–228). New York: Van Nostrand Reinhold.

Mark, M. M., Eyssell, K. M., & Campbell, B. (1999). The ethics of data collection and analysis. *New Directions in Evaluation, 82*, 47–56.

Marshall, C., & Rossman, G. B. (1989). *Designing qualitative research*. Newbury Park, CA: Sage.

Maxwell, J. A. (1998). Designing a qualitative study. In L. Bickman & D. J. Rog (Eds.), *Handbook of applied social research methods* (pp. 69–100). Thousand Oaks, CA: Sage.

McCollum, E. E., Trepper, T. S., Nelson, T. S., McAvoy, P. A., Lewis, R. A., & Wetchler, J. L. (1996). Participating in a couples therapy outcome study: Participants' views. *Contemporary Family Therapy, 18*, 607–617.

McKillip, J. (1998). Need analysis: Process and techniques. In L. Bickman & D. J. Rog (Eds.), *Handbook of applied social research methods* (pp. 261–284). Thousand Oaks, CA: Sage.

McLaughlin, J., & Jordan, G. (1999). Logic models: A tool for telling your program's performance story. *Evaluation and Program Planning, 22*, 65–72.

Millar, A., Simeone, R., & Carnevale, J. (2001). Logic models: A systems tool for performance management. *Evaluation and Program Planning, 24*, 73–81.

Mohr, L. B. (1995). *Impact analysis for program evaluation* (2nd ed.). Thousand Oaks, CA: Sage.

Morris, L. L., Fitz-Gibbon, C. T., & Freeman, M. E. (1987). *How to communicate evaluation findings*. Newbury Park, CA: Sage.

Orthner, D. K., & Bowen, G. L. (2004). Strengthening practice through results management. In A. R. Roberts & K. Yeager (Eds.), *Handbook of practice based research* (pp. 897–904). New York: Oxford University Press.

Owen, J. M., & Rogers, P. J. (1999). *Program evaluation: Forms and approaches*. London: Sage.

Patton, M. Q. (1987). *How to use qualitative methods in evaluation*. Newbury Park, CA: Sage.

Pinsof, W. M., & Wynne, L. C. (1995). The effectiveness and efficacy of marital and family therapy: Introduction to the special issue. *Journal of Marital and Family Therapy, 21*, 341–343.

Reneger, R., & Titcomb, A. (2002). A three-step approach to teaching logic models. *American Journal of Evaluation, 23*, 493–503.

Rosnow, R., & Rosenthal, R. (1988). Focused tests of significance and effect size estimation in counseling psychology. *Journal of Counseling Psychology, 35*(2), 203–208.

Rossi, P. H., Lipsey, M. W., & Freeman, H. E. (2004). *Evaluation: A systematic approach* (7th ed.). Thousand Oaks, CA: Sage.

Savaya, R. (1998). The potential and utilization of an integrated information system at a family and marriage counseling agency in Israel. *Evaluation and Program Planning, 21*, 11–20.

Scriven, M. (1997). Truth and objectivity in evaluation. In E. Chelimsky & W. R. Shadish (Eds.), *Evaluation for the 21st century: A handbook* (pp. 477–500). Thousand Oaks, CA: Sage.

Simmons, R., & Blyth, D. (1987). *Moving into adolescence*. New York: Aldine de Gruyter.

Stufflebeam, D. L. (2001). Evaluation models. *New Directions in Evaluation, 89*, 1–106.

Tebes, J., Kaufman, J., & Connell, C. (2003). The evaluation of prevention and health promotion programs. In T. P. Gullotta & M. Bloom (Eds.), *Encyclopedia of primary prevention and health promotion* (pp. 42–61). New York: Kluwer Academic/Plenum Press.

Thye, S. (2000). Reliability in experimental psychology. *Social Forces, 78*(4), 1277–1309.

Weiss, C. H. (1995). Nothing as practical as good theory: Exploring theory-based evaluation for comprehensive community initiatives. In J. P. Connell, A. C. Kubisch, L. B. Schorr, & C. H. Weiss (Eds.), *New approaches to evaluating community initiatives: Vol. 1. Concepts, methods, and contexts* (pp. 65–92). Washington, DC: Aspen Institute.

Witkin, B., & Altshuld, J. (1995). *Planning and conducting needs assessments: A practical guide*. Thousand Oaks, CA: Sage.

Witkin, B., & Altshuld, J. (1999). *From needs assessment to action: Transforming needs into solution strategies*. Thousand Oaks, CA: Sage.

PART IV

QUANTITATIVE METHODS

CHAPTER 16

Clinical Trials in Marriage and Family Therapy Research

KEVIN P. LYNESS
STEPHANIE R. WALSH
DOUGLAS H. SPRENKLE

> A properly planned and executed clinical trial is a powerful experimental technique for assessing the effectiveness of an intervention.
>
> —FRIEDMAN, FURBERG, AND DEMETS (1998, p. 2)

BACKGROUND

Introduction

Clinical trials are fast becoming the gold standard for clinical effectiveness research. As the field of marriage and family therapy (MFT) moves toward recognizing empirically supported treatments as the standard for treatment, clinical trials have become the sine qua non of empirical study (see Sprenkle, 2002). In order to show efficacy and effectiveness of a particular treatment, clinical trial methodology seems to be required. Researchers interested in establishing empirical support for their treatment model will need to meet the strict criteria for clinical trials discussed in this chapter. Of course, randomized clinical trials (RCTs) are based on the experimental design methodology (see Lyness & Sprenkle, 1996, for a detailed description of experimental design methods), and those research skills will serve the clinical trial researcher well.

Generally, in clinical trials, the researcher applies an intervention and observes the effect on an outcome (Cummings, Grady, & Hulley, 2001). Clinical trials can take many forms, including those without any comparison group (Meinert, 1986). More commonly, though, the methodological goal of a clinical trial is to compare an intervention group and a control group to determine differences in outcome; in the general form, clinical trials lack the rigorous controls needed to determine causality. RCTs are the most restrictive form of clinical trials, in that they involve the highest level of control over extraneous variables and are best suited to answering questions of clinical effectiveness. An RCT is a prospective study designed to compare the effect of an intervention against a control group (Friedman, Furberg, & DeMets, 1998). An RCT is "prospective" because it identifies a baseline time point from which to study participants. Once a baseline is established, an intervention is administered, and outcomes are assessed. Other characteristics of RCTs are that they employ randomization and use control and experimental groups. Essentially, the three basic elements to consider in RCT design are (1) an intervention and a control treatment, (2) an outcome measure to evaluate the treatments, and (3) randomization (Meinert, 1986). RCTs are conducted in many areas of study, including the medical, surgical, prevention, behavioral, and therapeutic fields (Friedman et al., 1998; Meinert, 1986), though the majority of the terminology and background comes from the medical field. For the purpose of this chapter, we conceptualize the clinical trial as an MFT intervention trial.

Philosophical Assumptions

Clinical trial research shares many of the philosophical assumptions of experimental methods in MFT (Lyness & Sprenkle, 1996). A clinical trial is experimental methodology applied to specific questions about effectiveness and efficacy of clinical intervention. There is an assumption that it is both desirable and possible to demonstrate evidence for positive outcomes.

Given its history in the medical field, many of the assumptions of clinical trial research are derived from medicine. One of the primary assumptions is that one treatment will be demonstrably better than another and will lead to measurably better outcomes. Given the move in MFT toward legitimizing our field by establishing empirically supported treatments, our field has adopted this assumption, at least in part (see Sprenkle, 2002).

There are some other assumptions of clinical trial research. The first is that RCTs are needed to establish the safety of our treatments (again, an assumption borrowed from the medical field, where treatments often have iatrogenic effects). RCTs developed out of the need to protect patients from harmful and ineffective treatments. Finally, as stated by Friedman and colleagues (1998), "Clinical trials are conducted because it is expected that they will influence practice" (p. 7).

Historical Roots and Development

Meinert (1986) gives an extensive history of the use of clinical trials in medicine, showing evidence of comparative examinations of treatments dating back to Biblical times, though Friedman and colleagues (1998) trace the evolution of clinical trials only to the 18th century. The first clinical trial that used a type of random assignment of participants to groups was reported in 1931 (see Friedman et al., 1998). One of the first books on clinical trials was published by Hill (1962). However, it has been in the last 40 years or so that "the clinical trial has emerged as the preferred method in the evaluation of medical interventions" (Friedman et al., 1998, p. 1).

In MFT, there has been a relatively long history of using experimental methods in testing research efficacy and effectiveness, though the use of the "clinical trial" terminology is relatively recent. In fact, experimental design is the classical quantitative research design and has been used in MFT research from the beginning. Whisman, Jacobson, Fruzzetti, and Waltz (1989) remark that a strength "of marital therapy research methodology is its legacy of elegant sophisticated experimental designs" (p. 177). Jacobson and his colleagues have probably used and published experimental methods more than any other MFT researchers (Jacobson, 1984; Jacobson & Addis, 1993; Jacobson & Baucom, 1977; Jacobson, Dobson, Fruzzetti, Schmaling, & Salusky, 1991; Jacobson et al., 1985, 1989; Jacobson, Follette, & Pagel, 1986; Jacobson, Schmaling, & Holtzworth-Munroe, 1987).

METHODOLOGY

A stage model of psychotherapy research proposed by Onken, Blaine, and Battjes (1997) highlights three essential building blocks in designing and conducting an RCT: (1) treatment development, (2) efficacy work, and (3) effectiveness research or transportability. The development of a treatment manual and a therapist rating scale to measure adherence to a specific model and intervention occur during Stage 1. In addition to adherence, the competence of the therapist is evaluated in the rating scale. The purpose of the treatment development phase is to ensure that the psychotherapeutic intervention to be delivered to couples or families is conducted in the same manner, and that the therapist providing the treatment has demonstrated competence and can adhere to the model of psychotherapy under investigation (Onken et al., 1997). According to Miklowitz and Hooley (1998, p. 425), there are several essential questions to address in the treatment manual:

- What are the core interventions that constitute the treatment?
- How does one address resistance(s) to the treatment approach?
- If patients get off track from the agenda, how does one get them back on?
- How is the treatment terminated?
- What referrals are made?

The second and third stages of the psychotherapy research model are conducting efficacy and effectiveness research in RCTs (Onken et al., 1997). Working definitions of "efficacy" and "effectiveness" are provided in a subsequent section of this chapter. The issue of the transportability of the intervention or clinical approach is addressed in the third stage of this model. "Transportability" is the ability to transport the psychotherapy intervention to the masses for clinical use (Onken et al., 1997). Stages 2 and 3 are discussed in the context of RCTs below.

In the field of MFT, an RCT is a research methodology used to test an intervention (e.g., a therapy model or component) in the context of couples and families. There are several essential elements needed to design and implement an RCT. The methodological goal of the RCT is to compare an intervention group and a control group to determine differences in outcome. RCTs have also been designed to compare two psychotherapy interventions and their outcomes. This is common when an established intervention exists and a researcher wants to compare a newly developed intervention to the existing intervention. In order to reach this goal, an appropriate study design is needed to address an a priori hypothesis. An "a priori hypothesis" is one that is clearly defined and stated in advance (Friedman et al., 1998). The hypothesis should indicate that the outcome produced by an intervention will differ in comparison to the outcome of a control or comparison treatment group. For example, one RCT in couple therapy compared emotionally focused therapy (EFT) to EFT with a communication training component (James, 1991). Another RCT compared EFT to systemic therapy (Goldman & Greenberg, 1992). Requirements for RCT treatments are outlined in Table 16.1. An RCT uses the same basic methodology as classical experimental design; that is, there are (at least) two groups (typically, treatment and control) and (at least) two times of measurement (pretest and posttest), though the terminology often used in RCTs differs from that used in experimental design (Lyness & Sprenkle, 1996).

RCTs are rarely conducted in isolation, because many study staff are needed to carry out the study protocol as characterized in Table 16.2. A study staff is usually assembled by the principal investigator (PI) to carry out the RCT. For instance, if we were to test the efficacy of an MFT intervention, we would expect that the PI may work alone or with coinvestigators to develop the research question specific to the intervention, the hypotheses, the study measures, and the design, and to plan for analyses to determine whether the intervention is efficacious. A coinvestigator may be included (i.e., a biostatistician) to assist with methodological and analysis procedures. Another important member of the study staff is the project manager, usually a master's-level clinician or researcher, who actively recruits and screens research participants, conducts the randomization, organizes and enters data for each follow-up interval, manages financial incentives for participants when grant funds are available, and works closely with the PI in monitoring the trial for adverse events (W. Denton, personal communication, September 19, 2003). In this particular example, several MFT practitioners will need to be involved as the treatment providers for the intervention, and the PI is responsible for providing the necessary training, supervision, and therapist adherence and competence checks throughout the treatment intervention.

Research Questions

RCT methodology is very specialized. There are only a few research questions that this methodology is designed to answer. RCT methodology can answer the following MFT research questions:

TABLE 16.1. Requirements for Treatment and Control Groups in MFT RCTs

1. The treatment and control provided must be distinguishable from one another.
2. The treatment and control must both be ethically justifiable.
3. The use of treatments must be relevant to the needs of couples and families in distress.
4. The treatment must be acceptable to the couples and families under study, and to practitioners making referrals to the study.
5. There should be "reasonable doubt" about the efficacy of the existing treatment to pursue the test condition.
6. The potential benefits of the test condition must outweigh the risks.
7. RCT treatment should be administered consistently and should be as close to real-world practice as possible.

Note. Data from Meinert (1986, p. 66).

TABLE 16.2. Study Protocol for an RCT

A. Background of study

B. Study objectives
1. Primary research question and outcomes
2. Secondary research question and outcomes
3. Hypotheses
4. Estimating and monitoring adverse effects of the treatment

C. Study design
1. Study population
   - Inclusion and exclusion criteria
2. Sample size estimates, power calculations
3. Participant enrollment
   - Informed consent
   - Assessment of eligibility for participation
   - Baseline examination
   - Method of intervention (randomization)
4. Intervention
   - Description of intervention
   - Measures of compliance
5. Follow-up visit description and schedule
6. Ascertaining response variables
   - Intervention training
   - Data collection
   - Quality control
7. Data analysis
   - Interim monitoring
   - Final analyses
8. Termination policy

D. Organization
1. Study investigators
   - Statistical or data-coordinating center
   - Labs
   - Clinical centers
2. Study administration
   - Steering committee
   - Data-monitoring committee
   - Funding organization

Note. Data from Friedman, Furberg, and DeMets (1998).

- Is X an efficacious treatment of _____?
- Is X an effective treatment of _____?
- Is intervention A more effective than intervention B in the treatment of _____?

In order to appreciate the impact of RCTs on the field of MFT, it is important to have a clear working definition of the terms "efficacy" and "effectiveness." These concepts are defined below, according to a published glossary of health outcome methodology:

Efficacy: How a treatment works in ideal circumstances, when delivered to selected patients by providers most skilled at providing it. Often demonstrated using randomized clinical trials with relatively restrictive selection criteria.

Effectiveness: How a treatment works under ordinary conditions by the average practitioner and delivery system for the typical patient. (Glossary, 2000, p. II-8)

Clearly, efficacy research and effectiveness research involve different procedures. For example, in MFT, efficacy research involves manualized treatments with protocols to maintain manual adherence and specific exploration of the skills of the providers, whereas effectiveness research does not necessarily involve the degree of manualization required for efficacy research. Effectiveness research seems to be of greatest interest to clinicians who are practicing in the field; as Sprenkle (2002) points out, there is a perceived research–practice gap that may be perpetuated by powerful third parties' insistence upon efficacy research.

Sampling and Selection Procedures

As the full name of the RCT approach suggests, a randomization procedure is used to assign research participants to a particular group. Randomization ensures that participants have an equal opportunity to be in the treatment or control group. Randomization in a clinical trial has three primary strengths: (1) limiting the bias of allocation of participants to the intervention or control group, (2) producing comparable treatment and control groups for testing intervention, and (3) validating statistical tests of significance (Friedman et al., 1998).

RCTs are, by their nature, comparisons of groups. As such, assignment of subjects to the various research groups is very important. Because the researcher is attempting to discover differences between groups due to a treatment (or comparison of treatments), these differences should be clearly due to the treatment, not due to extraneous factors. The groups should be equivalent before the treatment is given. Groups should be of similar or equal size, in order to meet the assumptions of many of the statistics used in analysis (Kazdin, 1994; Meinert, 1986). Randomization (specifically, "random assignment") is the mechanism used to distribute characteristics of the sample across groups.

Random assignment is one way to distribute "nuisance variables" across groups unsystematically, so that they do not interfere with interpretation of the findings of interest. Indirect (statistical) control involves the use of "covariates"—variables that systematically covary with the dependent variable (Winer, Brown, & Michaels, 1991). For example, a researcher may believe that age may make a difference in outcome, so the researcher uses age as a covariate. However, random assignment alone does not ensure equivalent groups in the short run. With small samples in particular, equivalence across groups may not be assumed (Kazdin, 1994). Use of larger samples (more than 40 subjects per group) or precise and rigorous preassignment blocking (see below) can increase confidence in group equivalence. Given small samples, pretests to compare groups are particularly necessary. Matching (through randomized block design) is another way of building the variable into the design. When the correlation between the matching variable and dependent variable is high (greater than .50 or .60), matching reduces the error term and increases the precision of the experiment

(Kerlinger, 1986). Matching should not preclude randomization; that is, randomized block designs should be used if matching is going to be used.

Preassignment blocking involves grouping subjects "into sets or blocks that are similar in the characteristic(s) of interest. . . . Subjects within each set or block of subjects are randomly assigned [to] conditions" (Kazdin, 1994, p. 35). Although randomized block designs were infrequently used in psychology research in the past (Keppel, 1982), blocked randomization is now a commonly used technique in clinical trials research (Cummings et al., 2001). To continue the example used above, it may be that age influences treatment outcome. Rather than simply using age as a covariate, the researcher may choose to create blocks of subjects matched on age prior to random assignment to treatment and control groups, particularly if the sample size is small; this will ensure comparability of age in the treatment and control groups.

However, matching does cause potential problems and should be used only when sample sizes are small. The variable on which the subjects are matched must be related substantially to the dependent variable, or the matching is "a waste of time" (Kerlinger, 1986, p. 289) and can even be misleading. Trying to match on more than one or two variables at the most results in lost subjects. Matching on more than three variables is almost impossible (Kerlinger, 1986). Each of these strategies (randomization, the use of covariates, matching) to control extraneous variables has strengths and weaknesses. Eliminating a variable as a variable (i.e., holding it constant across all groups) does eliminate that variable as a source of potential problems, but it reduces the ability to generalize; the researcher can only generalize to others with the same level of that variable. Randomization is the best way to control extraneous or supplementary variables (Kerlinger, 1986), and it is the only method of controlling all possible extraneous variables, but it requires larger sample sizes. Cummings and colleagues (2001) go so far as to say that "randomization is the cornerstone of a clinical trial" (p. 148), so it should be considered the best practice.

In order to generalize findings beyond the trial, the researcher should use "random selection" of subjects from a population. Random selection ensures that each person in the population has an equal chance of being selected for the study. With random selection, the researcher can justify *statistically* any generalizations made to the larger population (Keppel, 1982). However, most samples in MFT research are convenience samples; researchers cannot just select people at random to receive therapy. If previous research has shown similar results using subjects from different populations, it becomes easier to assume that those population differences are unimportant and that valid generalizations can be made (Keppel, 1982). However, caution should always be used in making generalizations beyond the treatment sample.

Sampling Biases

It is important to mention that sampling biases, or errors, can occur in RCTs. There are three main types of biases that can occur in the implementation of RCTs: "allocation," "response," and "assessment" bias. Allocation bias occurs when the study group assignment is influenced by the investigator's knowledge of treatment to be received. This bias may result in imbalances among the treatment groups and can potentially affect study outcomes (e.g., risk factors, lifestyle characteristics). Allocation bias can be prevented by using randomization. Response bias is most likely to occur when research participants know of their treatment assignment (i.e., treatment or control group) and they report according to their knowledge of their treatment assignment. The third type of bias is assessment bias, which occurs when staff members who work on the study are informed of the research participants' treatment assignment. Assessment bias can be prevented by a double-blind randomization procedure, in which treatment and control group assignments are coded to keep patients and study staff from knowing these assignments, so that measurement is not influenced. It is important to note, however, that in psychotherapy research it is difficult to conduct a single-blind study, and a double-blind study is almost impossible to consider in the design (Friedman et al., 1998; Meinert, 1986).

Power and Sample Size

Another important consideration in research design and sample selection is sample size: How large a sample will be needed to provide adequate power? According to Kazdin (1994), "a critical research issue is the extent to which an investigation can detect differences between groups when differences exist in the population" (p. 45). "Power" is the probability of rejecting the null hypothesis when it is false. Power is a function of the criteria set for statistical significance (alpha), sample size, and the "effect size," or the difference between the groups (Cohen, 1992). A large number of outcome studies provide weak tests, particularly in studies with small to moderate effect sizes, because they lack sufficient power (Kazdin, 1994). Meinert (1986) has criticized the clinical trial research for its "virtual disregard of power considerations" (p. 15).

Different types of studies are likely to yield different effect sizes. For example, comparisons of treatment groups and no-treatment control groups are likely to produce large effect sizes, while dismantling or comparative outcome studies are likely to produce smaller effect sizes. The smaller the effect size, the larger the sample needed to gain adequate power to detect differences. Given an alpha level, power level, and estimated effect size, we can calculate the needed sample size (in fact, given any three, we can calculate the fourth). Tradition places alpha at .05 and power at .80. Effect size can be estimated mathematically from previous studies (see Jacobson & Truax, 1991). Estimates of effect sizes can be obtained from published research, or from knowledge about the type of study being conducted. For a comparative outcome study, researchers would estimate a medium effect size of about .40 (Kazdin, 1994). Given these three (alpha = .05, power = .80, effect size = .40), researchers can use tables (e.g., Cohen, 1988) to look up the appropriate sample size, or can use a computer program designed to provide power analyses to get a sample size. Given the figures above, a sample of 40 subjects per group would be needed (Kazdin, 1994). Loosening the requirements on alpha or power, or increasing the effect size estimate, would lower the necessary number of subjects per group. Power analyses will become increasingly important in efforts to establish the effectiveness of MFT. Cohen (1992) states that "failure to subject your research plans to power analysis is simply irrational" (p. 329).

Variables

Experimental designs such as RCTs have three types of variables: "independent variables," "dependent variables," and "supplementary variables" (Winer et al., 1991). However, in most RCTs the dependent variables are termed "outcome variables," while the independent variable is simply the presence or absence of an intervention or the presence of competing interventions. Independent variables are variables that the researcher manipulates in order to produce change; they must vary either in kind or in magnitude (e.g., different type of treatment or different amount of treatment). Multiple independent variables may be used, and when they are, this allows the study of interaction effects among them. For example, it may be that age interacts with treatment type, such that Treatment A works best for people between 25 and 30 years old, while Treatment C works best for those over 55. A third level of independent variable could be added as well (e.g., gender). It is important to note, however, that with each added independent (or dependent) variable, the complexity of the design increases. Multiple-independent-variable designs are called "factorial designs" (Grady, Cummings, & Hulley, 2001; Keppel, 1982; Winer et al., 1991). In many factorial clinical trials, the researcher is attempting to answer multiple research questions by using a single cohort and multiple treatments (Grady et al., 2001), and variables such as age and gender are either seen as covariates or controlled through randomization. For example, a researcher may want to look at the efficacy of a narrative approach (Treatment A) versus a solution-focused approach (Treatment C) and would assign people to these different treatment groups in the same study, while controlling for age through covariation.

Outcome variables (i.e., dependent variables) are the outcome measures that should be affected by changes in the treatment (independent variables). To measure outcomes successfully, well-defined instruments are needed to accurately assess the intervention or treatment under study, and thus to determine the effect of this intervention or treatment. Experimental designs with a single outcome variable are considered "univariate," even if there are multiple treatments, while designs with multiple outcome variables are "multivariate" designs (Winer et al., 1991). The outcome variable chosen should be the variable that is most sensitive to the treatment condition (since the researcher is looking for change in the outcome variable due to the intervention). In addition, outcome variables should have small inherent variability between subjects (Winer et al., 1991). For example, in research exploring a model of couple therapy, the outcome measure (e.g., the Dyadic Adjustment Scale, or DAS) should not vary much between the subjects at pretest. At the beginning of the study, a group with homogeneous DAS scores will be more sensitive to changes brought about by an intervention. Smaller between-subject variability will increase the precision of estimation for parameters and increase the power of statistical tests. Outcome variables should also be chosen that are normally distributed, since many parametric statistics are based on the assumption of a normal distribution (Winer et al., 1991).

It is important to use a measure for outcome that is sensitive to increased therapeutic efficacy. Of course, "therapeutic efficacy" has been defined in many different ways. A researcher may want (1) to look at the "presenting problem" that a family came in with, and the improvement in that problem after intervention (Wynne, 1988); (2) to look at change in couple functioning from distressed to not distressed on a measure such as the DAS (Jacobson & Truax, 1991); (3) to look at objective symptom reduction (e.g., change in score on the Beck Depression Inventory); or (4) to use observational or behavioral measures of change in family functioning (Whisman et al., 1989).

Supplementary variables are often known as "nuisance variables." The control of these variables is necessary, because characteristics such as motivation and referral source (to name but a few), if uncontrolled, can lead to interference in interpreting group differences (Kazdin, 1994). The researcher can use direct (experimental) or indirect (statistical) methods to control for supplementary variables (Winer et al., 1991). Direct control involves the use of blocks (groups of subjects relatively equal on a supplementary variable) in a randomized block design, which holds the variable constant over all of the treatment groups, or the use of randomization (random assignment) across groups.

To summarize, the independent variable is typically the presence or absence of the treatment or intervention; dependent variables are the outcome measures that the researcher expects to be influenced by the intervention; and supplementary variables are those additional variables that may influence the outcome and can be controlled for through blocking or randomization.

Therapist Variables

The extent to which therapist differences may contribute to treatment outcome has probably been underemphasized in the literature on clinical trials (Sprenkle & Blow, 2004; Wampold, 2001). As Beutler, Malik, and Alimohamed (2004) state, "Unfortunately, standardizing the treatment has not eliminated the influence of the individual therapist on outcomes" (p. 245). This potential confound is highlighted when one considers the important issue of whether to use the same or different therapists to administer the various treatments in clinical trials. Both approaches have advantages and disadvantages. On the one hand, if different therapists administer the various treatments (e.g., forms of couple therapy), it is possible that differences in the abilities or effectiveness of the therapists, rather than differences in the actual treatments themselves, confound what is being measured. This is a potentially serious threat to validity, since there is ample evidence that therapists differ considerably in their effectiveness. In fact, in a major meta-analysis of the psychotherapy literature, Wampold (2001) asserts that therapist factors contribute more to the variance in psychotherapy outcome than do the differences among the treatments they are administering. Therefore, when different therapists provide treatments in a clinical trial, good scientists will ask whether the results are due to different treatments, to different therapists, or to an interaction between the two.

Another related threat to validity involves "allegiance" effects. Therapists vary not only in ability, but also in the extent to which they have an allegiance to (i.e., a commitment to, belief in, and/or passion about) the protocol they are administering. (If the therapists and investigators are not the same people, the allegiance of the investigators may have an additional impact on study results.) Wampold (2001) also provides considerable empirical evidence that allegiance effects may contribute more to outcome than differences among treatments may. If therapists using one model are true believers in that model, while therapists testing an alternative model are neutral about it, the former may get better results because of their passion and enthusiasm—independent of the value of the model itself. Once again, good scientists will ask whether the results are due to the treatment, to the allegiance, or to an interaction between the two.

On the other hand, if the same therapists are used to offer all treatments in the clinical trial, this choice is more likely to control for ability, since the same therapists will probably be consistent across treatments. However, this cannot necessarily be assumed, since some therapists may be effective with one treatment but not with another. Even more likely, some therapists may have varying allegiances toward the various protocols they are administering in the study. Perhaps some therapists are forced to administer treatment protocols that they find distasteful or not credible, while they have a strong allegiance to others. One could argue strongly that this is not a fair test of the disliked models.

Although there is no simple answer to this dilemma, it is clear that clinical trial research must find ways to control for therapist effectiveness and for allegiance effects (Sprenkle & Blow, 2004). If the same therapists are used to administer all treatments, investigators need to check that they are equally effective across conditions, and that they do not have differing allegiances that may confound the results. If different therapists are used to administer the alternative treatments, the therapists need to be matched on effectiveness and allegiance. If at all possible, multiple therapists should be used for each condition, and investigators should perform statistical analyses to see whether there are differences among therapists. It goes without saying that other therapist characteristics that could affect results (e.g., gender) also need to be examined and/or controlled.

Other Considerations That May Lead to Stronger Studies

Clinical trial research in MFT is stronger when the theoretical rationale for the interventions is grounded in basic (nonintervention) social science research that links family dynamics and problem behavior—for example, the link between teenage drug abuse and problematic parent–adolescent relationships. Using theoretically driven and empirically grounded interventions will help give the investigator a better sense of *why* change occurs, as opposed to simply knowing that a procedure works. Why an intervention works can also be determined through process research (see Bradley & Johnson, Chapter 14, this volume), which ideally will be an increasingly common component of clinical trials. Clinical trials are also stronger if they are a part of a programmatic research effort where one study builds on another. Finally, clinical trial results are more credible when they are replicated by independent investigators, especially those without strong allegiance to the method under investigation (Sprenkle, 2002).

Ethical Considerations in RCTs

General Considerations

Babbie (1986) discusses some of the most general ethical considerations in social science research. These are directly applicable to experimental designs in MFT outcome research, including RCTs. The first ethical principle is voluntary participation; that is, people have the right to refuse to participate in research projects and should not feel compelled to participate. In psychotherapy research, this is important because clients may feel that they must comply when their therapist, who is in a position of power, asks them to participate in their research. Informed consent is critical in ensuring that this principle is upheld and in making clear to potential participants the risks and benefits of participating or not participating in the research.

The second ethical principle is that research should do no harm to the participants. For this reason, it is unethical to assign people to groups that include negative life events. As such, control in research with these types of problems is compromised, and other control methods have to be used. This principle then brings into question the use of no-treatment control groups, where receiving no treatment may result in harm. This is discussed in more depth below. In addition, the identity of the participants in research needs to be protected, through either anonymity or confidentiality (the difference being that in an anonymous project the researcher him- or herself does not know the identity of the participants). MFT outcome research needs to take measures to protect the confidentiality of the participants. Professional organizations such as the American Association for Marriage and Family Therapy and the American Psychological Association have explicit codes of ethics for research.

Control Group Selection and Withholding Treatment

There are several ways to decide what type of control group to have. It is important to consider that denying or postponing treatment may be problematic; yet a no-treatment or waiting-list control group is often used. Alternatives to this include "treatment on demand" (TOD; Gurman & Kniskern, 1981), where clients in the comparison group are also assigned a therapist and told they can have access to therapy on demand, whenever they want a session. If such clients request more than a preset cutoff number of sessions, however, they will be dropped from the TOD condition. This design results in four groups: (1) clients (families or couples) receiving treatment; (2) TOD remainers who have not requested any sessions; (3) TOD remainers who have received fewer than the cutoff number of sessions; and (4) TOD dropouts who have received more than the cutoff number of sessions. Todd and Stanton (1983) criticize this design because of difficulties with self-selection: Clients themselves determine into which of Groups 2, 3, or 4 they fall. Although it is possible to make comparisons between Group 1 and a combination of 2, 3, and 4, this comparison is less than desirable. The advantage is that treatment is available for those who need it.

Another possible solution to withholding treatment is to compare parallel treatment groups (Todd & Stanton, 1983). In this design, the untreated control group is eliminated. This design can take two forms: (1) comparison between two or more equally valued treatments; or (2) an add-on or constructive design, where a new component is added to a previous treatment. In the first, the problem is determining whether the two treatments are truly equally valued. In the second, there may be an interaction between the new method and the existing treatment: They may add to one another or even cancel each other out, and the researcher will not be able to tell which is the case. In addition, it is difficult to make parallel groups truly parallel (Todd & Stanton, 1983). Finally, in both cases, if no differences are found between parallel groups, this may mean that they are equally effective or equally ineffective (Todd & Stanton, 1983). This design may be acceptable if previous research has shown that the researched treatment is better than a no-treatment control.

Another ethical consideration in clinical trials involves participant randomization (Chalmers, Black, & Lee, 1972; Shaw & Chalmers, 1970). Objections to RCTs usually relate to randomized group assignment, as stated by Friedman and colleagues (1998, p. 45):

> Many clinicians feel that they must not deprive a patient from receiving an new therapy or intervention which they, or someone else, believe to beneficial, regardless of the validity of

the evidence for that claim. The argument aimed at randomization is that in the typical trial it deprives about one half the participants [of] receiving the new and presumed better intervention.

Because RCTs are often used to understand possible benefits of a new intervention, researchers have argued that RCTs, when done well, can answer important questions about treatments. In MFT, this methodology can determine the effectiveness or efficacy of a treatment or intervention. However, if randomization is not conducted, the study design is weakened, diluting efforts to understand potential benefits of intervention because the treatment and control groups are less comparable (Friedman et al., 1998).

Data Collection Procedures

Data collection in RCTs can include face-to-face or telephone interviews, questionnaires, and examinations of participants (e.g., psychological, medical, or laboratory findings). In addition to these methods, medical or psychological records can be used in the trial (Friedman et al., 1998). In MFT research, participants usually complete a baseline questionnaire and/or interview before the intervention is conducted. This step is important because baseline measurement captures the status of a couple or family prior to the intervention. After the intervention is administered (e.g., psychotherapy), the couple or family complete a similar questionnaire to capture specific outcomes and change over time such as dyadic adjustment, couple communication, depression, or anxiety. All data should be stored in a secure location (e.g., a locked filing cabinet in the researcher's office). For computerized questionnaires, all data files should be password-protected. Furthermore, no identifying information about a couple or family should be attached to the data to protect the confidentiality of the research participants.

Data Analysis Procedures

"The simplest and often most useful analysis involves a comparison of the proportion of patients in the two treatment groups who have experienced the event of interest" (Meinert, 1986, p. 187). Of course, this quote seems more applicable to medical research, where investigators are interested in whether a treatment prevents people from dying. In most MFT research, the "event" is not measured in dichotomous terms. As a result, data analysis procedures for RCTs typically include analysis of variance (ANOVA) or analysis of covariance. ANOVA is the analysis of the difference between two groups: "analysis of variance is used when two or more means are compared to see if there are any reliable differences among them" (Tabachnick & Fidell, 1989, p. 37). Additional analysis may include multiple-regression modeling to explain or predict outcomes and to control for potential covariates (Kleinbaum, Kupper, & Muller, 1988). With multiple outcome variables, it is necessary to use a multivariate analysis of variance (MANOVA) instead of a series of univariate ANOVAs, particularly when the dependent variables are correlated. In MFT research, most outcome variables will be correlated. MANOVA takes this intercorrelation into account and controls for such correlations.

Whisman and colleagues (1989) make several data-analytic suggestions for improving MFT research. They suggest that attention be paid to the unit of analysis in analyzing couple data. If a married couple is the unit of analysis, how should one deal with individuals' scores on measures such as the DAS? Commonly, such scores are averaged, but that average may mask major discrepancies between the two spouses' scores. There are a number of alternatives, such as calculating the absolute difference between spouses' scores, using both spouses' scores as multiple dependent measures for the couple, and conducting analyses based upon the scores of the spouse who exhibits greater marital distress at the end of treatment (Baucom, 1983). Another question to be answered is this: Should a couple be defined as distressed if the *average* of the spouses' scores places them in the distressed range, or only if *both* spouses' scores fall in the distressed range (Whisman et al., 1989)? It is necessary to be aware of these questions when preparing data for analysis.

Survival analysis can also be used in MFT research. For example, Lawrence and Bradbury (2001) used survival analyses to link partner aggression and marital dysfunction. The analyses identified the survival or disruption of the marriage as outcome variables. Potentially, this approach to data analysis can provide a clearer understanding of relational predictors and outcomes.

Finally, there is the consideration of clinically significant change. Jacobson and Truax (1991) lay out a statistical approach to defining meaningful change in psychotherapy research. They make the point that even large effect sizes may not yield *clinically* significant results. Participants may have moved from being very dysfunctional to just being dysfunctional. If they are still dysfunctional, then treatment may not have been successful. Jacobson and Truax propose that for clinically significant change, "the level of functioning subsequent to therapy places that client closer to the mean of the functional population than it does to the mean of the dysfunctional population" (1991, p. 13). These authors also provide a "reliable change index" (p. 14), which is a measure of how much change has occurred as a result of therapy; this measure is particularly useful when the distributions of normal and dysfunctional populations overlap. (Refer to the Jacobson & Truax article for methods on calculating the reliable change index.)

Reporting

Generally, the findings from RCTs are reported in traditional research report format. The methods section should include sample characteristics, design of the study, treatment conditions, therapists, measures and assessment, administration and scoring procedures, hypotheses, and the data analysis strategy (Kazdin, 1994). The results section should provide information on the data analysis, including data screening, preliminary analyses, treatment effects, planned comparisons, and follow-up data (Meinert, 1986). The discussion section should describe the significance (or lack thereof) of the findings. Gurman, Kniskern, and Pinsof (1986) summarize recommendations for family therapy research reports. They recommend using the clinically significant change statistics developed by Jacobson (and refined by Jacobson & Truax, 1991). They also suggest going beyond reporting just group data, which can hide information relevant to clinicians. They suggest reporting the proportion of cases showing clinically significant improvement, clinically insignificant improvement, and clinically significant worsening for each outcome criterion measure. They also recommend reporting the breadth of treatment effects (shown as the number and percentage of change criteria on which each case improves, shows no change, or shows deterioration), presented as a series of frequency distributions. Whisman and colleagues (1989) note that very few studies in MFT publish exclusion criteria for participants, nor do they publish the number who were excluded. Since such exclusion limits the generalizability of the study, such criteria should be carefully specified and examined.

Cohen (1992) makes some suggestions for research reporting and design. First of all, Cohen recommends the principle that *"less is more,* except of course for sample size" (p. 316; emphasis in original). He suggests studying few independent variables and even fewer dependent variables. Because a great many variables in MFT research are correlated, the more investigators use, the more likely they are to have Type I error—rejecting the null hypothesis when in fact it is true. Large numbers of variables also tend to become redundant. Cohen notes too that the "less is more" principle applies to reporting of results. Four or five decimal places for statistics are not necessary in MFT research; so much detail is actually detrimental, because it creates clutter and distraction.

Cohen (1992) also recommends the principle "simple is better" (p. 318) in representation, analysis, and reporting of data. A picture is worth a thousand words, and graphic representations often make findings easier to understand. In fact, the act of diagramming findings may improve *researchers'* understanding of the data! Cohen recommends using the simplest statistic that will get the job done, but not simplifying at the expense of information (e.g., simplifying a factorial ANOVA by reducing all cell sizes to the size of the smallest through dropping cases). Finally, Cohen recommends being descriptive. Rich description will engage the audience and make the research more accessible and understandable.

Meinert (1986) devotes a chapter to preparing a clinical trial study for publication. Meinert suggests clear descriptions of the study population, the treatments used, design specifications (including methods of randomization, recruitment goals, etc.), patient safeguards taken, quality control procedures, and treatment-monitoring procedures (as well as reporting on treatment adherence). One common problem in presentation of clinical trials is the failure to provide sufficient detail in the methods section for readers to truly evaluate the research trial (Meinert, 1986).

DISCUSSION

Strengths and Weaknesses of the Methodology

Clearly, the greatest strength of this methodology is that, when statistically powered and conducted with rigor, RCTs can demonstrate the efficacy and effectiveness of MFT intervention. In addition, this methodological approach is powerful enough to determine comparisons between interventions. When done well, RCTs can inform patients, clinical providers, and other entities involved in health care (e.g., managed care, legislation efforts). RCTs have political implications for the future of MFT as the evidence-based practice movement gains momentum (see Denton & Walsh, 2001).

Although the strengths of this approach are obvious, it also has weaknesses that warrant consideration. Several issues involved in conducting RCTs may be perceived as obstacles. For example, RCTs tend to be very costly and time-intensive. Some of the factors that affect the costs of RCTs include (1) patient eligibility criteria, (2) sample size, (3) the time required to develop the protocol and data collection, (4) the outcome variable(s) defined to measure success of treatment, (5) the number of clinics and clinicians needed to facilitate the trial, (6) the intervention itself, (7) data collection frequency, (8) length of follow-up interval(s) and final assessment, (9) data analysis, and (10) study closeout (Meinert, 1986).

Another difficulty with this approach is that the MFT intervention tested should mirror real-world practice (this is particularly true for effectiveness research, as noted above). However, the uniformity striven for in the trial setting creates conditions that are often not part of real-world practice. For instance, a family therapist may abort a particular model of treatment during psychotherapy if he or she believes that it is having minimal desired effects or simply feels like using another approach. In order to measure treatment effectiveness, treatment manuals have been recommended strongly for family therapy research (Gurman & Kniskern, 1981). In marital therapy research, Jacobson has been noted as having strong treatment manuals (Whisman et al., 1989). Having a treatment manual, and measuring the therapists' adherence to the manual, constitute one way of assuring equal conditions for all subjects (important for reducing error variance). Unfortunately, however, most real-world therapy is not manualized. As therapists, we tailor our therapy to fit our clients, and it may be that each client receives a very different therapy from the same therapist. Indeed, Pinsof and Wynne (2000) argue that both efficacy research and effectiveness research suffer from a uniformity myth, since good real-world therapy is often a kind of disciplined improvisation.

Jacobson and colleagues (1989) looked into this. They compared "research-structured versus clinically flexible" (p. 173) treatments, and found at posttest that there were no differences in efficacy between the two. However, at a 6-month follow-up, the couples that received research-structured therapy were more likely to have deteriorated. On the other hand, Shadish, Ragsdale, Glaser, and Montgomery (1995) found in a large-scale meta-analysis that manualized laboratory research showed consistently higher effect sizes than clinic-based research. So, whereas manualized treatment provides better control and higher effect sizes, clinic-based treatment may have more real-world effectiveness. As researchers, we need to weigh the benefits of a structured therapy in reducing error variance (and increasing the sensitivity of our research) against the weakness of a potentially weaker treatment (which may mask real benefits of a flexible treatment). Although the structured, manualized treatment reduces error variance, it may also reduce experimental variance and may result in weaker research into the efficacy of the treatment as it is practiced. The debate on this topic continues (Jacobson et al., 1989; Shadish et al., 1995).

Other critics of clinical trial research point out that clinical trials promote homogeneity of treatment for problems that are typically not homogeneous (e.g., depression is often multicausal). Therefore, controlled clinical trials artificially reduce clients' options and do not pay sufficient attention to the unique nature of each client's problems. Furthermore, they create the erroneous assumption that therapy is something that is done by therapists to passive clients whose own contribution to the healing process is marginalized (Sprenkle, 2002).

Reliability and Validity

Reliability per se is not addressed in experimental designs and clinical trials, except as a means of reducing error variance. The more reliable the measures used, the less error variance is introduced in the design, and the more sensitive the analysis will be. Validity, however, is another story. Both internal and external validity are important considerations in clinical trials. In internally valid studies, findings are due to what researchers think they are (i.e., the treatment), and not to some other source. However, there are a number of common threats to internal validity, several of which are described in Table 16.3. History, maturation, testing, and selection can be controlled by random assignment to groups. Instrumentation can be controlled easily, either through maintaining the same instrumentation or through maintaining rigorous standards for coding if observation is being used. Statistical regression and mortality will have to be examined during analysis. Mortality should be reported and assessed as a potential threat.

External validity is a tougher criterion to satisfy (Kerlinger, 1986). By "external validity," we mean the representativeness or generalizability of the findings. Can these findings be applieds to all distressed married couples, for example? Or to all behavioral marital therapists? Caution is recommended in making sweeping claims as to the representativeness of findings, unless there is a similar demonstrated effect on multiple samples, or unless a random sample from the population of interest has been used.

Skills

Several skills are needed to design and carry out the multiple stages of RCTs. This type of design has many phases: (1) planning the study, assembling the study staff, and gaining institutional review board approval or the equivalent; (2) recruiting, screening, and randomizing participants; (3) administering the treatment or control intervention; (4) conducting follow-up when applicable; (5) closing out the study; (6) analyzing and

TABLE 16.3. Threats to Internal Validity

Threat	Definition
History	An event takes place between the pretest and posttest that is not the treatment of interest, but that affects the posttest scores.
Maturation	An effect may be due to the respondents' growing older, wiser, stronger, etc.
Testing	An effect may be due to the number of times participants' responses are measured.
Instrumentation	An effect may be due to a change in the measuring instrument between pretest and posttest.
Statistical regression	An effect may be due to respondents' being classified into experimental groups at, say, the pretest on the basis of pretest scores; however, if the measures are unreliable, high pretest scorers will score lower at posttest and low pretest scorers will score higher, resulting in regression to the mean and washing-out effects.
Selection	An effect may be due to differences between the groups when groups are not controlled.
Mortality	An effect may be due to different kinds of persons' dropping out of a particular treatment group.

Note. Data from Cook and Campbell (1979, pp. 51–52).

interpreting the data; and (7) disseminating the results to the field *and* to research participants (Friedman et al., 1998). Researchers must be able to create and implement each phase of the trial. Skills that are needed by researchers to conduct clinical trials include knowledge of experimental research methods, design, and analysis; organizational strengths; the ability to motivate clinicians to adhere to a particular model; supervision capabilities; and recruitment and retention strategies.

Clinicians are vital to the treatment intervention's development and implementation in RCTs. Skills needed by clinicians as providers in RCTs are knowledge of and strong adherence to the particular treatment model or intervention to be provided. Usually, in-depth training in the model and/or intervention is built into the study for clinicians, along with supervision to monitor theoretical competence and adherence. Clinicians have to be willing to adhere to the treatment modality; they must also be aware of adverse events that may arise during the course of the study (e.g., suicidality) and take action in addressing these events ethically with patients. Clinicians must report these events immediately to the PI, so that they can be addressed by the study's data-monitoring and safety board. The events should be reflected in the data, which may have implications for attrition or for adapting the intervention to better suit the needs of patients in the study.

Bridging Research and Practice

Clinicians can become involved in this particular methodology by providing the treatment under investigation to research participants. As previously mentioned, clinicians can be invaluable in tailoring interventions to specific populations under investigation, and they can work alongside researchers to develop and test specific treatments in MFT. The collaboration between clinicians and researchers is imperative in designing RCTs and in bridging the research and practice communities in MFT.

Future Directions

RCTs are greatly needed in MFT research. Many of the existing models of therapy in MFT have little or no evidence for their efficacy or effectiveness (Lebow & Johnson, 2000), but these models are widely used and practiced in the field. Future work should test the models of MFT that are broadly accepted as the standard of care in the field. Furthermore, RCTs should be conducted to develop evidence for varieties of MFT as efficacious and effective treatments for common psychiatric disorders (e.g., depression, anxiety, and substance abuse) and medical conditions (e.g., breast cancer). Rigorous trials in MFT have the potential to strengthen the field and the lives of patients by identifying and offering effective psychotherapy treatment. Conducting RCTs speaks to our integrity as a mental health profession, as we are challenged to provide the best possible treatment to couples and families. From a financial standpoint, RCTs are important in garnering payment for treatments that have demonstrated evidence for their effectiveness and efficacy in the era of managed care.

Although more clinical trials are needed in MFT, training programs in the field are potentially well suited to help clinicians identify and train in models that have received evidence for their effectiveness and efficacy. RCTs can be incorporated into clinical training through studying and practicing from treatment manuals in theory courses and supervision (McWey & Walsh, 2003). In addition to clinical training, advanced research training in experimental design, including RCTs, should be integrated into MFT training curricula to help clinicians interpret study findings and to help researchers conduct RCTs.

EXEMPLARS

Denton, W. H., Burleson, B. R., Clark, T. E., Rodriguez, C. P., & Hobbs, B. V. (2000). A randomized trial of emotion-focused therapy for couples in a training clinic. *Journal of Marital and Family Therapy, 26,* 65–78.

Henggeler, S. W., Rowland, M. D., Randall, J., Ward, D. M., Pickrel, S. G., Cunningham, P. B., et al. (1999). Home-based multisystemic therapy as an alternative to the hospitalization of youths in psychiatric crisis: Clinical outcomes. *Journal of the American Academy of Child and Adolescent Psychiatry, 38,* 1331–1339.

Jacobson, N. S., Dobson, K., Fruzzetti, A. E., Schmaling, K. B., & Salusky, S. (1991). Marital therapy as a treatment for depression. *Journal of Consulting and Clinical Psychology, 59,* 547–557.

Liddle, H. A., Dakof, G. A., Parker, K., Diamond, G. S., Barrett, K., & Tejeda, M. (2001). Multidimensional family therapy for adolescent drug abuse: Results of a randomized clinical trial. *American Journal of Drug and Alcohol Abuse, 27,* 651–688.

REFERENCES

Babbie, E. (1986). *The practice of social science research* (4th ed.). Belmont, CA: Wadsworth.

Baucom, D. H. (1983). Conceptual and psychometric issues in evaluating the effectiveness of behavioral marital therapy. *Advances in Family Intervention, Assessment and Theory, 3,* 91–117.

Beutler, L. E., Malik, M. L., & Alimohamed, S. (2004). Therapist variables. In M. J. Lambert (Ed.), *Bergin and Garfield's handbook of psychotherapy and behavior change* (5th ed., pp. 227–306). New York: Wiley.

Chalmers, T. C., Black, J. B., & Lee, S. (1972). Controlled studies in clinical cancer research. *New England Journal of Medicine, 287,* 75–78.

Cohen, J. (1988). *Statistical power analysis for the behavioral sciences* (2nd ed.). Hillsdale, NJ: Erlbaum.

Cohen, J. (1992). Things I have learned (so far). In A. E. Kazdin (Ed.), *Methodological issues and strategies in clinical research* (pp. 315–333). Washington, DC: American Psychological Association.

Cook, T. D., & Campbell, D. T. (Eds.). (1979). *Quasi-experimentation: Design and analysis issues for field settings.* Chicago: Rand McNally.

Cummings, S. R., Grady, D., & Hulley, S. B. (2001). Designing an experiment: Clinical trials I. In S. B. Hulley, S. R. Cummings, W. S. Browner, D. Grady, N. Hearst, & T. B. Newman (Eds.), *Designing clinical research* (2nd ed., pp. 143–155). Philadelphia: Lippincott Williams & Wilkins.

Denton, W. H., & Walsh, S. R. (2001). Competence and integrity: Ethical challenges for today and the future. In R. H. Woody & J. D. Woody (Eds.), *Ethics in marriage and family therapy.* Alexandria, VA: American Association for Marriage and Family Therapy.

Friedman, L. M., Furberg, C. D., & DeMets, D. L. (1998). *Fundamentals of clinical trials* (3rd ed.). New York: Springer.

Glossary. (2000). Health outcomes methodology. *Medical Care, 38*(Suppl. II), II-7–II-13.

Goldman, A., & Greenberg, L. (1992). A comparison of systemic and emotionally focused outcome studies. *Journal of Marital and Family Therapy, 15,* 21–28.

Grady, D., Cummings, S. R., & Hulley, S. B. (2001). Designing an experiment: Clinical trials II. In S. B. Hulley, S. R. Cummings, W. S. Browner, D. Grady, N. Hearst, & T. B. Newman (Eds.), *Designing clinical research* (2nd ed., pp. 157–174). Philadelphia: Lippincott Williams & Wilkins.

Gurman, A. S., & Kniskern, D. P. (1981). Family therapy process research: Knowns and unknowns. In A. S. Gurman & D. P. Kniskern (Eds.), *Handbook of family therapy* (pp. 742–775). New York: Brunner/Mazel.

Gurman, A. S., Kniskern, D. P., & Pinsof, W. M. (1996). Research on the process and outcome of marital and family therapy. In S. L. Garfield & A. E. Bergin (Eds.), *Handbook of psychotherapy and behavior change* (3rd ed., pp. 565–624). New York: Wiley.

Hill, A. B. (1962). *Statistical methods in clinical and preventive medicine.* New York: Oxford University Press.

Jacobson, N. S. (1984). A component analysis of behavioral marital therapy: The relative effectiveness of behavior exchange and communication/problem-solving training. *Journal of Consulting and Clinical Psychology, 52,* 295–305.

Jacobson, N. S., & Addis, M. E. (1993). Research on couples and couple therapy: What do we know? Where are we going? *Journal of Consulting and Clinical Psychology, 61,* 85–93.

Jacobson, N. S., & Baucom, D. H. (1977). Design and assessment of nonspecific control groups in behavior modification research. *Behavior Therapy, 8,* 709–719.

Jacobson, N. S., Dobson, K., Fruzzetti, A. E., Schmaling, K. B., & Salusky, S. (1991). Marital therapy as a treatment for depression. *Journal of Consulting and Clinical Psychology, 59,* 547–557.

Jacobson, N. S., Follette, V. M., Follette, W. C., Holtzworth-Munroe, A., Katt, J. S., & Schmaling, K. B. (1985). A component analysis of behavioural marital therapy: One-year follow-up. *Behavioural Research and Therapy, 23,* 549–555.

Jacobson, N. S., Follette, W. C., & Pagel, M. (1986). Predicting who will benefit from behavioral marital therapy. *Journal of Consulting and Clinical Psychology, 54,* 518–522.

Jacobson, N. S., Schmaling, K. B., & Holtzworth-Munroe, A. (1987). Component analysis of behavioral marital therapy: 2-year follow-up and prediction of relapse. *Journal of Marital and Family Therapy, 13,* 187–195.

Jacobson, N. S., Schmaling, K. B., Holtzworth-Munroe, A., Katt, J. L., Wood, L. F., & Follette, V. M. (1989). Research-structured vs. clinically flexible versions of social learning-based marital therapy. *Behaviour Research and Therapy, 27,* 173–180.

Jacobson, N. S., & Truax, P. (1991). Clinical significance: A statistical approach to defining meaningful change in psychotherapy research. *Journal of Consulting and Clinical Psychology, 49,* 12–19.

James, P. (1991). Effects of a communication training component added to an emotionally focused couples therapy. *Journal of Marital and Family Therapy, 17,* 263–276.

Kazdin, A. E. (1994). Methodology, design, and evaluation in psychotherapy research. In A. E. Bergin & S. L. Garfield (Eds.), *Handbook of psychotherapy and behavior change* (4th ed., pp. 19–71). New York: Wiley.

Keppel, G. (1982). *Design and analysis: A researcher's handbook* (2nd ed.). Englewood Cliffs, NJ: Prentice-Hall.

Kerlinger, F. N. (1986). *Foundations of behavioral research* (3rd ed.). New York: Holt, Rinehart & Winston.

Kleinbaum, D. G., Kupper, L. L., & Muller, K. E. (1988). *Applied regression analysis and other multivariable methods.* Boston: PWS-Kent.

Lawrence, E., & Bradbury, T. N. (2001). Physical aggression and marital dysfunction: A longitudinal analysis. *Journal of Family Psychology, 15,* 135–154.

Lebow, J., & Johnson, S. M. (2000). The "coming of age" of couple therapy: A decade review. *Journal of Marital and Family Therapy, 26,* 23–38.

Lyness, K. P., & Sprenkle, D. H. (1996). Experimental design in marriage and family therapy outcome research. In D. H. Sprenkle & S. M. Moon (Eds.), *Research methods in family therapy* (pp. 241–263). New York: Guilford Press.

McWey, L. M., & Walsh, S. R. (2003). *Student perceptions of evidence-based practice: The impact of a pilot curriculum in a marriage and family therapy doctoral program.* Manuscript submitted for publication.

Meinert, C. L. (1986). *Clinical trials design, conduct, and analysis.* New York: Oxford University Press.

Miklowitz, D. J., & Hooley, J. M. (1998). Developing family psychoeducational treatments for patients with bipolar and other severe psychiatric disorders: A pathway from basic research to clinical trials. *Journal of Marital and Family Therapy, 24,* 419–435.

Onken, L. S., Blaine, J. D., & Battjes, R. (1997). Behavioral therapy research: A conceptualization of a process. In S. W. Henggeler & R. Amentos (Eds.), *Innovative approaches for difficult-to-treat populations* (pp. 477–485). Washington, DC: American Psychiatric Press.

Pinsof, W. M., & Wynne, L. C. (2000). Toward progress research: Closing the gap between family therapy practice and research. *Journal of Marital and Family Therapy, 26,* 1–8.

Shadish, W. R., Ragsdale, K., Glaser, R. R., & Montgomery, L. M. (1995). The efficacy and effectiveness of marital and family therapy: A perspective from meta-analysis. *Journal of Marital and Family Therapy, 21,* 345–360.

Shaw, L. W., & Chalmers, T. C. (1970). Ethics in cooperative clinical trials. *Annals of the New York Academy of Sciences, 169,* 487–495.

Sprenkle, D. H. (2002). Editor's introduction. In D. H. Sprenkle (Ed.), *Effectiveness research in marriage and family therapy* (pp. 9–25). Alexandria, VA: American Association for Marriage and Family Therapy.

Sprenkle, D. H., & Blow, A. J. (2004). Common factors and our sacred models. *Journal of Marital and Family Therapy, 30,* 113–130.

Tabachnick, B. G., & Fidell, L. S. (1989). *Using multivariate statistics* (2nd ed.). New York: Harper & Row.

Todd, T. C., & Stanton, M. D. (1983). Research on marital and family therapy: Answers, issues, and recommendations for the future. In B. B. Wolman & G. Strickler (Eds.), *Handbook of family and marital therapy* (pp. 91–115). New York: Plenum Press.

Wampold, B. E. (2001). *The great psychotherapy debate: Models, methods, and findings.* Mahwah, NJ: Erlbaum.

Whisman, M. A., Jacobson, N. S., Fruzzetti, A. E., & Waltz, J. A. (1989). Methodological issues in marital therapy. *Advances in Behaviour Research and Therapy, 11,* 175–189.

Winer, B. J., Brown, D. R., & Michaels, K. M. (1991). *Statistical principles in experimental design* (3rd ed.). New York: McGraw-Hill.

Wynne, L. C. (1988). The "presenting problem" and theory-based family variables: Keystones for family therapy research. In L. C. Wynne (Ed.), *The state of the art in family therapy research: Controversies and recommendations* (pp. 89–108). New York: Family Process Press.

CHAPTER 17

Meta-Analysis in Family Therapy Research

KAREN S. WAMPLER
ALAN REIFMAN
JULIANNE M. SEROVICH

BACKGROUND

Definition and Importance

"Meta-analysis" is an empirical methodology for summarizing findings from different quantitative research studies on a given topic. It stands in marked contrast to the typical narrative review of literature, in which conclusions are based on a general summary of statistically significant and nonsignificant findings. In meta-analysis, a common metric known as "effect size," such as the product–moment correlation or the standardized difference between two groups—for example, $(M_e - M_c)/SD_{pooled}$—is used to represent a study finding. The study finding, as represented by this number, becomes a data point and can be used in any number of creative ways to statistically analyze what is known from many different research studies on a topic.

Meta-analysis is a precise and powerful way of providing information important to the field of marriage and family therapy (MFT) for any question on which multiple relevant quantitative studies have been conducted. Its purposes are to (1) summarize what is known; (2) assess the relations among study findings, variables, and methodology; (3) suggest recommendations for future research, including identifying areas in which little further research is needed; (4) develop and test models and theoretical propositions across samples; and/or (5) generate policy and practice implications (Carson, Schriesheim, & Kinicki, 1990; Durlak & Lipsey, 1991; Wampler, 1982a).

One important function of meta-analysis has been to summarize the effectiveness of psychotherapy. Rather than reading numerous separate studies, clinicians and policymakers can read a summary of the research that is couched in terms of easily understood numbers. Two examples of interest to MFT practitioners are the article by Lipsey and Wilson (1993), summarizing over 302 different meta-analyses of treatments in psychotherapy, prevention, and education, and the comprehensive meta-analysis by Shadish and colleagues (1993) of MFT outcome studies. More recently,

Shadish and Baldwin (2002) reviewed 20 meta-analyses that have been done on MFT intervention and prevention programs.

The information generated by a meta-analysis is often put in terms easily understood by clinicians. For example, Shadish and colleagues (1993) report an average effect size of .51, based on 71 studies comparing outcomes for those in MFT with controls. An effect size of .51 means that, on average, a client in MFT was better off than 70% of those in the control condition (Shadish et al., 1993). Clinicians might be interested in more specific questions as well, such as "On average, how effective is strategic therapy as compared with parent training for conduct disorder in children?" Such questions can also be addressed by meta-analysis (cf. Shadish & Sweeney, 1991).

Another reason that meta-analysis is so useful to the field of family therapy is the difficulty of conducting primary research on issues meaningful to clinicians and policymakers. Of necessity, family therapy research can be intensive and expensive, involving observational methodologies, extensive self-reports and interviews, and relatively small treatment and control samples. Small sample sizes mean that most family therapy research studies have low statistical power, making it harder to detect true differences when they do exist. In contrast, meta-analysis may be less important in a field such as demography, which can access a large volume of meaningful data through national telephone surveys or existing data archives. Given the complexity of the phenomena of interest in family therapy, the field of necessity depends on an *accumulation* of knowledge from studies involving relatively small samples and a wide range of methodological rigor. Evaluation of the relation of different types of methodological problems to study findings is included as part of a good meta-analysis and greatly helps the reader evaluate results.

Assumptions

As a quantitative methodology, meta-analysis rests on the same assumptions as quantitative research in general: that knowledge can be gained from scientific study of phenomena, and that quantifying or representing phenomena in terms of numbers is meaningful. It is assumed that knowledge integrated across a number of studies is superior to that from separate studies, and that the common metric used is meaningful. In essence, meta-analysis produces information that is far more general than that in an individual study. For example, scores for several different measures of marital satisfaction are likely to be reported in terms of standard deviation units, instead of more specific terminology (e.g., "The mean score on the Dyadic Adjustment Scale for this sample was 105").

Meta-analysis is a general methodology and is not associated with any one theory. Whether a particular meta-analysis is consistent with a particular theory, such as systems theory, will depend on the conceptualization the researcher has used to guide the meta-analysis. The most important and the most controversial assumption of meta-analysis is that the individual studies on which the meta-analysis is based have yielded meaningful and valid results. Critics have argued that meta-analysis produces a "garbage in, garbage out" problem and can make meaningless and invalid results look important by aggregating them across several studies (Michelson, 1985; Wanous, Sullivan, & Malinak, 1989). In their final overview chapter for the fifth edition of the influential *Handbook of Psychotherapy and Behavior Change*, Lambert, Garfield, and Bergin state that "Today the meta-analytic review is considered the gold standard for integrating research reports" (2004, p. 815), but go on to urge caution in the interpretation of results produced. Meta-analysts agree that the ultimate value of results rests on the validity of the individual studies included, and they have developed quantifiable ways to assess the impact of methodological inadequacies on study findings.

Historical Development

Although quantitative methods for combining results across studies have existed since the 1930s, the term "meta-analysis" was coined by Glass in 1976. The meta-analysis by Smith and Glass (1977) on the effectiveness of psychotherapy (later expanded into a book by Smith, Glass, & Miller, 1980) was the first widely cited study labeled "meta-analysis," even though other quantitative literature reviews had been published before the famous Smith and Glass meta-analysis. Meta-analysis is really a "family" of approaches to quantitative integration of research studies (Bangert-Drowns, 1986). Influential books (Cooper & Hedges, 1994; Glass, McGaw, & Smith, 1981; Hedges & Olkin, 1985; Hunter & Schmidt, 1990; Rosenthal, 1991; Wachter & Straf, 1990; Wolf, 1986) discuss important variations of meta-analysis.

Meta-analysis grew out of the increasing recognition that advancement of knowledge was relying much too heavily on the statistical significance test, which boils down findings to a "yes" or "no," resulting in the loss of much relevant information (Cohen, 1969; Rosnow & Rosenthal, 1989). Research information summarized and integrated in terms of the significance statistic, as in the traditional narrative review, obscures information on the magnitude of effects—information of critical interest to clinicians and other family practitioners. Overreliance on the statistical significance test results from exaggerated concern with Type I error (the probability of finding a significant difference when there is none) and the neglect of issues of statistical power and Type II error (the probability of finding no difference when there is one). This imbalance is the reason why most narrative reviews, based as they are on significance tests (yielding yes–no conclusions concerning whether any difference exists), reach much more conservative and less accurate conclusions about the impact of treatment than meta-analytic reviews that use effect size estimates. (For more extended discussions, see Beaman, 1991; Lipsey & Wilson, 1993; Rosenthal, 1991; Schmidt, 1992.)

The rapid development and acceptance of meta-analysis as a methodology can be seen in the large number of meta-analyses cited in the review of psychotherapy effectiveness and efficacy by Lambert and Ogles (2004), as well as in the Shadish and Baldwin (2002) review of meta-analyses specifically focused on MFT. Meta-analysis is well accepted by researchers and editors in many fields, particularly in medicine (Cook et al., 1993; Thompson & Pocock, 1991); psychotherapy, including MFT; and education. The number of meta-analyses in MFT has increased dramatically since Wampler (1982b) published the first meta-analysis in the field.

Articles specifically on the methodology of meta-analysis are also proliferating as meta-analytic techniques continue to become more complex and sophisticated. Indeed, Schmidt (1992) believes that some researchers will begin to specialize in meta-analysis rather than in primary research (individual research studies where data are collected directly from research participants). Although meta-analysis continues to have its critics, it has become more and more widely accepted as a crucial and valid methodology for the advancement of knowledge. Unfortunately, many researchers receive no training in meta-analytic techniques. Knowledge of the meta-analytic approach will be increasingly expected of both researchers and consumers of research.

METHODOLOGY

We have identified eight steps in performing a meta-analysis (Table 17.1). These steps are similar to those of a primary research study, but with a focus here on obtaining data from already completed research studies rather than directly from research participants. In the following sections, each step and the decisions associated with that step are discussed in turn.

Research Questions

The first step is to select an appropriate research question to test, based on a thorough knowledge of the research literature on a topic. The purpose of the research question may be description or hypothesis testing (Durlak & Lipsey, 1991). Here, we address three common types of research questions tested by meta-analysis.

To illustrate the steps used in meta-analysis, we use two examples throughout the methodology section: one based on differences between group means, and one involving correlations. The first example, experimental in nature, is outcome research on the Couple Communication (CC) Program, a four-session communication program for couples (Miller, Miller, Wackman, & Nunnally, 1991). Wampler (1982a) completed a meta-analysis of research on CC, as an illustration of the use of meta-analysis as a methodology. Examples from the original meta-analysis involving 20 studies (Wampler, 1982b) are used, as well as an update of that meta-analysis with an additional 15 studies (Butler & Wampler, 1999). CC research involves one common independent variable (the CC Program itself) and pre–post designs that are easy to conceptualize in terms of effect size. Examples of research questions for the CC meta-analysis were as follows: (1) How effective is the CC Program? (2) Does CC have a greater impact on women's or men's views of the couple relationship?

A contrasting correlational example is research on knowledge of HIV and AIDS, developed to test a model involving several different independent and dependent variables. In this study, the researchers were interested in the relationship between the independent variables of knowledge of HIV/AIDS and attitude toward HIV/AIDS, and the dependent variables of risky behavior and perceptions of vulnerability. Instead of investigating pre–post designs, this model seeks to condense extensive literature investigating the relationship between these variables.

TABLE 17.1. Steps in Performing a Meta-Analysis

- Step 1: Selection of an appropriate research question to test.
- Step 2: Identification of relevant studies.
- Step 3: Establishing criteria for inclusion and exclusion of studies.
- Step 4: Data collection and coding.
- Step 5: Data entry.
- Step 6: Determining and calculating the common metric.
- Step 7: Data analysis.
- Step 8: Report writing.

Effectiveness-of-Treatment Questions

Meta-analysis is a general methodology for integrating information across research studies, and as such is not limited to any particular type of question. A limitation on meta-analysis arises from the availability of basic research on a topic. For example, many family therapists would be interested in the question of the relative effectiveness of solution-focused as compared to problem-focused approaches to a problem, but a meta-analysis on such a question would not be appropriate, because insufficient primary research has been done on this topic.

Meta-analysis has been used most often to address the question of the effectiveness of some treatment. Information about differences between experimental and control groups on the outcome measure in terms of effect size is obtained and summarized across studies. Here effect size is simply the standardized difference between two groups—for example, $(M_e - M_c)/SD_{pooled}$. Meta-analysts can focus on issues ranging from very specific questions, such as "What is the impact of a team's calling into the therapy room?", to very general questions, such as "What is the effectiveness of MFT?"

Most of the meta-analyses completed in the area of MFT have been summaries of treatment effectiveness focused at the level of general questions, such as the overall impact of MFT (Hahlweg & Markman, 1988; Hazelrigg, Cooper, & Borduin, 1987; Shadish, 1992; Shadish et al., 1993) or of prevention programs (Butler & Wampler, 1999; Cedar & Levant, 1990; Giblin, Sprenkle, & Sheehan, 1985; Wampler, 1982b). A few have focused on specific disorders, such as drug abuse (Stanton & Shadish, 1997). (See Shadish and Baldwin, 2002, for a complete list of meta-analyses of MFT.) Closely related are meta-analyses of psychotherapy effectiveness in general, summarized in Lambert and Ogles (2004). Some examples of meta-analyses relevant to MFT, though not involving a comparison of treatments, are a review of the impact of witnessing domestic violence on children (Kitzmann, Gaylord, Holt, & Kenny, 2003) and an examination of the intergenerational transmission of couple violence (Stith et al., 2000).

Methodological Questions

Study quality is addressed in meta-analyses on substantive issues. Meta-analysis can also be used, however, to address a primarily methodological issue, such as the reliability and validity of a measure. For example, in a meta-analysis of primary research on a personality measure, a procedure was used to integrate results of factor analyses of the measure across several studies (Bushman, Cooper, & Lemke, 1991). In a more fine-grained analysis, Ambady and Rosenthal (1992) examined the accuracy of predictions based on length of behavioral observation and found that accuracy did not increase with longer period of time observed, suggesting that very brief observations can provide as much useful information as longer ones.

One of the most important uses of meta-analysis is to analyze and control for confounds that might be associated with psychotherapy outcome. In meta-analysis, research studies are coded for outcomes in terms of effect sizes and also for many other variables, such as type of sample, type of measures used, and investigator allegiance. These variables can then be entered into regression equations to assess the impact of these other "confounding" variables on study outcome. For example, research studies conducted under highly controlled conditions (such as university settings) with extensive supervision of therapists and use of a treatment manual generally have higher effect sizes than research studies conducted under more "real-world" conditions (Wampold, 2001). Thus it may not be the treatment itself that is producing the outcome, but other study qualities. Meta-analysis allows the identification and assessment of the importance of these other factors.

In addition, meta-analysis has allowed more sophisticated analyses of the impact of various problems in research methodology. As part of a summary of meta-analyses on psychological and educational treatments, Lipsey and Wilson (1993) included a meta-analysis of methodological biases that might lead to inflation of effect sizes. (For a more recent analysis by these authors of the effect of methodological factors on treatment effect sizes, see Wilson & Lipsey, 2001.) Although most methodological biases were found not to inflate effect sizes substantially, study designs using only one group (the experimental or treatment group) at pre- and posttest were found to have inflated effect sizes, compared with studies including both an experimental and a control group. Guidance on how to adjust effect sizes from repeated-measures designs and to integrate results from repeated-measures and independent-groups designs is now available (Dunlap, Cortina, Vaslow, & Burke, 1996; Morris & DeShon, 2002).

The usefulness of meta-analysis for examining methodological issues has barely begun to be exploited. Such recurrent methodological issues in MFT research as the similarity of constructs measured by different family measures, gender differences in perceptions of couple and family relationships, and the appropriateness of different family measures across cultures could be effectively addressed with meta-analysis. Such studies are important to the field of MFT and can offer valuable information to future researchers.

Theoretical Questions

Perhaps the most exciting use of meta-analysis—one that is being increasingly developed—is testing theoretical models (Cooper & Lemke, 1991). Meta-analysis can be used to test main effects (e.g., all couples will benefit from CC) as well as interactions (e.g., middle-class couples will benefit more from CC than working-class couples). Such interactions, in which the effect of the treatment on outcomes is examined within different levels of a third variable (in this case, socioeconomic status), are known as "moderator analyses," with the third variable being the moderator.

Generally, in meta-analysis focused on theory, the researcher develops a model and then tests the model by using meta-analytic techniques to summarize the evidence for each of the hypothesized relations. The correlation is usually the common metric used to summarize across studies (Rosenthal & Rubin, 1982). Providing a good example of meta-analysis used to test theory, Shadish and Sweeney (1991) present evidence for a model investigating moderators and mediators affecting MFT outcome.

Sampling and Selection Procedures

As in any methodology, there are few definitively correct answers in meta-analysis, but rather a series of choices that must be made, justified, and tested. A great deal of the controversy about meta-analysis has centered on the choice of studies to be included (high-quality vs. all, published vs. all) and the unit of analysis to use (study finding, study, subject).

Identification of Relevant Studies

Step 2, and a crucial part of meta-analysis, is identification of the population of relevant studies. The goal is to identify and sample studies in such a way that those studies included in the meta-analysis are an unbiased sample of the primary research studies available on a topic. In essence, the studies included in a meta-analysis must have something in common related to the research question. The "something in common" may be an independent variable (e.g., participation in a CC group), a dependent variable (e.g., knowledge of HIV/AIDS), a measure (e.g., use of the Family Adaptability and Cohesion Evaluation Scales), or a set of variables (e.g., all studies on strategic family therapy and conduct disorder).

As with any research process, the research question and the methodology constantly influence each other. For example, the researcher may not be able to locate enough studies on a particular topic, making the meta-analysis inappropriate for that research question. As relevant articles are identified and reviewed, the research question may need to be modified. For example, one possible question on the CC research is a comparison of the effectiveness of CC for middle-class and working-class couples. Unfortunately, not enough CC studies are available with data separated by social class for such a comparison to be made. Similarly, one of the problems in the knowledge of HIV/AIDS meta-analysis has been the lack of a common measure of knowledge. Comparing results of studies that used different measures is commonly referred to as the "apples-and-oranges" problem of meta-analysis.

In meta-analysis, the researcher strives to identify *all relevant research studies*. Sources are painstakingly searched manually and by computer. These include reference lists of relevant articles and book chapters; standard social science abstracts (*Psychological Abstracts, Sociological Abstracts*); compilations of unpublished material (the Educational Resources Information Center [ERIC], *Dissertation Abstracts International*); and other databases (*Social Science Citation Index*). Although computers and the Internet have helped immensely in identifying studies, there is no substitute for a thoughtful and dogged approach to the search process (including, inevitably, manual searches). The search may include contacting key researchers for references, and sometimes even for unpublished data. The care and time needed for this step are crucial to the quality of the meta-analysis. Sources vary widely in terms of identifying key studies. For example, Shadish, Doherty, and Montgomery (1989), in their search of the MFT outcome literature, identified 165 randomized controlled studies—many more than were included in other reviews and meta-analyses of the MFT outcome literature. Shadish and colleagues (1989) document the non-overlap of studies identified through different methods, and caution especially against relying solely on key word searches of bibliographic databases for identifying relevant studies.

CC EXAMPLE

CC research was fairly easy to locate. Manual and computer searches were made, using combinations of the keywords "couple," "communication," "enrichment," "marital/marriage," and "prevention." The major sources for research studies were *Psychological Abstracts* and *Dissertation Abstracts International*. The main developer of the program (Sherod Miller) was contacted and asked to identify research studies. *Social Science Citation Index* was searched, using a few early key articles on CC that most authors would cite. Some researchers were contacted directly because it was understood that they were engaged in CC research. This located some articles in press. Articles were obtained through interlibrary loan or the university library. Most CC research is in dissertations, and these were purchased from University Microfilms International at a relatively inexpensive per-item charge.

HIV/AIDS EXAMPLE

To identify relevant HIV/AIDS studies, PsycLIT, Sociofile, and ERIC were searched, using combinations of the keywords "AIDS," "HIV," "knowledge," "attitudes," "perceptions," and "behavior." In addition, *Dissertation Abstracts International* was searched for unpublished data, along with a thorough check of the reference sections of each of the articles found for presented papers and those in review.

Once a number of studies from the field to be meta-analyzed have been obtained, two preliminary statistical exercises might be considered. First, just as researchers are encouraged to do when conducting an ordinary (primary) research study, those beginning a meta-analysis may wish to evaluate the statistical power of their proposed analyses. Hedges and Pigott (2001) offer the following advice:

> No researcher wants to begin a meta-analysis project if there is little chance that the findings will prove useful. Power analyses conducted prior to a meta-analysis can provide the reviewer with the likelihood of finding a statistically significant result given the anticipated size of the overall effect, the number of studies included in a review, and the typical sample size within studies. (pp. 203–204)

Hedges and Pigott (2001) provide formulas and examples for determining the power of various statistical tests one might conduct within a meta-analysis.

Second, one might wish to examine the state of a body of literature via a framework called "cumulative meta-analysis" (Mullen, Muellerleile, & Bryant, 2001). By beginning with the earliest located study in a line of research and then adding studies one by one in chronological order, a meta-analyst can attempt to gauge whether and when two states of affairs have been reached. These are "sufficiency" (whether the existence of the phenomenon has been well established) and "stability" (whether additional studies would change the "aggregate picture" of the phenomenon).

Inclusion and Exclusion Criteria

Step 3 is determining which inclusion and exclusion criteria to use to select exactly which of the identified studies should be included in the meta-analysis. The key is to be *explicit* and to give a *rationale* for the choices made.

Basic criteria include (1) relevance to the research question; (2) sufficient similarity of variables, design, sample, and/or measures (the apples-and-oranges problem); (3) availability of the research report; (4) inclusion of appropriate and sufficient data and statistical findings in the research report; and (5) elimination of nonindependent data sets (e.g., two studies drawn from the same database). The researcher might add other specific criteria as well—for example, including only studies on distressed (clinical) populations, or only studies with data on more than one family member. Some may want to specify a relevant time period (e.g., only research done since 1990). Again, the researcher needs to defend each decision, just as the primary researcher would defend sampling decisions made in other types of research.

The validity of the conclusions reached in a meta-analysis depends on the quality of the primary research studies included. The predominant view in meta-analysis is to include studies with a range of methodological rigor and then systematically to assess the relation of various methodological problems to the meta-analysis results. Methodological features can be picked out, and for each, a moderator variable can be set up for that feature of research design. For example, effect sizes can be examined separately within randomized experiments and quasi-experiments. It is particularly important to include unpublished research studies, especially dissertations, and even studies completed but never published (sometimes called "file drawer data") (Cook et al., 1993; Rosenthal, 1991). Meta-analysts have provided clear evidence that effect sizes for published data are larger than effect sizes for unpublished data, because of a publication bias toward significant findings (Cook et al., 1993). Thus, if unpublished data are eliminated, effect size estimates are very likely to be inflated. Reifman (1999) reviewed all meta-analyses published in *Psychological Bulletin* (the leading source of meta-analyses in psychology) between 1996 and 1998 to see what methodological features authors had used as inclusion–exclusion criteria and moderators. This examination revealed a wide variety of methodological factors that had been taken into account. Whereas some features (e.g., measures having sufficient construct validity) were used exclusively as inclusion criteria, others were used for either inclusion or moderator purposes, depending on the preference of the authors.

Once other criteria are met, there are no set criteria in terms of number of studies to be included in a meta-analysis. In fact, the number of studies in each separate meta-analysis included in the Lipsey and Wilson (1993) review ranged from 5 to 475.

Data Collection and Coding Procedures

Once research studies are identified and evaluated in terms of inclusion and exclusion criteria, Step 4 is to obtain the data needed from each study. The most important data are the relevant effect sizes (see "Data Analysis Procedures," below). Additional data are coded describing the characteristics of the study. These variables will be used in describing the studies included in the meta-analysis, as well as in analyzing variables related to effect size. Particular variables differ according to the nature and purpose of the meta-analysis, but most include data related to (1) sample characteristics, (2) methodological quality, (3) independent variables, (4) dependent variables, and (5) moderator or mediator variables. Detailed information about measures must be included, along with appropriate numerical results.

To collect the data needed from each study, it is important to develop a detailed codebook specifying what and how data are to be collected. Many published meta-analyses will state that the codebook is available from the author. Texts on meta-analysis include examples as well. The codebook developed for the CC study is included in Appendix 17.1. It is divided into sections corresponding to study characteristics, ratings of methodological quality, and results in terms of effect sizes for each measure at pretest, posttest, and follow-up. The quality rating scale for the correlational meta-analysis to test a model of HIV/AIDS knowledge is included as Table 17.2.

TABLE 17.2. Quality Rating for Correlational Studies

Criteria	Points
Used established measures	5
Used multiple measures of dependent variable(s)	1
Multiple vantage points	1
Appropriate statistical analysis	5
Reported past reliability of measures	1
Reported current reliability of measures	2
Reported information on validity	2
Sufficiently describes measures	1
Sufficiently describes sampling	1
Sufficiently describes results	1
Accounted for response set bias	1
Replicability of procedures	1
Sufficient power/sample size	3
Tested for confounds; accounted for covariates	5
Total score (range = 0–30)	____

Shadish and Baldwin (2002) note that they have "several reservations about the routine use of any scale that results in a single number to represent study quality" (p. 359). Their major concern is with the heterogeneity of the types of attributes considered, such as internal and external validity, and whether a single score can accurately convey the strengths of a study. We feel that it is an arguable point whether study quality measures should be conceptualized as unitary, psychometric constructs (such as a measure of self-esteem) or as aggregations of attributes that do not necessarily have high internal consistency (such as socioeconomic status or life event stress scales). We do, however, endorse Shadish and Baldwin's call for the development of more sophisticated study quality scales, with an eye toward the dimensionality of such scales.

As with any data collection and coding task, training of coders and reliability checks are essential. It is important, therefore, for a second coder to retrieve data from at least a subset of studies, in order to document accuracy and interrater agreement. This is also important for ratings of methodological rigor. Information on interrater agreement should be reported as part of the methods section of the meta-analysis. Yeaton and Wortman (1993) have written about different ways to think about and calculate interrater agreement for a meta-analysis.

Step 5 is data entry. At this point, the meta-analyst usually enters the data into a computerized database. Meta-analysts have two options for data entry. One option is to enter the data into a computer program written specifically for meta-analysis (e.g., Johnson, 1993; Mullen, 1989; Shadish, Robinson, & Lu, 1999). These programs have limitations, but potential users may obtain a demonstration program from the publisher for a nominal fee to examine the program's utility. A second option is to enter the data into commonly used database programs or files created through statistical software.

Data Analysis Procedures

Determining and Calculating the Common Metric

After the data from each study are collected, coded, entered, and checked for accuracy and reliability, Step 6 is to determine and calculate the common metric to be used in combining data across studies. Again, there is no one correct common metric to use. The choice of the common metric depends on the type of meta-analysis and on the type of data produced at the level of the individual study finding.

Although there are numerous variations, the common metric used in most meta-analyses is either a standardized difference between group means (d), ($M_e - M_c$)/SD_{pooled}, for continuous dependent variables; the odds ratio (OR) for categorical dependent variables (e.g., completed treatment or not); or the product–moment correlation coefficient (r). The major sources on meta-analysis (Cohen, 1969; Glass et al., 1981; Hedges & Olkin, 1985; Rosenthal, 1991) provide formulas for computing the different measures of effect size, as well as formulas for converting different statistics (e.g., t, F, chi-square) into one of the basic types of common metric. Difference-between-means statistics can easily be converted to the product–moment correlation and vice versa (Rosenthal, 1991). Contrasts from analysis of variance can also provide information that can be converted into correlation-based effect sizes (Rosenthal, Rosnow, & Rubin, 2000). The computer programs available for meta-analysis (e.g., Johnson, 1993; Mullen, 1989; Shadish et al., 1999) are designed to convert different statistics into effect sizes, although the researcher can also use statistical packages such as SPSS and SAS to write the necessary computer programs.

The major sources on meta-analysis also contain ways of estimating the common metric when some information is missing (e.g., means are reported, but not standard deviations). This occurs somewhat often, unfortunately, but there are many ways to take the information available and convert it to an effect size. In other situations—for example, when results are only labeled "not significant"—the meta-analyst may choose to set the effect size to 0. This would seem to be most warranted when a study's sample size is large. With a large sample, even a small effect would tend to be significant, so one could be confident that a nonsignificant finding with a large sample truly had a small effect size. Again, the key is to be explicit about the decision rule and provide a rationale.

Interpreting Effect Sizes

How an effect size is interpreted depends on the common metric utilized for that particular study. Effect sizes are generally categorized as small, medium, or large. Studies using the r statistic produce effect sizes varying in magnitude from between +1.00 and −1.00, reflecting the range of a correlation. According to Cohen (1969), an effect size using the r statistic is considered large if above .50, medium at .30, and small at .10. When the standardized difference between two groups (d statistic) is used, however, effect sizes vary in magnitude from approximately +3.00 to −3.00, reflecting the normal curve. These are interpreted as being the difference between groups expressed as the percentage of a standard deviation, and are considered large if above .80, medium at .50, and small at .20 (Cohen, 1969). The formula is usually calculated so that a positive effect size indicates that the treatment group improved more than the control group. The interested reader might consult Cohen (1969, 1992) for additional information on statistical power interpretations.

Meta-analysts also generally test for whether mean effect sizes are significantly different from 0. As in the larger domain of statistical analysis, in recent years many meta-analytic researchers have been augmenting their tests of statistical significance with confidence intervals (CIs) around the mean effect sizes. CIs that exclude 0 (i.e., the low and high values of the obtained interval are either completely above 0 or completely below 0) are statistically significant (Rosenthal & DiMatteo, 2001). An important issue in this context that has received increasing attention is whether CIs—and inferences about the body of research summarized in a given meta-analysis, more generally—should be based on a "random-effects" or a "fixed-effects" model (Field, 2001; Rosenthal, 1995; Rosenthal & DiMatteo, 2001; Shadish & Baldwin, 2002).

In a random-effects model, studies are the unit of analysis, and so the issue is generalizing over studies in the "population" of studies. In a fixed-effects model, however, the studies of interest are "fixed" to those in the meta-analytic database, and inferences instead focus on new subjects who could be called to participate in the fixed set of existing studies. Field (2001) notes that "standard errors in the random-effects model are typically much larger than in the fixed case if effect sizes are heterogeneous, and therefore, significance tests of combined effects are more conservative" (p. 162). He argues further that "In reality the random-effects model is probably more realistic than the fixed-effects model on the majority of occasions (especially when the researcher wishes to make general conclusions about the research domain as a whole and not restrict his or her findings to the studies included in the meta-analysis)" (p. 162).

Unit of Analysis and Weighting

Before further analysis, data may be combined or weighted. It is rare that the unit of analysis is each separate effect size, because studies that use many measures would be weighted most heavily in the results of the overall meta-analysis, and the effect sizes for any one study are not independent. For example, the number of possible effect sizes generated for each CC study ranged from 1 to 14 for each type of contrast. To avoid this problem, some meta-analysts use the study itself as the unit of analysis, by combining into one all effect sizes within a study prior to proceeding with analyses across studies. Unfortunately, this means that much precision can be lost. A compromise alternative is to combine related effect sizes according to a few key constructs, thus limiting the number of effect sizes but still leaving more than one effect size per study. This alternative allows for meaningful flexibility and precise model testing, while still being responsive to the issues of independence and overall weighting of studies within the meta-analysis. If a set of multiple dependent variables has been used fairly consistently across studies (e.g., studies on couple relationship satisfaction have always used the Dyadic Adjustment Scale or number of treatment sessions attended as dependent variables), then one can conduct a separate meta-analysis on each dependent variable.

In the CC meta-analysis, for example, it would make sense to compute an effect size for self-report measures and a separate one for observational measures rather than combining effect sizes across all measures in a study. Before proceeding further, some meta-analysts weight the individual data points according to certain study criteria, while others do not. For example, one common weighting is by sample size, using the inverse of the variance (Hedges & Olkin, 1985, p. 81, Equation 10). Weighting for sample size is especially important for samples under 30. On the other hand, some meta-analysts will use unweighted effect sizes or correlations and then compare results by sample size. Others do not weight, but instead turn this issue into an empirical question—for example, comparing effect sizes for studies with random assignment to those without random assignment. (For discussions of the issue of weighting, see Durlak & Lipsey, 1991; Hedges & Olkin, 1985; Hunter & Schmidt, 1990; National Research Council, 1992; Rosenthal, 1991.)

Statistical Analyses of Research Questions

At this point, the meta-analyst is ready to move to Step 7: analyzing the data in terms of the research questions guiding the meta-analysis. Techniques specifically designed for meta-analysis have become increasingly sophisticated (Hedges & Olkin, 1985; Hunter & Schmidt, 1990). Careful consideration is given to meeting statistical assumptions, particularly those of homogeneity of variance.

As in a primary research study, statistical analysis moves from description (central tendency, variation, range, distribution) to analysis of the research questions in terms of independent and dependent variables, using analysis of variance and/or regression techniques (depending on how the research questions are stated). A unique aspect of meta-analysis is the opportunity it affords to perform statistical analyses related to methodological questions (e.g., comparing effect sizes for controlled vs. noncontrolled studies) as well as substantive questions (e.g., comparing effect sizes at posttest with those at follow-up).

Format for Reporting the Meta-Analysis

Step 8 is writing up the results of the meta-analysis. The format of an article reporting a meta-analysis is more similar to that for a quantitative study than that for a narrative review article. The introduction of the research question(s) and the relevant review of literature are followed by the methods section, the results section, and the discussion of results. The reference section often, but not always, includes two parts: one for those mentioned in the article, and a second for those research studies included in the meta-analysis itself.

Although the form and intent of each section of the report is the same as for a primary research study, the content differs. In the methods section, instead of describing a sample, the meta-analyst describes the identification and retrieval of studies, inclusion and exclusion criteria, and characteristics of the studies. The latter often includes a section on research participants as well (e.g., gender, age, socioeconomic status, race/ethnicity), but across all the studies involved, not study by study. Instead of measures, a description of how independent and dependent variables were grouped is included, along with a description of the means of calculating effect sizes. Measures of methodological adequacy are described, as are procedures to ensure accuracy and reliability of coding. The results section contains the statistical analyses across studies. The discussion section, as in any research report, contains an evaluation of results, connections back to the literature, and implications for research and practice (if in a clinical area).

For further information, see an article by Rosenthal (1995) on reporting meta-analyses.

DISCUSSION

Strengths and Weaknesses

Meta-analysis has clear advantages over a narrative review of the literature, including precision, objectivity, and replicability. The major summary of meta-analyses of treatment completed by Lipsey and Wilson (1993) is an example of the kind of power meta-analysis provides as a methodology. In one article, the results of 302 meta-analyses, themselves representing many research studies, are summarized in terms of effect size (the standardized difference between an intervention and a control group), in a straightforward manner that is easily translated into terms understood by clinicians. An extensive evaluation of these results is included that allows the reader to review the validity of the findings. Meta-analysis lessens the probability of Type II error by taking more information into account than simply whether results reach a certain level of statistical significance, avoiding the problems with narrative reviews and analyses that overemphasize avoidance of Type I error.

Meta-analysis is not as useful in less developed areas of research. Unfortunately, this includes several areas of interest to MFT practitioners. Until the primary research is conducted, many of the important questions will not be amenable to this methodology. Thus it is not a problem with the method, but rather a problem with the availability of basic research in the field. Of course, meta-analysis cannot be used to aggregate results across qualitative studies. Of necessity, meta-analysis focuses on general questions of broad interest, and lacks the detail that the reader might desire. For example, a detailed examination and description of individual measures and treatments are not usually included in a meta-analysis; nor are case examples or excerpts from transcripts illustrating the study findings.

Most problematic is that a meta-analysis, even one done poorly, can be very impressive and influential because the results are said to represent a large number of research studies and a large number of research respondents. Boiling down research in an area to a single number (say, a 70% rate of success) presents an obvious danger of being taken out of context and separated from the important cautions that should accompany such a statement. Because of its potent influence it is important—perhaps even more so than with primary research—for the consumer of meta-analyses to be able to look beyond the results and critically consider the meta-analytic methodology that generated them. Only such a careful and knowledgeable approach to meta-analytic research can help ensure that clinical and policy interpretations and conclusions neither misinterpret nor overstate the weight of meta-analytic findings. This, of course, speaks to the importance of educating researchers, clinicians, and policy-makers in the basics of meta-analytic research, just as we do now with primary research, so that they can be critical consumers.

Reliability and Validity

An important way to assess the quality of a meta-analysis, as with a primary research study, is the extent to which the authors make their methodology clear and explicit, so that the meta-analysis can be replicated. The reader should be able to evaluate the meta-analysis based on the information given in the research report. Important documentation criteria include reporting (1) procedures for retrieval of all relevant studies, (2) clear standards for study inclusion, (3) procedures for assessing accuracy and reliability of information retrieval from the individual studies, and (4) assessment of the relation of individual studies' methodological quality to the results of the meta-analysis.

It is important to remember that the validity of the meta-analysis ultimately rests on the quality of the individual research studies that are included. Again, this is why it is crucial for the meta-analyst to present data on how methodological characteristics of individual studies relate to the results of the meta-analysis.

Skills Needed

Conceptual and analytical skills are most important in meta-analysis. The researcher must be able to derive important questions from the existing literature and then determine how to organize the results of many studies in a way that is meaningful and clear. While paying attention to the details of individual studies, the meta-analyst cannot be caught up in detail. A meta-analysis also requires the attitude of a detective. It takes persistent, dogged, and creative effort to identify, locate, and obtain the studies that become the basis of a meta-analysis. The meta-analyst needs to maintain an objective attitude and be committed to reporting the results and evaluating them, regardless of outcome.

Basic training in both primary research and meta-analytic methods is important to the researcher undertaking meta-analysis. The meta-analyst must thoroughly review and critically evaluate each primary research study. The extensive literature on meta-analysis as an approach, and the number of examples of meta-analysis, make it possible for someone trained in primary research to undertake a meta-analysis, although specific training in meta-analysis will help to ensure detailed knowledge of the various approaches to the technique and the possibilities for its use.

Bridging Research and Practice

As with any research, the results of a meta-analysis provide information to help a clinician in decision making, but do not provide answers as to how to treat a particular couple or family. As Thompson and Pocock (1991) state in reference to the usefulness to physicians of meta-analyses of clinical trials, meta-analysis does not provide simple answers to "complex clinical problems" (p. 338).

Meta-analysts provide important information on broad issues to clinicians and policymakers. Probably the most important function of meta-analysis is to integrate, summarize, and evaluate the results of a large number of individual studies in a way that is accessible to practitioners. By "boiling down" results into a few findings expressed in the metric of effect size or correlation, the meta-analysis provides an accessible and effective overview. Effect size can be translated into terms easily understood and evaluated by clinicians. For example, knowing that attending four sessions of the CC Program, on average, produced an effect size of .52 means that, on average, couples completing CC were half a standard deviation more improved in terms of relationship satisfaction than control couples not attending CC.

Other methods are being developed to translate effect sizes into terms meaningful to clinicians. Rosenthal and Rubin (1982) developed the "binomial effect size display," which puts effect sizes in terms of the proportion of control and treatment subjects above a specified level on an outcome variable. This type of analysis works best for outcomes that are naturally dichotomous (divorcing or not, continuing treatment or not), or for variables that have a widely accepted cutoff (e.g., scoring below a specific level on a particular couple satisfaction measure is considered distressed). It is also possible to put results in cost–benefit terms (Durlak & Lipsey, 1991).

Future Directions

To date, meta-analysis has been used in MFT only to evaluate overall treatment effectiveness. As more research is conducted, this function of meta-analysis will continue to be important. More evidence is needed for the basic effectiveness of MFT as opposed to other approaches. Unfortunately, in many areas, use of meta-analysis will have to await further basic research. In others, however, enough research is already available to make meta-analysis appropriate. For example, family psychoeducational approaches to severe mental illness (e.g., major depression or bipolar illness), spouse-aided therapy, and family therapy for adolescent conduct disorder are already good candidates for meta-analysis. There is sufficient new research in other areas, such as family approaches to drug and alcohol treatment, to justify updates of existing meta-analyses.

Meta-analysis is also useful for looking at components of therapy, conditions under which therapy is more or less successful, fit between problem type and therapy, and characteristics of the therapist and training related to outcome. The analysis by Shadish and Sweeney (1991) is an excellent example. Finally, meta-analysis can be effectively used now to evaluate methodological issues in MFT research, particularly the validity of different observational and self-report measures of couple and family functioning.

EXEMPLARS

Useful summaries of meta-analytic work, which also offer useful guidance, continue to be published by leading practitioners of the technique (Rosenthal & DiMatteo, 2001; Shadish & Baldwin, 2002). Exemplary meta-analyses on family therapy and other related types of intervention also continue to be published. Five are listed below.

Dunn, R. L., & Schwebel, A. I. (1995). Meta-analytic review of marital therapy outcome research. *Journal of Family Psychology, 9*, 58–68.

Franklin, C., Grant, D., Corcoran, J., Miller, P., & Bultman, L. (1997). Effectiveness of prevention programs for adolescent pregnancy: A meta-analysis. *Journal of Marriage and the Family, 59*, 551–567.

Pitschel-Walz, G., Leucht, S., Bauml, J., Kissling, W., & Engel, R. R. (2001). The effect of family interventions on relapse and rehospitalization in schizophrenia: A meta-analysis. *Schizophrenia Bulletin, 27*, 73–92.

Stanton, M. D., & Shadish, W. R. (1997). Outcome, attrition, and family–couples treatment for drug abuse: A meta-analysis and review of the controlled, comparative studies. *Psychological Bulletin, 122*, 170–191.

Stith, S. M., Rosen, K. H., Middleton, K. A., Busch, A. L., Lundeberg, K., & Carlton, R. P. (2000). The intergenerational transmission of spouse abuse: A meta-analysis. *Journal of Marriage and the Family, 62*, 640–654.

ACKNOWLEDGMENT

We appreciate the assistance of Mark H. Butler and Judy A. Kimberly.

REFERENCES

Ambady, N., & Rosenthal, R. (1992). Thin slices of expressive behavior as predictors of interpersonal consequences: A meta-analysis. *Psychological Bulletin, 111,* 256–274.

Bangert-Drowns, R. L. (1986). Review of developments in meta-analytic method. *Psychological Bulletin, 99,* 388–399.

Beaman, A. L. (1991). An empirical comparison of meta-analytic and traditional reviews. *Personality and Social Psychology Bulletin, 17,* 252–257.

Bushman, B. J., Cooper, H. M., & Lemke, K. M. (1991). Meta-analysis of factor analyses: An illustration using the Buss–Durkee hostility inventory. *Personality and Social Psychology Bulletin, 17,* 344–349.

Butler, M. H., & Wampler, K. S. (1999). A meta-analytic update of research on the Couple Communication Program. *American Journal of Family Therapy, 27,* 223–237.

Carson, K. P., Schriesheim, C. A., & Kinicki, A. J. (1990). The usefulness of the "fail-safe" statistic in meta-analysis. *Educational and Psychological Measurement, 50,* 233–243.

Cedar, B., & Levant, R. F. (1990). A meta-analysis of the effects of parent effectiveness training. *American Journal of Family Therapy, 18,* 373–384.

Cohen, J. (1969). *Statistical power analysis for the behavior sciences.* New York: Academic Press.

Cohen, J. (1992). A power primer. *Psychological Bulletin, 112,* 155–159.

Cook, D. J., Guyatt, G. H., Ryan, G., Clifton, J., Buckingham, L., Willan, A., et al. (1993). Should unpublished data be included in meta-analyses? *Journal of the American Medical Association, 269,* 2749–2753.

Cooper, H. M., & Hedges, L. (Eds.). (1994). *Handbook of research synthesis.* New York: Russell Sage Foundation.

Cooper, H. M., & Lemke, K. M. (1991). On the role of meta-analysis in personality and social psychology. *Personality and Social Psychology Bulletin, 17,* 245–251.

Dunlap, W. P., Cortina, J. M., Vaslow, J. B., & Burke, M. J. (1996). Meta-analysis of experiments with matched groups or repeated measures designs. *Psychological Methods, 1,* 170–177.

Durlak, J. A., & Lipsey, M. W. (1991). A practitioner's guide to meta-analysis. *American Journal of Community Psychology, 19,* 291–332.

Field, A. P. (2001). Meta-analysis of correlation coefficients: A Monte Carlo comparison of fixed- and random-effects methods. *Psychological Methods, 6,* 161–180.

Giblin, P., Sprenkle, D., & Sheehan, R. (1985). Enrichment outcome research: A meta-analysis of premarital, marital and family interventions. *Journal of Marital and Family Therapy, 11,* 257–271.

Glass, G. (1976). Primary, secondary and meta-analysis of research. *Education Researcher, 5,* 3–8.

Glass, G., McGaw, B., & Smith, M. (1981). *Meta-analysis in social research.* Beverly Hills, CA: Sage.

Gurman, A. S., & Kniskern, D. P. (1978). Research on marital and family therapy: Program, perspective, and prospect. In S. Garfield & A. Bergin (Eds.), *Handbook of psychotherapy and behavior change: An empirical analysis* (2nd ed., pp. 817–901). New York: Wiley.

Hahlweg, K., & Markman, H. J. (1988). Effectiveness of behavioral marital therapy: Empirical status of behavioral techniques in preventing and alleviating marital distress. *Journal of Consulting and Clinical Psychology, 56,* 440–447.

Hazelrigg, M. D., Cooper, H. M., & Borduin, C. M. (1987). Evaluating the effectiveness of family therapies: An integrative review and analysis. *Psychological Bulletin, 101,* 428–442.

Hedges, L. V., & Olkin, I. (1985). *Statistical methods for meta-analysis.* Orlando, FL: Academic Press.

Hedges, L. V., & Pigott, T. D. (2001). The power of statistical tests in meta-analysis. *Psychological Methods, 6,* 203–217.

Hunter, J. E., & Schmidt, F. L. (1990). *Methods of meta-analysis: Correcting error and bias in research findings.* Newbury Park, CA: Sage.

Johnson, B. T. (1993). *D-Stat: Software for the meta-analytic review of research literatures.* Hillsdale, NJ: Erlbaum.

Kitzmann, K. M., Gaylord, N. K., Holt, A. R., & Kenny, E. D. (2003). Child witnesses to domestic violence: A meta-analytic review. *Journal of Consulting and Clinical Psychology, 71,* 339–352.

Lambert, M. J., Garfield, S. L., & Bergin, A. E. (2004). Overview, trends, and future issues. In M. J. Lambert (Ed.), *Bergin and Garfield's handbook of psychotherapy and behavior change* (5th ed., pp. 805–821). New York: Wiley.

Lambert, M. J., & Ogles, B. M. (2004). The efficacy and effectiveness of psychotherapy. In M. J. Lambert (Ed.), *Bergin and Garfield's handbook of psychotherapy and behavior change* (5th ed., pp. 139–193). New York: Wiley.

Lipsey, M. W., & Wilson, D. B. (1993). The efficacy of psychological, educational, and behavioral treatment. *American Psychologist, 48,* 1181–1209.

Michelson, L. (1985). Editorial: Introduction and commentary. *Clinical Psychological Review, 5,* 1–2.

Miller, S., Miller, P., Wackman, D., & Nunnally, E. W. (1991). *Couple Communication.* Littleton, CO: Interpersonal Communication Programs.

Morris, S. B., & DeShon, R. P. (2002). Combining effect size estimates in meta-analysis with repeated measures and independent-groups designs. *Psychological Methods, 7,* 105–125.

Mullen, B. (1989). *Advanced BASIC meta-analysis.* Hillsdale, NJ: Erlbaum.

Mullen, B., Muellerleile, P., & Bryant, B. (2001). Cumulative meta-analysis: A consideration of indicators of sufficiency and stability. *Personality and Social Psychology Bulletin, 27,* 1450–1462.

National Research Council. (1992). *Combining information: Statistical issues and opportunities for research.* Washington, DC: National Academy Press.

Reifman, A. (1999, August). *Taking study quality into account in meta-analysis: A review.* Paper presented at the 107th Annual Convention of the American Psychological Association, Boston.

Rosenthal, R. (1991). *Meta-analytic procedures for social research.* Newbury Park, CA: Sage.

Rosenthal, R. (1995). Writing meta-analytic reviews. *Psychological Bulletin, 118,* 183–192.

Rosenthal, R., & DiMatteo, R. M. (2001). Meta-analysis: Recent developments in quantitative methods for literature reviews. *Annual Review of Psychology, 52,* 59–82.

Rosenthal, R., Rosnow, R. L., & Rubin, D. B. (2000). *Contrasts and effect sizes in behavioral research: A correlational approach.* New York: Cambridge University Press.

Rosenthal, R., & Rubin, D. B. (1982). Comparing effect sizes of independent studies. *Psychological Bulletin, 92,* 1165–1168.

Rosnow, R. L., & Rosenthal, R. (1989). Statistical procedures and the justification of knowledge in psychological science. *American Psychologist, 44,* 1276–1284.

Schmidt, F. L. (1992). What do data really mean?: Research findings, meta-analysis, and cumulative knowledge in psychology. *American Psychologist, 47,* 1173–1181.

Shadish, W. R. (1992). Do family and marital psychotherapies change what people do?: A meta-analysis of behavioral outcomes. In T. D. Cook, H. Cooper, D. S. Cordray, H. Hartman, L. V. Hedges, R. J. Light, et al. (Eds.), *Meta-analysis for exploration: A casebook* (pp. 129–208). New York: Russell Sage Foundation.

Shadish, W. R., & Baldwin, S. A. (2002). Meta-analysis of MFT interventions. In D. H. Sprenkle (Ed.), *Effectiveness research in marriage and family therapy* (pp. 339–370). Alexandria, VA: American Association for Marriage and Family Therapy.

Shadish, W. R., Doherty, M., & Montgomery, L. M. (1989). How many studies are in the file drawer?: An estimate from the family/marital psychotherapy literature. *Clinical Psychology Review, 9,* 589–603.

Shadish, W. R., Montgomery, L. M., Wilson, P., Wilson, M. R., Bright, I., & Okwumabua, T. (1993). Effects of family and marital psychotherapies: A meta-analysis. *Journal of Consulting and Clinical Psychology, 61,* 992–1002.

Shadish, W. R., Robinson, L., & Lu, C. (1999). *ES: A computer program and manual for effect size calculation.* St. Paul, MN: Assessment Systems Corporation.

Shadish, W. R., & Sweeney, R. B. (1991). Mediators and moderators in meta-analysis: There's a reason we don't let dodo birds tell us which psychotherapies should have prizes. *Journal of Consulting and Clinical Psychology, 59,* 883–893.

Smith, M. L., & Glass, G. V. (1977). Meta-analysis of psychotherapy outcome studies. *American Psychologist, 32,* 752–760.

Smith, M. L., Glass, G. V., & Miller, T. I. (1980). *The benefits of psychotherapy.* Baltimore: Johns Hopkins University Press.

Stanton, M. D., & Shadish, W. R. (1997). Outcome, attrition, and family–couples treatment for drug abuse: A meta-analysis and review of the controlled, comparative studies. *Psychological Bulletin, 122,* 170–191.

Stith, S. M., Rosen, K. H., Middleton, K. A., Busch, A. L., Lundeberg, K., & Carlton, R. P. (2000). The intergenerational transmission of spouse abuse: A meta-analysis. *Journal of Marriage and the Family, 62,* 640–654.

Thompson, S. G., & Pocock, S. J. (1991). Can meta-analyses be trusted? *Lancet, 338,* 1127–1130.

Wachter, K. W., & Straf, M. L. (Eds.). (1990). *The future of meta-analysis.* New York: Russell Sage Foundation.

Wampler, K. S. (1982a). Bringing the review of literature into the age of quantification: Meta-analysis as a strategy for integrating research findings in family studies. *Journal of Marriage and the Family, 44,* 1009–1023.

Wampler, K. S. (1982b). The effectiveness of the Minnesota Couple Communication Program: A review of research. *Journal of Marital and Family Therapy, 8,* 345–355.

Wampold, B. E. (2001). *The great psychotherapy debate: Models, methods, and findings.* Hillsdale, NJ: Erlbaum.

Wanous, J. P., Sullivan, S. E., & Malinak, J. (1989). The role of judgment calls in meta-analysis. *Journal of Applied Psychology, 74,* 259–264.

Wilson, D. B., & Lipsey, M. W. (2001). The role of method in treatment effectiveness research: Evidence from meta-analysis. *Psychological Methods, 6,* 413–429.

Wolf, F. M. (1986). *Meta-analysis: Quantitative methods for research synthesis.* Beverly Hills, CA: Sage.

Yeaton, W. H., & Wortman, P. M. (1993). On the reliability of meta-analytic reviews: The role of intercoder agreement. *Evaluation Review, 17,* 292–309.

APPENDIX 17.1. CODEBOOK FOR
COUPLE COMMUNICATION (CC) STUDIES

Identification

STUDY IDENTIFICATION NUMBER _____

YEAR OF PUBLICATION _____

FORM OF PUBLICATION ____
- 1. Dissertation
- 2. Journal article
- 3. Book or book chapter
- 4. Unpublished manuscript
- 5. Other

Sample

MARITAL STATUS ____
- 1. Married
- 2. Engaged
- 3. Other

SETTING ____
- 1. Urban
- 2. Suburban
- 3. Rural
- 4. University
- 5. Unspecified/general
- 6. Mixed

DISTRESS LEVEL ____
- 1. General population
- 2. Distressed
- 3. Not distressed

SOCIOECONOMIC STATUS ____
- 1. Middle-class
- 2. Working-class
- 3. Mixed

RACE/ETHNICITY ____
- 1. Nonminority
- 2. Minority
- 3. Mixed
- 4. Unspecified

- 4. Mixed
- 5. Unspecified

Methodology

STUDY DESIGN ____
- 1. CC only, pre–post
- 2. CC plus control, pre–post
- 3. CC plus comparison, pre–post
- 4. CC plus control plus comparison, pre–post
- 5. CC only, pre–post–follow
- 6. CC plus control, pre–post–follow
- 7. CC plus comparison, pre–post–follow
- 8. CC plus control plus comparison, pre–post–follow

TYPE OF COMPARISON GROUP ____
- 1. Growth/enrichment group
- 2. Behavior training
- 3. Communication skills/other
- 4. Concurrent CC
- 5. Sex therapy
- 6. Relationship Enhancement (RE)

LENGTH OF FOLLOW-UP IN MONTHS ____

TYPE OF CC ____
- 1. Standard, described
- 2. Standard, not described
- 3. Modified

Note: Leave blank if missing or not applicable

NATURE OF ASSIGNMENT TO CONDITION ____
- 1. Random
- 2. Matched, then random/stratified random
- 3. Not random
- 4. Not specified

(continued)

Quality Ratings

(Based on Gurman & Kniskern, 1978, pp. 820–821)
    1. Controlled assignment to conditions (5 points) ____ . ____
    2. Pre–post measurement (5 points) ____ . ____
    3. Independent variable not contaminated, experience level, therapist per treatment group, competence (5 points) ____ . ____
    4. Appropriate statistical analysis (1) ____ . ____
    5. Follow-up: none (0), 1–3 mos. (.5), +3 mos. (1) ____ . ____
    6. Treatments equally valued (1) ____ . ____
    7. Treatment carried out as planned: presumptive evidence (.5), clear evidence (1) ____ . ____
    8. Multiple change indices used (1) ____ . ____
    9. Multiple vantage points in assessing outcome (1) ____ . ____
    10. Outcome not limited to only identified patient (1) ____ . ____
    11. Data on concurrent treatment: none or equivalent across groups (1), mention but no documentation (.5) ____ . ____
    12. Equal treatment length across conditions (1) ____ . ____
    13. Outcome allows for both positive and negative change (1) ____ . ____
    14. Therapist–investigator nonequivalence (1) ____ . ____
    15. Sufficient power/sample size (1) ____ . ____
    16. Dropouts/attrition followed (1), followed and analyzed (2) ____ . ____
    17. Check on equivalence of groups (1) ____ . ____
TOTAL QUALITY SCORE ____ . ____

Effect Sizes

FOR EACH EFFECT SIZE:
ID ____
EFFECT SIZE NUMBER ____
TYPE ____
    01. CC only, pre–post
    02. CC only, pre–follow
    03. CC plus control, pre–post
    04. CC plus control, pre–follow
    05. CC plus control, post only
    06. CC plus control, follow only
    07. CC plus comparison, pre–post
    08. CC plus comparison, pre–follow
    09. CC plus comparison, post only
    10. CC plus comparison, follow only
DOMAIN OF MEASURE ____
    01. Observation of marital interaction (B)
    02. Self-report of relationship satisfaction (R)
    03. Self-report of communication (C)
    04. Self-report of other relationship quality (OR)
    05. Self-report of individual quality (OI)
    06. Other (O)
EFFECT SIZE ____ . ____
SAMPLE SIZE ON WHICH EFFECT SIZE IS BASED
CC ____   CONTROL ____   COMPARISON ____

CHAPTER 18

Economic Evaluation Methodology for Family Therapy Outcome Research

DAVID P. MACKINNON

BACKGROUND

You are the administrative and research director of the Sunnyside Family Therapy Clinic (SFTC) in a large metropolitan area. The clinic is rather large, with a clinical staff of 40 and an administrative/support staff of 8. You have been having trouble getting reimbursements from several local managed care operators for several of your treatment programs. You suspect that the managed care administrators do not understand or appreciate family therapy as an alternative therapy modality.

Specifically, you have a family violence treatment program that you feel is far superior to the individual family violence treatment program at rival Darkside Therapy Clinic (DTC). DTC is about half the size of SFTC in terms of personnel, clients, and physical premises. You want to approach the local managed care administrators with justification for reimbursing your family domestic violence program. What are you going to do?

In these times of rising health care costs and increasingly scarce resources, policymakers, insurance companies, employee assistance programs, and individuals are demanding that services be not only effective, but cost-effective as well. The continuing national debate on health care reform stems in part from the overwhelming cost of adequate, effective health care. The health care industry and consumers who pay for treatment are justifiably interested in knowing both whether a prescribed treatment works and whether it is worth the cost.

Mental health care is no different from other health care areas: The field needs to justify its existence. Managed care providers are seeking mental health care services that can prove their effectiveness (Aderman, Bowers, Russell, & Wegmann, 1993). Third-party reimbursers are particularly concerned with cost-effectiveness. Third-party payers must know that treatment is both *outcome*-effective and *cost*-effective.

339

With more effective treatment in the present, clients will be less likely to need future treatment, which will reduce future third-party payments. If treatment for a particular presenting problem with a specific population can be reduced to a cost per treatment hour, the third-party payer can determine and promote the most cost-effective treatment modality. In addition, if treatment benefits can be measured against treatment costs to determine the net treatment benefit of each modality, third-party payers can promote treatments with the greatest overall net benefit.

Family therapy is one of several treatment modalities available to address mental health difficulties that occur in families. We know that with certain populations family therapy works (Sprenkle, 2002), but generally we do not know whether family therapy is cost-effective. Although our understanding of this issue is improving, little attention has been paid to economic evaluation in family therapy

Due to the general lack of attention to economic evaluation issues in mental health research, and the increasing concern about the scarcity of available resources to pay for mental health services, several have emphatically called for the inclusion of economic evaluations in mental health research (Kiesler, 1980; Maynard, 1993a, 1993b). Leitch (1993) specifically exhorts family therapy researchers to add cost analyses to their research, while former editors of two of the major family therapy journals have called for the inclusion of cost-effectiveness analyses in family therapy outcome research (Sprenkle & Bailey, 1995; Steinglass, 1996). Pinsof and Wynne (1995a, 1995b), as *Journal of Marital and Family Therapy* guest editors, identified the inclusion of cost analyses in family therapy outcome research as one of the critical next steps in family therapy research. Lastly, family therapy researchers have gathered four times in the last decade (1996, 1999, 2000, and 2001) to discuss the future of family therapy research. Each conference identified economic evaluations as vital not only to the funding of future research, but to the justification of the field of family therapy. The purpose of this chapter is to prepare researchers for the inclusion of economic evaluations in their research.

History of Economic Evaluations

Levin (1975) indicates that modern economic evaluation methodologies were first used by the military. He cites decision making about public works in the first half of the 20th century as the reason these methodologies were developed. He points out that according to the Flood Control Act of 1936, the Army Corp of Engineers was required to certify whether or not water resource projects were feasible, based on a ratio of benefits to costs. Techniques for measuring both the direct and indirect societal benefits and costs of flood control projects were identified, and then methods for assigning a monetary value to these benefits and costs were established. The ratio of benefits to costs was used to allocate public funds in such a way as to maximize the public's investment in these types of projects. As both the benefits and costs were monetarily valued, the first economic evaluation methodology developed was "cost–benefit analysis" (CBA) (Levin, 1975).

Not all allocation decisions could realistically and reliably apply CBA, however, because not all benefits could be converted into monetary terms. Thompson and Fortess (1980) point to the military's attempts in the early 1960s to evaluate weapons systems as the impetus for developing a different economic evaluation methodology. The difficulty in determining a monetary value for the extent of target destruction and/

or loss of human life led to considering the number of targets destroyed a more appropriate evaluation measure. The movement to nonmonetary measures of outcome for economic decision making became known as "cost-effectiveness analysis" (CEA) (Levin, 1975).

Since the 1960s, economic evaluation techniques have been utilized in a variety of fields and disciplines. The field of industrial economics is credited with input into the development of economic evaluation techniques (Panzetta, 1973). Competitive marketplaces force decision makers to constantly evaluate the allocation of scarce financial, physical, and human resources to maximize returns on investments. Levin (1975) also points to the fields of health care and personnel training as contributors to the development of economic evaluation techniques and utilization

The development of economic evaluation methodology in the mental health field varies greatly by segment. A number of mental health studies have presented full economic evaluations (e.g., studies of various living situations for persons with severe mental illnesses). Unfortunately, when it comes to the psychotherapy segment of the mental health field, the attention paid to economic evaluation of any kind has been significantly absent (Krupnick & Pincus, 1992). And worse yet, family therapy is clearly behind the fields of psychiatry and individual clinical psychology in the development and implementation of these important methodologies.

Previous Economic Evaluation Methodology Studies

Only two attempts have been made in the published family therapy literature to articulate economic evaluation methodology (Pike & Piercy, 1990; Pike-Urlacher, Mackinnon, & Piercy, 1996). Pike and Piercy (1990) presented the Office of Technology Assessment's (1980a) 10 general steps to conducting CEA, while Pike-Urlacher and colleagues (1996) reiterated these general steps in the context of a more thorough review of the concept of cost analyses in family therapy outcome research.

Most psychological economic evaluation research refers to the work of Yates (1985, 1996, 1997, 1999, 2000; Yates & Newman, 1980), a clinical psychologist who has published extensively in the area of economic evaluation methodology and application to clinical research. Others (Aos, Phipps, Barnoski, & Lieb, 2001; Weisbrod, 1981; Weisbrod, Test, & Stein, 1980; Wortman, 1983) also present methodologies for CBA and CEA that are relevant to family therapy researchers.

Other works not related to the field of family therapy give thorough presentations of economic evaluation methodology. These include publications by the Centers for Disease Control and Prevention (1995), Drummond, Stoddart, and Torrance (1987), and the Office of Technology Assessment (1980a, 1980b). The Centers for Disease Control and Prevention (1995) guide, specifically written for researchers in the public health prevention–effectiveness field, presents a systematic approach to gathering CBA, CEA, and "cost–utility analysis" (CUA) data. The Drummond and colleagues book is designed to be a nontraditional textbook that concentrates on practical methodological issues and applications.

The background papers from the Office of Technological Assessment (1980a, 1980b) were intended to supplement an Office of Technological Assessment report titled *The Implications of Cost-Effectiveness Analysis of Medical Technology*. These supplemental reports, especially the 1980a paper, provide significant descriptions of economic evaluation methodology.

METHODOLOGY

The case has been made for the importance of economic evaluation to the future of the family therapy field (McCollum & Stith, 2002, O'Farrell & Fals-Stewart, 2003; Pinsof & Wynne, 1995a; Sprenkle & Bailey, 1995; Steinglass, 1996). What we need today is a step-by-step explanation of how to structure economic evaluations in order to incorporate these analyses into family therapy outcome research. Several critical issues that will determine the value and usefulness of the cost analysis results must be addressed in the formative stages of research design. In the absence of a thorough, systematic approach to economic evaluation design, the results will have little to no value for anyone but the researcher(s). The first objective of this chapter is to clearly identify the issues that must be addressed *before* any kind of methodologically sound economic evaluation can be undertaken and to provide an example of how to handle the identified issues. Table 18.1 outlines the areas/steps to be addressed. The order is as important as the content, since subsequent decisions are greatly influenced by preceding decisions. Some of the steps are intuitively obvious and represent universally sound research practices, while other steps are unique to economic evaluations.

This chapter is intended both for researchers who are planning to include cost analyses in their outcome effectiveness research and for evaluators of research who are looking toward determining the applicability and marketability of the research findings. Those to whom these clinicians and researchers wish to "sell" their research results are generally well schooled in the ways of economic evaluations. It is imperative then that family therapy researchers elevate their understanding of economic evaluations to the level of the "buyers" of the research findings, in order to compete in the arenas where heretofore family therapists have struggled to be included. Family therapists must learn the language of those who make key economic decisions about the future of mental health care treatment (Steinglass, 1996). The research design issues discussed are critical to gaining the credibility family therapists want.

Formulate the Question

The goal of economic evaluation research is to provide relevant or pertinent information for making decisions that lead to increased utilization of family therapy services. At the outset of economic evaluations, researchers must address a number of issues.

TABLE 18.1. Study Design Issues

- Formulate the question.
  - Identify the problem area.
  - Define the audience.
  - Specify the objectives.
  - Link the objectives to interventions.
  - Operationalize the problem or question.
  - Specify the perspective.
  - Select the time frame and analytic horizon.
- Select the analytic method.
- Identify marginal and/or incremental analysis needs.
- Identify all relevant costs and benefits.
- Address time value of money with discounting.
- Address uncertainty with sensitivity analysis.

The target audience, study perspective, and analytic method are among the key issues that are critical not only to the nature of the analysis, but to the interpretation and usefulness of the results as well. Therefore, certain steps in cost analysis research design must precede other steps in order to ensure the results' relevance.

Identify the Problem Area

Consistent with most research methodology, the first step is to identify the problem area (Office of Technology Assessment, 1980a). Initially, the objective is to decide very broadly which family problem area (e.g., substance abuse, juvenile delinquency, family violence, etc.) will be the focus of treatment in the study. This starting place may be so self-evident and automatic that it is overlooked as a separate design step. What is different about this initial step is the recommendation to resist going beyond selecting the general problem area until other research design steps are completed.

Example. Throughout this discussion of methodology, each section will end with the section's issues being applied to the scenario presented at the beginning of the chapter. The family problem area identified in the opening scenario is family violence. In a real-world situation, the specific kind of family violence will need to be identified.

Define the Audience

The second, and most important, step in the study design is to select a target audience (Centers for Disease Control and Prevention, 1995). The identified audience of study findings is the driving force behind the study design (Halpern, 1977). The interests of the target audience will influence the study objectives, questions asked, perspective, time frame, analytic method, and relevancy of certain costs and benefits. In other words, the objectives of a target audience will drive the goals of the service being delivered, which will in turn affect the effectiveness measures that will be used to evaluate the treatment (Menninger, 1977; Spivack, St. Clair, Siegel, & Platt, 1975; Weinstein, 1986).

In order for the research results to be relevant, a party-at-interest or "consumer" of the study findings who will benefit from the results must be identified (Glass & Goldberg, 1977). It is difficult to imagine researchers undertaking research that they believe to be irrelevant, but how often does research "fill the gaps" in the literature while providing no information to assist decision makers in their resource allocation tasks? The goal of economic analysis research is to provide information relevant to or pertinent to making these decisions. Family therapy researchers need to produce information that leads to decisions increasing the utilization of family therapy services.

For the research results to lead to a benefit, the interests of the research consumer must be known, so that the findings answer the questions the consumer is asking. For example, a managed care company will be significantly more interested in reducing mental health claims in relation to premium revenues than in the cost of improving family satisfaction. This is not to say that family satisfaction is not important, but to managed care administrators who want to maximize profits and keep their jobs, claims information will be a lot more compelling. Family therapy researchers must not take the "If you build it, they will come" attitude, but must have a target audience in mind as research studies are designed.

Target audiences can be defined in several ways. Column 1 of Table 18.2 lists several family therapy research consumers to whom research results may be directed. The

TABLe 18.2. Target Audiences

Family therapy research consumers	Possible areas of interest
Individuals	Out-of-pocket payments, alternative uses of time, productivity, relational functioning, quality of life . . .
Immediate families	Out-of-pocket payments, alternative uses of time, relational functioning, quality of life . . .
Extended families	Alternative uses of time, relational functioning . . .
Employers	Productivity, health care premium payments, absenteeism . . .
Reimbursers (managed care organizations, insurance companies)	Claims vs. premium payments received, member retention . . .
Providers (health maintenance organizations, preferred provider organizations, clinics, hospitals)	Staff requirements, facilities expenses, hospitalization, community image . . .
Immediate community • Schools • Police • Fire department	Attendance, academic performance, school behavior . . . Vandalism, incarceration, staffing . . . Arson, firefighting equipment, staffing . . .
Government	See "Immediate community" areas of interest as related to tax implications, overall societal costs and benefits that translate into social programs, image/re-electability . . .
Society	Overall societal costs and benefits that translate into quality of life, tax implications . . .

Centers for Disease Control and Prevention (1995) suggest that consumers are generally either policy decision makers or program decision makers. They indicate that policy decision makers are typically elected officials and agency heads who make broad decisions about the availability and/or viability of treatment modalities such as family therapy. Program decision makers are those who make decisions about resource allocation among and within various therapy interventions. There are also direct purchasers of family therapy, such as individual families who select the treatment modality and treatment provider. The more specific researchers can be about the target audience, the better the research design will be in leading to more relevant results.

Example. In the scenario at the beginning of the chapter, the target audience will be the local managed care company's administrators.

Specify the Objectives

Once the problem area has been selected and a target audience has been identified, the third task is to specify the objectives of the study. The question answered in this step is

"What specifically will be measured in the study?" Once the target audience is defined, the information of interest to that audience can be determined.

Column 2 of Table 18.2 lists possible areas of interest to the listed family therapy research consumers. Notice that different parties-at-interest are likely to be interested in different information, as they are generally making vastly different resource allocation decisions. Selecting the target audience thus influences the composition of the information that will be useful, and thereby drives the objectives of the study.

Wortman (1983) points out that setting study objectives raises several problems. Measurement is one common problem. He suggests that certain areas of interest may be very difficult to quantify and measure. For example, individual families may be interested in improving the quality of family life, but determining an appropriate measure of quality of family life will be difficult.

Wortman also points out that most audiences have multiple areas of interest, which can lead to multiple study objectives. He encourages researchers to focus on the most important dimensions of the target audience's areas of interest. Of course, to focus on the most important dimensions, researchers have to know what the target audience's most important areas of interest are. It is therefore imperative that the researchers interview representatives of the target consumers, in order to clearly identify the information that will be relevant. The study objectives can then be tailored to the audience's interests.

Example. Managed care administrators, the selected target audience in the opening scenario, are known to be interested in increasing profits by reducing claims in relation to premium revenues. The objective of the study then will be to demonstrate that overall mental health claims are reduced.

Link the Objectives to the Interventions

Once the problem area, the target audience, and the study objectives have been determined, specifying one or more interventions that will achieve the objectives is the next step. Family therapy researchers may have already decided what form of family treatment the study will be evaluating, but the appeal here is to ask this question: "What are all the alternative interventions that could achieve the study objective in the selected problem area?" The economic evaluations being proposed here are intended to be comparative analyses between alternative courses of resource allocation. Cost-effectiveness always involves a comparison to something, even if the alternative is a "do-nothing" control (Aos et al., 2001; French, Zarkin, & Bray, 1995; Office of Technology Assessment, 1980b).

The purpose of this step is to articulate the competing courses of action that will achieve each stated objective. Researchers should assume that the target audience is a good steward of its resources, and that it knows (or will know) its available resource choices. It is best then to be as thorough as possible in identifying the alternative means to achieve the stated objectives. It is "smart business" to acknowledge competitors rather than deny their existence. The consumers of family therapy research are well aware that other treatment modalities can achieve the same or similar therapeutic results, and it is important to account for these competing alternatives in the design of the study question.

On the other hand, caution must be taken to avoid making the study too cumbersome. When reducing the number of alternatives, researchers should include programs that are considered representative of the broader set of alternatives (Wortman, 1983). Also, when choosing among similar interventions, researchers should make an effort to select interventions that are believed to be most effective (Wortman, 1983). If a program is not effective in the first place, it makes no difference whether or not it is cost-effective (Drummond et al., 1987). Typically, economic evaluations in the mental health field are add-ons or follow-ups to efficacy studies. Again, discussing the objectives and the interventions to be compared with representatives of the target audience will ensure usefulness of the study results. Achieving methodology "buy-in" from members of the target audience at the beginning of a study is clearly better than trying to convince them of the findings' relevancy after the study is completed.

Example. Having talked with one national managed care administrator and one local managed care administrator, you know that they believe only individual treatment programs to be effective with family violence, and that they believe the DTC to be a representative program of this modality. Therefore, this study will compare claims data between the SFTC family violence program and the DTC individual violence program.

Operationalize the Problem or Question

The next step is to develop a well-constructed, clear study question. Well-constructed study questions address the issues and needs of the target audience (Centers for Disease Control and Prevention, 1995). This is familiar territory for most researchers, who regularly design study questions to answer these specific questions: "Who? Did what? To whom? Where? When? How often? With what result? In comparison to what alternatives?" Clearly indicating the treatment protocol and the comparison protocols is not new, but building the study question with the previously described steps will ensure the relevance of the findings.

Good cost analysis questions involve comparisons and the viewpoint(s) from which the comparison is being made (Drummond et al., 1987). Questions like "Is family therapy worth it?" and "How much does it cost to run an adolescent day treatment program?" raise important issues and provide accounting and management information, but fail to address comparisons and viewpoints.

Good cost analysis questions examine benefits *and* costs. Questions like "Is Treatment X with families presenting with substance abuse issues more effective than treatment Y for the same population?" provide some good information, but not on cost-effectiveness data.

Good cost analysis questions also emphasize specificity. Questions like "Is Treatment X more cost-effective than Treatment Y? are pertinent to cost analyses, but lack the specificity of questions such as "Does Treatment X reduce health care claims more than Treatment Y?" Although the latter question is better than the preceding question, incremental benefits of one treatment over the other are not addressed and should be.

Example. An acceptable question for the opening scenario is "Are total family mental health claims lower with SFTC's family violence program than with DTC's violence program?" Each of the components of the question (i.e., total family mental health claims, SFTC's family violence program, and DTC's violence program) will then need to be clearly articulated. Family mental health claims are likely to be defined as the claims made on the local managed care organization.

Specify the Perspective

Once the study question is formulated, the next step is to define the study's perspective (Centers for Disease Control and Prevention, 1995). The study perspective determines which costs and benefits are relevant to the study. In other words, not all costs and benefits that can be measured need to be measured, depending on the perspective selected. As previously outlined in Table 18.2, a study that is being conducted from the perspective of an employer will be oriented to gathering different information than a study whose perspective is that of a referral network. Health care providers and health care reimbursers will normally be interested in different types of costs and benefits. The perspective then guides the various kinds of information (costs and benefits) that will be gathered during the study (Glass & Goldberg, 1977; Masters, Garfinkel, & Bishop, 1978; Weinstein, 1986).

The "Specify the perspective" step is especially important to family therapy researchers. From these researchers come the arguments that family "pathology" is a systemic phenomenon and that the effects/benefits of psychotherapy will also be systemic. The implication is that to be consistent with family therapy's theoretical roots, familial (immediate and extended), transgenerational, community, and societal costs and benefits must be considered when the effects of psychotherapy are being analyzed. The concept of perspective in economic evaluation gives family therapists the opportunity to argue to the world and competing professions that costs and benefits broader than the individual and his or her clinician must be part of the evaluation structure. It is interesting to note that in the psychology and psychiatry cost-effectiveness literature (Krupnick & Pincus, 1992), these concepts are well accepted and expected. Pinsof and Wynne (1995a) point out that the most important contribution family therapy can make to economic analyses of mental health services is a systems approach.

Researchers may find that their selected target audience has several perspectives, due to the various constituencies to whom its members must respond. A local hospital administration is likely to want information that relates to the internal costs of providing services, in order to make decisions about facilities and financial resources. This same hospital administration is also likely to be interested in community costs and benefits for marketing purposes. A study with this hospital administration in mind will be taking two perspectives: an internal hospital perspective and a community/society perspective. Well-constructed study questions make identifying the study perspective or perspectives a rather simple task.

On the other hand, studies that incorporate a societal perspective are among the most complicated to execute effectively. The societal perspective requires analyzing all benefits of an intervention (regardless of who receives them) and all costs of an intervention (regardless of who pays them). Typically, audiences that are interested in the societal perspective are making societal resource allocation decisions (Centers for Disease Control and Prevention, 1995), such as a local government agency's allocating tax dollars to community services.

When researchers are considering the societal perspective, the term "opportunity cost" is often used. Opportunity costs represent the resources not available to society because of a client's condition (Centers for Disease Control and Prevention, 1995). For example, when a person is unable to work because of his or her own condition or that of a spouse, society loses the benefit of that person's contribution to the overall workforce. The loss of productivity is considered an opportunity cost and should be included in an economic evaluation from a societal perspective. Other types of opportunity costs include volunteer time, services provided by trainees, and alternative uses for equipment and/or facilities being utilized for a particular program. When calculating opportunity costs, one approximates the monetary value of the resource (French et al., 1995; Office of Technological Assessment, 1980b).

Example. The perspective of the scenario proposed at the beginning of this chapter is that of the managed care company. In conversations with the managed care administrators, they have indicated that decisions about recommended treatment for family violence will be made on strictly economic grounds. This means that relevant costs and benefits will be focused on claims data.

Select the Time Frame and Analytic Horizon

The last step in formulating the question is to specify the time frame of the intervention and the analytic horizon of the intervention effects (Centers for Disease Control and Prevention, 1995). The time frame of the analysis is the period of time during which the specific therapeutic programs are being administered. In other words, in the context of family therapy research, the time frame refers to the period when the actual therapy is taking place. It can be defined as either the number of therapy sessions or a period of time during which therapy occurs. Generally, the time frame seems well understood and articulated in family therapy outcome research.

It is important to identify a time frame that is long enough to encompass all the therapeutic activity. Family therapists have long argued that handling relational problems in the context of the system in which the problems emerge is better and more efficient than dealing with one family member's symptoms after another sequentially over a longer period of time. It makes sense to attach a systemic perspective to the defined intervention period in economic evaluations. The time frame of analysis, to maintain consistency between systemic and individual forms of treatment, must take into consideration therapeutic treatment of all family members—whether it occurs simultaneously or sequentially.

The analytic horizon is the period over which the costs and benefits of the therapeutic interventions are realized. The analytic horizon is usually longer than the time frame, since the effects of the treatment continue long after the therapy is over. The key analytic horizon question is "For how long will the benefits that were initially observed and attributed to the therapeutic intervention continue to be attributed to the treatment?" For example, for how long does a family that presents with an alcohol abuse problem benefit from treatment that results in alleviation of the alcohol abuse? Analytic horizon decisions need to be explicit, so that recipients of the study findings can evaluate the reasonableness of the assumptions.

Example. The SFTC treatment program runs for 20 weekly sessions, while the DTC treatment program runs for 36 weekly sessions. The time frame of analysis for the SFTC treatment program will be the 20 weeks of family therapy. Likewise, the time frame of analysis for the DTC treatment program will be 36 weeks of individual treatment.

The family has been defined as the unit of analysis. For purposes of determining the analytic horizon, this means that the costs and benefits related to the particular programs will be gathered on a family basis. Preliminary data indicate that frequently, as an abusing family member changes, other family members exhibit behaviors that cause them to interact with mental health professionals. In the SFTC treatment program, these auxiliary behaviors occur simultaneously with the family therapy and are dealt with in the context of the family treatment. In the DTC treatment program, these auxiliary behaviors occur during and after the individual treatment. In fact, it appears that family members of the originally presenting individual are seeking treatment for up to 1 year after the end of the initial individual's treatment. You should expect to continue to gather cost data for the DTC treatment program for at least a year and a half. The benefits of both treatment programs are expected to last a lifetime. The managed care company, on the other hand, has indicated that it is interested in claims reductions in the 2-year period after the end of treatment. The analytic horizon will then be approximately 2 years and 36 weeks from the start of treatment.

The study question should now be formulated, with the problem area, target audience, objectives, interventions, operational details, perspective, time frame, and analytic horizon clearly outlined. Because it is a well-constructed study, its expected results will be useful to the decision makers to whom they will be delivered. For purposes of evaluating previously completed economic evaluations, all of these areas ought to be articulated and evident in the write-ups. Whereas the preceding steps set the stage for economic evaluations, the next steps are specifically related to doing economic evaluations.

Select the Analytic Method

As previously mentioned, the basic tasks of economic evaluation in family therapy outcome research are to identify, measure, value, and compare the costs and benefits of alternative therapy treatment modalities. Drummond and colleagues (1987) suggest that this description of the economic evaluation leads to a classification system for the various types of cost analyses, based on two key questions: (1) "Is there a comparison of two or more alternative therapy initiatives?" (2) "Are both costs and consequences (benefits) of the alternatives being examined?" Figure 18.1 represents the matrix based on these two key questions.

Ideally, the most informative and thorough economic evaluation is the full economic evaluation, or the lower right quadrant of Figure 18.1. Since the ideal is not always possible, it is beneficial to know the characteristics of the partial economic evaluations. In the absence of comparisons of treatment modalities, the findings are strictly descriptive. When either costs *or* consequences (benefits) are being evaluated, rather than costs *and* consequences (benefits), and there are no alternative comparisons, the analysis is labeled either an "outcome description" or a "cost description." Outcome descriptions examine and report only the benefits of a single treatment program. An example would be a study reporting that for a particular solution-focused family therapy modality, the Dyadic Adjustment Scale score improves 20%. Cost descriptions examine and report only the costs of a single treatment program. A study reporting that the cost of the solution-focused family therapy at ABC Family Clinic is $5,700 per family is an example of a cost description. An economic evaluation is labeled a "cost–outcome description" when costs and consequences of a single treatment program are being evaluated but not compared to other program costs and consequences. An example would be research determining that for $5,700 per family, the solution-focused

Are both costs and consequences (benefits) of the therapeutic alternatives examined?			
		NO		YES

		Examines only consequences	Examines only costs	
Is there comparison of two or more therapeutic alternatives?	NO	PARTIAL EVALUATION Outcome description	Cost description	PARTIAL EVALUATION Cost–outcome description
	YES	PARTIAL EVALUATION Efficacy or effectiveness evaluation	Cost analysis	FULL ECONOMIC EVALUATION Cost minimization analysis Cost effectiveness analysis Cost–benefit analysis Cost–utility analysis

FIGURE 18.1. Distinguishing characteristics of economic evaluations. From Drummond, Stoddart, and Torrance (1987, p. 8). Copyright 1987 by Oxford University Press. Reprinted by permission.

family therapy at ABC Family Clinic improves the Dyadic Adjustment Scale score 20%.

It is possible to perform an economic evaluation involving a comparison of two or more therapeutic alternatives, but not to examine both costs and benefits. If a comparison of consequences or benefits of at least two therapy modalities occurs in a study without consideration of costs, the study is labeled an "efficacy evaluation" or "effectiveness evaluation." An example of an efficacy study would be one determining that the solution-focused family therapy at ABC Family Clinic is more effective than the narrative family therapy at XYZ Community Clinic, on the basis of the ABC treatment's achieving a 20% improvement in the Dyadic Adjustment Score and the XYZ treatment's only achieving a 10% improvement. When costs of two or more therapy alternatives are compared without a corresponding benefits comparison, the evaluation is labeled a "cost analysis." A study reporting that the solution-focused family therapy at ABC Family Clinic is less costly ($5,700 per family) than XYZ Community Clinic's narrative family therapy ($6,500 per family) would be an example of a cost analysis.

None of the preceding analyses meets the criteria of a full economic evaluation. All provide information, but none of the nature that would assist a decision maker in allocating scarce resources. Full economic evaluations examine both cost and benefits while simultaneously comparing them to alternative therapy programs. A full economic evaluation provides decision makers with information necessary to choose between competing alternatives. As they are adequately and thoroughly described elsewhere (Aos et al., 2001; Centers for Disease Control and Prevention, 1995; Drummond et al., 1987; Office of Technological Assessment, 1980b; Pike & Piercy, 1990; Pike-Urlacher et al., 1996; Yates, 1985, 1996, 1997, 1999, 2000), the following are only brief descriptions of the key full economic evaluations that are important to family therapy outcome research.

"Cost-minimization analysis" (CMA) is the simplest full economic evaluation method and is actually very similar to the previously described cost analysis. CMA involves comparing alternative treatments that are assumed to produce substantially identical results. This assumption is based on empirical evidence. (Cost analysis ignores the effects or benefits of treatment and disregards evidence about the nature of the treatment outcomes.) With the assumption of identical effects, the focus of CMA is on the costs necessary to achieve the consequences. In other words, benefits are considered irrelevant for evaluation purposes, and the objective is to find the alternative treatment modality that minimizes costs. As in all full economic evaluations, costs in CMA are measured in dollars. An example of CMA results would be identical to the cost analysis results outlined earlier, but identical therapy outcomes would be explicitly assumed. The disadvantage of CMA is that the assumption about identical outcomes can seldom be made.

CEA, mentioned earlier in this chapter, is probably the best-known method of economic evaluation and the most widely reported. Costs are again measured in dollars, while no effort is made to assign monetary value to benefits or outcomes. Instead, the unit of measure for benefits is a single effect of interest that is common to both or all alternatives, but is achieved to differing degrees between alternatives. Examples of CEA benefits would include reduced number of inpatient hospital days, increased days without violence, reduced symptomatology, increased family satisfaction, fewer days absent from work, and lower health care claims. CEA combines the cost of implementing an intervention with the effectiveness of the intervention. Comparisons are usually made on the basis of cost per unit of effect/benefit (e.g., a particular alcohol treatment program achieves 1 day of sobriety for $1,200, vs. another program that achieves 1 day of sobriety at a cost of $1,500). Sometimes, the CEA comparisons are made on the basis of effects per unit of cost (e.g., days of sobriety per dollar spent).

CEA is most often used when one wants to choose the most cost-effective strategy from a set of alternative strategies that produce a common effect. Note that if a common effect can be identified between two programs, even though the programs have little or nothing in common, they can be evaluated by CEA. The disadvantage of CEA is that if a common effect cannot be found, CEA cannot be used. For example, if a clinic has to make a decision between building a play therapy room and hiring additional clinicians to staff the growing program for battered women, CEA cannot be used to provide useful information.

CBA, also mentioned earlier, addresses the shortcomings of CEA by attempting to value both costs and benefits in monetary terms. In doing so, CBA permits researchers to compare treatment modalities with singular or multiple benefits that are not necessarily common to both or all alternatives. Expressing benefits in dollars also allows for comparisons of treatment effects that vary in degree. CBA is most often used when the outcomes of the alternative treatments are not the same and cannot be reduced to a single common effect. The preceding decision about building the play therapy room versus staffing the program for battered women can be addressed by CBA, since the unit of measure (dollars) will be common to both alternatives. Program funding decisions often require CBA findings. The results of CBA are usually expressed as net monetary benefits (i.e., treatment benefits minus treatment costs). For example, researchers may find that the play therapy room will produce a $4,000 net benefit, whereas the program for battered women will generate a $5,000 net benefit. Sometimes CBA findings are expressed as a net benefit ratio (i.e., total benefits divided by total costs). The advantage of the net monetary benefit calculation is that a researcher has an absolute dollar amount with which to evaluate a program. The researcher can determine whether the benefits exceed the costs by a sufficient amount to warrant continuing the program.

The advantage of the net benefit ratio is that the relative magnitude of the benefits to each dollar of cost is provided. If, for example, the net benefit ratio for the battered-women's program is 4:1, and for the play therapy room the ratio is 2:1, every dollar of cost spent on the battered-women's program will result in $4 of benefits. On the other hand, every dollar spent on the play therapy room will achieve $2 of benefits. Parties-at-interest can conclude that they will get twice as much value for each dollar spent on the battered-women's program as they would for the play therapy room. Program efficiency may be revealed by the net benefit ratio, but the absolute benefit requires the net monetary benefit. A strong argument can be made for reporting both measures.

The disadvantage of CBA is the difficulty in assigning monetary values to various health states and outcomes. For example, valuing the averting of pain and suffering is extremely difficult, but this may be an important outcome of family therapy. Lives saved or physical difficulties avoided because of treatment are also benefits that present measurement difficulties and controversy.

CUA, mentioned briefly earlier, is a variation of both CEA and CBA that attempts to address the difficulties of CBA. Again, as in all economic evaluations, cost are measured in dollars. As in CBA, benefits can be singular or multiple, can be common or not common to the alternative treatments, and can occur in varying degrees. But as in CEA, the benefits are measured and converted to a common effect called "quality-adjusted life years." The concept of utility captured by CUA is that specific levels of health status, or improvements in health status, have value relative to other levels of health. In other words, efforts are made to rank-order and then quantify a series of levels of health, in order to state for comparison purposes that one level of health treatment outcome is better than another. CUA measures and quantifies these values by soliciting preferences of individuals or segments of society for various levels of health or health outcomes. These quality-of-life preferences are then combined with the expected years of life to determine quality-adjusted life years. CUA is most appropriate when the quality of life is the most important factor in the target audience's decision criteria. The major drawback to using CUA in family therapy research is that the existing quality-of-life scales are primarily oriented to physical health states and not to mental or relational health states. It is a technique that is relatively new and is just being applied to a variety of new health care research.

The purpose of the "Select the analytic method" step is to determine which method of economic evaluation is appropriate for each study question being asked. As all full economic evaluations measure and value costs in monetary terms, the focus is on the nature and comparability of the benefits. If the treatment effects are substantially the same in nature but differ in magnitude, CEA is the appropriate choice. If the treatment effects are significantly different in both nature and magnitude, CBA is the appropriate choice. If the treatment effects are primarily oriented to improving quality of life, CUA is the preferred evaluation method.

Example. The question developed in the "Frame the question" section has focused on reducing managed care mental health claims as a result of the alternative therapy treatments. As there are economic implications for the managed care company in both the number of claims (e.g., staffing and administrative costs for the managed care company) and the dollar amount of total claims, both the number and the dollar amount of mental health claims will be of interest to the managed care company. The number of claims as a benefit is substantially the same for both treatment modalities, but is expected to differ in magnitude. Therefore, a CEA will be conducted for this part of the study. On the other hand, the total claims in dollars as a benefit will lead to a CBA's being conducted for the second part of the study.

Identify Marginal and/or Incremental Analysis Needs

The next step in setting up an economic evaluation is to consider whether or not the study question requires marginal and/or incremental analysis (Centers for Disease Control and Prevention, 1995). When the evaluation is intended for the purpose of deciding whether or not to make an investment to expand a particular treatment program, "marginal analysis" is the appropriate methodology to follow. The basic premise of marginal analysis is that evaluations of program expansions should not take into consideration costs that already exist. Only new costs ought to be considered with the new benefits that will be derived from the expanded program (Kee, 1994). If the new costs/investments are averaged with the existing program costs and benefits, the true effect of the program expansion will be diluted, and a possibly wrong investment decision will be made.

When the analysis is intended for the purpose of a family therapy clinic deciding whether or not to make an investment in a new treatment program, "incremental analysis" is the appropriate methodology to follow. Like marginal analysis, incremental analysis refers to focusing on the new investment and expected added benefits instead of adding the new investment and benefits with existing program costs and benefits. Again, the evaluation focus needs to be on the new, incremental costs and benefits.

When the wrong methodology is used to analyze program expansions or new program additions, there can be quite a difference in the evaluation findings and resultant decision. Table 18.3 provides a hypothetical example of how marginal and incremental analyses can produce different results from those obtained by simply averaging total costs and benefits. The scenario presented in Table 18.3 is about a decision a particular family therapy clinic needs to make about either investing in a program expansion or developing a whole new therapy treatment protocol as an adjunct to its

TABLE 18.3. Marginal and Incremental Analysis Examples

Treatment protocol	Clinically significant improvement on the CTS (# of individuals)	Costs (U.S. $)	Cost to outcome (cost per successful treatment—U.S. $)
1. Family therapy (40 clinicians)	50	200,000	4,000
2. Family therapy (50 clinicians)	60	225,000	3,750
3. Marginal analysis results	10	25,000	2,500
4. Family therapy plus drug tx.	70	336,000	4,800
5. Incremental analysis results	20	136,000	6,800

Note. CTS, Conflict Tactics Scale, which is often used in domestic violence evaluations.

existing program. Specifically, Table 18.3 presents data regarding whether this family therapy clinic ought to expand its existing domestic violence program by hiring an additional 10 therapists or to start a new testosterone-regulating drug treatment program as an add-on to the existing domestic violence program. The analysis outcome measure is the number of individuals who show clinically significant improvement on the Conflict Tactics Scale. The objective of the study is to determine which alternative investment more efficiently and effectively minimizes cost per outcome. As the outcome measure is identical for both alternatives but varies in degree, a CEA is the appropriate form of analysis. The first alternative, expanding the current program by 10 therapists, is outlined on lines 1, 2, and 3. When marginal analysis is used, the hypothetical cost of adding 10 clinicians is $2,500 (line 3) per successful outcome, rather than the average cost of $3,750 (line 2). The second alternative, adding a testosterone-regulating drug treatment program as an add-on program to the existing domestic violence program, is outlined on lines 1, 4, and 5. When incremental analysis is used, the hypothetical cost of adding the drug treatment program is $6,800 (line 5) per successful outcome, rather than the average cost of $4,800 (line 4). The comparative analysis then is between the $2,500 cost per successful outcome achieved by adding clinicians and the $6,800 per successful outcome achieved by adding a new drug therapy program. The first alternative is substantially the more effective of the two alternatives. Although the average costs calculated on lines 2 and 4 would have rendered the same relative results, the difference between the two alternatives appears much smaller than it actually is. It is not uncommon for cost averaging to result in no benefit being realized, when in fact the incremental benefit is significant for the incremental dollars invested.

Example. As there are no expanded or additional programs being considered in the opening scenario, neither marginal or incremental analysis is appropriate.

Identify All Relevant Costs and Benefits

The next step in the design of economic evaluations is to identify all of the relevant costs and benefits that will be included in the analysis. Up to this point in the study design, costs and benefits have been described as broad concepts that will require specification and quantification. Measurement and valuation are relatively straightforward concepts for those costs and benefits that are regularly assigned monetary values, such as therapists' time or facilities' rent, but often costs and benefits do not have associated monetary values and must have values imputed to them. The act of assigning values to these costs and benefits is often more art than science. Other sources (Centers for Disease Control and Prevention, 1995; Drummond et al., 1987; Levin, 1975; Mackinnon, 1998; Office of Technology Assessment, 1980b) provide thorough discussions of the various ways to go about determining the appropriate values of these costs and benefits.

"Relevancy" of specific costs and benefits depends on the selected study perspective (Centers for Disease Control and Prevention, 1995; Yates, 1985). As previously outlined, different perspectives necessitate collecting different cost and benefit data. In this step, all the costs and benefits relevant to the perspectives chosen, associated with the alternative treatment programs being compared, and contextually relevant to the study question being asked are identified. It is likely that not all the costs and benefits identified as relevant can or should be measured and valued, but the starting point is a list of all relevant costs and benefits (Drummond et al., 1987). From this cost–benefit inventory (Centers for Disease Control and Prevention, 1995), decisions can be made about the importance, magnitude of impact on the overall analysis, and difficulty of measurement and valuation. Decisions to exclude various relevant costs and benefits ought to be articulated in the study write-up, allowing recipients of the study findings to make their own judgments. Likewise, decisions to include specific costs and benefits should be articulated for the same evaluation purposes. Any cost or benefit that is believed to have a significant impact on the final results ought to be included, even if its measurement or valuation requires estimation.

Costs can be categorized in several ways. Drummond and colleagues (1987) suggest that costs are best thought of as resources being used up. As such, they identify two types or categories of costs that are relevant to family therapy: (1) organizing and operating costs, and (2) costs borne by clients and their families. Organizing and operating costs are associated with delivering the treatment program; they include therapist professional time, rent, equipment, and utilities. These costs are also referred to as "inputs" or "resources" for the intervention (Centers for Disease Control and Prevention, 1995).

Some of the costs borne by clients and their families are the out-of-pocket expenses incurred by the family members who are in treatment, as well as the value of other resources that are used to assist in the therapeutic process. Whereas out-of-pocket expenses are easily identified as monetary payments by family members toward the process of therapy (e.g., transportation expenses and child care), other resources in this category requiring attention are the opportunity costs, such as lost work time (a productivity loss) due to the treatment program. Some (Drummond et al., 1987) believe that psychological costs (e.g., pain and suffering of family members) ought to be measured and included in the assessment of costs borne by the client families.

Drummond and colleagues (1987) organize benefits into three categories: (1) changes in physical, social, and emotional functioning; (2) changes in resource use; and (3) changes in the quality of life of the client family members. The first category is traditionally the focus of outcome studies, where the emphasis is on objectively measuring the effects of treatment on client family members' physical, social, and emotional functioning. These changes refer to functioning ability rather than to the significance or value of the functioning.

The second category, changes in resource use, refers to both the client family members and their activities, and the broader societal sector. Client families experience benefits from therapy beyond functioning, in areas such as increased leisure time and reduced expenditures (e.g., on alcohol and drugs). These are benefits that can and should be measured and valued.

Resource use changes occur in the broader societal sector as well. A successful family violence program will reduce law enforcement requirements for both personnel and facilities. Successful alcohol abuse treatment programs positively affect law enforcement, hospital emergency rooms, vehicle insurance companies, and so forth. These resource use benefits must be considered when identifying relevant costs and benefits. If a benefit is determined relevant, attempts should be made at measurement and valuation.

The last category of benefits refers to the significance placed on the various functioning changes that occur as result of therapy. Consideration must be given to the relative value of a particular return to family functioning. Although such a value is difficult to quantify, we ought to recognize its existence. For example, a family that was previously debilitated because of a patriarchal, autocratic system but has reorganized on a more gender-equal, empowering basis has gained a lot more than just "functioning better." Attempts must be made to capture this "something extra."

In summary, from the various possible costs and benefits, a list of costs and benefits relevant to the study question is compiled. Each cost or benefit on the list is then reviewed for significance (i.e., the perceived magnitude of impact on the overall analysis), measurement viability (i.e., ability to reasonably measure the cost or benefit), and valuation possibility (i.e., likelihood that a valuation method can be determined). Typical costs included in family therapy outcome research are therapist fees, rent, supplies, and administrative overhead, while typical benefits include workplace productivity and reduced medical costs. The reasons for inclusion and the methodologies for measurement and valuation must be articulated in the study write-up. Exclusions of relevant costs and benefits should be justified in the write-up as well.

Example. As the objective of the managed care company in the opening scenario is to reduce overall claims, both the costs and benefits revolve around the claims data at the managed care company. SFTC family therapy claims and DTC individual therapy claims paid over the therapeutic time frame will be considered costs in this study. As previously indicated, both the number and total dollar amount of family mental health claims are considered benefits important to measure, because they specifically address the study question.

Address Time Value of Money with Discounting

The next step is to consider the effects of costs and benefits occurring at different times over the analytic horizon, and to make plans for addressing these "timing differences" in the analysis. According to the "time value of money" principle, a specific amount of money received today is worth more to the recipient than a like amount received at some later date. The reason is that the recipient can take what is received today and invest it. Having the invested (original) amount plus the earned interest is obviously worth more than receiving the original amount at the future date. The time value of money suggests that the recipient will be indifferent to receiving the original amount today or receiving the original amount plus interest at the future date. Monetary outflows (payments) can be viewed the same way but in the reverse. We would all rather make monetary outlays later rather than sooner, which also reflects the time value of money.

In the context of family therapy outcome research, benefits received today are assumed to be worth more than benefits received at a later date, and costs paid today are assumed to be more "costly" than costs paid in the future. The dilemma that must be addressed is how to compare a dollar of today's cost or benefit with a dollar of cost or benefit at a later date, since these dollars have different values. The business and economic communities solved this problem long ago with the concept of "discounting," whereby the future costs and benefits are adjusted by formula to allow for comparisons in the present. Discounting provides the opportunity to evaluate in the present a program's total costs and benefits, even though many of these costs and benefits will be realized in the future.

In structuring outcome research, it is important to recognize the timing of costs and benefits. Therefore, when cost and benefit data are gathered, the timing of the data relative to other data needs to be recorded, along with the actual data. Figure 18.2 is a hypothetical chart that addresses both relevant costs and benefits and the timing of their occurrence.

Discounting methodology is complicated and dependent on choosing appropriate formulas and factors. The details of discounting and all the issues surrounding this valuation issue are beyond the scope of this chapter, but are thoroughly outlined by others (Aos et al., 2001; Centers for Disease Control and Prevention, 1995; Drummond et al., 1987; Mackinnon, 1998; Pike-Urlacher et al., 1996).

Example. A chart similar to Figure 18.2 will be set up to record costs and benefits over the analytic horizon (2 years and 36 weeks).

Address Uncertainty with Sensitivity Analysis

Uncertainty and assumptions abound in economic evaluations. Decisions about the relevancy of certain costs and benefits are often based on assumptions. Although discounting and valuation methodologies have not been thoroughly addressed in this chapter, they are based more on assumptions than on fact. Whenever assumptions are essential to variable valuation, it is very important to test how changes in these assumptions affect the variable valuations and, in turn, the overall analysis results (Aos et al., 2001; Centers for Disease Control and Prevention, 1995). This assumption testing is known as "sensitivity analysis." It is appropriate to perform such testing on all aspects of economic evaluations, in order to determine the extent to which the findings are subject to variability. Sensitivity analysis is a common practice in the business world and will be expected by most target audiences of family therapy economic evaluations.

Sensitivity analysis can show that the study results are very dependent on certain assumptions that are tenuous at best. Varying these tenuous assumptions allows researchers and recipients of the study results to see how much influence these assumptions will have on the final results. Sensitivity analysis can either enhance the validity of the findings or reveal that the "true" results lie in a range too broad for meaningful conclusions to be drawn.

Costs and benefits	Month 1	Month 2	Month 3	Month 4	Month 5
Costs:					
Therapist fees	−20,000	−20,000	−20,000		
Total facilities cost	−1,000	−1,000	−1,000		
Transportation cost	−467	−467	−466		
Total costs	−21,467	−21,467	−21,466		
Benefits					
Increased productivity				10,000	20,000
Reduced need for hospitalization	50,000	50,000	50,000		
Total benefits	50,000	50,000	50,000	10,000	20,000

FIGURE 18.2. Hypothetical costs and benefits chart.

If, for example, the study includes the cost of therapists delivering a certain modality of treatment, an assumption about the therapists' fees will probably be made. It is appropriate in the final analysis to run the economic evaluation several times, using higher and lower therapist fee rates, to determine how sensitive the findings are to changes in therapist fees. Reporting these sensitivity findings allows the readers of the findings to determine whether therapists in their geographic location with their average fee schedules are likely to have the same economic outcome as presented in the findings.

Although uncertainty can be minimized, it must not be ignored in either the analysis or the presentation of study results. The full disclosure of assumptions and estimates is what allows the recipients of the study results to evaluate for themselves the usefulness of the study's conclusions. Others have discussed the various types of sensitivity analyses (Aos et al., 2001; Centers for Disease Control and Prevention, 1995; Drummond et al., 1987; Mackinnon, 1998; Office of Technology Assessment, 1980a; Pike-Urlacher et al., 1996).

Example. The proposed cost and benefit data in the opening scenario are relatively assumption-free. The discounting, on the other hand, will entail selecting a discount factor, which will be subject to speculation and assumptions. Information on market interest rates should be gathered in the study design phase, in order to generate a range of discount factors for sensitivity analysis use later in the study.

DISCUSSION

Summary of Economic Evaluations in Family Therapy Research

Few family therapy studies have reported full economic evaluation data, using Drummond and colleagues' (1987) categorizations of economic evaluations. The following studies are presented as family therapy research, to the extent that each incorporates some element of treatment in which two or more family members are included simultaneously.

Langsley, Pittman, Machotka, and Flomenhaft (1968) are credited with the first attempt at incorporating economic evaluations in the family therapy research field (Pike-Urlacher et al., 1996). They compared the costs of a standard inpatient treatment protocol for mentally ill patients who were traditionally hospitalized to those of a short-term, family-centered crisis therapy model that they had developed. Their study was designed to present just the costs of the alternative treatments, and thus it can be labeled a partial economic evaluation or a cost analysis (Drummond et al., 1987). Unfortunately, the perspectives and bases on which the costs of the alternative programs were different for each program, making the comparisons irrelevant. The standard treatment program costs were derived from direct cost data, whereas the family-centered therapy program costs were annual budget indirect costs. It was unclear who incurred the latter costs, or even whether they were ever incurred. In addition, many systemic costs were not addressed, while discounting and sensitivity analysis were ignored.

Azrin (1976) studied an alcohol treatment model that introduced an expanded treatment unit (i.e., a unit that included other family and/or community members). He measured the reduction in staff contact hours per client when clients participated in treatment with more community reinforcement. As with other studies, the cost data were severely limited, and benefits were not combined with the cost data for comparison purposes. Discounting and sensitivity analysis were not addressed in the findings presented.

Christensen, Johnson, Phillips, and Glascow (1980) compared individual and group behavioral family therapy and attempted to report the cost-effectiveness of each. They used only average professional time spent with each family to determine the cost figures per treatment modality. Numerous systemic cost areas were ignored, and the measured benefits (i.e., outcome measures) were not compared with the costs. Again, discounting and sensitivity analysis were not addressed in the findings presented.

Tarrier, Lowson, and Barrowclough (1991) evaluated the hypothesis that in spite of the increase of costs related to adding a behavioral family therapy component to the traditional treatment of schizophrenia, the overall costs (hospitalization, medication, and contact with mental health professionals) would be reduced. Only direct costs were gathered for two treatment alternatives studied. Broader systemic family costs were not addressed. The findings were not discounted, and sensitivity analysis was not conducted.

Although they did not specifically examine a family therapy treatment model, Chamberlain and Reid (1991) studied a specialized foster care program for youth who had been previous psychiatric hospital patients. Family therapy with each youth and his or her family was a small component of the program. Again, a partial economic evaluation was conducted, as only costs were reported. Costs beyond the direct program costs were not evaluated. Discounting and sensitivity analysis issues were not addressed.

Kinney, Haapala, and Booth (1991) reported on Homebuilders, the Tacoma, Washington, program that provides intensive in-home services for families where there is a high potential for out-of-home foster care placement of a difficult child, although this also is not a true family therapy program. They compared the Homebuilders program to more traditional foster care. The authors addressed just program costs and then only some of those costs. Benefits were not considered in relation to the costs. Bishop and McNally (1993) also reported on the Homebuilders program and provided cost data based on a reduction of average psychiatric hospital stays. Total cost savings were estimated for the number of hospital days saved by participating in the Homebuilders program. The key cost index, the cost of a hospital day, represented the cost of a general hospital day in the area rather than the cost of a psychiatric hospital day. There was no control group to validate the hospital stay estimate for a non-Homebuilders program family. Broader systemic costs were not gathered or identified, and again, discounting and sensitivity analysis were not performed.

Henggeler, Melton, and Smith (1992) looked at family preservation in juvenile offender families when comparing multisystemic therapy to traditional incarceration models of dealing with juvenile delinquency. As in previously described studies, systemic family costs were ignored, discounting was not addressed, and sensitivity analysis was not conducted.

Mikkelsen, Bereika, and McKenzie (1993) looked at a short-term mentoring program that included a family therapy component as an alternative to psychiatric hospitalization for children and adolescents. Only the costs of these treatment programs were considered; data on benefits, which were collected, were not combined with the cost data to present a full economic evaluation. The results were not adjusted for the time value of money (i.e., discounting), nor were they subjected to sensitivity analysis.

Cunningham, Bremner, and Boyle (1995) compared a large-group, community-based parent training program with a clinic-based, individual parent training program. Costs were measured and reported, but there was no attempt to connect them with the program benefits. The authors did a good job of identifying a number of the costs associated with the respective programs. Unfortunately, they did not specify the study perspective from which the analysis was taking place, so the measured costs and benefits might or might not be relevant to the recipients of the study results. These results also lacked discounting and sensitivity analysis.

Simmons and Doherty (1995) presented a cost description (Drummond et al., 1987) of the average cost of marital therapy. This form of partial economic evaluation does not attempt to compare costs with benefits, or to compare therapeutic alternatives with other treatment modalities. Simmons and Doherty surmised that marital therapy was less expensive than divorce proceedings, but they only appealed to common assumptions about the cost of divorce for comparison purposes. No attempts were made to gather costs of marital therapy beyond the clinician fees. There were no benefits data, so costs and benefits could not be combined for analysis. Likewise, discounting and sensitivity analysis were not conducted.

Schoenwald, Ward, Henggeler, Pickrel, and Patel (1996) compared the costs of multisystemic therapy to those of the usual outpatient local state-sponsored programs for adolescents with substance abuse or dependence. Full economic evaluation was not conducted, but a well-documented cost analysis was reported. A difference from other studies was that a sensitivity analysis was conducted to assess the impact of treatment cost variations on the initial findings. As in other studies, however, the study perspective was not clearly identified, and discounting and systemic costs and benefits were not addressed.

Sexton and Alexander (2000) compared the cost data of functional family therapy, short-term (30-day) detention, and longer-term (90-day) residential treatment for delinquent and violent adolescents. They presented a basic cost analysis rather than a full economic evaluation. The study perspective, discounting, sensitivity analysis, and systemic costs and benefits were not addressed.

A few family therapy studies have attempted to incorporate full economic evaluations. Cardin, McGill, and Falloon (1985) described a family therapy study incorporating CBA and CEA. Cardin and colleagues evaluated family management in the context of community care of schizophrenia versus individual management. They did an excellent job of outlining the differences between CBA and CEA, as they conducted both types of analysis. The authors identified the relevant direct and indirect costs and benefits that ought to be measured, and then demonstrated how to collect the data. They did not discount their findings, however, nor did they conduct a sensitivity analysis to test the robustness of their findings.

Lipsey (1984) presented an adjusted CBA for a family-based juvenile delinquency prevention program. He designed a study to determine returns on investments in juvenile delinquency prevention programs by measuring both the direct costs of the program and the cost savings associated with preventing future acts of delinquency. The cost savings consisted of the direct costs of an arrest times an estimate of the number of arrests saved due to the prevention program, plus a valuation of the effect of an act of juvenile delinquency on potential victims times an estimate of the number of acts of juvenile delinquency saved due to the prevention program. Lipsey divided the cost savings by the program costs to generate a cost differential or a cost–benefit ratio. He then performed two operations on the cost differential. First, since a prevention program was offered to both "at-risk" youth and "not-at-risk" youth simultaneously, he adjusted the cost differential by a ratio of an estimated delinquency risk times a historical rate of success of delinquency prevention programs ("success" being defined as at-risk youth choosing not to engage in future delinquent acts). He wanted to deflate the results to reflect the actual impact of the program, which would be overstated when not-at-risk youth were included. Second, Lipsey conducted extensive sensitivity analysis to test the breadth of the results. The time value of money was not addressed, nor were systemic benefits (i.e., cost savings) beyond the victims. This study does represent a fine example of CBA and sensitivity analysis.

An excellent example of CEA is the analysis by Holder, Longabaugh, Miller, and Rubonis (1991) of the cost-effectiveness of alcoholism treatments. These researchers compared both the costs and the effectiveness of multiple alcohol treatment modalities. Holder and colleagues generated a matrix of evidence-based effectiveness (good, fair, indeterminate, no, and insufficient evidence) and costs (minimal, low, medium-low, medium-high, and high), and plotted various treatments (e.g., brief motivational counseling, Alcoholics Anonymous, behavior contracting, marital behavioral therapy, and psychotropic medication). The description and methodology for collecting cost data were excellent. The stated objective of this study was to create a relative comparison of cost effectiveness of treatment modalities, rather than to provide an accurate computation of the cost of each treatment modality. The study perspective was not overtly discussed, but the methodology leads the reader to the researchers' intent. Discounting, sensitivity analysis, and systemic costs and effects were not considered.

O'Farrell and colleagues (1996b) conducted an economic evaluation of behavioral couple therapy with and without relapse prevention sessions for persons with alcoholism and their spouses. This study presented both CBA and CEA, with excellent explanations and rationales of the costs and benefits measured and valued. The perspective of the study was not clearly defined, but several perspectives could be accommodated in the data collected and presented. Costs and benefits beyond program, hospital, halfway house, and jail costs and cost savings were not addressed for the CBA. The effectiveness data (percentage of days abstinent and couple Marital Adjustment Test scores) gathered for the CEA also ignored systemic effects. Moreover, discounting and sensitivity analysis issues were not addressed. Still, in spite of the gaps in this study's analysis, it is one of the most thorough economic evaluations presented in couple and family therapy research.

O'Farrell and colleagues (1996a) also conducted an economic evaluation in conjunction with their comparison of behavioral couple therapy plus individual treatment, interactional couple therapy plus individual treatment, and individual therapy alone for alcoholism. As in the preceding study, O'Farrell and colleagues presented both CBA and CEA. Their explanations for the measured costs and benefits were excellent. Also as in the preceding study, the perspective was not specifically identified, and systemic costs and benefits were not measured. Discounting and sensitivity analysis continued to be absent as well.

In Fals-Stewart, O'Farrell, and Birchler's (1997) analysis of behavioral couple therapy and individually based treatment with substance-abusing male patients, they conducted both CBA and CEA. They were very thorough in their description of the study design and the justifications of the various costs and benefits measured. Unlike other researchers, they identified a study perspective. As in other studies, however, discounting, sensitivity analysis, and systemic costs and benefits were not addressed.

Aos and colleagues (2001) conducted the most complete CBA on crime offender treatment to date. They looked at the economics of various programs designed to reduce crime from the perspective of taxpayers and crime victims. Included in their analyses was functional family therapy. Aos and colleagues did not conduct the original efficacy research, but took studies published in the last 25 years and applied sound CBA methodology to them. Not only was the target audience identified, but the study perspective was made clear as well. The descriptions of costs and benefits and the techniques of gathering them were well articulated. Unlike the authors of all other studies discussed here, Aos and colleagues attempted to capture societal/systemic costs and benefits. Although the attempt was substantial and not completely quantifiable, they provided thorough explanations of their assumptions and estimates. Marginal and incremental costs were also evaluated, in addition to discounting. Lastly, sensitivity analysis was conducted on the findings to determine how robust they were. All family therapy researchers conducting economic evaluations ought to review this presentation before starting their research.

French and colleagues (2002) conducted a thorough CEA of adolescent drug treatment as a part of the Cannabis Youth Treatment Study. Using the methodology developed by French, Dunlap, Zarkin, McGeary, and McLellan (1997), these researchers compared the cost effectiveness of two family-based treatments (multidimensional family therapy and family support network) with the National Treatment Improvement Study data. Costs and benefits were well defined, as were the collection methodologies. Although not specifically discussed, the study perspective was clear. Attempts to gather systemic data, discounting, and sensitivity analysis were not undertaken.

Sheidow and colleagues (in press) compared the cost of multisystemic therapy and hospitalization for youths in psychiatric crisis. These researchers conducted a very complete CEA, with excellent discussions of the costs to be measured, the methodology of data collection, and their results. Although a target audience was not specifically identified, the study perspective was addressed. Discounting, sensitivity analysis, and systemic costs and benefits were not discussed.

Future Directions

The intent of this chapter is to outline the integration of economic evaluation study design methodology with family therapy outcome research. Not unexpectedly, several study design issues arise that ought to be discussed and debated among family therapy researchers. The following is a brief listing of these issues.

The first area that needs additional exploration is that of target audiences. Who constitute the target audiences on whom family therapy research should focus? Are there high-priority audiences that should be addressed before others? As Table 18.2 suggests, there are several broad categories of target audiences. Ideally, researchers should determine in greater specificity and detail who these audiences are.

Once a more thorough effort is made to identify appropriate target audiences for family therapy research, the question "What information is relevant to each potential target audience?" needs to be addressed. The greater the understanding of what data various audiences want when making resource allocation decisions, the more readily study questions can be designed to deliver relevant, useful information.

Defining a target audience for study findings raises the issue of research bias. In spite of the importance of identifying a target recipient of the research results, does such a determination potentially contaminate the research? How do we protect against designing studies to find the findings we want? Any cost accountant knows that in spite of sensitivity analysis to test assumptions, economic evaluations can be structured to deliver any results a researcher wants if he or she knows how to "work the numbers." In taking the approach that our economic evaluation has a specific audience in mind and the study results are to assist in a resource allocation decision, are we really becoming salespersons rather than researchers? Finally, what safeguards or standards need to be developed to ensure the integrity of family therapy economic evaluation research?

A basic premise in full economic evaluations is that alternative forms of treatment are being compared. What if there is no cooperative opportunity to do a comparative analysis? In other words, there are likely to be times when data are not readily available for competing treatment modalities. What do we researchers do in this instance? Is there a way to collect competing programs' data without their specific cooperation? What form should economic evaluations take if the data are not forthcoming? It may be possible to force the issue by repeatedly presenting family therapy cost–outcome descriptions and challenging competing treatment modalities to do the same. Several of the target audiences may take up the cause and request the same information. Nonetheless, it is important to decide proactively how we will proceed with economic evaluation in the absence of competing treatment data.

The implications of family therapy's systemic perspective on economic evaluations also need to be explored. In setting up a study, how far from the immediate presenting family ought costs and benefits to be collected? When the target audience is interested in the economic effects of treatment on "the family," decisions must be made about what "the family" is and what information ought to be collected. What is the appropriate analytic horizon? In other words, when should the effects of family therapy be deemed to be indistinguishable from all other life experiences? Despite our strong beliefs that relational patterns, both positive and negative, are transferred from generation to generation, how do we gather data in a timely manner to prove or disprove, family therapy's multigenerational effectiveness and cost-effectiveness? Assuming that as researchers we must determine and value future costs and benefits because of the systemic and generational effects of therapy, how do we do it? What data need to be collected now in order to extrapolate to the future?

The ethics of economic evaluation research need to be addressed as well. Data collection standards ought to be reviewed as we family therapy researchers attempt to gather information that we may have previously ignored. What are the ethical issues connected with a target audience's funding of economic evaluation research? Should funding standards be set, and if so, by whom? As economic evaluation data are written up, are there ethical issues in the way findings are presented? Since numbers can readily be manipulated to say anything anyone wants, standards should be addressed. It may also be appropriate to set guidelines for the information that ought to be included in reports of findings, so that overall credibility is established, enhanced, and maintained with the targeted recipients of our research results.

Lastly, it is appropriate to explore gender, racial, and cultural biases that may be inherent in economic evaluation methodology. There is a void in the literature in all fields regarding potential biases in economic evaluation. It would be consistent with our efforts as family therapists to promote respect and dignity for all humankind to address potential biases in this methodology before anyone else does.

CONCLUSIONS

In these times of increasingly scarce resources, economic evaluations in family therapy research are important to the long-term viability of the field as a whole. Those who pay for the treatment family therapists provide are interested in both the effectiveness and cost-effectiveness of treatment. Effectiveness and efficacy studies show that in many instances family therapy is more effective than competing treatment modalities. Presently, family therapy studies that report full economic evaluation findings are becoming more common, but still lag behind those in other therapy research fields.

This chapter presents a systematic approach for designing a full economic evaluation as part of or as a follow-up to family therapy outcome research. In designing an economic evaluation study question, all the issues outlined must be addressed in the order in which they are presented in this chapter. This methodological imperative ensures the integrity of the results and thereby the usefulness of the findings to the decision-making recipients of the study. The success of economic evaluations in family therapy outcome research is dependent on the resulting information's relevancy to a particular decision-making process. The study design phase of economic evaluations is critical to ensuring that the research findings are relevant and useful. Care taken at the beginning of this process will pay significant dividends in the end.

EXEMPLARS

Aos, S., Phipps, P., Barnoski, R., & Lieb, R. (2001). *The comparative costs and benefits of programs to reduce crime* (Document No. 01-05-1201). Olympia: Washington State Institute for Public Policy.

Cardin, B., McGill, C. W., & Falloon, I. R. H. (1985). An economic analysis: Costs, benefits, and effectiveness. In I. R. H. Falloon (Ed.), *Family management of schizophrenia: A study of clinical, social, family, and economic benefits*. Baltimore: Johns Hopkins University Press.

French, M. T., Roebuck, M. C., Dennis, M. L., Diamond, G., Godley, S. H., Tims, F., et al. (2002). The economic cost of outpatient marijuana treatment for adolescents: Findings from a multi-site field experiment. *Addiction, 97*(Suppl. 1), 84–97.

Holder, H., Longabaugh, R, Miller, W. R., & Rubonis, N. V. (1991). The cost effectiveness of treatment for alcoholism: A first approximation. *Journal of Studies on Alcohol, 52*(6), 517–536.

Lipsey, M. W. (1984). Is delinquency prevention a cost effective strategy?: A California perspective. *Journal of Research in Crime and Delinquency, 21*(4), 279–302.

REFERENCES

Aderman, J., Bowers, M., Russell, T., & Wegmann, N. (1993, October). *Making the cut: Family therapists and managed care*. Panel discussion presented at the annual conference of the American Association for Marriage and Family Therapy, Anaheim, CA.

Aos, S., Phipps, P., Barnoski, R., & Lieb, R. (2001). *The comparative costs and benefits of programs to reduce crime* (Document No. 01-05-1201). Olympia: Washington State Institute for Public Policy.

Azrin, H. G. (1976). Improvements in the community reinforcement approach to alcoholism. *Behaviour Research and Therapy, 14*, 339–348.

Bishop, E. G., & McNally, B. (1993). An in-home crisis intervention program for children and their families. *Hospital and Community Psychiatry, 44*, 182–184.

Cardin, B., McGill, C. W., & Falloon, I. R. H. (1985). An economic analysis: Costs, benefits, and effectiveness. In I. R. H. Falloon (Ed.), *Family management of schizophrenia: A study of clinical, social, family, and economic benefits*. Baltimore: Johns Hopkins University Press.

Centers for Disease Control and Prevention. (1995). *A practical guide to prevention effectiveness: Decision and economic analysis*. Springfield, VA: U.S. Department of Commerce, National Technical Information Service.

Chamberlain, P., & Reid, J. B. (1991). Using a specialized foster care treatment model for children and adolescents leaving the state mental hospital. *Journal of Community Psychology, 19*, 266–276.

Christensen, A., Johnson, S. M., Phillips, S., & Glascow, R. E. (1980). Cost effectiveness in family therapy. *Behavior Therapy, 11*, 208–226.

Cunningham, D. E., Bremner, R., & Boyle, M. (1995). Large group community-based parenting programs for families of preschoolers at risk for disruptive behavior disorders: Utilization, cost-effectiveness, and outcome. *Journal of Child Psychology and Psychiatry, 36*, 1141–1159.

Drummond, M. F., Stoddart, G. L., & Torrance, G. W. (1987). *Methods for the economic evaluation of health care programmes*. New York: Oxford University Press.

French, M. T., Dunlap, L. J., Zarkin, G. A., McGeary, K. A., & McLellan, A. T. (1997). A structured instrument for estimating the economic cost of drug abuse treatment: The Drug Abuse Treatment Cost Analysis Program (DATCAP). *Journal of Substance Abuse Treatment, 14*, 1–11.

French, M. T., Roebuck, M. C., Dennis, M. L., Diamond, G., Godley, S. H., Tims, F., et al. (2002). The economic cost of outpatient marijuana treatment for adolescents: Findings from a multi-site field experiment. *Addiction, 97*(Suppl. 1), 84–97.

French, M. T., Zarkin, G. A., & Bray, J. W. (1995). A methodology for evaluating the costs and benefits of employee assistance programs. *Journal of Drug Issues, 25*(2), 451–470.

Glass, N. J., & Goldberg, D. (1977). Cost–benefit analysis and the evaluation of psychiatric services. *Psychological Medicine, 7*, 701–707.

Halpern, J. (1977). Program evaluation, systems theory, and output value analysis: A benefit/cost model. In R. D. Coursey (Ed.), *Program evaluation for mental health*. New York: Grune & Stratton.

Henggeler, S. W., Melton, G. B., & Smith, L. A. (1992). Family preservation using multisystemic therapy: An effective alternative to incarcerating serious juvenile offenders. *Journal of consulting and Clinical Psychology, 60*, 953–961.

Holder, H., Longabaugh, R., Miller, W. R., & Rubonis, N. V. (1991). The cost effectiveness of treatment for alcoholism: A first approximation. *Journal of Studies on Alcohol, 52*(6), 517–536.

Kee, J. E. (1994). Benefit–cost analysis in program evaluation. In J. S. Wholey, H. P. Hatry, & K. E. Newcomer (Eds.), *Handbook of practical program evaluation*. San Francisco: Jossey-Bass.

Kiesler, C. A. (1980). Mental health policy as a field of inquiry for psychology. *American Psychologist, 35*, 1066–1080.

Kinney, J., Haapala, D., & Booth, C. (1991). *Keeping families together: The Homebuilders model*. New York: Aldine de Gruyter.

Krupnick, J. L., & Pincus, J. A. (1992). The cost-effectiveness of psychotherapy: A plan for research. *American Journal of Psychiatry, 149,* 1295–1305.

Langsley, D. G., Pittman,F. S., III, Machotka, P., & Flomenhaft, K. (1968). Family crisis therapy: Results and implications. *Family Process, 7*(2), 145–158.

Leitch, L. (1993, May–June). Judgment day for health care. *Family Therapy Networker,* pp. 65–68.

Levin, H. M. (1975). Cost-effectiveness analysis in evaluation research. In M. Guttentag & E. L Struening (Eds.), *Handbook of evaluation research.* Beverly Hills, CA: Sage.

Lipsey, M. W. (1984). Is delinquency prevention a cost effective strategy?: A California perspective. *Journal of Research in Crime and Delinquency, 21*(4), 279–302.

Mackinnon, D. (1998). *Economic evaluations in marital and family therapy outcome research: Methodologies and applications.* Unpublished doctoral dissertation, Purdue University.

Masters, S., Garfinkel, I., & Bishop, J. (1978). Benefit–cost analysis in program evaluation. *Journal of Social Science Research, 2,* 19–93.

Maynard, A. (1993a). Are mental health services efficient? *International Journal of Mental Health, 22*(3), 3–32.

Maynard, A. (1993b). Cost management: The economist's viewpoint. *British Journal of Psychiatry, 163*(20), 7–13.

McCollum, E. E., & Stith, S. M. (2002). Leaving the ivory tower: An introduction to the special section on doing marriage and family therapy research in community agencies. *Journal of Marital and Family Therapy, 28*(1), 5–7.

Menninger, R. W. (1977). Psychiatric treatment: What is quality and how do you measure it? *Bulletin of the Menninger Clinic, 41,* 181–190.

Mikkelsen, E. J., Bereika, G. M., & McKenzie, J. C. (1993). Short-term family-based residential treatment: An alternative to psychiatric hospitalization for children. *American Journal of Orthopsychiatry, 63,* 28–33.

O'Farrell, T. J., Choquette, K. A., Cutter, H. S. G., Brown, E., Bayog, R., McCourt, W., et al. (1996a). Cost–benefit and cost-effectiveness analyses of behavioral marital therapy as an addition to outpatient alcoholism treatment. *Journal of Substance Abuse, 8,* 145–166.

O'Farrell, T. J., Choquette, K. A., Cutter, H. S. G., Brown, E., Bayog, R., McCourt, W., et al. (1996b). Cost–benefit and cost-effectiveness analyses of behavioral marital therapy with and without relapse prevention sessions for alcoholics and their spouses. *Behavior Therapy, 27,* 7–24.

O'Farrell, T. J., & Fals-Stewart, W. (2003). Alcohol abuse. *Journal of Marital and Family Therapy, 29*(1), 121–146.

Office of Technology Assessment. (1980a). *The implications of cost-effectiveness analysis of medical technology: Background Paper 1. Methodological issues and literature review.* Washington, DC: U.S. Government Printing Office.

Office of Technology Assessment. (1980b). *The implications of cost-effectiveness analysis of medical technology: Background Paper 3. The efficacy and cost effectiveness of psychotherapy.* Washington, DC: U.S. Government Printing Office.

Panzetta, A. F. (1973). Cost–benefit studies in psychiatry. *Comprehensive Psychiatry, 14*(5), 451–455.

Pike, C. L., & Piercy, F. P. (1990). Cost effectiveness research in family therapy. *Journal of Marital and Family Therapy, 16,* 375–388.

Pike-Urlacher, C. L., Mackinnon, D. P., & Piercy, F. P. (1996). Cost-effectiveness research in family therapy. In D. H. Sprenkle & S. M. Moon (Eds.), *Research methods in family therapy* (pp. 365–387). New York: Guilford Press.

Pinsof, W. M., & Wynne, L. C. (1995a). The effectiveness and efficacy of marital and family therapy: An empirical overview, conclusions, and recommendations. *Journal of Marital and Family Therapy, 21*(4), 341–343.

Pinsof, W. M., & Wynne, L. C. (1995b). The effectiveness and efficacy of marital and family therapy: Introduction to the special issue. *Journal of Marital and Family Therapy, 21*(4), 585–613.

Schoenwald, S. K., Ward, D. M., Henggeler, S. W., Pickrel, S. G., & Patel, H. (1996). Multisystemic therapy treatment of substance abusing or dependent adolescent offenders: Costs of reducing incarceration, inpatient and residential placement. *Journal of Child and Family Studies, 5*, 431–444.

Sexton, T. L., & Alexander, J. F. (2000, December). Functional family therapy. *Juvenile Justice Bulletin*, pp. 1–7.

Sheidow, A. J., Bradford, W. D., Henggeler, S. W., Rowland, M. D., Halliday-Boykins, C., Schoenwald, S. K., et al. (in press). Treatment costs for youths in psychiatric crisis: Multisystemic therapy versus hospitalization. *Psychiatric Services.*

Simmons, D. S., & Doherty, W. J. (1995). Defining who we are and what we do: Clinical practice of marriage and family therapists in Minnesota. *Journal of Marital and Family Therapy, 21*, 3–16.

Spivack, G., St. Clair, C. H., Siegel, J., & Platt, J. (1975). Differing perspectives on mental health evaluation. *American Journal of Psychiatry, 132*, 1295–1299.

Sprenkle, D. H. (Ed.). (2002). *Effectiveness research in marriage and family research.* Alexandria, VA: American Association for Marriage and Family Therapy.

Sprenkle, D. H., & Bailey, C. E. (1995). Editors' introduction. *Journal of Marital and Family Therapy, 21*(4), 339–340.

Steinglass, P. (1996). Family therapy's future. *Family Process, 35*(4), 403–405.

Tarrier, N., Lowson, K., & Barrowclough, C. (1991). Some aspects of family interventions in schizophrenia: II. Financial considerations. *British Journal of Psychiatry, 159*, 481–484.

Thompson, M. W., & Fortess, E. E. (1980). Cost-effectiveness analysis in health program evaluation. *Evaluation Review, 4*(4), 549–568.

Weinstein, S. M. (1986). Cost-effectiveness analysis in mental health. *Canadian Journal of Community Mental Health, 5*(1), 77–88.

Weisbrod, B. A. (1981). Benefit cost analysis of a controlled experiment: Treating the mentally ill. *Journal of Human Resources, 16*(4), 543–568.

Weisbrod, B. A., Test, M. A., & Stein, L. I. (1980). Alternative to mental hospital treatment: II. Economic benefit–cost analysis. *Archives of General Psychiatry, 37*, 400–405.

Wortman, P. M. (1983). Evaluation research: A methodological perspective. *Annual Review of Psychology, 34*, 223–260.

Yates, B. T. (1985). Cost-effectiveness analysis and cost–benefit analysis: An introduction. *Behavioral Assessment, 7*, 207–234.

Yates, B. T. (1996). *Analyzing costs, procedures, processes, and outcomes in human services.* Thousand Oaks, CA: Sage.

Yates, B. T. (1997). Formative evaluation of costs, cost-effectiveness, and cost–benefit: Toward cost procedure process outcome analysis. In L. Bickman & D. Rog (Eds.), *Handbook of applied social research methods.* Thousand Oaks, CA: Sage.

Yates, B. T. (1999). *Measuring and improving cost, cost-effectiveness, and cost–benefit for substance abuse treatment programs.* Rockville, MD: National Institute on Drug Abuse,

Yates, B. T. (2000). Cost–benefit analysis and cost-effectiveness analysis. In A. Kazdin (Ed.), *Encyclopedia of psychology.* Washington, DC: American Psychological Association.

Yates, B. T., & Newman, F. L. (1980). Approaches to cost-effectiveness analysis and cost–benefit analysis of psychotherapy. In G. Vanderbos (Ed.), *Psychotherapy: Practice, research, policy.* Beverly Hills, CA: Sage.

CHAPTER 19

Approaches to Prediction

CORRELATION, REGRESSION, AND CLASSIFICATION TECHNIQUES

DOUGLAS K. SNYDER
LAUREL F. MANGRUM

BACKGROUND

Philosophical Assumptions

In many ways, scientific understanding of couples and families progresses in a manner similar to children's knowledge of their surrounding world. Like a child's first impression of a parent, science begins with an awareness of some phenomenon not yet understood but sensed to be important for further exploration. Exploration leads to efforts to refine the ability to recognize and define instances of occurrence and nonoccurrence, and this ability promotes efforts to quantify. Like the child's insight that parents provide nurturance, science progresses with the recognition that certain phenomena go hand in hand; the occurrence of one denotes the likelihood of the other, the absence of one the improbability of the other. It is this recognition of covariation between events that precedes the last stage of understanding, reflected in the ability to influence or control one phenomenon by manipulating another. Thus awareness leads to exploration, exploration to measurement, measurement to observation of covariation, and covariation to manipulation and influence.

We do not mean to imply by this proposed progression that marital and family dynamics are either singular or unidirectional. Most phenomena are influenced by multiple other phenomena, and directions of influence are often recursive: *A* affects *B*, and *B* affects *A*. Nor does this progression acclaim quantitative approaches to the exclusion of qualitative ones; Cavell and Snyder (1991) have argued elsewhere that both play critical roles in the generation and verification of knowledge. Indeed, efforts to delineate covariation with quantitative techniques often proceed best when the phenomena selected for study have been identified through intensive qualitative methods. Rather, we propose that prediction strategies based on correlation and related procedures provide a useful bridge between observation of existing phenomena—whether qualitatively or quantitatively based—and attempts to modify the same.

Historical Roots and Development

Science based on covariation is as timeless as civilization. The recognition that seasons covary with celestial patterns prompted early astronomy as a basis for predicting optimal occasions for planting. Quantitative techniques emphasizing covariation took hold in the behavioral sciences in the late 1800s with the efforts of Sir Francis Galton, an English biologist, to establish an anthropometric laboratory in order to accumulate a systematic body of data on individual differences. Galton (1888), whose interest lay in the heritability of physical and simple psychological functions, suggested principles of the correlation coefficient as a method of expressing the extent to which two variables covary. Karl Pearson (1896), Galton's student, operationalized the product–moment correlation coefficient, now known as the "Pearson r." The investigation of individual differences and covariation of abilities in both Europe (Binet & Simon, 1905; Spearman, 1910) and the United States (Cattell, 1890; Terman, 1916; Thurstone, 1947) anticipated advanced correlational techniques of multiple-regression analysis and factor analysis, which were already well established by 1950. It was Terman's initial interest in individuals with distinguished intellectual abilities that subsequently led to his use of correlation in a study of psychological factors predicting marital happiness (Terman, 1938).

METHODOLOGY

Overview

In this chapter, we emphasize the use of correlation and related techniques to examine factors contributing to marital distress and couples' response to marital therapy. Throughout our discussion, we draw heavily on examples linking depression and relationship difficulties. Our emphasis on depression and marital unhappiness derives partly from convenience (specifically, our previous research efforts in this area) and partly from the literature. The co-occurrence of depressed affect and marital distress has been examined from a broad range of theoretical perspectives and correlational techniques. Numerous studies have identified marital distress as a vulnerability factor, precipitant, concomitant, consequence, and potentiator of depression (cf. Beach & Gupta, 2003; Whisman & Uebelacker, 2003). For example, in evaluating the association between marital distress and psychiatric disorders in an epidemiological sample of 2,538 married persons, Whisman (1999) noted that compared to nondistressed partners, maritally distressed individuals were 3.2 times more likely to experience major depression and 5.7 times as likely to experience dysthymia. Depression in one or both spouses has been found to predict poorer response to marital therapy (Sher, Baucom, & Larus, 1990; Snyder, Mangrum, & Wills, 1993); similarly, marital distress is associated with a slower recovery in treatment for depression (Goering, Lancee, & Freeman, 1992) and a greater likelihood of relapse (e.g., Hooley & Teasdale, 1989; Whisman, 2001).

Our presentation of methodology is divided into two major sections. The first section, reviewing basic techniques, begins with a brief discussion of the kinds of data lending themselves to correlational analysis. Assumptions underlying correlation, techniques of computation, and associated interpretive issues are examined at length, because these also apply to more advanced techniques derived from correlation. The relation of correlation to prediction is examined via simple linear regression. "Third variables" affecting correlation coefficients are discussed in terms of moderator and suppressor variables and from the perspective of partial correlations. These concepts are extended to the technique of multiple-regression analysis, involving two or more predictors. The second major section introduces more advanced techniques used in prediction. Canonical-correlation analysis offers an approach for relating multiple predictors to multiple criteria. Multiple-discriminant-function (MDF) analysis relates multiple predictors to a single criterion measured on a nominal or ordinal scale. Finally, cluster analysis is described as a method of classifying individuals into distinct groups, based on their similarity across multiple dimensions. Throughout our presentation, the emphasis is on conceptual rather than statistical understanding of these research methodologies.

Basic Techniques

Measurement Levels and Distributions

What measurement characteristics are important to consider in correlation? Variables can typically be considered as being measured at one of four levels, each progressively more demanding in terms of data requirements and more generous in terms of potential analytic procedures (Stevens, 1946). At the simplest level are "nominal" scales, by which events are grouped into discrete classes for which no assumptions regarding order or distance are made; examples include classifying individuals by ethnicity or marital status. At the next level are "ordinal" scales, by which individuals are grouped into discrete classes presumed to reflect rank order; examples include classifying individuals by socioeconomic status (low, middle, high) or by family life stage (childless, oldest child less than 5 years old, and so on). Lacking in ordinal scales is information about the "distance" or degree of difference between categories.

"Interval-level" scales imply not only that classes are ordered by rank, but also that the distances between categories are defined in terms of fixed and equal units. Examples include typical measures of relationship satisfaction, such as the Dyadic Adjustment Scale (DAS; Spanier, 1976) or the Marital Satisfaction Inventory—Revised (MSI-R; Snyder, 1997). Interval-level scales may be discrete (e.g., indicating level of marital happiness by circling 1 of 7 points on a scale anchored by "extremely unhappy" on one end and "extremely happy" on the other) or continuous (e.g., indicating level of marital happiness along the same scale by marking an "X" anywhere along the line). Finally, "ratio-level" scales have all the properties of interval-level scales plus a meaningful "zero point" inherently defined by the measurement scheme and construct. Examples of ratio-level scales include length of marriage or number of agreements expressed during a 5-minute discussion. Ratio-level scales permit proportional comparisons (e.g., a husband may express twice as many agreements as his wife), whereas interval-level scales do not (e.g., one would not describe a wife as being "twice as maritally happy" as her husband).

Levels of measurement have important implications for the kinds of analytic procedures that can be applied to the data. For example, assessing covariation between variables measured along nominal or ordinal scales requires nonparametric approaches (e.g., chi-square or rank-order correlations), whereas variables measured using interval- or ratio-level scales lend themselves to more powerful parametric approaches, including product–moment correlation (Pearson r) and regression. Variables measured as dichotomies present special consideration in correlation and related techniques, depending on whether the underlying construct is viewed as dichotomous (e.g., using "husband" and "wife" to reflect gender) or continuous (e.g., using "divorced" vs. "still married" to reflect effectiveness of marital therapy). For most correlational procedures, dichotomies can be treated as interval-level measures.

In addition to level of measurement, different approaches to assessing covariation make different assumptions about the manner in which observations on some variable are "dispersed" or distributed around the center of those observations. For example, the Pearson correlation coefficient assumes that each of the two variables being related are continuous, and that measurement error for each is normally distributed; normal distributions are those reflecting the familiar "bell-shaped" curve. Variables whose distributions deviate significantly from normality may require less powerful, non-parametric approaches to examining covariation.

Correlation

CONCEPTUAL BASIS

At its simplest level, correlation denotes the extent to which two variables "co-relate" or covary. For example, do high levels of depressed affect go hand in hand with high levels of marital distress? It is important to emphasize that correlation reflects only association, not causality. For example, depression may contribute to marital distress, or marital distress may contribute to depression, or each may contribute to the other, or each may be influenced by some third variable or set of variables, or all of these things may be true. The propensity to attribute causality to correlational findings constitutes probably the most frequent and conceptually most problematic interpretive error in the use of correlation and related techniques.

Correlations can be depicted graphically, as in Figure 19.1. In this example, individuals are each measured on two variables: depression (abbreviated in this and other figures as DEP) and global marital distress (abbreviated in the figures as GDS). For each variable, the distribution of subjects' scores can be summarized by using two statistics: (1) a measure of central tendency (typically the arithmetic mean), and (2) a measure of dispersion (typically the variance or standard deviation). In Figure 19.1, each circle or sphere denotes the variability of subjects on the corresponding variable. The covariability of observations, or covariance (i.e., the extent to which high scores on one variable systematically denote either high or low scores on the other), is indicated by the area of the two circles' overlap.

Pearson's product–moment correlation is simply a "standardized" index of covariation that ranges from -1.0 to $+1.0$. If two variables have a correlation of 1.0, then high scores on one variable covary perfectly with high scores on the other; if they have a correlation of -1.0, then high scores on one variable covary perfectly with low scores on the other. In either case, the two circles in Figure 19.1 would overlap completely. By contrast, a correlation of .00 would indicate a complete absence of covariation between the two variables, and their corresponding circles in Figure 19.1 would not overlap at all. The amount of overlap depicted between depression (DEP) and global marital distress (GDS) in Figure 19.1 denotes a correlation of approximately .60.

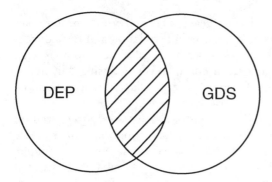

FIGURE 19.1. Simple correlation between depression (DEP) and global marital distress (GDS).

According to the guidelines suggested by Cohen (1988), correlations of approximately .40, .25, and .10 can be regarded as reflecting "large," "medium," and "small" effects, respectively. However, the strength of association between two variables is best inferred not by the correlation coefficient itself, but rather by the *squared* correlation coefficient. Specifically, the squared correlation between two variables reflects the percentage of variance (variability of observations about the mean) in one variable that can be explained or predicted by knowledge of individuals' variance (or variability in scores) in the other variable. In Figure 19.1, if the correlation between DEP and GDS is .60, then 36% of the variability in individuals' scores on the depression measure can be explained by their scores on the measure of global marital distress. (Similarly, 36% of the variability in marital distress can be predicted by individuals' scores on depression.)

The squared correlation coefficient constitutes the most prevalent but fairly rigorous interpretation regarding the *meaningfulness* (rather than statistical significance) of one's findings. (For contrasting views, see Abelson, 1985, and Ozer, 1985.) For example, correlations approaching .70 in absolute magnitude explain only half the variance (49%) in one variable from another; more common correlations in the research literature, ranging from .30 to .40, permit explanation or prediction of only 10% to 15% of the variability in one variable from the other.

ASSUMPTIONS

What requirements should the data satisfy before correlational techniques are used? Nunnally and Bernstein (1994) list three assumptions underlying use of the Pearson product–moment correlation. First, the relation between the two variables should be monotonic (consistently positive or consistently negative), and preferably linear (see Figure 19.2). Although prediction models can be derived for nonlinear relations, the Pearson *r* is not appropriate to these situations. For example, Figure 19.3 depicts a hypothetical curvilinear relation between level of family functioning and level of cohesion or intrafamily attachments (ranging from disengaged at one extreme to enmeshed at the other), where optimal family functioning occurs at a middle range of attachment. In this example, level of family functioning can be predicted perfectly from level of attachment; yet the two variables would still obtain a Pearson *r* of .00. Alternative methods exist for assessing curvilinear relations (e.g., polynomial regression or log transformation of variables; see Pedhazur, 1997).

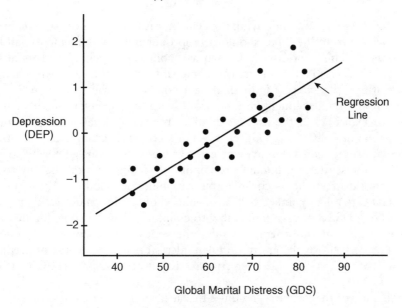

FIGURE 19.2. Simple linear regression, predicting depression (DEP) from global marital distress (GDS).

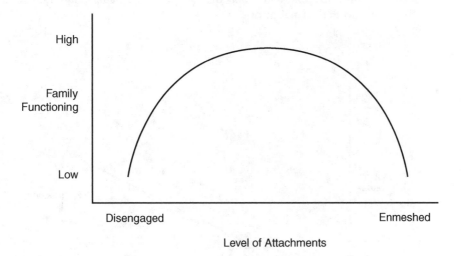

FIGURE 19.3. Hypothetical curvilinear relation between level of family functioning and level of intrafamily attachments.

A second assumption underlying the Pearson r is that errors of estimate in predicting one variable from the other should be approximately the same across all levels of both variables. (This condition is known as "homoscedasticity," and its absence as "heteroscedasticity.") Prediction error is depicted by the distance between actual sample observations (depicted by individual data points) and the regression line for predicting scores on the dependent variable from scores on the independent variable. For example, in Figure 19.2, the average error in predicting levels of depression (DEP) from global marital distress (GDS) remains fairly constant throughout the entire range of GDS (with some increase in average error at higher levels of GDS). By contrast, in Figure 19.4, the scatterplot linking probability of seeking marital therapy to level of global marital distress shows considerable variability across the range of GDS. Low levels of GDS are reliably linked to low likelihood of seeking marital therapy, whereas high levels of GDS relate less predictably to couples' behavior; some highly distressed couples may enter marital therapy, while others may pursue divorce. A common regression line derived for the entire sample underestimates the degree of predictability from low scores on GDS and overestimates the degree of predictability from high scores on GDS.

Finally, use of the Pearson r assumes that measurement error affecting each of the variables must be normally distributed; that is, differences between measured levels of a construct and the true, underlying levels of the construct for individuals in the sample must have a normal distribution. This also implies that the construct underlying each measure is presumed to be continuous. When all three assumptions—linearity, homoscedasticity, and normality—are met, the two variables being related are said to reflect a "bivariate normal distribution."

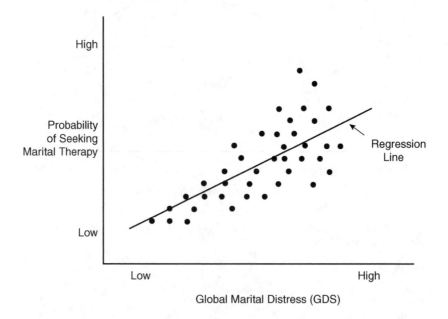

FIGURE 19.4. Scatterplot reflecting heteroscedasticity. The average error in predicting probability of seeking marital therapy is greater at higher levels of global marital distress (GDS).

Fortunately, inferences drawn from the Pearson r are fairly robust to violations of these assumptions. That is, moderate degrees of skewness, nonlinearity, or heteroscedasticity may not greatly affect the magnitude of r or its interpretation. However, when clear violations of these assumptions exist, or when data reflect ordinal- rather than interval-level measurement, alternative approaches to examining covariation should be used. These are summarized in Table 19.1. For example, the phi coefficient (ϕ) is used when both variables are dichotomous (e.g., gender and employment). Although ϕ and r are computationally equivalent, ϕ can be expected to underestimate the value of r that would have been obtained from continuous data that have been dichotomized. The point–biserial correlation (r_{pb}) is used when one variable is dichotomous and the other is continuous. Like ϕ, r_{pb} is computationally equivalent to r. However, whereas both ϕ and r can reach values of 1.0, the maximum size of r_{pb} between a dichotomous variable and a normally distributed variable is about .80 (Nunnally & Bernstein, 1994).

Alternative correlation coefficients have been proposed as estimates of the Pearson r in cases where the two underlying (latent) variables are presumed to be continuous, but one or both of the measures of these variables has been dichotomized (e.g., expressed emotions have been coded as positive or negative). In the case of one continuous and one dichotomized measure, the biserial correlation (r_{bis}) can be computed; in the case of two dichotomized measures (reflecting two continuous constructs), the tetrachoric correlation (r_{tet}) can be used. Generalizations of these two coefficients (polyserial and polychoric correlations) have been developed for use in cases where continuous constructs have been measured with three or more categories. In general, polyserial and polychoric correlations (including r_{bis} and r_{tet}) will always be somewhat higher than values of r derived from the same data. These estimates may or may not be accurate, and should be used only with caution and with clear justification.

Finally, two alternative correlation coefficients should be considered in cases where the data reflect ordinal- rather than interval-level data. The Spearman rho (ρ) and Kendall tau (τ) coefficients are used when observations on two variables reflect rank order without implied equal distance between adjacent ranks. Both coefficients assume a relatively large number of categories and relatively few tied observations (ranks) on each variable. Spearman's ρ provides a closer approximation to the Pearson r than Kendall's τ when the number of categories is large and the number of tied ranks is small (i.e., the data are more or less continuous). Kendall's τ is more appropriate when a fairly large number of cases have been classified into a relatively small number of categories. (When a small number of categories have been measured for each variable at a nominal rather than ordinal level of measurement, the chi-square [χ^2] statistic should be used.) Although both ρ and τ can range from –1.0 to +1.0, the absolute value of Kendall's τ tends to be smaller than that of Pearson's r.

INTERPRETIVE ISSUES

Several properties of data can render interpretation of correlation coefficients difficult or inappropriate. For example, we have already noted that the absolute magnitude of r is likely to be compromised to the extent that the two variables (1) are noncontinuous in measurement, (2) have nonsimilar distributions, or (3) are related in nonlinear fashion. An additional factor potentially contributing to spuriously low correlations involves restricted range of observations. In general, such restricted range may result

TABLE 19.1. Measurement Characteristics and Assumptions Underlying Selection among Alternative Statistics Reflecting Degree of Association

Statistic	First variable		Second variable		Comments[a]
	Measure	Construct	Measure	Construct	
Pearson r	Interval or ratio	Continuous	Interval or ratio	Continuous	Assumes bivariate normal distribution
Spearman rho (ρ)	Ordinal	Continuous	Ordinal	Continuous	Approximates r when number of tied ranks is small
Kendall tau (τ)	Ordinal	Continuous	Ordinal	Continuous	Preferred when number of tied ranks is large
Phi (ϕ)	Dichotomy	Dichotomy	Dichotomy	Dichotomy	Underestimates r when data are dichotomized
Point–biserial (r_{pb})	Dichotomy	Dichotomy	Interval or ratio	Continuous	Maximum value = .80
Biserial (r_{bis})	Dichotomy	Continuous	Interval or ratio	Continuous	May overestimate r
Tetrachoric (r_{tet})	Dichotomy	Continuous	Dichotomy	Continuous	May overestimate r
Chi-square (χ^2)	Nominal	Nominal	Nominal	Nominal	Also appropriate for ordinal-level measures

[a] See text for clarification of comments.

from methodological limitations in either measurement or sampling. Measurement sources of restricted range occur when the measuring technique is insufficient to adequately reflect the construct variation that is actually present in the sample. For example, if one wished to examine the relation of spousal differences in personality style to global marital accord in a nonclinic sample, the Minnesota Multiphasic Personality Inventory–2 (MMPI-2; Butcher, Dahlstrom, Graham, Tellegen, & Kaemmer, 1989) would be a poor instrument to use, because its construction is oriented toward individual differences in psychopathology rather than variation in personality style within the nonpathological spectrum. Most scores for a nonclinical sample could be expected to cluster at the low end of MMPI-2 scales.

Sampling sources of restricted range emerge when respondents are selected in such a way as to minimize potential covariation between the two variables of interest. For example, if one wished to examine the relation of individual psychopathology to couples' response to marital therapy, then initially excluding couples where one or both partners exhibit a thought disorder, severe personality disorder, or substance abuse could be expected to limit variability on measures of psychopathology—and consequently the covariability (correlation) between these measures and any measure of treatment outcome.

We have noted that the squared correlation coefficient provides the best index for evaluating the strength of the relation between two variables, and hence the correlation's meaningfulness. Meaningfulness differs from statistical significance; with a sufficiently large sample ($n > 100$), a correlation of only .20 (and explaining less than 5% of the variance in one variable from the other) may be statistically significant (i.e., not due to chance) at a probability level of $p < .05$. Similarly, one should avoid discussing the "difference" between correlations based on (1) their absolute magnitude, or (2) one correlation reaching statistical significance and the other not. In citing the difference between two correlations, one should first determine their statistically significant difference by using Fisher's (1921) r-to-z transformation, described in most intermediate-level statistics texts (see also Kashy & Snyder, 1995).

Finally, the ease with which correlations can be computed, and the tendency of researchers to examine large numbers of variables, require consideration of errors in statistical inference. Specifically, a Type I error involves falsely concluding that a correlation is significant; the probability of such an error is set by the "alpha" or probability level (denoted by p) adopted for hypothesis testing. Citing a correlation as significant at $p < .05$ implies that there is a 5-in-100 chance that the correlation has reached statistical significance due to chance alone (i.e., sampling error), rather than resulting from true covariation between the two variables in the population of interest. If one were to correlate the scores for husbands on 15 variables with the scores for wives on these same variables, a correlation matrix with 105 unique correlations would result. Suppose 10 of these reach statistical significance at $p < .05$. Given that we could expect approximately 5 of the 105 correlations to reach significance by chance alone, which 5 of the 10 significant correlations should we attribute to covariation generalizable to the population of interest, and which 5 to chance? Unfortunately, there is no way to determine the answer to this question.

A method of controlling overall Type I errors when one is computing numerous correlations is to split the sample in half, compute the same correlation matrices for both halves, and then consider only those correlations that are replicated across split-half samples. If one were to use a probability level of $p < .05$ in each sample, the likelihood that a correlation between the same two variables will be significant *by chance* in both samples is roughly .0025 (less than 3 out of 1,000 and considerably less than 1 out of 100). The benefits of replicating results across independent samples cannot be overstated.

Regression

CONCEPTUAL BASIS

How does correlation relate to prediction? Whereas a correlation expresses the direction and strength of relation between two variables, it does not by itself permit predicting an *individual's* score on one measure from that person's score on the other. The method one uses to accomplish this is simple linear regression.

In discussing correlation, we have described a hypothetical relation between individuals' level of depression (DEP) and global marital distress (GDS), where the two variables have a correlation of $r = .60$. Given this relation, how can spouses' level of depressed affect be predicted from level of marital distress? Regression analysis requires the following information: (1) the means and standard deviations of the distributions of scores for each variable; (2) the correlation between the two variables; and (3) the individual's score on the marital distress measure from which to predict that person's score on the depression measure. If marital distress and depression are represented by X and Y, respectively, then predicting an individual's level of depression (Y') from his or her level of marital distress (X) can be fairly easily computed from the following:

$$Y' = r_{XY}(s_Y / s_X)(X - \overline{X}) + \overline{Y}$$

where Y' is the predicted level of depression; r_{XY} = the correlation between depression (Y) and marital distress (X); s_Y and s_X are the standard deviations of Y and X, respectively; and $\overline{Y}$ and $\overline{X}$ are the means of Y and X, respectively. This formula is much simplified if one uses standardized z-scores for each of the two variables. The advantage of z-scores is that they constitute a simple linear transformation of raw scores, have a mean of 0 and standard deviation of 1, and can be interpreted relative to the unit-normal distribution. If z_X equals the individual's standardized score on X and z_Y' equals the predicted standardized score on Y, then:

$$z_Y' = r_{XY}z_X$$

INTERPRETIVE ISSUES

Figure 19.2 shows a scatterplot of scores from a small sample of couples on standardized measures of depression (DEP) and of global marital distress (GDS). The bivariate distribution of these scores reflects a correlation between these two variables of approximately .60. The line passing through this distribution reflects the best-fitting line for predicting levels of depression from marital distress, where "best fit" minimizes the sum of squared distances from each point to the line (commonly called the "least-squares solution"). This line is defined by the regression formula cited earlier. From Figure 19.2, one can observe that a score of 50 on GDS predicts a standardized score

of approximately –1 on DEP, equivalent to the 15th percentile of individuals' scores
on the depression measure; similarly, a score of 80 on GDS predicts a standardized
score of approximately +1 on DEP, equivalent to roughly the 85th percentile of individuals' scores on the depression measure.

Several features of prediction from regression analysis are worth noting. First,
when the correlation between two measures is ± 1.0, the relative distance of the predicted criterion score from the mean of the criterion measure will be precisely equal to
the relative distance of the predictor score from the mean of the predictor measure. For
example, with a correlation of $r = 1.0$, if a wife's marital distress score were at the 85th
percentile for that measure, then her predicted depression score would also be at the
85th percentile. Second, the lower the absolute magnitude of the correlation between
two measures, the closer the predicted criterion score will be to the mean of the criterion measure, compared to the distance of the individual's score on the predictor measure relative to the mean of the predictor variable. The tendency of predicted scores,
Y', to converge on the mean of the criterion measure was termed "*reversion*" by
Galton and was the basis of Pearson's identifying the product–moment correlation as
the "*r*" coefficient. Thus, with a correlation of $r = .60$, if a wife's marital distress score
were at the 85th percentile, her predicted depression score would only be at the 73rd
percentile. Third, if the correlation between two variables is 0, the best prediction of
an individual's score on the criterion measure is the *mean* of the criterion measure, regardless of that individual's score on the predictor measure.

Finally, given a correlation between two variables with absolute magnitude less
than 1.0 and the inevitability of some error in predicting Y' from X, one can specify a
level of confidence that an individual's actual criterion score is within some interval
bounding the predicted criterion score. The statistic used to establish this "confidence
interval" is the standard error of estimate, defined as follows:

$$s_{est(Y)} = s_Y \sqrt{1 - r^2_{XY}}$$

One could state with approximately 68% confidence of accuracy that the actual criterion score should fall within $\pm 1 s_{est(Y)}$ of the predicted criterion score, and with approximately 95% confidence that the actual criterion score should fall within $\pm 2\, s_{est(Y)}$ of the
predicted criterion score.

Third Variables

MODERATOR VARIABLES

How can correlations between two variables be influenced by individuals' scores on
some other variable? When the correlation between a predictor variable (X) and a criterion measure (Y) varies systematically as a function of some third variable (M), that
third variable is termed a "moderator" variable. The effect of a moderator variable is
depicted in Figure 19.5. Again, as in Figure 19.1, the overall covariability between depression (DEP) and global marital distress (GDS) is reflected by the overlap between
the two circles, reflecting variability in individuals' scores on each respective measure.
In Figure 19.5, we have indicated husbands' and wives' scores on each measure by the
letters H and W, respectively. Although an equal number of H's and W's appear in
each circle, the area of these two measures' overlap (representing covariability) is de-

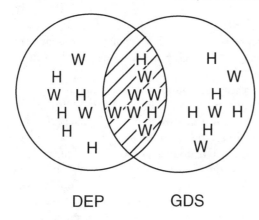

FIGURE 19.5. Gender as a moderator variable. The relation between depression (DEP) and global marital distress (GDS) is stronger for wives (W) than for husbands (H).

termined primarily by wives' scores (the W's). In this example, the overall correlation between depression and global marital distress for the combined sample of husbands and wives would underestimate the correlation between these two measures for wives alone, and would overestimate the correlation between these two measures derived separately for husbands.

Moderator effects are quite common. In fact, this example reflects recent findings that the temporal path from marital distress to depression is stronger for women than for men (Kiecolt-Glaser & Newton, 2001). Although common moderators include such sociodemographic indices as gender, age, ethnicity, marital status, and socioeconomic status, *any* variable (including discrete behavioral observations or indirectly measured psychological constructs) can function as a moderator variable. Moderator variables are identified most readily by testing for the statistical significance of differences between correlations of predictor to criterion measures for two or more subgroups (e.g., husbands vs. wives).

If one were to graphically depict the scatterplot of individuals' scores on criterion and predictor measures for subgroups defined by some moderator variable (e.g., distinguishing scores for husbands and wives by H and W, as in Figure 19.6), moderator effects would be noted from regression lines' having unequal slope. Finally, in multiple-regression analysis, moderator effects are reflected by significant prediction from "interaction terms" between two or more predictors. Typically, one investigates potential moderator effects for variables hypothesized on the basis of theory, clinical experience, or previous research as possibly influencing the covariability between predictor and criterion variables for different subgroups.

SUPPRESSOR VARIABLES

How can we reduce error in predicting from correlations? When two variables are imperfectly correlated, some variability in individuals' scores on the predictor variable X does not systematically covary with variability in individuals' scores on the criterion variable Y. Therefore, if we were to use simple linear regression to predict scores on Y from scores on X, there would be some error in our prediction, due to variance in X uncorrelated with variance in Y. In Figure 19.1, the portion of the circle denoting variance in GDS (global marital distress) that does not overlap with the circle denoting variance in DEP (depression) constitutes error in predicting DEP from GDS.

One method of improving our prediction of depression from global marital distress is to find some third variable (S) that correlates with the portion of GDS that constitutes error (i.e., that portion of GDS that does not overlap [correlate] with DEP). Such a variable is termed a "suppressor" variable, because its effect is to covary out or suppress the portion of variability in a predictor measure that is irrelevant to prediction of the criterion. Figure 19.7 provides an example of such a suppressor variable. In this example, the suppressor variable is marital commitment (COM), reflecting the extent to which an individual has an emotional stake in maintaining the marriage. As depicted in Figure 19.7, commitment (COM) is significantly (and negatively) correlated with marital distress (GDS), but uncorrelated with depression (DEP). If depression covaries with some portion of marital distress that is *not* related to level of marital commitment, then we can improve our prediction of depression by first subtracting (covarying out) from GDS the portion of global distress that covaries with commitment. Improvement in prediction occurs because, of the remaining (residual) variance in GDS, proportionately more covaries with depression (DEP) than does the total variability in GDS; that is, we have subtracted out (suppressed) nonpredictive variance in GDS. The prediction equation will have the following general form:

$$DEP = b_1 GDS - b_2 COM + c$$

where b_1 and b_2 denote some weighting (regression coefficients) of the two predictor variables GDS and COM, respectively; and c denotes some value of a constant.

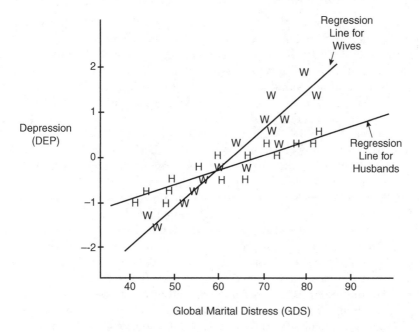

FIGURE 19.6. Separate regression lines showing a stronger relation in predicting depression (DEP) from global marital distress (GDS) for wives (W) than for husbands (H).

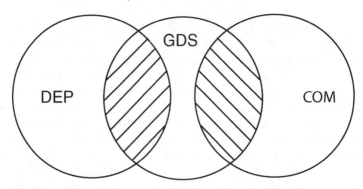

FIGURE 19.7. Commitment as a suppressor variable. A portion of the error in global marital distress (GDS) in predicting depression (DEP) is suppressed by controlling for commitment (COM).

Suppressor variables are identified in multiple-regression analysis when significant standardized weights are given to some variable correlating minimally with the criterion variable and significantly with one or more predictor variables. It bears noting that the absolute magnitudes of these correlations and standardized weights (regression coefficients) are important, rather than their direction (valence), because the direction of the correlations is an artifact of the manner in which the measurement instrument is scored.

PARTIAL AND SEMIPARTIAL CORRELATIONS

Up to this point, we have emphasized primarily "zero-order" correlations—that is, the unadjusted or simple correlations between two variables, ignoring (i.e., not controlling for) the effects of any third variable. By contrast, "partial" correlations provide an index of the association between two variables, X and Y, while adjusting for the effects of one or more additional variables on *both* X and Y. "Semipartial" correlations provide an index of the association between two variables, X and Y, while adjusting for the effects of one or more additional variables on *either* X or Y, but not both variables.

For example, Figure 19.1—discussed earlier—depicts the zero-order (or simple) correlation between depression (DEP) and global marital distress (GDS), which we have described as being approximately .60. By comparison, Figure 19.8A depicts the intercorrelations or overlap among three variables: depression (DEP), global marital distress (GDS), and attribution of marital difficulties to one's own behavior (AOB). Each of the three variables is shown to be correlated (to varying degrees) with each of the remaining two. Consider the situation where the zero-order correlation between GDS and AOB and between AOB and DEP is approximately .30. To what extent does attributing marital difficulties to one's own behavior (AOB) correlate with depression (DEP) *after* controlling for covariance of both variables with global distress (GDS)? The partial correlation of AOB with DEP, controlling for GDS, can be derived via formulae provided by Pedhazur (1997, p. 176). If one literally covers up that area in both DEP and AOB overlapping with the circle denoting variance in GDS, one observes that the remaining portion of DEP overlapping with AOB is relatively small (see Figure 19.8B); in this case, the partial correlation equals .16. The semipartial correlation of

AOB with DEP, controlling only for the covariance of GDS with AOB but not with DEP, is only slightly smaller (.13) (see Figure 19.8C).

Partial and semipartial correlations facilitate an understanding of suppressor variables. For example, if in Figure 19.7 the correlation of depression (DEP) with global marital distress (GDS) is .60 and the correlation of global distress with marital commitment (COM) is .50, the semipartial correlation of global marital distress with depression, controlling for effects of commitment to retaining one's marriage, increases to .69. Similarly, as we will see shortly, partial and semipartial correlations provide the key to understanding multiple-regression analysis.

Multiple Regression

CONCEPTUAL ISSUES

What techniques permit us to combine information from several variables to predict some criterion? For example, can prediction of spouses' depressed affect from their level of marital distress be improved by considering other potential contributing factors? Multiple regression is a general statistical procedure for investigating the relation of a single criterion variable to two or more predictor variables. Multiple regression can be used to derive the best linear prediction equation from some set of predictor variables and to evaluate the overall accuracy of that equation. It can also be used to control for possible confounding effects of one or more variables to evaluate the predictive contribution from some other specific variable or set of variables. Finally, multiple regression can be used to discover structural relations among complex multivariate data sets.

Essentially, the objective of multiple linear regression (or multivariate prediction) is to identify multiple predictors associated with different or unique components of criterion variance. This objective will be met to the extent that predictors are significantly correlated with the criterion and minimally correlated with each other. The correlation between a criterion variable and the linear composite of predictor variables derived from multiple-regression analysis is called the multiple correlation (R); the square of the multiple correlation, R^2, denotes the total proportion of criterion variance explained by the linear combination of predictor variables.

Figure 19.8, discussed earlier from the perspective of partial correlation, also provides an example for considering multiple regression. In attempting to predict individuals' scores on the criterion measure of depression (DEP), multiple regression will ordinarily select as the *first* predictor the variable that has the highest zero-order (simple) correlation with the criterion—in this case, global marital distress (GDS), which has a correlation of .60 with depression. If two or more additional predictors remain, multiple regression will then ordinarily select as the *next additional* predictor the variable that has the highest partial correlation with the criterion, controlling for the effects of the first predictor (GDS) on both the criterion and remaining possible predictors. As noted earlier, the partial correlation between depression and attributing marital difficulties to one's own behavior, controlling for global marital distress, is only .16— which may or may not add significantly to predictive accuracy beyond prediction from marital distress alone.

Multiple regression becomes decidedly more complex when three or more predictor variables are considered, as depicted in Figure 19.9. In this example, two addi-

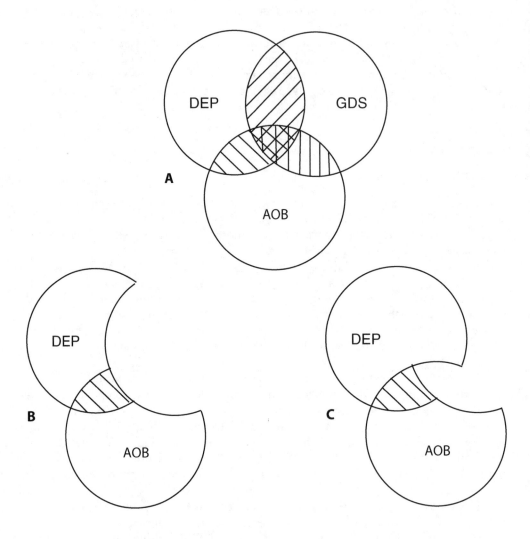

FIGURE 19.8. (A) Relations among depression (DEP), global marital distress (GDS), and attribution of marital difficulties to one's own behavior (AOB). DEP correlates with GDS at $r = .60$; DEP and GDS both correlate with AOB at $r = .30$. (B) The partial correlation of DEP with AOB is lower ($r = .16$) after controlling for the correlation of both variables with GDS. (C) The semipartial correlation of DEP with AOB is also lower ($r = .13$) after controlling only for the correlation of AOB with GDS.

tional variables are available as potential predictors of depression—namely, life event stressors (LES) and attribution of marital difficulties to the partner's behavior (APB). Consider the situation in which life event stressors are correlated with depression at .15, and attribution of marital difficulties to the partner's behavior is uncorrelated with depression but is correlated with attribution of marital difficulties to one's own behavior at .60. GDS would ordinarily be selected as the first predictor of DEP, because of its highest zero-order correlation with the criterion. Although AOB has the next highest zero-order correlation with DEP (.30), LES would probably be selected as the second predictor—because its partial correlation with DEP, controlling for GDS (.19), is higher than AOB's partial correlation with DEP, controlling for GDS (.16).

If these three predictors were the only ones being considered, their order of entry into the multiple-regression equation would probably be GDS first, then LES, and then AOB (presuming that all added significantly to the prediction of depression). However, as depicted in Figure 19.9, attribution of marital difficulties to the partner's behavior (APB) acts as a suppressor variable, in that it subtracts out that portion of variance in AOB not related to the criterion—perhaps a general tendency to attribute marital problems to both partners' behavior. In this example, the partial correlation of AOB with DEP, controlling for effects of both GDS *and* APB, would be .20. Thus, in a

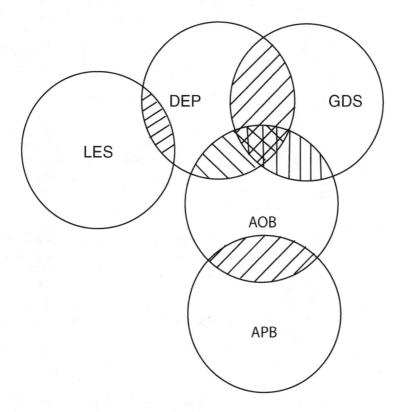

FIGURE 19.9. Multiple linear regression reflects covariation between the criterion (depression [DEP]) and multiple predictors (global marital distress [GDS], life event stressors [LES], and attribution of marital difficulties to one's own behavior [AOB]), including suppressor variables (attribution of marital difficulties to partner's behavior [APB]).

regression equation selecting the best combination of three predictors, the variables entered might be GDS, AOB, and APB (weighted negatively)—with LES subsequently being entered as the fourth predictor.

PROCEDURAL ISSUES

The results of multiple regression depend not only on the correlations of predictors with the criterion and with other predictors, but also on decisions regarding the specific procedures used in the regression analysis. For example, the Statistical Package for the Social Sciences (SPSS, Inc., 2003) requires a series of decisions regarding various options for conducting multiple regression. The first decision involves the method of entering predictors into the prediction equation. Three basic options exist: (1) forced entry of all possible predictors, to examine their cumulative predictive accuracy; (2) controlled entry of subsets of predictors in hierarchical fashion, to test specific hypotheses; and (3) stepwise entry or deletion of predictors, based solely on covariance structure among predictors and criterion.

Forced entry of all predictor variables is used when the investigator has no specific hypotheses regarding subsets of predictors and wishes to examine the overall utility of predictor variables considered in their entirety. For example, one might be interested in the overall relation between the five personality dimensions measured by the NEO Personality Inventory—Revised (NEO-PI-R; Costa & McCrae, 1992) and the Global Distress (GDS) scale of the Marital Satisfaction Inventory—Revised (MSI-R; Snyder, 1997) as an index of the relation between personality and marital functioning. The squared multiple correlation between the GDS scale of the MSI-R and the regression equation incorporating ideal weightings of the five NEO-PI-R scales would provide the best measure of this relation.

Hierarchical entry is used when one wants to test specific hypotheses regarding some subset of possible predictors. For example, if an important hypothesis concerns the effects of marital distress (GDS) on depression (DEP) *after* the effects of life events (LES) have already been accounted for, one would compare (1) the squared multiple correlation (R^2) for the regression equation predicting DEP with LES entered first and GDS second, to (2) the R^2 for the equation with LES entered alone.

Stepwise entry of predictors is used when the investigator wishes to derive an optimal prediction equation, using the smallest possible set of the strongest combination of predictors. Several stepwise procedures are possible: (1) forward inclusion, in which predictors are added if they satisfy certain statistical criteria determined by the investigator; (2) backward exclusion, in which predictors are eliminated one by one (again, on the basis of specified statistical criteria) from a regression equation that initially includes all predictors; and (3) forward inclusion combined with deletion of variables no longer meeting predetermined statistical criteria at each successive step. The most common of these stepwise procedures is the first (forward inclusion).

If selecting stepwise procedures for the regression analysis, the investigator must specify criteria for entering or deleting predictors from the regression equation. The first criterion specifies the maximum number of predictor variables to be selected (e.g., the best 3 of 10). The second criterion specifies the minimum F ratio that must be computed in a test for significance of a regression coefficient if that variable is to be included in the next step. The third criterion specifies what proportion of variance in a potential predictor, *not* explained by predictors already selected for the regression equation, that is required when that predictor is considered for possible inclusion. Most statistical packages have default values for these statistical criteria, so that the user can execute stepwise regression without specifying these criteria; however, default values tend to be very liberal toward inclusion of predictor variables with minimal incremental predictive utility, leading to a number of interpretive difficulties concerning results.

INTERPRETIVE ISSUES

Multiple-regression analysis constitutes an important statistical tool for developing prediction models, testing specific prediction hypotheses, and enhancing overall predictive accuracy. However, use of multiple regression requires familiarity with the assumptions and limitations of the technique, which have a bearing on interpretation of results (see Nunnally & Bernstein, 1994, pp. 185–193).

First, because of their complexity, reporting of multivariate results requires attention to both their applicability and verification by the informed consumer. When one is presenting results of multiple-regression analysis, both standardized and unstandardized weights should be presented; standardized weights permit interpretation of the relative contribution of predictor variables to some linear function, while unstandardized weights provide the means for actually computing linear composites without transforming predictor variables to standardized scores.

Second, multiple linear regression makes all the same assumptions as correlation and simple regression—namely, that the bivariate distributions between predictors (and between predictors and the criterion) satisfy the conditions of linearity, homoscedasticity, and normality. In addition, multiple regression is optimized when predictor variables are relatively independent (i.e., uncorrelated). When two or more of the predictor variables are highly intercorrelated (e.g., $>.80$)—a condition termed "multicollinearity"—then derivation of the regression equation may not be possible; if calculation of the equation does proceed, results may be highly unreliable from one sample to another.

Third, in addition to multicollinearity, the likelihood of unreliable results increases when (1) the ratio of subjects to predictor variables is relatively small (e.g., $<5:1$); (2) predictors are selected without careful consideration of theory or previous empirical findings; or (3) nonlinear solutions (e.g., exponential or log transformations of predictor variables) are used that capitalize on chance covariation between predictors and the criterion. An important means of guarding against spurious (chance) findings involves cross-validating the results of a multiple-regression equation derived from one sample by applying the same equation to an independent sample and assessing the amount of shrinkage in the squared multiple correlation (R^2). Another means of minimizing chance findings involves using stringent criteria for entering and retaining predictor variables in a stepwise procedure.

Finally, it is critical that the standardized weights (regression coefficients or "beta" weights) applied to predictor variables not be interpreted as reflecting the "importance" of predictor variables *outside the context of multivariate prediction*. When predictor variables are highly correlated relative to their correlation with the criterion, regression coefficients may be poorer indicators of predictors' importance than zero-order (simple) correlations may be. A more useful concept than importance in evaluating a multiple-regression equation concerns predictor variables' "uniqueness." The uniqueness of a specified predictor variable is the difference in R^2 when (1) all predictors are included in the regression equation, versus when (2) the predictor in question is excluded from the equation.

Advanced Techniques

Canonical-Correlation Analysis

CONCEPTUAL ISSUES

Suppose one wants to relate multiple predictors to multiple criteria simultaneously. For example, one might wish to examine the relation of marital distress to children's adjustment, using scales from the MSI-R (Snyder, 1997) as predictors and scales from the Personality Inventory for Children—Revised (PIC-R; Wirt, Lachar, Klinedinst, & Seat, 1984) as criteria. Canonical correlation permits such prediction by combining elements of both regression analysis and factor analysis. We have noted that multiple-regression analysis permits consideration of multiple predictor variables and their intercorrelations in predicting some single criterion variable. Canonical correlation differs from multiple regression in that, rather than relating two or more predictor variables to one criterion variable, canonical analysis examines the relation(s) of two or more predictor variables to two or more criterion variables. Factor analysis is a statistical procedure for reducing some set of variables to a smaller number of dimensions by examining the correlations or shared variance among those variables. Canonical-correlation analysis differs from factor analysis in that, whereas the latter generates linear combinations of variables to account for as much variance as possible *within one* set of variables, canonical analysis generates linear combinations of variables to explain the maximum amount of covariance *between two* sets of variables.

Objectives of canonical-correlation analysis can be depicted graphically as in Figure 19.10. In this example, five predictor scales from the MSI-R (Conflict over Child Rearing [CCR], Dissatisfaction with Children [DSC], Affective Communication [AFC], Problem-Solving Communication [PSC], and Disagreement about Finances [FIN]) have been related to three criterion scales from the PIC-R (Social Skills [SSK], Academic Achievement [ACH], and Delinquency [DLQ]). Canonical analysis first forms two linear combinations, one of the predictor variables and one of the criterion variables, by differentially weighting them so that the maximum possible correlation between them is obtained. This correlation constitutes the first canonical correlation or canonical variate. As depicted in Figure 19.10, the first canonical variate reflects a strong relation between a predictor composite made up of marital communication difficulties (AFC and PSC) and FIN and a criterion composite made up primarily of deficits in SSK

Canonical analysis then partials out variance in each variable accounted for by the first pair of linear combinations, and forms a second pair of linear combinations that provides the maximum possible correlation between remaining (residual) variance in each variable; this second correlation constitutes the second canonical correlation. In this example (see Figure 19.10), the second canonical variate reflects a strong relation between a predictor composite made up of spousal conflict over child rearing (CCR) and dissatisfaction with children (DSC), and a criterion composite determined primarily by deficits in social skills (SSK), delinquent behavior (DLQ), and—to a lesser extent—academic difficulties (ACH). The number of canonical correlations that can

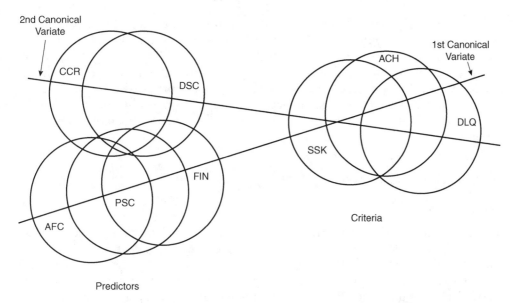

2nd Canonical
Variate

1st Canonical
Variate

Predictors

Criteria

FIGURE 19.10. Canonical-correlation analysis. Two canonical variates account for covariation between five predictor measures reflecting dimensions of marital satisfaction (Conflict over Child Rearing [CCR], Dissatisfaction with Children [DSC], Affective Communication [AFC], Problem-Solving Communication [PSC], and Disagreement about Finances [FIN]) and three criterion measures reflecting dimensions of child adjustment (Social Skills [SSK], Academic Achievement [ACH], and Delinquency [DLQ]).

be derived in canonical analysis is one fewer than the smaller of (1) the number of predictors, or (2) the number of criteria. In the present example, the maximum number of canonical correlations that can be derived is two (one fewer than three).

INTERPRETIVE ISSUES

A major advantage of canonical-correlation analysis is its ability to examine intricate relations among multiple sets of variables typical of theories concerning family systems. However, interpretation of canonical correlations is more complex than interpretation of multiple correlations from regression analysis. First, the meaning of squared canonical correlations differs from the meaning of squared multiple correlations in regression. Because canonical correlations reflect covariation of linear combinations of predictor and criterion variables, one could obtain a large canonical correlation if one predictor variable were highly correlated with only one criterion variable, even if the total variability among predictors were only marginally related to the total variability among criteria. Fortunately, "redundancy analysis" (Stewart & Love, 1968) provides a means for determining the proportion of the total variance in a set of criterion variables accounted for by the total variance in a set of predictor variables for each successive canonical correlation. The overall proportion of variance in a criterion set accounted for by a predictor set is then reflected by the sum of redundancy indices across all possible canonical variates.

Second, interpretation of the underlying constructs reflected by canonical variates is rendered difficult by the complexity of linear combinations on *both* sides of the prediction equation. Furthermore, although the overall variability in a criterion set accounted for by variability in a predictor set may be fairly stable across samples, the canonical weighting of specific variables comprising each canonical correlation may be highly unstable. Therefore, cross-validation is even more critical to interpretation in canonical analysis than in multiple-regression analysis, due to sample-specific covariation.

Multiple-Discriminant-Function Analysis

CONCEPTUAL ISSUES

Regression analysis techniques are restricted to situations in which the prediction criterion involves a continuous interval-level variable (e.g., extent of depressed affect or relationship dissatisfaction). What can we do if this requirement is not satisfied? When the criterion variable involves nominal-level measurement (e.g., distinguishing among individuals from different ethnic groups or among intact, separated, and divorced couples), regression procedures can no longer be used. Multiple-discriminant-function (MDF) analysis is a statistical procedure for distinguishing among individuals who constitute two or more groups. Whereas regression techniques lead to prediction of individuals' scores along some continuous interval-level measure, MDF techniques emphasize classification of individuals into a relatively small number of discrete groups. MDF analysis can also be used where scores on an interval-level criterion are related in nonlinear fashion to the predictors (e.g., where optimal family functioning occurs at intermediate levels of attachment between family members, and scores at either end of the attachment continuum [very high or very low] reflect impaired functioning).

Consider, for example, a situation in which we would like to identify predictors of couples' response to marital therapy. Potential predictors of treatment outcome in a hypothetical data set might include the following measures obtained at the beginning of treatment: (1) global marital distress (GDS); (2) commitment to the marriage (COM); (3) additional life event stressors (LES); (4) attribution of marital difficulties to the partner's behavior (partner blame) (APB); and (5) attribution of marital difficulties to one's own behavior (self-blame) (AOB). In this example, MDF analysis can be used either for prediction (classification) or for delineating complex multivariate relations reflected in group differences (theory exploration). As an example of the former, MDF analysis might be used to identify predictors of treatment response in order to predict outcome (or alter treatment strategy) among a new sample of couples entering therapy. Alternatively, results of the MDF analysis might be used to examine hypotheses regarding the role of relationship attributions in contributing to or maintaining marital distress.

In MDF analysis, the investigator identifies a set of predictor variables hypothesized to provide a basis for distinguishing among groups or classes of individuals. The investigator then derives one or more weighted linear combinations of predictor variables (these combinations are the multiple discriminant functions, or MDFs) that optimally discriminate among groups. The maximum number of MDFs that can be derived is either (1) one less than the number of groups; or (2) equal to the number of predictor variables, if there are more groups than variables. After the first function has been determined, each successive function attempts to explain (predict) group differences not already accounted for by previous discriminant functions.

Consider again the example in which MDF analysis is used to predict treatment outcome from measures of marital distress, commitment, life event stressors, partner blame, and self-blame. Figure 19.11 depicts the hypothetical results of this analysis, where treatment outcome is reflected in spouses' classification into one of three groups: (1) divorced (D), (2) unhappily married (U), and (3) happily married (H). In this example, two MDFs have been derived to distinguish among these three criterion groups. The first function (MDF-1) is determined primarily by weights given to three predictor variables: global distress (GDS), life event stressors (LES), and partner blame (APB). Individuals' composite scores on this first function discriminate primarily between happily married spouses and those who have either divorced or are unhappily married. Scores on MDF-1 above 0 identify all of the divorced and most of the unhappily married individuals, and scores below 0 identify all of the happily married spouses. However, scores on MDF-1 do not distinguish well between distressed spouses who remain married and those who divorce; for example, with a score of 1 on this function, subjects are about as equally likely to end their marriage as to remain unhappily married.

In Figure 19.11, a second function (MDF-2) has been derived by giving weight primarily to two predictor variables: commitment (COM) and self-blame (AOB). Like MDF-1, this second function distinguishes between divorced and happily married individuals. However, unlike MDF-1, MDF-2 also distinguishes fairly well between di-

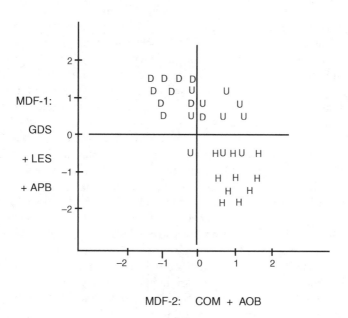

FIGURE 19.11. Classification of happily married (H), unhappily married (U), and divorced (D) couples via multiple-discriminant-function (MDF) analysis. Predictor variables include global marital distress (GDS), life event stressors (LES), attribution of marital difficulties to partner's behavior (APB), commitment (COM), and attribution of marital difficulties to one's own behavior (AOB).

vorced and distressed married spouses. Among maritally distressed individuals, those low on commitment and self-blame (below a score of 0 on this second function) are likely to divorce, whereas those high on commitment and self-blame (above a score of 0 on MDF-2) are more likely to retain their marriage.

PROCEDURAL ISSUES

In conducting MDF analysis, the investigator must first decide how to measure or categorize the criterion variable. For instance, in the example considered earlier, we could have combined divorced with unhappily married couples and retained happily married couples as a separate category, to form two groups distinguished primarily by level of relationship distress; alternatively, we could have combined unhappily and happily married couples, retaining divorced couples as a separate category, to form two groups distinguished by marital status. In addition, depending on our sample, we might instead identify a fourth group of separated but nondivorced couples. Results of the MDF analysis will depend on which two-group, three-group, or four-group classification scheme for the criterion variable we select. Given a sufficient number of valid predictors, then the larger the number of criterion groups, the larger the number of functions that may be derived, and the more complicated the interpretation of results will be.

As in multiple-regression analysis, the objective of selecting predictor variables in MDF analysis is to choose the smallest number of predictors that maximally distinguish among groups and minimally correlate with each other. The larger the number of correlated predictors, then the more unstable (unreliable) will be the weights given to predictor variables defining the MDFs and the interpretations given to these functions. Potential predictor variables should be selected on the basis of theory, previous research, or their relative statistical independence (low intercorrelations).

Also as in mutiple-regression analysis, the results of MDF analysis depend in part on the specific procedures and criteria used for entering and retaining predictor variables in each successive function. For example, all potential predictors could be entered simultaneously if the objective of the analysis is to delineate structural relations among predictors as they relate to the criterion for theoretical purposes. Alternatively, several stepwise procedures for entering predictor variables are available; these differ primarily in (1) methods used to compute the distances among groups, and (2) criteria for determining the statistical significance of predictor variables' incremental predictive utility. As with multiple-regression procedures, the default values for selection criteria set by many statistical packages are quite liberal, often leading to inclusion of marginally useful and unreliable predictors in the MDFs. Users of these statistical routines should consider options for defining more conservative inclusion criteria.

In addition to deriving MDFs, most statistical packages provide the option of applying results to the original sample (or an independent cross-validation sample) to determine the percentage of cases correctly classified by these discriminant functions. Plotting of cases along the functions, as done in Figure 19.11, can facilitate interpretation of results—particularly when only two or three functions have been derived.

INTERPRETIVE ISSUES

Unlike multiple-regression analysis, in which a single linear composite predictor equation is derived, MDF analysis may produce multiple predictive equations (functions).

An initial interpretive task involves deciding how many functions should be considered; both statistical significance and interpretive meaningfulness enter into this decision. Procedures exist for determining the proportion of criterion variance explained by any given MDF relative to the complete set of MDFs, as well as the proportion of MDF variation explained by group membership.

Interpretive meaningfulness may also be evaluated by considering the theoretical implications of predictor variables weighted highly on a particular function. Standardized MDF weights assigned to predictor variables (called "standardized coefficients") denote the relative contribution of each variable to that function. They also possess the nice feature of producing MDF scores having a mean of 0 and standard deviation of 1, so that any individual's score on the MDF can be easily translated into percentile rank (by using a table of z-scores for the unit-normal distribution).

As in regression and canonical analysis, individual MDF coefficients must be interpreted *within the context of multivariate prediction*; they do not necessarily denote the relative strength of predictors that would be observed in univariate prediction. In addition, as with canonical-correlation analysis, MDF analysis becomes increasingly complex as the number of functions increases. Moreover, the likelihood that weights assigned to individual predictors will reflect chance covariation increases as (1) the numbers of predictor variables, criterion groups, and functions increase; and (2) the number of subjects in the sample of derivation decreases. As with other multivariate procedures, cross-validation of results in an independent sample is highly desirable.

Cluster Analysis

CONCEPTUAL ISSUES

Cluster analysis is a procedure for identifying subgroups of individuals within some larger group or population (Aldenderfer & Blashfield, 1984). Cluster analysis sorts individuals into groups by using their scores on two or more variables, such that individuals in any given group are more similar to each other than to individuals in other groups. The most common use of cluster analysis is to develop a typology or classification system by which new cases may be sorted, based on their similarity to defined types. For example, efforts to expand the *Diagnostic and Statistical Manual of Mental Disorders* (American Psychiatric Association, 2000) to include distinctions among marital and family disorders reflect the belief that homogeneous subgroups exist within the broader population of couples and families seeking treatment. The identification of these discrete diagnostic categories is thought to be important, because these subgroups may vary not only in their presenting symptoms, but potentially in both the underlying causes and optimal treatment of their difficulties.

Although cluster analysis is similar to factor analysis in that they are both data reduction techniques, the methods apply different approaches to reduction. Factor analysis is used to reduce a larger number of *variables* to a smaller number of factors or dimensions that describe these variables. By contrast, cluster analysis is used to reduce a larger number of *individuals* to a smaller number of groups or clusters that capture the most important similarities and differences among these persons on observed variables. Cluster analysis also differs from MDF analysis, in that the latter uses two or more variables to predict group membership among individuals whose classification is already known (e.g., spouses who divorce vs. remain married following marital therapy), whereas cluster analysis uses individual differences along two or more variables to create homogeneous groups within a larger sample or population whose underlying group structure is unknown.

Once groups have been quantitatively defined via cluster analysis, group differences may then be explored further on variables or constructs separate from those initially used to define the groups. Examination of the subgroups on these independent criterion variables provides a new understanding of additional characteristics that may distinguish members assigned to different clusters. For example, as with classification schemes developed for individual emotional and behavioral disorders, persons clustered into distinct groups based on various facets of current marital dysfunction may be found to differ as well along measures reflecting potential causal mechanisms, current emotional or physical well-being, or response to various intervention strategies.

For example, consider a large sample of individuals pursuing treatment for difficulties in their sexual relationship. Previous research suggests that sexual difficulties often coexist with nonsexual relationship difficulties (Regev, O'Donohue, & Avina, 2003), and that both sexual and nonsexual relationship difficulties often coexist with depression (Michael & O'Keane, 2000). Given these research findings, sorting individuals into groups based on the relative prominence of marital, sexual, and emotional distress may improve our conceptual understanding of contributing risk factors and our capacity for differential assessment and intervention. Figure 19.12 depicts hypothetical results for individuals whose scores on independent measures of marital, sexual, and emotional distress have been subjected to cluster analysis. Group 1 reflects individuals who exhibit both sexual and nonsexual marital distress. General relationship enhancement emphasizing communication and positivity may be critical for individuals in this group prior to intervention strategies targeting specific sexual complaints. By contrast, Group 2 reflects individuals with primary sexual difficulties and only modest marital unhappiness, combined with better-than-average emotional functioning. Such persons may be particularly suitable for traditional sex therapy or may warrant screening for physical factors contributing to their sexual complaints. Finally, Group 3 reflects individuals with prominent sexual and emotional distress and only modest nonsexual relationship complaints. For these individuals, psychosocial and pharmacological treatments targeting depression or related emotional features may constitute an important adjunct to more focused sex therapy.

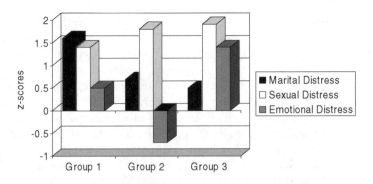

FIGURE 19.12. Classification via cluster analysis of individuals seeking treatment for sexual difficulties into three groups based on marital, sexual, and emotional distress.

PROCEDURAL ISSUES

Cluster analysis begins when the researcher selects those variables hypothesized on the basis of theory or previous research to distinguish among individuals in some optimal fashion. Ideally, as with other multivariate procedures discussed earlier, the variables should be relatively independent. Transformation of variables to a common metric (e.g., z-scores) facilitates subsequent interpretation of their relative contribution to defined subgroups. Numerous alternative clustering techniques are available that differ in the method of cluster formation. In agglomerative hierarchical clustering, each person is initially considered a separate cluster, and individuals are then combined into progressively larger groups until all individuals constitute one large cluster. By contrast, in divisive clustering, all individuals are first grouped into one large cluster, and clusters are then divided at each successive step into smaller units until the desired number of clusters is achieved. In practice, agglomerative clustering procedures are more commonly used than divisive procedures.

Cluster-analytic procedures also vary in terms of (1) how individuals or clusters are compared, and (2) what measure of similarity or distance is used. For example, in the single-linkage or "nearest-neighbor" method, individuals are placed in clusters if at least one member of the existing cluster is of the same level of similarity as the individual being considered. Alternatively, in the complete-linkage or "furthest-neighbor" method, individuals are included in an existing cluster if the individual is within a specified level of similarity to *all* members of that cluster. The average-linkage-between-groups method rests within these two extremes by computing an average of the similarity of an individual and all cases in an existing cluster when determining cluster membership. Another approach, known as "Ward's method," works by minimizing variance within clusters relative to variance between clusters. Within these and other methods, distance or similarity may be computed by various indices, such as the Pearson correlation or squared Euclidean distance.

An important consideration when one is choosing among these various methods of cluster analysis is that different clustering algorithms produce different results when applied to the same data. For example, the average-linkage method tends to produce clusters with approximately the same variance, whereas Ward's method tends to create clusters of relatively equal sizes (number of individuals per group). By comparison, the single-linkage method tends to form "elongated" cluster solutions characterized by one very large group and several very small residual groups, whereas the complete-linkage method tends to create a higher number of compact groups composed of highly similar cases.

INTERPRETIVE ISSUES

The first step in interpreting the results of cluster analysis involves determining the number of clusters to retain. Although no definitive criteria exist for this determination, several approaches are common. First, the number of preferred clusters may sometimes be apparent from visual inspection of the "dendogram," which graphically depicts the progression of the clustering process from each case representing its own group to all individuals composing a single group; however, such inspection is highly subjective and susceptible to biases of the researcher. A more quantitative approach involves plotting "fusion" coefficients, reflecting the relative distance of groups being joined at each successive stage of the clustering process; similar to a "scree plot" in factor analysis, the plot of fusion coefficients may indicate a significant jump reflecting the merger of two relatively dissimilar clusters.

An important hazard of cluster-analytic procedures involves their ability to misidentify or create clusters in data sets in which no subgroup structure exists. The use of a large sample of individuals relative to a small number of variables on which to cluster, as well as the selection of variables based on theory or previous research, reduces but does not eliminate the potential to wrongly "detect" clusters when none exist in reality. Hence it is critical to evaluate both the reliability and validity of a classification system derived from cluster analysis. Reliability can be assessed by using independent or split-half samples to replicate findings, or by using a variety of "bootstrapping" procedures (Efron & Tibshirani, 1994) to examine multiple replications across resampled subsets. The validity of the classification system should be assessed by examining group differences across independent criteria *other than* those variables originally used in deriving the clusters. For example, regarding the groups depicted in Figure 19.12, one could evaluate the extent to which the three groups also vary in family life stage, previous history of either individual or marital therapy, response to different treatments, and so forth.

DISCUSSION

Correlation itself is a simple concept. Some things go hand in hand; they covary. The techniques reviewed here, ranging from simple correlation to more complex multivariate procedures, all stem from this basic interest in describing how fluctuation in one phenomenon relates to fluctuation in another.

Correlational techniques can become more complex because of issues concerning how we measure the things we're interested in, how many things we're predicting to and from, how predictors overlap and influence each other, how many observations we're able to obtain, how well these observations reflect other situations of interest, and how much we're able to make use of what we discover.

Issues of Sampling

Throughout our presentation, we have noted three issues regarding the sample of individuals for whom data are collected: size, range, and representativeness. Because of the potential for multivariate techniques to capitalize on chance covariation among predictor and criterion variables, it is critical that the sample be large relative to the total number of variables being considered. Subject-to-variable ratios of 10:1 are encouraged, with 5:1 being a minimum standard. At the same time that large samples contribute to the stability of findings, they also enable relatively small correlations to reach statistical significance. Consequently, one should consider the meaningfulness of correlations (reflected in r^2 or R^2), as well as their statistical significance.

The ability of two variables to covary depends in part on the degree of variability in each independently. When the range of observations on one or both variables is restricted, the observed correlation between them may underestimate their true correlation in the larger population. Restricted range may result either from inadequate measurement techniques or from inadequate sampling.

However, it is also critical that the sample be representative of the population to which findings will be applied. If the sample of application has a restricted range, than generalizing a correlation derived from a sample with unrestricted range to the sample with restricted range will lead to faulty conclusions. For example, although depression and marital distress covary in the general population, they may not correlate as strongly among couples entering marital therapy, where levels of marital distress tend to be restricted to moderate or high levels.

Issues of Reliability and Validity

Considerations of sample size relate directly to issues of reliability. Using multivariate correlational procedures in studies with low subject-to-variable ratios will inevitably lead to unstable results. Even where the overall magnitude of relation between criterion and predictors remains stable, the weights assigned to individual predictors may vary considerably across samples. The problems of unstable weights are magnified when multiple linear composites are derived, as in canonical-correlation or MDF analysis, or when predictor variables are highly intercorrelated (the problem of multi-collinearity).

The reliability of findings also suffers from "fishing expeditions," where an investigator searches for significant correlations in a relatively large matrix without specifying prior to the analysis which correlations are predicted to reach significance and in which direction. For example, even a relatively small matrix of intercorrelations among 10 variables produces 45 unique correlations, 2 or more of which may be expected to reach statistical significance at $p < .05$ by chance alone. Cross-validation of findings across split-half samples greatly reduces the likelihood of attributing meaningfulness to chance findings.

Even reliable (replicable) findings may not be valid; that is, they may not really mean what investigators believe they mean (or may not represent what investigators propose them to represent), and thus may not generalize to some intended application. There are numerous sources of compromised validity. First, an investigator must identify variables likely to correlate with other variables of interest, based on theory, prior research, or subjective experience; inadequate selection of constructs may compromise either prediction strategies or efforts to delineate structural relations of theoretical relevance. Second, once relevant constructs are identified, the investigator needs to select appropriate measures of those constructs—a task that can only be accomplished by examining what those measures have previously been shown to relate to on an empirical basis.

Third, the validity of findings depends on the appropriateness of the statistical procedures applied to the data. For example, variables with bivariate distributions departing significantly from requirements of normality, linearity, and homoscedasticity may require alternative statistical procedures from those reviewed here. In addition, specific criteria and procedures adopted in multivariate correlational techniques may be inappropriate to either the measures, the sample, or intended application of results.

Finally, the meaningfulness of multivariate correlational techniques often depends on the extent to which linear composites of variables (as in multiple-regression, canonical-correlation, or MDF analysis) lend themselves to unambiguous interpretation. Unfortunately, it is not uncommon for investigators to seize upon the weights of one or two variables meeting their theoretical bias for "labeling" a canonical variate or MDF, while ignoring significantly weighted variables not meeting their bias. The proportion of variance in linear composite scores accounted for by all predictor variables contributing to that composite should be carefully considered.

Issues of Application

Misinterpretation of correlations as reflecting causal relations constitutes the most common abuse of correlational techniques. Covariation demands further explanation. The functional relation between two related phenomena—that is, the extent to which one variable influences another—must always be established by observing effects of controlled manipulation.

The second most common error in using multivariate techniques is to interpret weights assigned to predictor variables as reflecting their relative importance separate from the multivariate prediction context. We have noted in our discussion that a predictor variable correlating highly with the criterion may receive no weight in a multivariate analysis because of its overlap with other predictors, whereas another predictor correlating not at all with the criterion may receive a strong weighting because of its role as a suppressor variable. An implication of this principle is that univariate (simple or zero-order) correlations should always be presented along with multivariate results. Also, as we have noted earlier, when one is presenting results of multiple-regression or MDF analysis, both standardized and unstandardized weights should be given.

Despite these limitations, multivariate correlational techniques provide powerful tools for exploring and discovering important relations among variables of interest. Even simple correlation allows us to confirm or disconfirm the relatedness of two phenomena that *appear* informally to co-relate, and to establish the magnitude of this relation. More sophisticated multivariate procedures permit hypothesis testing of the relative importance of specific factors in the context of related factors through hierarchical approaches to data analysis.

In addition to articulating criteria for including and retaining predictor variables in any given analysis, the meaningfulness of predictors should be communicated by presenting information about the change in R and R^2 resulting from inclusion of any specific predictor. In canonical-correlation and MDF analysis, the percentage of criterion variance explained by each linear composite should be specified.

Graphic presentation of results can dramatically facilitate their interpretation. Plots of simple regression lines, with confidence bands for prediction indicated by including lines reflecting $\pm 1 s_{est(Y)}$, effectively depict the nature of the bivariate distribution as well as prediction accuracy. In MDF analysis, plots of cases on respective functions both indicate accuracy of classification and enhance interpretation of the functions' utility in distinguishing among specific criterion groups.

Finally, when correlational techniques are intended to facilitate clinical intervention as well as theoretical understanding, methods should be used to maximize efficient application of results. For example, an investigator could make available a simple spreadsheet on floppy disk or on the Internet, in which clinicians or other consumers could enter subjects' raw scores on measures, and the spreadsheet would compute predicted criterion scores, confidence intervals for estimated scores, and interpretive guidelines for score ranges.

Future Directions

We have begun this chapter by suggesting that correlational techniques provide an important bridge between observation of two or more phenomena and efforts to modify the same. We have noted that considerable research has established the linkage of depressed affect and marital conflict, although the precise nature of this complex relation remains unclear. As with other areas of correlational research involving marital and family dynamics, findings relating depression to marital discord have led to new treatment approaches aimed at the co-occurrence of these two clinical concerns and experimental investigations of these treatments' efficacy (Beach & Gupta, 2003). We anticipate that other correlational studies of couples and families regarding other clinical phenomena will similarly facilitate development and validation of more effective intervention approaches (Snyder & Whisman, 2004).

Various texts provide good introductions to multivariate correlational techniques (e.g., Grimm & Yarnold, 1995, 2000); others offer more detailed presentations of these same procedures (e.g., Pedhazur, 1997; Stevens, 2002). Similarly, several statistical packages provide excellent discussions of multivariate procedures for the unsophisticated user, including SAS (SAS Institute, 2004) and SPSS (SPSS, Inc., 2003); both provide software for personal computers as well as mainframe applications and are well documented in supplemental resources (e.g., Der & Everitt, 2001; George & Mallery, 2002).

More sophisticated multivariate prediction techniques are being developed on a regular basis. Others already developed in the agricultural, economic, and physical sciences are finding their way into the behavioral sciences. While we expect new techniques to become available, we anticipate increasing use of such well-established techniques as multiple-regression analysis and MDF analysis by marital and family researchers. Finally, we anticipate that future investigators will retain a keen appreciation for the application of their findings in the typical clinical setting. Conscientious efforts must be made to bridge research and practice. These include development of theory with explicit implications for overt operations of assessment and intervention, use of measures accessible to the modal clinician, and translation of complex multivariate findings into specific applications.

EXEMPLARS

Basic Techniques

Regression (Including Moderator and Suppressor Variables)

Addis, J., & Bernard, M. (2002). Marital adjustment and irrational beliefs. *Journal of Rational-Emotive and Cognitive Behavior Therapy, 20*, 3–13.—This study examined the relation of irrational beliefs and emotional traits (anxiety, curiosity, anger) to levels of marital satisfaction. Correlational and multiple-regression analyses indicated the importance of individual partners' emotional traits and accompanying irrational beliefs in marital adjustment and dissatisfaction. "Self-downing" and need for comfort were the dimensions of irrational thinking most strongly related to marital dysfunction. Both anger and anxiety, but neither curiosity nor communication skills, distinguished individuals experiencing versus not experiencing marital problems.

Heim, S. C., & Snyder, D. K. (1991). Predicting depression from marital distress and attributional processes. *Journal of Marital and Family Therapy, 17*, 67–72.—This study examined the interaction between marital distress and spouses' attributions and expectancies regarding the marital relationship in predicting depressive symptoms. The best single predictor of depression for both sexes was a measure of disaffection, reflecting emotional distance and alienation in the marriage. Prediction of wives' depression in multiple-regression analyses was enhanced by measures of overt marital disharmony, attribution of causality for relationship difficulties to their own behavior, and failure to attribute difficulties to their husbands' behavior.

Advanced Techniques

Canonical-Correlation Analysis

Fisher, L., Nakell, L. C., Terry, H. E., & Ransom, D. C. (1992). The California Family Health Project: III. Family emotion management and adult health. *Family Process, 31*, 269–287.—This study explored the broad patterning of interrelationships between family emotion management and adult health. Ratings of husband–wife behavior were made during each of three 10-minute emotion management interaction tasks designed to elicit emotional themes of loss, intimacy, or conflict. In canonical-correlation analyses, the couple ratings demonstrated significant associations with health scores for both husbands and wives for the intimacy and conflict tasks, but not for the loss task. In general, couple overt emotional aversiveness was negatively associated with husbands' health, and couple emotional avoidance/distance was negatively associated with wives' health.

Multiple-Discriminant-Function Analysis

Carrère, S., Buehlman, K. T., Gottman, J. M., Coan, J. A., & Ruckstuhl, L. (2000). Predicting marital stability and divorce in newlywed couples. *Journal of Family Psychology, 14*, 42–58.—In a longitudinal study with 95 newlywed couples, an MDF analysis of data from an oral history interview predicted with 87% accuracy those couples whose marriages remained intact or had broken up 4–6 years later; the oral history data also predicted with 81% accuracy those couples who remained married or divorced 7–9 years later.

Cluster Analysis

Ridley, C. A., Wilhelm, M. S., & Surra, C. A. (2001). Married couples' conflict responses and marital quality. *Journal of Social and Personal Relationships, 18*, 517–534.—Using cluster analysis methods, this study sought to identify married couples' conflict response profiles, and to relate these conflict profiles to appraisals of marital quality. Spouses completed measures of aggressive, withdrawing, and problem-solving responses occurring during conflict episodes, as well as indices of marital quality. Cluster analyses of married dyads' conflict responses generated four profiles—two symmetrical ("distancing couples" and "engaging couples") and two asymmetrical ("distancing husbands" and "distancing wives"). Results indicated that couples endorsing different conflict profiles could be distinguished by their level of marital adjustment.

REFERENCES

Abelson, R. P. (1985). A variance explanation paradox: When a little is a lot. *Psychological Bulletin, 97*, 129–133.

Aldenderfer, M. S., & Blashfield, R. K. (1984). *Cluster analysis*. Thousand Oaks, CA: Sage.

American Psychiatric Association. (2000). *Diagnostic and statistical manual of mental disorders* (4th ed., text rev.). Washington, DC: Author.

Beach, S. R. H., & Gupta, M. (2003). Depression. In D. K. Snyder & M. A. Whisman (Eds.), *Treating difficult couples: Helping clients with coexisting mental and relationship disorders* (pp. 88–113). New York: Guilford Press.

Binet, A., & Simon, T. (1905). Methodes nouvelles pour le diagnostic du niveau intellectuel des anormaux. *Annee Psychologique, 11,* 191–244.

Butcher, J. N., Dahlstrom, W. G., Graham, J. R., Tellegen, A., & Kaemmer, B. (1989). *Manual for the Minnesota Multiphasic Personality Inventory–2.* Minneapolis: University of Minnesota Press.

Cattell, J. M. (1890). Mental tests and measurements. *Mind, 15,* 373–380.

Cavell, T. A., & Snyder, D. K. (1991). Iconoclasm versus innovation: Building a science of family therapy—Comment on Moon, Dillon, and Sprenkle. *Journal of Marital and Family Therapy, 17,* 167–171.

Cohen, J. (1988). *Statistical power analysis for the behavioral sciences* (2nd ed.). Hillsdale, NJ: Erlbaum.

Costa, P. T., & McCrae, R. R. (1992). Normal personality assessment in clinical practice: The NEO Personality Inventory. *Psychological Assessment, 4,* 5–13.

Der, G., & Everitt, B. S. (2001). *Handbook of statistical analyses using SAS* (2nd ed.). Boca Raton, FL: CRC Press.

Efron, B., & Tibshirani, R. J. (1994). *An introduction to the bootstrap.* Boca Raton, FL: CRC Press.

Fisher, R. A. (1921). On the "probable error" of a coefficient of correlation deduced from a small sample. *Metron, 1* Part 4), 3–32.

Galton, F. (1888). Co-relations and their measurement. *Proceedings of the Royal Society, 45,* 135–145.

George, D., & Mallery, P. (2002). *SPSS for Windows step by step: A simple guide and reference, 11.0 update* (4th ed.). Upper Saddle River, NJ: Pearson Allyn & Bacon.

Goering, P. N., Lancee, W. J., & Freeman, J. J. (1992). Marital support and recovery from depression. *British Journal of Psychiatry, 160,* 76–82.

Grimm, L. G., & Yarnold, P. R. (1995). *Reading and understanding multivariate statistics.* Washington, DC: American Psychological Association.

Grimm, L. G., & Yarnold, P. R. (2000). *Reading and understanding more multivariate statistics.* Washington, DC: American Psychological Association.

Hooley, J. M., & Teasdale, J. D. (1989). Predictors of relapse in unipolar depressives: Expressed emotion, marital distress, and perceived criticism. *Journal of Abnormal Psychology, 98,* 229–235.

Kashy, D. A., & Snyder, D. K. (1995). Measurement and data analytic issues in couples research. *Psychological Assessment, 7,* 338–348.

Kiecolt-Glaser, J. K., & Newton, T. L. (2001). Marriage and health: His and hers. *Psychological Bulletin, 127,* 472–503.

Michael, A., & O'Keane, V. (2000). Sexual dysfunction in depression. *Human Psychopharmacology: Clinical and Experimental, 15,* 337–345.

Nunnally, J. C., & Bernstein, I. H. (1994). *Psychometric theory* (3rd ed.). New York: McGraw-Hill.

Ozer, D. J. (1985). Correlation and the coefficient of determination. *Psychological Bulletin, 97,* 307–315.

Pearson, K. (1896). Mathematical contributions to the theory of evolution: Regression, heredity, and panmixia. *Philosophical Transactions of the Royal Society of London, 187A,* 253–318.

Pedhazur, E. J. (1997). *Multiple regression in behavioral research: Explanation and prediction* (3rd ed.). Belmont, CA: Wadsworth.

Regev, L. G., O'Donohue, W., & Avina, C. (2003). Sexual dysfunction. In D. K. Snyder & M. A. Whisman (Eds.), *Treating difficult couples: Helping clients with coexisting mental and relationship disorders* (pp. 181–200). New York: Guilford Press.

SAS Institute. (2004). *SAS System 9 user's guide*. Cary, NC: Author.

Sher, T. G., Baucom, D. H., & Larus, J. M. (1990). Communication patterns and response to treatment among depressed and nondepressed maritally distressed couples. *Journal of Family Psychology, 4*, 63–79.

Snyder, D. K. (1997). *Manual for the Marital Satisfaction Inventory—Revised*. Los Angeles: Western Psychological Services.

Snyder, D. K., Mangrum, L. F., & Wills, R. M. (1993). Predicting couples' response to marital therapy: A comparison of short- and long-term predictors. *Journal of Consulting and Clinical Psychology, 61*, 61–69.

Snyder, D. K., & Whisman, M. A. (2004). Treating distressed couples with coexisting mental and physical disorders: Directions for clinical training and practice. *Journal of Marital and Family Therapy, 30*, 1–12.

Spanier, G. B. (1976). Measuring dyadic adjustment: New scales for assessing the quality of marriage and similar dyads. *Journal of Marriage and the Family, 38*, 15–28.

Spearman, C. (1910). Correlation calculated from faulty data. *British Journal of Psychology, 3*, 271–295.

SPSS, Inc. (2003). *SPSS Version 12.0 user's guide*. Chicago: Author.

Stevens, J. P. (2002). *Applied multivariate statistics for the social sciences* (4th ed.). Mahwah, NJ: Erlbaum.

Stevens, S. S. (1946). On the theory of scales of measurement. *Science, 103*, 677–680.

Stewart, D., & Love, W. (1968). A general canonical correlation index. *Psychological Bulletin, 70*, 160–163.

Terman, L. M. (1916). *The measurement of intelligence*. Boston: Houghton Mifflin.

Terman, L. M. (1938). *Psychological factors in marital happiness*. New York: McGraw-Hill.

Thurstone, L. L. (1947). *Multiple factor analysis*. Chicago: University of Chicago Press.

Whisman, M. A. (1999). Marital dissatisfaction and psychiatric disorders: Results from the National Comorbidity Survey. *Journal of Abnormal Psychology, 108*, 701–706.

Whisman, M. A. (2001). Marital adjustment and outcome following treatments for depression. *Journal of Consulting and Clinical Psychology, 69*, 125–129.

Whisman, M. A., & Uebelacker, L. A. (2003). Comorbidity of relationship distress and mental and physical health problems. In D. K. Snyder & M. A. Whisman (Eds.), *Treating difficult couples: Helping clients with coexisting mental and relationship disorders* (pp. 3–26). New York: Guilford Press.

Wirt, R. D., Lachar, D., Klinedinst, J. K., & Seat, P. D. (1984). *Multidimensional description of child personality: A manual for the Personality Inventory for Children* (1984 rev. by D. Lachar). Los Angeles: Western Psychological Services.

PART V

ADVANCED QUANTITATIVE METHODS

CHAPTER 20

Multilevel Growth Modeling in the Context of Family Research

MARGARET K. KEILEY
NINA C. MARTIN
TING LIU
MEGAN DOLBIN-MacNAB

BACKGROUND

Change or growth is a fundamental premise of many, if not most, therapeutic modalities. Clients often enter therapy seeking resolution to situations they consider problematic or undesirable—hoping for decreases in levels of stress, for example, or increases in personal power, strength, or esteem. Change can be especially complicated in the context of the family, as multiple individuals are involved in simultaneous change processes, sometimes in concert with one another and sometimes in conflict. In addition, change can occur on multiple levels, affecting individuals within a family or influencing the family as a whole. Because family therapists are often the catalysts of such change, they are interested not only in clients' and family members' patterns of growth or change during the course of therapy, but also in whether or not change is sustained over the long term or even continues after therapy has ended. Those who engage in research about the family are particularly attuned to these changes; they seek not only to measure what clients' and family members' course of development looks like over time, but also to assess what predicts that development. For example, do individuals and family members get better over time, do they get worse, or do they stay the same? Why do some clients and family members change or grow differently from others, and what makes some get better whereas others get worse? Indeed, these two major questions—what change looks like over time, and what predicts that change—are fundamental to understanding whether or not many therapeutic modalities (and, indeed, many therapists) are successful. They are also the two fundamental questions that underlie the statistical methodology of multilevel growth modeling.

Prior to the 1980s, answering complex questions about growth such as the ones posed above was difficult, and efforts to do so were often fraught with confusion. In recent years, statisticians and methodologists have developed a class of statistical methods and accompanying computer programs that make answering those questions easier. In the course of developing these methods and programs, however, the terminology surrounding growth and the modeling of growth has become confusing. "Individual growth modeling," "multilevel modeling," "growth mixture modeling," "random-coefficient modeling," and "hierarchical linear modeling" have all been used to describe the analysis of growth or change over time. In this chapter, we use the term "multilevel growth modeling" to describe the process of modeling growth over time. We discuss both models that incorporate only manifest or single indicators of growth (whether in single or multiple domains), and models that incorporate multiple measures of change via a latent-variable approach to growth modeling. For example, models with a single indicator of Externalizing behavior (one domain) from the Child Behavior Checklist (CBCL; Achenbach, 1991) could be fitted to examine the growth of these behaviors. Alternatively, a single model could be fitted to examine simultaneously the growth in CBCL Externalizing and Internalizing behaviors (two domains). Models also can be fitted to examine the growth in a latent construct (e.g., depression) that is measured by several indicators at each time point. We note, however, that all of these growth models are inherently multilevel models—modeling, at a minimum, change both between and within individuals (i.e., two-level models)—and as such can also be referred to as "hierarchical models," indicating the nested within/between, or hierarchical, structure of the data. These models incorporate, or contain a mix of, both fixed effects (e.g., estimated parameters) and random effects (e.g., variance components), leading to the nomenclature of "mixed models" or "random-coefficient models." These distinctions will become clearer throughout this chapter. In addition, we hope to clarify what multilevel growth modeling is, how it can be conducted with methods that are currently available, and how the results can be interpreted. In the process, we focus on examples from family and couple research to illustrate the concepts and process of growth modeling and demonstrate its usefulness and applicability within the field of family research.

METHODOLOGY

Requirements for Multilevel Growth Modeling

In order to model change over time, multiple waves of data are necessary. The more waves the better, but at least three waves are required to begin to model patterns of growth. Two waves of data (e.g., pretest and posttest data) can be used to assess change, but are not sufficient to model the *shape* of the change trajectory over time. For example, in Figure 20.1, Person 1 and Person 2 have the same values of marital satisfaction at the beginning of treatment (Time 1) and the end of treatment 9 weeks later (Time 2), but their growth trajectories are very different and cannot be captured with just the two time points. If the researcher had only collected data about marital satisfaction at pre- and posttreatment, he or she would not be able to illustrate or examine the very different experiences that each respondent had during treatment. The researcher would also have to assume with only pre- and posttreatment data that growth between those two points was linear (i.e., it went up, went down, or stayed the

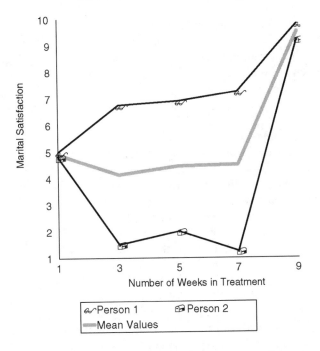

FIGURE 20.1. Individual- versus mean-level growth trajectories of two hypothetical respondents on the level of marital satisfaction through 9 weeks of marital therapy.

same). On the other hand, because the researcher has collected data at each of the 9 weeks under study, patterns of growth other than those conforming to a straight line can be considered. The collection of multiple waves, though a necessary condition of multilevel growth modeling, is not sufficient for the proper estimation of change, however. Once collected, multiple-wave data must be analyzed in such a way as to incorporate both the average level of change at each time point (illustrated by the gray line in Figure 20.1) and each individual's pattern of change (the dark lines in Figure 20.1). We return to this point later in the discussion of the estimation procedures of multilevel growth modeling.

A second requirement for the study of change is a meaningful or useful metric for time. For example, an investigator who is examining change in the therapeutic alliance with clients over the course of treatment might use session number to denote time (e.g., Time 1 = Session 1, Time 2 = Session 2, etc.). If, however, the time between sessions was variable across clients (e.g., Session 2 occurred 1 week after Session 1 for Client 1 but 3 weeks after Session 1 for Client 2), the meaning of the session numbers would be different for each client. In this case, a more appropriate coding of time would be in weeks. The proper coding of time is not always immediately apparent; researchers should rely on both theory and previous research to determine the best metric for demonstrating change. In addition, the timing of the waves of data collection should be considered carefully during the design phase of the study. For example, if the researcher hypothesizes that changes in therapeutic alliance are more likely to occur at the beginning of the treatment, he or she may decide to collect data more frequently in the early phases of treatment (e.g., every week for 5 weeks) and to space the later data collection times further apart (e.g., every month for the remainder of sessions). Again, however, the investigator should take care to allow theory and previous research to guide the decision about when to measure respondents. If change in therapeutic alliance occurs more rapidly at the end of treatment, for example, a data collection schedule that is frequent in the early stages and subsequently intermittent would cause the researcher to miss important information about the course of change in therapeutic alliance.

Finally, the outcome under study must change or develop systematically over time. Such change may be linear, nonlinear, increasing, decreasing, or even discontinuous (e.g., it may grow upward, drop off, then grow upward again), but it must occur. The outcome variable itself does not have to conform to a continuous distribution, however; recent advances have allowed for modeling change over time in categorical as well as continuous outcomes (e.g., Muthen & Muthen, 2000). Regardless of the distributional properties of the outcome, the metric of the outcome variable must be preserved over time. That is, the measure of the outcome must be equatable at each time point, such that systematic change can be observed and will have the same meaning and interpretation at every assessment point. Ideally, the same measure should be used for the outcome variable at each time point. As an aside, it is important to note that this equatability cannot be achieved by standardizing the variable, since doing so eliminates the original metric and confounds the evaluation of change. Often both raw and standardized scores are available for many common measures, such as the CBCL. The raw scores should be used, because the standardized scores are usually percentile scores, which obscure change over time.

In addition to being equatable across time, the outcome must be measured validly and reliably across occasions of measurement. As with any statistical analysis, without valid and reliable measures of change, much of the variance we are trying to explain will be due simply to error. A discussion of the construction and availability of valid and reliable measures for various outcomes is beyond the scope of this chapter; it should be noted, however, that, as in many fields, problems related to measurement often plague family researchers. At a minimum, investigators should incorporate in the design phase of their studies measures that have demonstrated validity and reliability, while also contributing to the ongoing effort to develop even better measures of family processes and other constructs centrally related to the field of family research.

Exploratory Growth Analysis

In order to illustrate the steps of multilevel growth modeling, we now introduce a secondary data analysis of a study of drug abuse treatments. The original study as designed by Lewis (1990) compared the effects of three forms of treatment (couple therapy, individual therapy focused on couple issues, and standard drug treatment) on the reduction in drug use among 123 women of childbearing years with drug addictions and their partners (i.e., husbands or significant others). The women and their partners were randomly assigned to each of the three groups for 3 months of treatment. In our secondary analysis of these data (Keiley, Liu, & Dolbin-MacNab, 2004), we found no effect of the type of treatment on the drug use or relational functioning of the women and their partners. Thus we collapsed the data across the three groups, and we consider in this chapter the effect of treatment per se (regardless of type) for all 123 women. Accordingly, our two research questions for this illustration of multilevel growth modeling are as follows: (1) Was treatment of any type related to change in women's self-reported drug use, as measured by the Addiction Severity Index (ASI; McLellan et al., 1988)? (2) What variables might predict this change? As family researchers, we are also interested in whether changes in women's self-reported drug use were related to changes in their partners' self-reported drug use (i.e., an examination of growth in two domains). For the sake of simplicity, however, we examine first the changes in self-reported drug use for the women. We return later to the potential relation between the women's changes and their partners' changes.

The average age of the women in the study across all conditions was 33 years (SD = 7) and ranged from 18 to 73 years. The mean number of years of education for these women was 12 years (SD = 2), equivalent to a high school diploma. Years of education ranged from 8 to 20, indicating that some in the sample had not completed high school, whereas others had completed graduate education. Approximately 66% of the sample had 12 or fewer years of education. The majority of the women in the sample (62%) were unemployed at the time of the study. The mean annual income was $13,436 ($SD$ = $19,187), and 58% reported an income of $10,000 or less. Eighty-two percent of the sample were self-identified as European American; the remainder were Hispanic, Native American, African American, and Asian. Prior to beginning treatment, the women and their partners completed a variety of questionnaires (Time = 0). Follow-up assessments were at 3, 6, 12, and 18 months after the pretreatment assessment (Time = 0.25, 0.5, 1, and 1.5 years).

For the analyses presented here, we focus on an outcome measure of drug use—the ASI Drug Use scale (McLellan et al., 1988), used in the original study. The ASI assesses problem severity in the area of drug and alcohol use. In the following analyses, we use only the Drug Use scale; high scores indicate more severe drug addiction. We use as a predictor of drug use whether or not a woman used intravenous (IV) drugs (46% of women were thus classified at the beginning of the study). Accordingly, we can refine our original two research questions: (1) Did women's self-reported use of drugs on the ASI change over time? (2) Were those changes related to women's IV drug use?

The first step in fitting growth models to data should include the appropriate exploratory analyses. Singer and Willett (2003) devote an entire chapter to these exploratory techniques; we present a few of these techniques here. Accordingly, after examining all variables in our analysis for distributional properties and other features, we examined the empirical growth trajectories of the outcome (ASI) for each of the individuals in our sample. As we examined the plots of the outcome versus time for each sample member, we sought to determine whether they shared a common functional form. In this exploratory stage, imposing a smooth trajectory over the series of points can often illuminate this common form. Most graphics programs allow the "smoothing" of a line by selecting a curve or other functional form to join the points (e.g., in Harvard Graphics, it is the "curve" option). In Figure 20.2a, we present examples of the smoothed empirical growth trajectories for six randomly chosen individual women in the study of women with drug addictions described above. The application of this "smoothing function" then led to the question of whether the data points defined a linear or a nonlinear trajectory. We began by adopting the simplest functional form, the linear trajectory, and fitted a linear regression line to each individual respondent's data. Though we could have used a regression procedure via statistical software to fit a linear model to each individual and plotted the resulting trajectories, we used the auto-

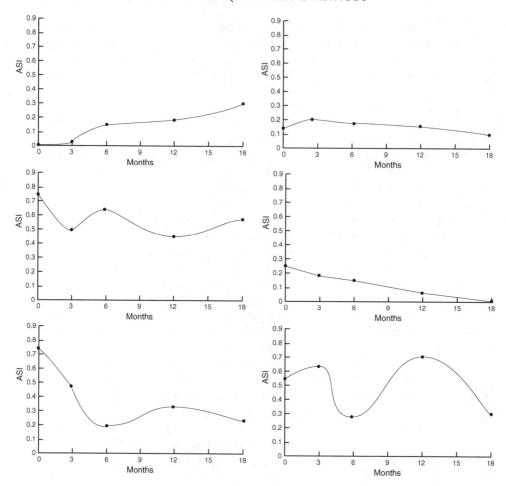

FIGURE 20.2a. Smoothed empirical growth trajectories for six women in the study of women with drug abuse.

mated procedure in our graphics program to fit these individual models for display purposes only in this initial exploratory stage. Figure 20.2b includes examples of these straight-line trajectories for the same six randomly chosen women illustrated in Figure 20.2a. In so doing, we sought to determine, by this preliminary visual inspection, whether the linear form captured the general shape of the individual trajectories of the sample respondents. In our examination of all of the straight-line trajectories for all of the women in the sample, we concluded tentatively that any nonlinear component that appeared in the data might be nothing more than measurement error. We were able later to confirm this conclusion more formally by testing whether a quadratic or other form would fit the data better than a linear model. (Please see Singer & Willett, 2003, for information about these tests.)

As a second stage in our initial exploratory data analysis, we examined a plot of women's mean self-reported ASI scores across the five time points (see Table 20.1). A plot of the mean ASI scores across time enabled us to determine whether we had cho-

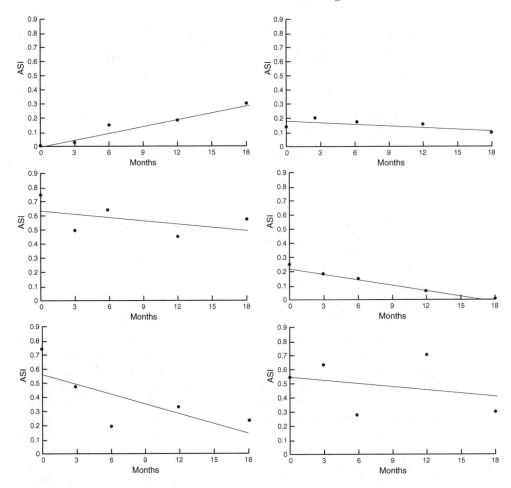

FIGURE 20.2b. Linear growth trajectories fitted to the observed data for the same six women as in Figure 20.2a.

sen the most appropriate, yet simplest, functional form for the growth model. As Figure 20.3 indicates, the plot of mean ASI scores, representing the sample average growth trajectory, appeared linear; this confirmed the conclusion that we drew in our examination of the individual empirical trajectories for each woman. Accordingly, two parameter estimates—a fitted intercept and a fitted slope—would describe the initial status and the rate of change, respectively, of self-reported drug use on the ASI for each woman in the sample. Before we describe our multilevel growth model for this sample, we describe its various components.

The Multilevel Model of Change

In the background section, we have posed two questions: "How does change occur over time?" and "What predicts the differences among people in their changes?" These questions are about change on two different levels. The first question asks us to de-

TABLE 20.1. Average Scores on the Urinalysis and the Addiction Severity Index (ASI) Drug Use Scale at Each Assessment (Time from Beginning of Treatment in Parentheses)

Variable	Mean	SD
ASI		
Pretreatment (0 years)	0.18	0.12
Posttreatment (0.25 years)	0.10	0.11
3-month follow-up (0.50 years)	0.08	0.11
6-month follow-up (1.00 years)	0.09	0.12
12-month follow-up (1.50 years)	0.05	0.08
Urinalysis		
Pretreatment (0 years)	0.11	0.12
Posttreatment (0.25 years)	0.09	0.12
3-month follow-up (0.50 years)	0.10	0.13
6-month follow-Up (1.00 years)	0.10	0.12
12-month follow-Up (1.50 years)	0.09	0.13

Note. n = 123.

scribe how each person changes over time. We want to know about change within each person. For example, is an adolescent in a treatment program for reducing delinquent behavior increasing, decreasing, or remaining the same in his or her delinquent behavior over time? The second question asks how these changes differ across people. We want to know the differences in change or growth between people. For example, do the adolescents in the delinquency treatment program differ from person to person in some systematic way? Are girls, for example, changing more rapidly than boys? To answer these two kinds of questions about within- and between-person change, we need a multilevel statistical model.

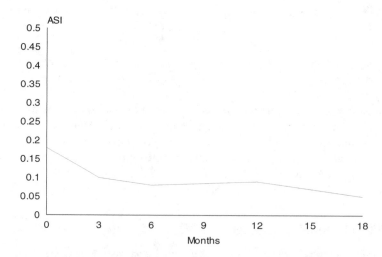

FIGURE 20.3. Plot of mean scores for the women's self-report of drug use on the ASI for the five time points (*n* = 123).

Level 1 Model of Individual Change

In our example of women with drug abuse, we decided, based on examination of both individual plots and a means plot, that their changes in self-reported drug use over time seemed, on average, to be linear. It is the "Level 1" component of the multilevel model, sometimes called the "individual growth model," that describes this individual change over time. This linear, Level 1 model is represented below:

$$\text{ASI}_{it} = [\pi_{0i} + \pi_{1i}(\text{Time}_{it})] + [\varepsilon_{it}] \tag{1}$$

We are hypothesizing that in the population from which this sample was drawn, ASI_{it}—the value of self-reported drug use (ASI) for each woman i at time t—is a linear function of the woman's time in treatment and follow-up (Time_{it}). In other words, we are positing that a straight line adequately represents each woman's true change in self-reported drug use over time, and that any deviations from linearity are the result of random measurement error (ε_{it}). The structural part of Equation 1, the true scores, is represented by $[\pi_{0i} + \pi_{1i} (\text{Time}_{it})]$, while the stochastic part, the random-measurement-error scores, is represented by $[\varepsilon_{it}]$. We are assuming that all of the women have the same algebraic form of change over time, but not the same trajectory. That is, each woman will have an intercept, π_0, and a slope, π_1, representing her trajectory, as well as a residual, ε_t, at each time point that describes the deviation of her actual scores at each time point from the predicted scores represented by the fitted linear trajectory. Thus π_{0i} is the ith woman's true initial status before treatment; π_{1i} is the ith woman's true rate of change over time; and ε_{it} is the set of residuals-per-time terms, such that ε_{i1} is the ith woman's residual at Time 1, ε_{i2} is the ith woman's residual at Time 2, and so on. This set of residuals, ε_{it}, represents the differences between the ith woman's observed trajectory and her true trajectory at each time point. We have called these residuals "random measurement error," but it is also possible that some of this variance might be explained by other time-varying predictors. (See Curran & Willoughby, 2003, for an explanation of how to fit models that incorporate time-varying predictors.) Our growth model, then, provides estimates of the initial status and growth rate of self-reported drug use for all individuals in the sample, thus revealing the "underlying true growth trajectory of each person" in the sample (Willett, 1990, p. 636). In the simplest form of this model, a simple error structure for ε_{it} is assumed, such that each ε_{it} is normally distributed, with a mean of 0 and a variance of σ^2 (such that the errors are uncorrelated across time for any given subject) (Bryk & Raudenbush, 2002). Most statistical packages for growth modeling allow for the examination of the residuals to verify these assumptions. Alternative error structures, which do not assume that the error terms are uncorrelated over time, can also be specified. See Singer and Willett (2003) for more information about how to model error structure.

The representation of time in the Level 1 growth model is often recentered (i.e., a constant is subtracted from each observed value of time) to facilitate interpretation of the intercept parameter. In our example, we did not have to recenter time, because the beginning of time was set at pretreatment as Time = 0. Thus we could already meaningfully interpret the intercept in Equation 1 to be the time when treatment started. The later values of time (0.25, 0.5, 1, and 1.5 years) denote the number of years from pretreatment assessment. Centering time so that the intercept is interpretable may make sense in the context of other studies. For example, if we were assessing adolescents' math achievement from Grade 7 to Grade 12 and hypothesized a linear trajectory, we might fit the following model using a recentered version of time:

$$Y_{ij} = [\pi_{0i} + \pi_{1i}(\text{Grade}_{ij} - 7)] + [\varepsilon_{ij}] \tag{2}$$

In this case, centering time (here denoted by "Grade") by subtracting a constant of 7 from each observed value of grade results in an intercept that now refers to the true value of the outcome, Y, at a particular grade—here, Grade 7. If the constant that is subtracted represents the first wave of data collection in the study, the intercept may also be referred to as an individual's true "initial status." The choice of whether to recenter the time variable and what constant to use in so doing is dependent upon the kinds of interpretive statements the researcher wishes to make about the data. Alternatively, in many studies, the interpretation of the intercept may be meaningless if time is not recentered. In the example above, time/grade left in its uncentered form would force the intercept to be interpreted as the value of math achievement (the outcome) at Grade 0—a nonsensical value in the context of this study.

In both examples above, the only predictor in the Level 1 model is time; individual growth parameters are allowed to differ across people, thus providing information about within-person change. That is, a growth model is fitted to every individual's data and an intercept and slope are estimated for each individual. Each person's intercept and slope describe his or her within-person change trajectory. To examine differences in change between people, we must examine the Level 2 model.

Level 2 Growth Model of Interindividual Differences in Change

Multilevel growth modeling incorporates not only change at the individual level, or intraindividual change, but also data about the average change trajectory in the population and the variability around that average trajectory. It is the "Level 2" component of the multilevel model that captures this kind of information. The Level 2 component model reexpresses the intercept and slope parameters from the Level 1 model to provide information about the means and variances of intercept and slope parameters across all individuals. In other words, the "group difference," or the *between-individual*, Level 2 model, conceptually incorporates the intercept (i.e., level) and slope (i.e., growth rate) parameters of the within-individual, Level 1 growth model as *outcomes*. It can include various characteristics of the individual (e.g., treatment status, IV drug use, or parental depression) as *predictors*.

$$\text{ASI}_{it} = [\pi_{0i} + \pi_{1i}(\text{Time}_{it})] + [\varepsilon_{it}] \qquad [\text{Level 1}] \tag{1}$$

$$\left. \begin{array}{l} \pi_{0i} = \gamma_{00} + \zeta_{0i} \\[2mm] \pi_{1i} = \gamma_{10} + \zeta_{1i} \end{array} \right\} \qquad \begin{array}{c} \\[2mm] [\text{Level 2}] \end{array} \begin{array}{c} (3) \\[2mm] (4) \end{array}$$

In the intercept component of the Level 2 model (Equation 3), the intercept for each individual, π_{0i}, is a sum of the average of the intercepts, γ_{00}, plus the deviations of the individual from this average, ζ_{0i}. In the slope component (Equation 4), the slope for each individual, π_{1i}, is a sum of the average of the slopes, γ_{10}, plus the deviations of the individual from this average, ζ_{1i}. The parameters γ_{00} and γ_{10} above are the fixed effects of the Level 2 model, reflecting the average initial status and average rate of change, respectively, across all individuals. The error terms in the Level 2 model, ζ_{0i} and ζ_{1i}, reflect deviations around the average slope and intercept parameters, respectively. Their variances ($\sigma_{\zeta 0}^2$ and $\sigma_{\zeta 1}^2$) and their covariance ($\sigma_{\zeta 10}$) are the random effects of the Level 2 model, reflecting the individual variability that exists around the estimates of average initial status and average rate of change. If variability exists around these estimates, we can then seek to predict this variability with our substantive predictor, IV drug use (or with other relevant substantive predictors).

In this part of the analysis, then, a model is fitted to the data in which "group differences" can account for "some of the observed variation in the parameters of individual change [π_{0i} and π_{1i}]" (Coie, Terry, Lenox, Lochman, & Hyman, 1995, p. 703). In the present example, we are interested in the relation between IV drug use and the parameters of individual change (i.e., our second research question).

The pair of between-individual models that predict the level and growth rate parameters of the individual women and include IV drug use as a group-characteristic predictor would be written as follows:

$$\pi_{0i} = \gamma_{00} + \gamma_{01} \cdot \text{IV drug use} + \zeta_{0i} \tag{5}$$

$$\pi_{1i} = \gamma_{10} + \gamma_{11} \cdot \text{IV drug use} + \zeta_{1i} \tag{6}$$

In Equation 5, γ_{00} represents the average *level* of drug use for women who did not use IV drugs before treatment, and γ_{01} represents the relationship between IV drug use and initial status (i.e., the increment or decrement in the initial level of drug use associated with using IV drugs). In Equation 6, γ_{10} represents the average *growth rate* for women who did not use IV drugs, and γ_{11} represents the relationship between IV drug use and the average growth rate (i.e., the differential in the growth rate) associated with IV drug use. The residuals, ζ_{0i} and ζ_{1i}, represent random effects with variances $\sigma_{\zeta 0}^2$ and $\sigma_{\zeta 1}^2$, respectively, and covariance $\sigma_{\zeta 10}$. These residuals, then, indicate the extent to which variability in the level and growth rates of drug use are not fully explained by the included between-individual characteristics (here, IV drug use). That is, they tell us the population residual variance in the true initial status and the true rates of change, controlling for IV drug use. The covariance tells us about the relationship between the slopes and intercepts, controlling for IV drug use. For this analysis, the same assumptions are made about these Level 2 residuals as for the Level 1 residuals: a mean of zero with a normal distribution and an unknown variance and covariance. These Level 2 residuals can also be examined to ensure that the assumptions are met.

Though discussion of the separate "parts" of a fitted growth model in terms of within-individual and between-individual components allows for a relatively simple explication of the various components of the model (as above), the model actually fitted to the data (in the process of multilevel growth modeling) simultaneously includes the parameters of *both* the within-individual and between-individual models. This complete multilevel model, then, simultaneously addresses questions of both individual and group change; in so doing, the multilevel growth model goes beyond traditional analysis-of-variance methods of examining change by enhancing information about group mean change (Willett, 1988). In the current example, the multilevel model that combines the Level 1 and Level 2 models (as explicated above) yields the following:

$$ASI_{it} = [\gamma_{00} + \gamma_{01} \cdot \text{IV drug use}] + [\gamma_{10} + \gamma_{11} \cdot \text{IV drug use}] \cdot \text{Time}_{it} + [\zeta_{0i} + \zeta_{1i} + \varepsilon_{it}] \qquad (7)$$

The Level 1 residual variance and the Level 2 error variance–covariance matrix are the total variance components of the combined, multilevel model.

Fitting the Multilevel Growth Model

ESTIMATION

A number of statistical packages include routines for fitting growth models, such as Mplus (Muthen & Muthen, 1998); LISREL (Joreskog & Sorbom, 1996); Proc Mixed within the SAS program (SAS Institute, 2001); Amos (Arbuckle, 1995); Hierarchical Linear Models (Bryk & Raudenbush, 2002); and Mx (Neale, Boker, Xie, & Maes, 1999), which is free on the Internet (*http://griffin.vcu.edu/mx*). These programs vary along such dimensions as flexibility and capability, user-friendliness, and even expense. For the current example, we have used maximum-likelihood estimation in Mplus to obtain the parameter estimates. Likelihood estimation procedures, whether using restricted or full information, allow for the inclusion of respondents who have missing values on the outcome (and on the predictors at Level 2) at various time points, provided that the data are missing at random. Since restricted- and maximum-likelihood methods do differ in the interpretation of the resultant fit statistics, however, the researcher is advised to be aware of the default method of estimation used by his or her chosen software. For a discussion of maximum-versus restricted-likelihood estimation procedures, see Singer and Willett (2003).

MODEL FIT

The question of how to assess model fit for growth models is dependent in part on the program used to fit the models. Some programs (Mplus, Mx, Amos, LISREL) include a variety of fit indices, while others include fewer (e.g., SAS Proc Mixed). For example, most programs provide a deviance statistic, the –2 log likelihood statistic, denoted as –2LL. To indicate "good fit," we would like to have a deviance statistic that is small with a nonsignificant *p*-value. Two other criteria—the Akaike information criterion (AIC) and the Bayesian information criterion (BIC), which correct the deviance statistic for the number of parameters or for the sample size—can also be used to assess model fit. These criteria can be compared even across models that are not nested. Smaller absolute values of the AIC and BIC indicate better model fit.

INTERPRETING THE ESTIMATED PARAMETERS OF THE FITTED GROWTH MODEL

To illustrate how to interpret the estimated parameters, we have first fitted the unconditional growth model (with no predictors), represented as follows in its multilevel form:

$$ASI_{it} = [\gamma_{00} + \gamma_{10} \cdot \text{Time}_{it}] + [\zeta_{0i} + \zeta_{1i} + \varepsilon_{it}] \qquad (8)$$

In Table 20.2, we present the parameter estimates from this fitted unconditional growth model. All estimation software includes estimates of the fixed effects (the estimated means of the intercepts and slopes across the entire sample of respondents) and the random effects (the estimated variances of the intercepts and slopes across the respondents and the covariance of the intercepts with the slopes). In addition, programs include various statistics (e.g., t-statistics, z-statistics) and p-values that allow hypothesis tests to be conducted on all of the parameter estimates to determine whether the estimates are different from 0. In general, these statistics are obtained by dividing the parameter estimate by the standard error of that estimate. For example, in Table 20.3, we obtain the t-statistic for the estimate of the intercept by dividing the estimate (.193) by its standard error (.019), giving us 10.04. The p-value for this t-statistic can be determined by examining a table of the percentiles of the t-distribution that can be found in any statistics book. Luckily, most programs used for growth modeling provide t-statistics and associated p-values.

Just as in simple regression analysis, we have interpreted the parameter estimates by first writing the fitted equation from the unconditional model, substituting into the equation the estimates in Table 20.2:

$$A\hat{S}I = .193 - .065(\text{Time}) \tag{9}$$

(The "little hat" over ASI in this equation and those that follow indicate this is a fitted, or estimated, equation.) The t-statistics for the average initial status and average rate of change indicate that both of these estimates are significantly different from 0. In other words, on average, the women began their drug use trajectories significantly above 0 and reported that they declined significantly in their drug use over time. We can illustrate this on-average trend by plotting the trajectory for a prototypical woman in the sample, substituting into Equation 9 the values of time (0, 0.25, 0.5, 1, 1.5 years) (Figure 20.4). In this figure and the remaining figures, we have transformed the representation of time that we have used for estimation (years) into its representation as months for ease of interpretation. From this figure we can see that, on average, women reported significantly lower drug use both after treatment and at follow-up. We can also interpret the estimated covariance ($\hat{\sigma}^2_{10} = -.007$, $t = -1.96$, $p < .05$) between the true initial status and true rate of change. Combined with the two variances, we can convert this covariance to a correlation ($r = -.56$). This negative correlation indicates a significant relation between women's initial status of drug use and their rates of change: Women who reported lower drug use prior to treatment had more rapid rates of change through follow-up, and vice versa.

TABLE 20.2. Estimates of the Unconditional Growth Model

Parameter	Fixed effects: Means		Random effects: Variances	
	Estimate (SE)	t-statistic	Estimate (SE)	t-statistic
Initial status	.193 (.019)	10.04***	.028 (.006)	4.35***
Rate of change	−.065 (.012)	−5.39***	.009 (.005)	1.80~

Note. $n = 123$.
~$p < .10$; *** $p < .001$.

TABLE 20.3. Results of Fitting a Taxonomy of Growth Models for Change in the ASI for Women with Drug Abuse

	Parameter	Unconditional model: Estimate (SE)	Conditional model: Estimate (SE)
Fixed effects			
Initial status, π_{0i}			
Intercept	γ_{00}	.193 *** (.019)	.095*** (.022)
IV drug use	γ_{01}		.236*** (.032)
Rate of change, π_{1i}			
Intercept	γ_{10}	−.065*** (.012)	−.035** (.016)
IV drug use	γ_{11}		−.066** (.023)
Variance components			
In initial status	σ_0^2	.028*** (.006)	.015** (.005)
In rate of change	σ_1^2	.009~ (.005)	.009~ (.005)
Covariance	σ_{01}	−.007~ (.004)	−.005 (.003)
Deviance		184.19	119.97
AIC		299.36	160.86
BIC		259.99	110.24

Note. n = 123.
~$p < .10$; **$p < .01$; ***$p < .001$.

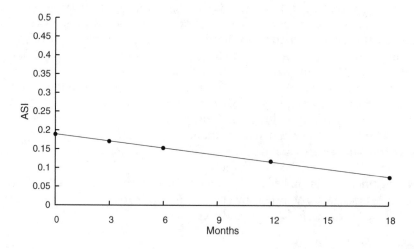

FIGURE 20.4. Plot of the fitted trajectory for a prototypical woman's self-reported drug use on the ASI over five time periods (n = 123).

EXAMINING THE VARIANCE COMPONENTS OF THE FITTED GROWTH MODEL

In order to answer our second question, "What might predict the differences among women in their changes?," we must first determine whether, indeed, the women in the sample differed significantly from one another in either their beginning levels of drug use or their rates of change. In order to do that, we have examined the random effects, or the variance components, of the fitted model. The variance estimates in Table 20.2 summarize the population heterogeneity in the true intercept and true slope. In other words, the variance of the true initial status ($\sigma_{\zeta 0}^2$) describes the scatter of the π_{0i} around the estimate of the average true initial status, and the variance of the true rate of change ($\sigma_{\zeta 1}^2$) describes the scatter of the π_{1i} around the estimate of the average true rate of change. In our case, because both of the variance estimates are different from 0 (the slope variance is marginally different from 0), we can conclude that the women varied significantly from one another in both their initial status and rate of change. That is, not all women began at the same starting level of reported drug abuse, and not all changed in the same way over time. We can then predict these variances by including predictors in the model at Level 2.

Fitting the Multilevel Conditional Growth Model

We have fitted the multilevel conditional model (here, a model with one Level 2 predictor) in the same manner as we have fitted the unconditional model. In order to determine whether IV drug use is a significant predictor of the variance in the intercepts (π_{0i}) and slopes (π_{1i}) of the ASI, we must conduct a difference-in-deviance-statistics test. In this case, we must constrain the effects of IV drug use on the intercepts and slopes to be 0 and refit the model, examining the resultant fit statistics (i.e., examining a model with and without the predictor IV drug use). In our example, after refitting the appropriate models and comparing their deviance statistics, we have determined IV drug use to be a significant predictor of the variance in the intercepts and slopes of the ASI.

INTERPRETING THE PARAMETER ESTIMATES OF THE FITTED
CONDITIONAL GROWTH MODEL

In Table 20.3, we present results for both our unconditional and conditional growth models. We then interpret the parameter estimates by again writing the fitted multilevel equation:

$$\text{A}\hat{\text{S}}\text{I} = [.095 + .236 \cdot \text{IV drug use}] + [-.035 - .066 \cdot \text{IV drug use}] \cdot \text{Time} \qquad (10)$$

As Table 20.3 indicates, the significance levels of the average initial status, the average rate of change, and the effects of IV drug use on the average initial status and average rate of change indicate that all of these estimates are significantly different from 0. As with our Level 1 model, the best way to understand the Level 2 model is to plot trajectories for individuals whose values on the various predictors in the model identify them as "prototypical," or representative of the population from which the sample was drawn. In this case, we are interested in a woman who used IV drugs (IV drug use

= 1) and in one who did not (IV drug use = 0). We have substituted these values into Equation 10:

$$\text{When IV drug use} = 0,\ \hat{ASI} = [.095 + .236 \cdot 0] + [-.035 - .066 \cdot 0] \cdot \text{Time}, \quad (11)$$
$$\text{or } \hat{ASI} = .095 - .035 \cdot \text{Time}$$

$$\text{When IV drug use} = 1,\ \hat{ASI} = [.095 + .236 \cdot 1] + [-.035 - .066 \cdot 1] \cdot \text{Time}, \quad (12)$$
$$\text{or } \hat{ASI} = .331 - .101 \cdot \text{Time}$$

These two fitted equations (11 and 12) indicate that, on average, women who used IV drugs had a higher initial status ($\hat{ASI}$ =.331) than women who did not use IV drugs ($\hat{ASI}$ = .095). In addition, the former women had a more rapidly decreasing trajectory ($\hat{ASI}$ = −.101) than the latter women ($\hat{ASI}$ = −.035). These differences between the two groups are illustrated in Figure 20.5. We have substituted the values for time (0, 0.25, 0.50, 1.00, 1.50 years) into each of the two equations (11 and 12) and plotted the trajectories for these prototypical women. In our example, we have used a dichotomous predictor, which makes choosing "substantively interesting" values and identifying "prototypical" individuals straightforward. If a predictor is continuous, prototypical plots might be constructed by substituting into the equations the 25th- and 75th-percentile values of the variable, the mean value, or the mean value plus or minus one standard deviation. The choice of plotting values will depend on the particular variable(s) whose effects are to be illustrated and the distribution of the variable(s) in the sample; as the label implies, "prototypical" individuals should be not represent extreme cases at the far edges of a variable's distribution. Figure 20.5 illustrates the finding that women who used IV drugs reported beginning their trajectories significantly

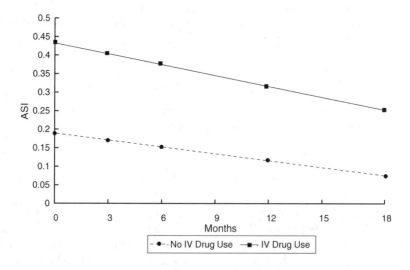

FIGURE 20.5. Plot of the fitted trajectories for two prototypical women's self-reported drug use on the ASI over five time periods—one for a woman who used IV drugs prior to treatment, and one for a woman who did not (*n* = 123).

higher than did those women who did not use IV drugs. In addition, the self-reported trajectories for women who used IV drugs declined significantly more rapidly than did those for women who did not use IV drugs. An examination of the covariance of the initial status with the slope of ASI ($\hat{\sigma}^2{}_{10}$ = –.005, n.s.), now, controlling for IV drug use, indicates no relationship between where a woman started on the ASI and her later trajectory. That is, once ASI is controlled for IV drug use, we can conclude that a woman who began high or low on the ASI might have a declining, increasing, or stable trajectory.

OUTCOME VARIATION EXPLAINED BY THE PREDICTOR

Having determined that our Level 2 predictor is a significant addition to the model, we would like to be able to quantify how much of the variance in the intercept and slope parameters we have explained by including this predictor. Most growth-modeling software provides some form of pseudo-R^2 statistic or provides the information needed for the user to construct this statistic. Some base the computation on the squared correlation between the observed and predicted values of the outcome. Others construct a pseudo-R^2 statistic or a proportional-reduction-in-variance statistic from the variance components, using a formula similar to the one presented below for the residual variance in the intercept of ASI after being predicted by IV drug use:

$$\text{Pseudo-}R^2{}_{\zeta 0} = \frac{\hat{\sigma}^2{}_0(\text{unconditional growth model}) - \hat{\sigma}^2{}_0(\text{condtional growth model})}{\hat{\sigma}^2{}_0(\text{unconditional growth model})}, \text{ or } \quad (13)$$

$$\text{Pseudo-}R^2{}_{\zeta 0} = (.028 - .015)/.028 = .46$$

In other words, in this case, 46% of the variation in the intercepts of ASI has been explained by adding IV drug use to the model. Using the same formula in regard to the slopes, we can determine that IV drug use predicts 10% of the variation in the slopes of ASI. In a similar manner, estimates of the reduction in variance associated with the addition of further variables to the model can be generated. (For more on the uses of and caveats related to the pseudo-R^2 statistic, see Singer & Willett, 2003.)

EXAMINING THE VARIANCE COMPONENTS OF THE FITTED
CONDITIONAL GROWTH MODEL

The variance estimates in Table 20.3 for the conditional model summarize the population heterogeneity in the true intercept and true slope, controlling for IV drug use. In other words, the estimate of the variance of the true initial status ($\hat{\sigma}^2{}_0$) describes the scatter of the π_{0i} around the estimate of the mean true initial status, and the estimate of the variance of the true rate of change ($\hat{\sigma}^2{}_1$) describes the scatter of the π_{1i} around the estimate of the mean true rate of change, controlling for the predictor (IV drug use). In our case, both of these variance estimates are different from 0, and we can conclude even after controlling for IV drug use that the women varied in both their initial status and rate of change. That is, although IV drug use is a significant predictor of the variance in both the initial status and growth of ASI-reported drug use, significant variation still exists in the intercept ($\hat{\sigma}^2_0 = .015$, $p < .01$) and slope ($\hat{\sigma}^2_1 = .009$, $p < .10$) after the inclusion of this predictor. Additional predictors may then account for differences in women's varying initial levels and patterns of growth, now controlled for IV drug use. Though we do not proceed further with the inclusion of additional predictors in the model in the current example, the logical "next steps" for analyses would include determining the effects on the intercept and slope variance of other variables in which a researcher is interested.

Cross-Domain Analysis of Change

We now continue with our example of women with drug abuse, but add another domain in which change might occur. In so doing, we construct a cross-domain, or multiple-domain, analysis of change. Cross-domain analyses of change may be especially relevant to the field of family research, in which investigators are often interested in the relationships between reports of multiple constructs, or domains, by a single family member (e.g., growth in mother-reported family cohesion vs. growth in mother-reported family conflict) or between reports of the same single construct by different family members (e.g., mother's report of family cohesion vs. child's report of family cohesion). In the present example, our research question in relation to cross-domain change is how a woman's self-report of drug use (Domain 1) would compare with her urinalysis report of drug use (Domain 2) over this same period of time. The analysis of an individual's urine serves as an objective measure of whether the individual has recently used drugs. The drugs that are screened in a urinalysis include cocaine, methadone, amphetamines, barbiturates, benzodiazepines, opiates, PCP, and cannabis. High urinalysis scores indicate more drugs within an individual's system. In addition, we continue to examine the predictor of IV drug use to determine its effect on the growth parameters in each domain. In a cross-domain analysis, then, we are no longer interested in change in just one domain (here, women's self-report of drug use), but in two domains (here, self-report of drug use and urinalysis report of drug use). We are interested in questions such as these:

1. Was true initial status on self-reported drug use positively related to true initial status on the urinalysis? That is, did women who report high drug use prior to treatment also have high urinalysis scores, and vice versa?
2. Was the true rate of change in self-reported drug use related positively to the true rate of change in urinalysis scores? That is, did women who showed a rapid downward trajectory in self-reported drug use also show a rapid downward trajectory in urinalysis scores, and vice versa?
3. Was the true initial status of self-report related negatively to the true slope of urinalysis? In other words, did women who started high on self-reported drug use have a more rapid decrease in their urinalysis scores than did women who started low on self-report, and vice versa?
4. Was the true initial status on the urinalysis score negatively related to the true slope of the self-reported scores?

These complex questions can be addressed in a multiple-domain growth model, in which we model change in both domains simultaneously.

Unconditional Multiple-Domain Growth Model

The unconditional multiple-domain Level 1 and Level 2 growth models for the current example are represented as follows:

$$\text{ASI}_{it} = [\pi^A_{0i} + \pi^A_{1i}(\text{Time}_{it})] + [\varepsilon^A_{it}] \qquad \text{[Level 1]} \qquad (14)$$

$$\pi^A_{0i} = \gamma^A_{00} + \zeta^A_{0i} \qquad (15)$$
$$\qquad \text{[Level 2]}$$
$$\pi^A_{1i} = \gamma^A_{10} + \zeta^A_{1i} \qquad (16)$$

$$\text{Urin}_{it} = [\pi^U_{0i} + \pi^U_{1i}(\text{Time}_{it})] + [\varepsilon^U_{it}] \qquad \text{[Level 1]} \qquad (17)$$

$$\pi^U_{0i} = \gamma^U_{00} + \zeta^U_{0i} \qquad (18)$$
$$\qquad \text{[Level 2]}$$
$$\pi^U_{1i} = \gamma^U_{10} + \zeta^U_{1i} \qquad (19)$$

The superscripts "A" and "U" in the models above indicate which growth parameters are from the model for the ASI and which are from the model for the urinalysis scores, respectively. These models have been fitted simultaneously in a cross-domain growth analysis. Most available growth-modeling software programs facilitate multiple-domain modeling. In this example, fitting the cross-domain model yields estimates for the unconditional model, as presented in Table 20.4.

INTERPRETING THE FITTED UNCONDITIONAL GROWTH MODEL

As in our single-domain analysis previously presented, we write the fitted growth equations:

$$\hat{\text{ASI}} = .205 - .063\text{Time}_t \qquad (20)$$

$$\hat{\text{Urin}} = .233 + .002\text{Time}_t \qquad (21)$$

The model statistics, as presented in Table 20.4, indicate that the average true initial status for the ASI, the average true rate of change for the ASI, and the average true initial status for the urinalysis are significantly different from 0. The average true slope for the urinalysis is 0 in the population; no change exists in the trajectory for the urinalysis. On average, then, women began their drug use trajectories (both ASI and urinalysis) significantly above 0, but they reported a significant decline in their drug use on the ASI over time, while their urinalysis scores remained stable. We can illustrate these findings by plotting the trajectory for a prototypical woman in the sample. By substituting into Equations 20 and 21 the values of time (0, 0.25, 0.50, 1.00, and 1.50 years), we can plot the resulting average growth trajectories (Figure 20.6). We present these plots in two separate figures, because the metrics of the outcome scales differ. Again, we have translated the time in years to time in months in constructing the prototypical plots. From the figures of the two trajectories, we can see that, on average, these women reported significantly lowered drug use after treatment, whereas their urinalysis scores did not exhibit this trend. Findings such as these might then lead the researcher to investigate why the women self-reported lowered drug use after treat-

TABLE 20.4. Results of Fitting a Taxonomy of Growth Models for Change in the ASI and Change in Urinalysis for Women with Drug Abuse

	Parameter	Unconditional model: Estimate (*SE*)	Conditional model: Estimate (*SE*)
Fixed effects			
Initial status, π^{A}_{0i}			
Intercept	γ^{A}_{00}	.205*** (.019)	.098*** (.022)
IV drug use	γ^{A}_{01}		.236*** (.032)
Rate of change, π^{A}_{1i}			
Intercept	γ^{A}_{10}	−.063*** (.012)	−.035** (.032)
IV drug use	γ^{A}_{11}		−.060** (.023)
Initial status, π^{U}_{0i}			
Intercept	γ^{U}_{00}	.233*** (.019)	.125*** (.021)
IV drug use	γ^{U}_{01}		.236*** (.031)
Rate of change, π^{U}_{1i}			
Intercept	γ^{U}_{10}	.002 (.013)	.003 (.013)
IV drug use	γ^{U}_{11}		— —
Variance components			
In initial status	$\sigma^{A}_{0}{}^{2}$	.031*** (.006)	.017*** (.005)
In rate of change	$\sigma^{A}_{1}{}^{2}$	.001** (.005)	.011** (.005)
In initial status	$\sigma^{U}_{0}{}^{2}$	.027*** (.006)	.012** (.004)
In rate of change	$\sigma^{U}_{1}{}^{2}$	.010 (.008)	.011 (.007)
Covariances	$\sigma^{A}_{0}{}^{A}_{1}$	−.009** (.003)	−.005~ (.003)
	$\sigma^{A}_{0}{}^{U}_{0}$	.030*** (.005)	.016*** (.003)
	$\sigma^{A}_{1}{}^{U}_{0}$	−.009*** (.002)	−.005** (.002)
	$\sigma^{A}_{0}{}^{U}_{1}$	−.001 (.003)	−.003 (.002)
	$\sigma^{A}_{1}{}^{U}_{1}$	.003** (.001)	.004** (.001)
	$\sigma^{U}_{0}{}^{U}_{1}$	.010** (.003)	.007** (.003)
Deviance		408.06	353.01
AIC		667.40	538.82
BIC		577.41	552.11

Note. n = 123.
~*p* < .10; **p* < .01; ***p* < .001.

ment but showed no change on what might be considered a more objective measure of drug use, the urinalysis report. Was the treatment actually ineffective, although the women perceived that it worked? Were the women in this sample simply misrepresenting the truth about treatment in reporting its effects? Were the findings similar for all three forms of treatment in this study? Would the partners' drug use trajectories display similar patterns? Depending on the various predictors that investigators have chosen to measure, questions such as these, and others, can be answered in the context of multiple-domain growth analyses.

As we have done with the single-domain growth analysis, we can also interpret the estimated covariances reported in Table 20.4 by converting them into correlations; most growth-modeling programs provide these estimated correlations among the true initial status and true rate of change for each of these domains, however. Here, the correlation between the intercepts and slopes of the ASI ($\hat{r} = -.46$, $p < .01$) suggests that women who reported lower drug use prior to treatment had more rapid rates of change through follow-up, and vice versa, controlling for change in urinalysis. The correlation between intercepts and slopes of urinalysis ($\hat{r} = .58$, $p < .01$) denotes that women who started lower on their urinalysis reports prior to treatment had less rapid change in their urinalysis trajectory over time, and vice versa, controlling for change in ASI. The intercepts of ASI and urinalysis are highly correlated ($\hat{r} = .98$, $p < .001$), suggesting that, at least at pretreatment, the self-report and test results for drug use were similar: Women who reported using a large amount of drugs also tested high for drug use on the urinalysis, and vice versa. The slopes of the ASI and the urinalysis are also correlated but at a lower level ($\hat{r} = .31$, $p < .01$), indicating that, on average, women with increasing trajectories of ASI-reported drug use also had slightly increasing trajectories on their urinalysis, and vice versa. We have to remember, however, that, on average, the trajectories of urinalysis were the same across all women; that is, we find no significant variance in the slopes of the urinalysis ($\hat{\sigma}^{U_0 2} = .010$, n.s.). Interestingly, though, on average, women scoring high on the urinalysis drug use measure at pre-

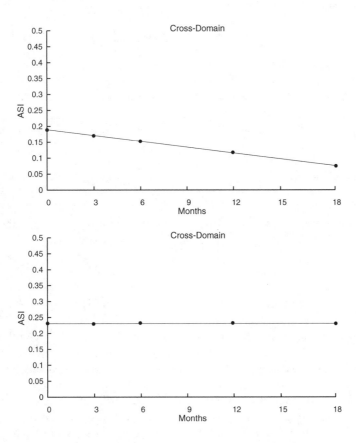

FIGURE 20.6. Plots of the fitted trajectories for a prototypical woman's self-reported drug use (ASI) and urinalysis results over five time periods ($n = 123$).

treatment had less rapid rates of change on the ASI over time, and vice versa ($\hat{r} = -.49$, $p < .001$), whereas the opposite was not true. This finding provides some evidence that women who were using a lot of drugs at pretreatment, based on the urinalysis, were reporting more of a decline in their drug use than were women who were not as heavily involved with drugs at pretreatment. The urinalysis trajectories of women were not related to their ASI scores at pretreatment ($\hat{r} = -.05$, n.s.). Again, this finding is partly due to the absence of variance in the slopes of the urinalysis; women were stable over time in their trajectories. They differed in their trajectories only in their initial status on the urinalysis report at pretreatment.

We find significant variance remaining in the intercept and slope of ASI ($\hat{\sigma}^A_0{}^2 =$ .031, $p < .001$, and $\hat{\sigma}^A_1{}^2 = .001$, $p < .01$, respectively) and the intercept of urinalysis ($\hat{\sigma}^U_0{}^2 = -.009$, $p < .001$); therefore, we are interested in fitting a conditional growth model predicting these variances with IV drug use. Because we have found no variance in the slope of urinalysis, we do not examine predictors in relation to this parameter.

Conditional Multiple-Domain Growth Model

Our conditional model can be represented at Level 1 and Level 2 as follows:

$$\text{ASI}_{it} = [\pi^A_{0i} + \pi^A_{1i}(\text{Time}_{it})] + [\varepsilon^A_{it}] \qquad \text{[Level 1]} \qquad (22)$$

$$\pi^A_{0i} = \gamma^A_{00} + \gamma^A_{01} \cdot \text{IV drug use} + \zeta^A_{0i} \qquad (23)$$
$$\text{[Level 2]}$$
$$\pi^A_{1i} = \gamma^A_{10} + \gamma^A_{11} \cdot \text{IV drug use} + \zeta^A_{1i} \qquad (24)$$

$$\text{Urin}_{it} = [\pi^U_{0i} + \pi^U_{1i}(\text{Time}_{it})] + [\varepsilon^U_{it}] \qquad \text{[Level 1]} \qquad (25)$$

$$\pi^U_{0i} = \gamma^U_{00} + \gamma^U_{01} \cdot \text{IV drug use} + \zeta^U_{0i} \qquad (26)$$
$$\text{[Level 2]}$$
$$\pi^U_{1i} = \gamma^U_{10} + \gamma^U_{11} \cdot \text{IV drug use} + \zeta^U_{1i} \qquad (27)$$

We can also represent these equations in combined multilevel form, substituting the Level 2 parameters into the Level 1 models and rearranging the terms as follows:

$$\text{ASI}_{it} = [\gamma^A_{00} + \gamma^A_{01} \cdot \text{IV drug use}] + [\gamma^A_{10} + \gamma^A_{11} \cdot \text{IV drug use}] \cdot \text{Time}_{it} + [\zeta^A_{0i} + \zeta^A_{1i} + \varepsilon^A_{it}] \quad (28)$$

$$\text{Urin}_{it} = [\gamma^U_{00} + \gamma^U_{01} \cdot \text{IV drug use}] + [\gamma^U_{10} + \gamma^U_{11} \cdot \text{IV drug use}] \cdot \text{Time}_{it} + [\zeta^U_{0i} + \zeta^U_{1i} + \varepsilon^U_{it}] \quad (29)$$

The results from fitting this model appear in Table 20.4. As with our single-domain fitted growth model, we have substituted substantively interesting values for the predictor IV drug use (0, 1) and plotted our fitted model across the five time points (0, 0.25, 0.50, 1.00, 1.50 years). These fitted plots are presented in the two panels of Figure 20.7—one for each domain, representing the different metric of ASI versus IV drug use. As in Figure 20.5, these panels indicate that women who used IV drugs began their ASI trajectories significantly higher than did those women who did not use IV drugs, and vice versa, controlling for urinalysis. In addition, the trajectories for women who used IV drugs declined significantly more rapidly than did those for women who did not use IV drugs, and vice versa, controlling for change in urinalysis.

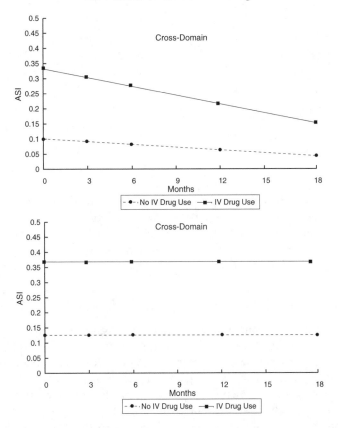

FIGURE 20.7. Plots of the fitted trajectories for two prototypical women's self-reported drug use (ASI) and urinalysis results over five time periods—one for a woman who used IV drugs prior to treatment, and one for a woman who did not ($n = 123$).

The urinalysis trajectories for the women using IV drugs also began at higher levels than did those for the women not using these drugs, controlling for ASI—but whether or not the women used IV drugs, their urinalysis trajectories were stable, on average, over time.

When we examine the correlations (constructed from the covariances) among the growth parameters for ASI and urinalysis, little changes from the unconditional model. On average, the correlation between the intercept of ASI and the slope is now of lower magnitude than before ($\hat{r} = -.27$, $p < .10$), as is the correlation between the intercepts of ASI and urinalysis ($\hat{r} = .56$, $p < .001$). The correlation between the slope of ASI and initial status on the urinalysis measures is also diminished ($\hat{r} = -.28$, $p < .01$). These correlations can be interpreted similarly to those reported for the unconditional model (above), with the exception that these relations are now conditional upon IV drug use.

As family researchers, we might also be interested in comparing the changes in these women's drug use (self-reported or urinalysis) to the changes in drug use for their partners. In this case, the unconditional growth model would be a multiple-domain model in which the two domains are women's drug use and partners' drug use:

$$\text{ASI}^W_{it} = [\pi^W_{0i} + \pi^W_{1i}(\text{Time}_{it})] + [\varepsilon^W_{it}] \qquad [\text{Level 1}] \qquad (30)$$

$$\pi^W_{0i} = \gamma^W_{00} + \zeta^W_{0i} \qquad\qquad\qquad (31)$$
$$\qquad\qquad\qquad\qquad\qquad [\text{Level 2}]$$
$$\pi^W_{1i} = \gamma^W_{10} + \zeta^W_{1i} \qquad\qquad\qquad (32)$$

$$\text{ASI}^P_{it} = [\pi^P_{0i} + \pi^P_{1i}(\text{Time}_{it})] + [\varepsilon^P_{it}] \qquad [\text{Level 1}] \qquad (33)$$

$$\pi^P_{0i} = \gamma^P_{00} + \zeta^P_{0i} \qquad\qquad\qquad (34)$$
$$\qquad\qquad\qquad\qquad\qquad [\text{Level 2}]$$
$$\pi^P_{1i} = \gamma^P_{10} + \zeta^P_{1i} \qquad\qquad\qquad (35)$$

The superscript "W" denotes the unconditional model for the women, and the superscript "P" denotes the one for the partners. The conditional growth models in which IV drug use is a predictor would be fitted simultaneously in the same manner as the cross-domain conditional model illustrated above. The definition of the second "domain," however, has now changed.

More Complex Growth Models

In addition to single-domain and multiple-domain growth models, more complex growth models can also be fitted. For example, if we had data at several time points for both male and female adolescents on their conduct-disordered behaviors during and after family treatment, and if we believed that the pattern of change in these behaviors might differ across gender, we could conduct one of two analyses. In one analysis, we could enter gender as a covariate in a single-domain growth model of conduct-disordered behaviors. This analysis would be similar to the one illustrated above for the women who used IV drugs and those who did not. What might be more useful, however, might be a second kind of analysis in which we fit a multiple-group model and test for parameters that differ across gender. By so doing, we would be conducting a test of the interaction between the change process and group membership. To complete this second type of analysis, the growth model is fitted simultaneously to the data for each group, and a series of equality constraints are imposed and tested to determine the invariance of the parameter estimates as a function of group membership (i.e., male vs. female). (For more information on how to conduct this kind of analysis via structural equation modeling, see Keiley, Dankoski, MacNab, & Liu, Chapter 21, this volume.) Results from this type of analysis might indicate, for example, a different effect of family treatment for males than for females. That is, we might find that the average initial status in conduct-disordered behaviors is the same for male and female adolescents, but that the rate of decrease in these behaviors is more rapid for females than for males, indicating a stronger effect of family treatment for girls than for boys. If we had both a treatment and control group for this same study, we could examine differences across treatment groups by conducting a similar multiple-group analysis, but this time imposing and testing for equality of parameter estimates across the treatment and control groups. In addition, if we had a large enough sample, we could essentially conduct all of these analyses simultaneously, testing for differences across both the treatment and control groups and across male and female adolescents (a four-group model).

In essence, then, complex analyses involving two or more groups can be conducted if the sample size is sufficient. The relevance to family research of these kinds of complicated models is clear: We are often interested in the effect of a family treatment versus a control condition, for example, on different families or on different members within the same family. Analyses involving more than two groups can be used to answer these kinds of questions, as well as others. For more detailed information about fitting these types of models, see Curran and Willoughby (2003) and Muthen and Muthen (1998).

Another more complex form of growth modeling is second-order growth modeling. For example, if we have multiple indicators of a construct—such as the Control scale from the Family Environment Scale (Moos & Moos, 1986), the Firm Control scale from the Children's Report of Parental Behavior Inventory (Schaefer, 1965), and the Parenting Scale (Arnold, O'Leary, Wolff, & Acker, 1993)—we could form a latent factor or variable, Family Control/Discipline, on which these three observed variables load. We could then examine the change in the latent variable across the time periods, rather than change in three domains represented by the three separate measures. Curran and Willoughby (2003) and Khoo and Muthen (2000) provide additional detailed information about fitting second-order growth models. In regard to family research, second-order growth models can be especially beneficial. Within any field of research, the use of multiple measures to create a single construct increases the precision and reliability of measurement within a study. Within the family research field in particular, given the myriad measures of family environment and other family indicators that exist, the ability to combine those measures into fewer and more reliable higher-order latent constructs via second-order growth models may be especially useful.

Finally, though we have presented only two-level growth models in all of the examples used in this chapter, we note that researchers also can estimate models with more than two levels. For example, an investigator might be interested in change over time in siblings' perception of the family environment. In this case, the Level 1 and Level 2 models are as before: Change over time within individual siblings is the Level 1 model, and differences between these growth parameters due to sibling differences constitute the Level 2 model. An additional level also exists, however, since groups of siblings are "nested" within, or belong to, the same family. In this example, then, the family represents a third level of the growth hierarchy. A three-level model fitted to the data would indicate the amount of variance in changes over time in children's perceptions of the family environment that is due to within-individual sibling differences over time (Level 1), the amount that is due to between-sibling differences (Level 2), and the amount that is due to between-family differences (Level 3). These types of models can quickly become quite complex, given the multiple levels of estimation; however, they can be extremely useful in those situations in which the nesting of individuals within higher-order groups, such as families or schools, is of central relevance to the research questions under investigation. The reader is referred to such sources as Singer and Willett (2003) and Bryk and Raudenbush (2002) for additional information on fitting growth models with three or more levels.

SUMMARY AND CONCLUSIONS

In this chapter, we have presented an overview of the use of multilevel growth modeling (also known as "growth mixture modeling," "random-coefficient modeling," and "hierarchical linear modeling") in the context of family research. In addition, we have illustrated how to conduct a growth analysis (both single- and multiple-domain), from exploratory procedures to the actual fitting and interpretation of the multilevel models of change. In the process, we have demonstrated that the methodology of multilevel growth modeling is useful within any field, but may be especially beneficial to family researchers, given the nature of research questions within this field. Due to space limitations, however, our overview has been necessarily cursory, and we encourage the reader to go beyond this introduction to learn more about the methodology of multilevel growth modeling. Several excellent resources exist for gaining additional knowledge about the use of this method, and some resources go so far as to furnish actual data examples that provide practice in application (e.g., Singer & Willett, 2003). In addition, many software developers often conduct workshops about longitudinal methods, and these workshops can also be an excellent source of information about growth modeling. We have included the websites of several developers in the list of references.

We encourage the use of sophisticated methods such as multilevel growth modeling when such methods may be the only appropriate way to answer particular research questions. Ultimately, however, we caution the researcher to develop sound and intelligent research questions, so that investigations are driven by theory and not by available software or statistical methods. It is our hope that this chapter's overview of and introduction to multilevel growth modeling have acquainted the reader with the value of these methods in his or her own research, have illustrated the basic steps in fitting such models, and have encouraged the reader to explore the topic more deeply in furthering the field of family research.

EXEMPLARS

DeGarmo, D. S., Patterson, G. R., & Forgatch, M. S. (2004). How do outcomes in a specified parent training intervention maintain or wane over time? *Prevention Science*, 5, 73–89.

Garber, J., Keiley, M. K., & Martin, N. (2002). Developmental trajectories of adolescents' depressive symptoms: Predictors of change. *Journal of Consulting and Clinical Psychology*, 70, 79–95.

Keiley, M. K., Bates, J., Dodge, K., & Pettit, G. (2000). A cross-domain analysis: Externalizing and internalizing behaviors during 8 years of childhood. *Journal of Abnormal Child Psychology*, 28(2), 161–179.

Keiley, M. K., Howe, T., Dodge, K., Bates, J., & Pettit, G. (2001). Timing of abuse: Group differences and developmental trajectories. *Development and Psychopathology*, 13, 891–912.

REFERENCES

Achenbach, T. M. (1991). *Manual for the Child Behavior Checklist/4–18 and 1991 Profile*. Burlington: University of Vermont, Department of Psychiatry.

Arbuckle, J.L. (1995). *Amos for Windows: Analysis of moment structures* (Version 3.5) [Computer software]. Chicago: SmallWaters. (Available at *http://www.smallwaters.com*)

Arnold, D. S., O'Leary, S. G., Wolff, L. S., & Acker, M. M. (1993). The Parenting Scale: A measure of dysfunctional parenting in discipline situations. *Psychological Assessment*, 5(2), 137–144.

Bryk, A. S., & Raudenbush, S. W. (2002). *Hierarchical Linear Models: Applications and data analysis methods* (2nd ed.). Thousand Oaks, CA: Sage.

Coie, J. D., Terry, R., Lenox, K., Lochman, J., & Hyman, C. (1995). Childhood peer rejection and aggression as predictors of stable patterns of adolescent disorder. *Development and Psychopathology, 7,* 697–713.

Curran, P. J., & Willoughby, M. T. (2003). Implications of latent trajectory models for the study of developmental psychopathology. *Development and Psychopathology, 15,* 581–612.

Joreskog, K. G., & Sorbom, D. (1996). *LISREL 8: User's reference guide.* Chicago: Scientific Software International.

Keiley, M. K., Liu, T., & MacNab, M. (2004). *Longitudinal analysis of couple-focused treatment for drug-abusing women.* Manuscript in preparation.

Khoo, S. T., & Muthen, B. (2000). Longitudinal data on families: Growth modeling alternatives. In J. Rose, L. Chassin, C. Pressson, & J. Sherman (Eds.), *Multivariate applications in substance use research* (pp. 43–78). *Mahwah, NJ: Erlbaum.*

Lewis, R. A. (1990). *Couple-focused therapy for drug abusing women* (NIDA grant application). West Lafayette, IN: Purdue University.

McLellan, A. T., Luborsky, L., Cacciola, J., Griffith, J., McGahan, & O'Brien, C. P. (1988). *Guide to the Addiction Severity Index: Background, administration, and field testing results.* Rockville, MD: U.S. Department of Health and Human Services.

Moos, R. H., & Moos, B. S. (1986). *Family Environment Scale manual* (rev. ed.). Palo Alto, CA: Consulting Psychologists Press.

Muthen, B. O., & Muthen, L. K. (2000). Integrating person-centered and variable-centered analysis: Growth mixture modeling with latent trajectory classes. *Alcoholism: Clinical and Experimental Research, 55,* 882–891.

Muthen, L. K., & Muthen, B. O. (1998). *Mplus user's guide.* Los Angeles: Muthen & Muthen. (Available at *http://www.statmodel.com*)

Neale, M. C., Boker, S. M., Xie, G., & Maes, H. H. (1999). *Mx: Statistical modeling* (5th ed.). Richmond, VA: Medical College of Virginia, Department of Psychiatry.

SAS Institute. (2001). *Statistical analysis system.* Cary, NC: Author. (Available at *http://www.sas.com*)

Schaefer, E. S. (1965). A configural analysis of children's reports of parent behavior. *Journal of Consulting Psychology, 27,* 552–557.

Singer, J. D., & Willett, J. B. (2003). *Applied longitudinal data analysis: Modeling change and event occurrence.* New York: Oxford University Press.

Willett, J. B. (1988). Questions and answers in the measurement of change. In E. Rothkopf (Ed.), *Review of research in education (1988–89)* (pp. 345–422). Washington, DC: American Educational Research Association.

Willett, J. B. (1990). Measuring change: The difference score and beyond. In H. J. Walberg & G. D. Haertel (Eds.), *The international encyclopedia of educational evaluation* (pp. 632–637). New York: Pergamon Press.

CHAPTER 21

Covariance Structure Analysis

FROM PATH ANALYSIS
TO STRUCTURAL EQUATION MODELING

MARGARET K. KEILEY
MARY DANKOSKI
MEGAN DOLBIN-MacNAB
TING LIU

BACKGROUND

Covariance structure analysis (CSA) has become one of the most useful and powerful tools for answering the complex questions that arise within the field of family research. Does family economic health have an influence on a parent's levels of depression, and ultimately on an adolescent's behavior in school? Do the 40 items on an instrument developed to measure family cohesion and conflict resolution actually measure these two constructs? As with most methodologies that are available to address complicated research questions, the method itself has been somewhat difficult to understand and to apply. The objective of this chapter is to provide a comprehensive, yet coherent, overview of the types of analyses that can be conducted via CSA.

In general, CSA is an extension of regression analysis and path analysis that includes components from factor analysis and classical test theory. In order to facilitate the reader's understanding of both the theoretical and practical aspects of CSA, we present the various "tools" in the CSA "toolkit," from the most basic (path analysis) to the more advanced (multiple-group CSA). We also illustrate confirmatory factor analysis (CFA) and structural equation modeling (SEM). However, in order to begin this journey into CSA, we first need to define covariance, since CSA (as its full name indicates) is the analysis of covariance structures.

What Is Covariance?

In data analysis, we usually summarize the relationship between two variables by estimating a correlation. To summarize the relationship among all of the variables in any analysis, we usually estimate a correlation matrix. In CSA, we summarize bivariate relationships by estimating covariances and summarizing these relationships in a covariance matrix. As previously mentioned, CSA is the analysis of *covariance* structures, not *correlation* structures. Correlations are covariances from which the metric of the measure has been removed; thus you can compare one correlation with another, because they are all in the common standardized metric of having a mean of 0 and a standard deviation of 1.00. Covariances contain more information about variables than do correlations; they include information about the metric in which the variable is measured. In most statistical analyses, more information is better! Basically, a covariance is an "unstandardized" correlation. Correlation matrices contain the correlations among the variables in the off-diagonal positions, and the diagonal elements are 1.00 (see Table 21.1). In a covariance matrix, the off-diagonal positions contain the covariances of the variables, and the diagonal elements are the variances of those variables.

If you extract the square root of the variance of a variable, you obtain the standard deviations of that variable. For example, in Table 21.1, the square root of the variance of the outcome variable ($\sqrt{.17}$) is .41, which is the standard deviation of the outcome variable. Similarly, the square root of the variance of the question predictor ($\sqrt{.07}$) is .26, which is the standard deviation of that variable. In order to obtain the correlation of a pair of variables, you divide the covariance of the two variables by the product of the standard deviations of each of the two variables. For example, the correlation of the outcome with the question predictor is the covariance of the two variables (.05), divided by the product of the standard deviations of the two variables (.41 • .26 = .1066); 05 divided by .1066 is .47. In other words, you "standardize" the covariance to obtain the correlation. When you divide the covariance by the standard deviations, you remove the metric of the covariance and are left with the "standardized" correlation; this is easier to interpret than a covariance is, because correlations can be compared to one another. But the covariance matrix contains more information about the relationships among variables than the correlation matrix does. For example, in Table 21.1, the covariance matrix for those three variables contains three covariances and three variances for a total of six pieces of information, while the correlation matrix for those same variables only contains three correlations for a total of three pieces of information! Now that we have this understanding of covariance, we can move on to describe the various "tools" in the CSA "toolkit."

TABLE 21.1 Correlation and Covariance Matrix for an Outcome, a Question Predictor, and a Control Predictor

	Correlation matrix				Covariance matrix		
	Outcome	Question predictor	Control predictor		Outcome	Question predictor	Control predictor
Outcome	1.00			Outcome	.17		
Question	.47	1.00		Question	.05	.07	
Control	−.03	.03	1.00	Control	−.01	.01	.16
SD	.41	.26	.40				

Note. n = 168.

METHODOLOGY

Path Analysis with CSA

Multiple regression is a statistical technique for investigating relationships among one outcome and several predictors. But why limit an investigation to just one outcome? In family research, we are often interested in how multiple predictors are related simultaneously to multiple outcomes, resulting in multiple residuals. For example, we might be interested in investigating how marital and sexual satisfaction (two outcomes) are predicted by differentiation of self and adult attachment (two predictors). We can answer this research question by conducting a multivariate regression analysis in which we allow differentiation of self and adult attachment to predict marital and sexual satisfaction (see Figure 21.1). We may want to extend this analysis by investigating whether the effects of adult attachment and differentiation of self on our two outcomes are mediated by sexual communication (Timm & Keiley, 2004) (see Figure 21.2). In this case, not only do we have more than one outcome (sexual satisfaction, marital satisfaction, and sexual communication), but we are allowing one of those outcomes (sexual communication) to predict the two other outcomes (sexual and marital satisfaction). Traditionally, path analysis has been used to conduct analyses in which one outcome predicts another outcome. However, when the techniques available in most statistical programs (SAS, SPSS, etc.) are used, path analysis can be difficult to conduct. With CSA, path analyses are much simplified.

To illustrate path analysis, we describe a study in which we used this form of CSA to answer our research question of whether the relationship among marital satisfaction, emotional support, and sexual communication is mediated by sexual satisfaction. For the purposes of this chapter, we only present a portion of the entire analysis (see Dolbin-MacNab & Keiley, 2004). The researchers collected data from 205 married men ($n = 100$) and women ($n = 105$) who were not married to each other. The mean age of participants was 38 years ($SD = 10.76$, range = 19–84). Eighty-two percent of

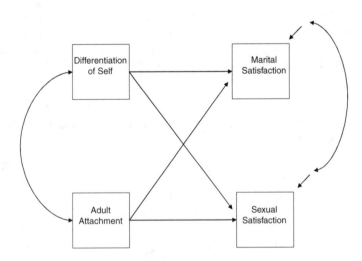

FIGURE 21.1. Hypothesized model of marital and sexual satisfaction predicted by differentiation of self and adult attachment.

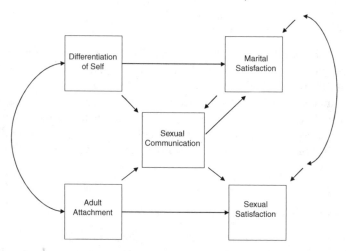

FIGURE 21.2. Hypothesized model of marital and sexual satisfaction predicted by adult attachment and differentiation of self as mediated by sexual communication.

the participants reported that they were still in their first marriage, while 18% were in a subsequent marriage (second, third, etc.). The mean length of marriage was 13 years (*SD* = 10.03, range = 1–54). Approximately one-quarter of the sample had been married 5 or fewer years, and 48% had been married for fewer than 10 years. Participants reported a mean number of 2.3 children (including adoptive, foster, step-, and biological children) (*SD* = 1.84, range = 0–13). In terms of racial/ethnic background, the majority of the sample was white (86%). Participants were also relatively well educated; that is, the majority of the sample reported at least a bachelor's degree (60%). Reflecting the participants' high level of education, the majority of the sample (45%) earned an annual income of $50,000 or higher. Thirteen percent of the sample reported an income of less than $20,000 per year.

The measure of emotional support in this study was the Quality of Relationships Inventory (QRI; Pierce, 1994). This self-report questionnaire contains 25 items. High QRI scores reflect higher levels of perceived relationship support and lower levels of perceived conflict. In this study, Cronbach's alpha for the QRI was .92. The Sexual Communication Satisfaction Scale (SCSS; Wheeless, Wheeless, & Baus, 1984) is a 22-item self-report questionnaire that was used to assess sexual communication. On this scale, high scores represent a higher level of satisfaction with the communication about sexual behavior that occurs within an intimate relationship. In the present study, the Cronbach's alpha for the SCSS was .94. Sexual satisfaction was measured with the Global Measure of Sexual Satisfaction subscale of the Interpersonal Exchange Model of Sexual Satisfaction Questionnaire (Lawrance & Byers, 1992, 1995, 1998). After the five items of this subscale are summed, high scores reflect a more positive assessment of the sexual relationship. In this study, the Global Measure of Sexual Satisfaction had a Cronbach's alpha of .96. Finally, the Kansas Marital Satisfaction Scale (KMSS; Schumm, Scanlon, Crow, Green, & Buckler, 1983) was used to assess marital satisfaction. Creating an average scale score for the three items on the KMSS leads to an overall score. High scores reflect greater marital satisfaction. In the present study, the Cronbach's alpha for the internal consistency of the KMSS was .96.

Preliminary Steps in Path Analysis

The first step in conducting any of the types of CSA in this chapter (including path analysis) is to conduct a univariate analysis of the data, checking for miscodings, skewed distributions, missing data, and unusual data points that might influence the parameter estimates. In addition, since the methods in this chapter assume linearity among the variables, a bivariate analysis should be conducted as well, including an examination of scatterplots to determine whether the relationships that will be modeled are indeed linear. For a full discussion of multivariate normality and its assessment, see Bollen (1989).

Developing a Path Diagram

The second step in any CSA is to create a path diagram to represent the hypotheses (see Figure 21.3). The convention in CSA is that observed variables are represented as squares. Note that the subscript "p" on each variable indicates that each person in the sample has a score on each of these variables. Therefore, both our predictors or "exogenous" variables (emotional support, X_{1p}, and sexual communication, X_{2p}) and our outcomes or "endogenous" variables (sexual satisfaction, Y_{1p}, and marital satisfaction, Y_{2p}) have a subscript "p." In CSA, exogenous variables are variables whose "causes" exist outside the model, while endogenous variables are influenced by variables within the model.

In a path diagram, single-headed arrows (gammas, $\gamma_{11}, \gamma_{12}, \gamma_{21},$ and γ_{22}, and beta, β_{21}) represent the hypothesized pathways between variables, while the double-headed arrows (phi, ϕ_{21}) represent the hypothesized covariances. We also provide for unexplained variation in our outcomes by including residuals, which are the short, angled arrows (zetas, ζ_{1p} and ζ_{2p}) pointing to the outcomes. (Researchers using covariance

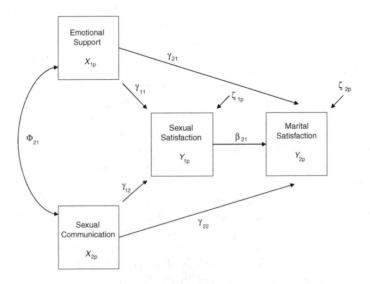

FIGURE 21.3. Hypothesized model of marital satisfaction predicted by emotional support, and sexual communication as mediated by sexual satisfaction ($n = 205$).

structure analysis become very familiar with the Greek alphabet!) The path diagram in Figure 21.3 represents the hypothesized relationships among the observed variables in our model. Because we have 4 variables, the covariance matrix that will be analyzed will have 6 covariances and 4 variances. In our analysis, we will also input the 4 means of all the variables. Thus our sufficient statistics for fitting this hypothesized model contain the 14 pieces of information in Table 21.2 (6 covariances, 4 variances, and 4 means). CSA fits the model to the sufficient statistics in order to estimate the parameters in the fitted model. Our hypothesized model (Figure 21.3) contains 14 unknown parameters (4 variances and 4 means for the observed variables, 5 regression coefficients for the pathways, and 1 covariance between our exogenous variables) that will be estimated by the statistical program we use. Two of the variances that will be estimated—those for marital satisfaction and sexual satisfaction—are actually the residual variances ζ_{1p} and ζ_{2p}.

Statistical Programs

The third step in conducting path analysis is to choose the program you will use to analyze your data. Several user-friendly CSA and SEM programs now exist. You might investigate LISREL (Joreskog & Sorbom, 1996); Mplus (Muthen & Muthen, 1998); EQS (Bentler, 1995); or Mx (Neale, Boker, Xie, & Maes, 1999), which is free on the Internet (*http://griffin.vcu.edu/mx*). Some of the statistical programs are fairly expensive, but are well worth the cost if you plan to investigate complex questions with complex data. If you are also interested in conducting longitudinal analyses, these programs can also be used for growth modeling (see Keiley, Martin, Liu, & Dolbin-MacNab, Chapter 20, this volume). After writing your computer program and reading in the data (which should consist of either a covariance matrix and a set of means or the raw data), you will obtain output. The output from most statistical packages contains a variety of information: (1) the estimates of the unknown parameters (regression coefficients, variances and covariances related to the variables and residuals, and means); (2) the standard errors of the estimates; (3) the ratio of the parameter estimate to the standard error of that estimate (*t*-values, *z*-scores, etc.); and (4) a *p*-value to indicate the level at which you can or cannot reject the null hypothesis about the parameter's estimate being 0 in the population. In addition, most statistical programs give you

TABLE 21.2. Estimated Covariance Matrix and Means for the Investigation of Marital Satisfaction Predicted by Emotional Support, and Sexual Communication as Mediated by Sexual Satisfaction

	Marital satisfaction	Sexual satisfaction	Emotional support	Sexual communication
Marital satisfaction	191.042			
Sexual satisfaction	101.282	160.618		
Emotional support	11.128	6.161	1.420	
Sexual communication	20.616	24.440	1.650	8.011
Means	33.896	35.369	5.201	10.284

Note. n = 205.

a means to evaluate whether your hypothesized model fits the data and some information about the residuals. However, before interpreting the estimated parameters and drawing conclusions about your findings, you should examine model fit.

Model Fit

Similar to nonstandardized regression coefficients in multiple regression, the nonstandardized estimates from fitting our hypothesized model in Figure 21.3 that we present in Figure 21.4 cannot be interpreted directly, since they are not in a common metric. In Figure 21.4, we present these nonstandardized parameter estimates, along with the common model-fitting indices in CSA. One of the primary indices of model fit is the chi-square (χ^2) statistic, with its related p-value and degrees of freedom. It is important to understand what the χ^2 statistic summarizes. In CSA, the sufficient statistics (which in our case contain 14 pieces of information) are fitted to the hypothesized model in Figure 21.3. In our hypothesized diagram, we are estimating 14 parameters. The difference between the number of pieces of information that exist in your sufficient statistics and the number of unknown parameters you will estimate are the degrees of freedom for the model fit—in our example, 14 − 14, or 0 degrees of freedom. We have used all of our degrees of freedom and cannot add any more paths to our model. Once the program fits the hypothesized model, the parameter estimates in this fitted model are used to recover the fitted (or predicted) covariance matrix and mean vector. This set of values is often contained in the residual analysis section of the output provided by the specific statistical program you are using. We can compare this predicted covariance matrix and mean vector with the observed covariance matrix and

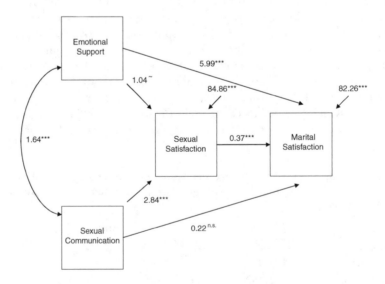

FIGURE 21.4. Nonstandardized estimates of the fitted model of marital satisfaction predicted by emotional support, and sexual communication as mediated by sexual satisfaction ($n = 205$). *Note.* ~$p < .10$; ***$p < .001$. $\chi^2 = 86.57$, $df = 2$, $p = .00$; TLI = .28, CFI = .71, RMSEA = .46 (.00), SRMR = .12.

mean vector, to see how well we have done in recovering the observed matrix and vector. When we do this, we are asking how well the fitted model replicates reality. If the observed and predicted covariance matrix and mean vector are very similar, then we have "good" model fit. If they are not similar or are very discrepant, then we have "lousy" fit.

The χ^2 goodness-of-fit statistic summarizes the total discrepancy between the observed and predicted covariance matrix and mean vector. The χ^2 statistic's p-value and degrees of freedom help you determine whether you can or cannot reject the null hypothesis, "The model fits the data in the population." For CSA, you are hoping *not* to reject the null hypothesis. In our case, the χ^2 statistic is 0, with 0 degrees of freedom and a p-value of 1.00. According to the usual convention, we would fail to reject the null hypothesis of model fit. Our model fits the data. Because the χ^2 statistic is very sensitive to sample size, when you evaluate the fit of your model with a large sample, the χ^2 statistic will often be significant, indicating that your model does not fit the data. To deal with this dilemma, other fit indices have been created to take into consideration the effect of sample size on fit statistics. A Tucker–Lewis (or non-normed fit) index (TLI), a comparative fit index (CFI), and a goodness-of-fit index (GFI) between .90 and 1.00 indicate "good" model fit. These indices tell you how much better your model fits than a baseline model—usually the independence model (a model in which all observed variables are uncorrelated). With any of these fit indices, you should report the specific index, the degrees of freedom, and the p-value. In addition to the fit indices already mentioned, the root mean square error of approximation (RMSEA) can be used to assess model fit. The RMSEA takes into account the error of approximation in the population and the precision of the fit measure itself. In other words, RMSEA measures this discrepancy per degree of freedom, thus providing a fit index that is relatively independent of sample size. A RMSEA that is close to 0 also indicates that your model fits the data. The RMSEA is often given with a p-value that tests the null hypothesis, "The RMSEA is 0 in the population." Again, you do *not* want to reject the null hypothesis. Report the RMSEA and its associated p-value. The standardized root mean square residual (SRMR) can also be used to assess model fit and should be less than .05. The SRMR is the average of the raw residuals that have been standardized to a mean of 0 and a standard deviation of 1.00. In the current example, the TFI is 1, the CFI is 1, the RMSEA is 0 ($p = 1.00$), and the SRMR is 0. According to these fit statistics as well as the χ^2 statistic, our model fits the data. We cannot reject the null hypothesis of model fit. In recent years, there has been a proliferation in the development of fit indices. For more information about model fit and these numerous fit indices, see Bollen (1989). For the purposes of illustrating path analysis, we have a model that fits.

Fitting and Testing Nested Models: The Delta Chi-Square Test

Before we interpret the coefficients from our fitted model, we can test one other model to determine whether sexual communication might be considered a partial mediator of the relationship between our exogenous predictors and our endogenous outcome. To test this model, we eliminate two paths from our path diagram (see Figure 21.5). To test mediation completely, we would need to follow the outline in Baron and Kenny (1986). However, by comparing the models in Figure 21.4 and Figure 21.5, we will be

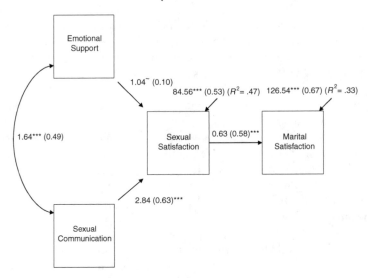

FIGURE 21.5. Non-standardized estimates of the fitted model of marital satisfaction predicted by sexual satisfaction, and sexual satisfaction predicted by emotional support and sexual communication ($n = 205$). *Note.* $\sim p < .10$; $***p < .001$. $\chi^2 = 86.57$, $df = 2$, $p = .00$; TLI = .28, CFI = .71, RMSEA = .46 (.00), SRMR = .12. Standardized estimates are in parentheses.

able to illustrate the delta chi-square ($\Delta\chi^2$) test for the purposes of this chapter. In fitting the model in Figure 21.5, we still have 14 pieces of information, but now we are estimating only 12 parameters. Thus the degrees of freedom for this model are 2. We can see from the fit statistics in Figure 21.5 that this model does not fit as well as our first model. However, we can use the $\Delta\chi^2$ test to compare these models to each other. As with other statistical techniques, we can use a difference in the goodness-of-fit statistic to compare nested models[1] and to test complex simultaneous hypotheses. For instance, in our example, if sexual satisfaction did in fact partially mediate the relationship between emotional support, sexual communication and the outcome, marital satisfaction, we would expect that the paths between the exogenous predictors (sexual communication, emotional support) and the outcome (marital satisfaction) would actually be 0. Using the $\Delta\chi^2$ test, we can in fact test whether by not estimating these two paths—constraining them to 0 simultaneously—they are indeed 0 in the population. In our example, we will compare the "full" model with all the paths estimated (Figure 21.4) to the "reduced" or constrained model (Figure 21.5), in order to test the null hypothesis that the regression coefficients are 0 simultaneously in the population. After constructing the $\Delta\chi^2$ statistic ($\chi^2_{\text{Figure 21.5}} - \chi^2_{\text{Figure 21.4}} = \Delta\chi^2 = 86.57 - 0.00 = 53.52$, for

---

[1] Nested models are defined by two characteristics: (1) They are fitted on the same sample of data. That is, if, as you add a variable to the model, you lose some respondents because they have missing values on that variable, the first model is not nested within the second model. (2) The "reduced" model (the one with fewer parameters) must be obtainable from the "full" model by setting constraints on the "full" model. That is, you must be able to fit the "reduced" model by setting some parameters to 0.

$\Delta df = 2$) and comparing it to a critical value of χ^2 ($\hat{\alpha} = .05$, $df = 2$), which is 5.99, we can decide whether to reject the null hypothesis or not. In our case, because the $\Delta\chi^2$ statistic is greater than the critical value of χ^2, we can reject this null hypothesis; that is, the two paths are not 0 in the population. Based on this result, we can conclude that the model shown in Figure 21.4 represents reality better than does the model shown in Figure 21.5.

Before we interpret the coefficients from the model in Figure 21.4, we would like to show how the $\Delta\chi^2$ test can help you in testing many different kinds of hypotheses. Of course, your research question and your exploration of existing theory and research should be used to guide your analysis of additional hypotheses. For example, with the current example, we could test whether the paths between the two exogenous predictors (emotional support, sexual communication) and sexual satisfaction are equal. In this case, the "full" model would still be the one in Figure 21.4; the "reduced" model would be one with the same number of paths, but two of them would be constrained to be equal. Thus the degrees of freedom for this "reduced" model would only differ from the degrees of freedom in Figure 21.4 by 1. We estimate both paths, but constrain them to be equal, requiring that we only estimate one parameter and use it for both paths. Although this is just one specific example, many other kinds of hypotheses can be tested. Now that we have compared models and tested our hypotheses about those models, we can interpret the coefficients from the model in Figure 21.4.

Interpreting Parameter Estimates

All of the regression coefficients that have been estimated in Figure 21.4 can be interpreted as though they are regular regression coefficients. For example, we can state that when we control for all the other variables in the model, for a 1-unit difference in sexual communication, a 2.84 difference in sexual satisfaction exists. When you are using this form of interpretation, it is important that the scales of your variables have meaning. If they are meaningless, you cannot really interpret the coefficients or compare them to each other.[2] One of the ways that has been developed to ease the difficulty of including different scales with different metrics into the same model is the use of standardized coefficients. When all of the variables in the model are standardized to unit variance, you obtain standardized coefficients, which are correlations. In Figure 21.6, we present our full model with standardized coefficients. Now we can compare the effects of the exogenous variables on the endogenous variables across the measures.

In this final fitted model, emotional support is related more strongly to marital satisfaction ($\hat{r} = .52$) than is sexual communication ($\hat{r} = .05$),[3] controlling for all else in the model. However, sexual communication is related more strongly to sexual satisfac-

---

[2] If you are using a standardized scale that has its own scoring manual, score the scale as directed. But, if not, one of the ways that you can make your scale meaningful is to create an average scale score. For example, if you have a 10-item scale that is answered on a Likert scale of 1–5, you might be tempted just to sum the scores across the 10 items, giving you a scale that would range from 10 to 50. A better idea would be to sum the items and divide by the number of items. This process gives you a scale of 1–5 that has the same meaning as the original scale does.

[3] The "little hat" over r indicates an estimated, or fitted, value.

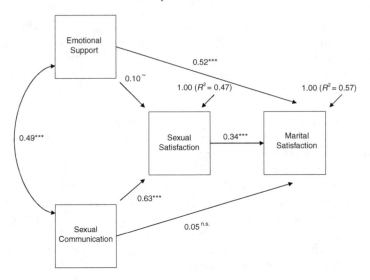

FIGURE 21.6. Standardized estimates of the fitted model of marital satisfaction predicted by emotional support, and sexual communication as mediated by sexual satisfaction (n = 205). *Note.* ~p < .10; ***p < .001. χ^2 = 0, df = 0, p = 1.000; TLI = 1, CFI = 1, RMSEA = .00 (1.00), SRMR = .00.

tion ($\hat{r}$ = .63) than is emotional support ($\hat{r}$ = .10), again, controlling for all else in the model. In fact, it appears that sexual satisfaction, which relates to marital satisfaction ($\hat{r}$ = .34), might partially mediate the relationship of sexual communication with marital satisfaction. However, mediation would have to be tested by fitting a series of other models, as outlined in Baron and Kenny (1986). We have predicted 57% of the variation in marital satisfaction and 47% of the variation in sexual satisfaction with all of the variables in the model. We may also want to note that our exogenous predictors, emotional support and sexual communication, are also related to each other ($\hat{r}$ = .49). In interpreting this model, it is important that we steer clear of using "causal" language. Because our data are cross-sectional data, we cannot say that high emotional support causes higher marital satisfaction, controlling for all else in the model, and vice versa. These paths are correlational paths, not causal paths. True causality can only be determined through the use of longitudinal methods and experimental designs.

Structural Equation Modeling with CSA

Introducing Latent Constructs and Measurement Error

Figure 21.7 represents a structural equation model (SEM) that we will fit by using CSA. (Note that from this point on, we use "SEM" to mean either "structural equation *modeling*" or "a structural equation *model*.") This figure is somewhat different from the figures we presented in our discussion of path analysis. In the previous figures, we have only included observed variables. In this figure, we distinguish between underlying constructs or latent variables (denoted by circles) and the observed variables or indicators (denoted by squares) that measure them. The assumption that we make in using latent constructs is that the latent construct causes its indicators to take on specific values. For example, in Figure 21.7, we assume that a person's true score on a Tolerance factor (see below) is latent or hidden, and that this latent or hidden construct underpins the person's actual functioning and drives that person's observed indicators (X_{1p} to X_{5p}). Hence we denote the relationship between the construct and its indicators with single-headed arrows from the construct to the observed indicators. The indicators of any construct are fallible measures of a construct's true value. We are able to distinguish the construct's true value from its indicators' values by allowing the presence of measurement error. In Figure 21.7, the small arrows (δ_{1p} to δ_{5p}) pointing toward the observed indicators (X_{1p} to X_{5p}) from the sides of the squares opposite to the latent construct represent the measurement error in each observed variable. As in path analysis, the subscript "p" on each observed variable indicates that every person has a score on each of these variables, but now each person also has a measure-

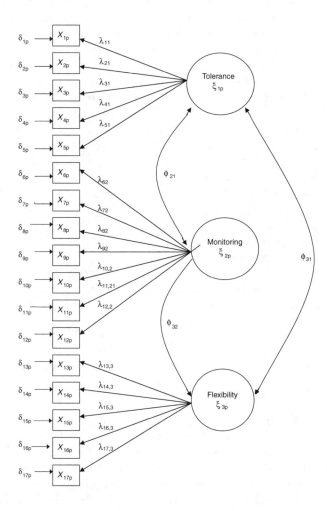

FIGURE 21.7. Hypothesized CFA model for the 17 items of the Abbreviated Affect Regulation Scale as indicators of three latent variables, Tolerance, Monitoring, and Flexibility ($n = 207$).

ment error for each item. In addition, each person has a score on the latent variable that is indicated with the subscript "p." The representation of a construct (true scores) being measured by the indicators (observed scores) and measurement error (error scores) describes the "measurement model" of an SEM.

Implicit in traditional analyses such as multiple regression, multiple analysis of covariance, and factor analysis, among others, is the assumption that all the variables are measured without error (i.e., that they are infallible). In reality, all measured variables contain random error. For example, measurement error in predictors results in bias in the parameter estimates. Measurement error in an outcome results in underestimation of the strength of the relationships. In either case, our inferences to the population will be incorrect. One of the major strengths of SEM with CSA is its ability to use each construct's multiple indicators to tease apart the variances of our observed measures into two variance components—"true" variance (represented by latent constructs) and error/stochastic variance (represented by the small arrows denoting error). Removal of the error variance prior to examining the relationships among our constructs allows us to model the "true" variances of the latent constructs and the "true" covariance structure among several latent constructs.

As family researchers, we are often interested not in the relationships among our observed measures, but in the relationships among the "true" values or hidden constructs that underlie those measures. In addition, we are often interested in the relationships among several of these constructs. For example, we may be interested in whether drug use is related to sexual and marital satisfaction in a sample of married women. Our research question is about the underlying true relationship among these three constructs, but we have collected data that measure the values of the indicators. To answer our research question, we must remove the measurement error from these indicators to examine the underlying true relationships among drug abuse, sexual satisfaction, and marital satisfaction.

In Figure 21.7, the three latent constructs with their indicators and measurement errors compose the "measurement model" of an SEM. The double-headed arrows between the latent constructs represent the expected set of interrelationships among the constructs. This portion of the model is the "structural model" of an SEM. Every SEM is composed of a measurement model that distinguishes the constructs from the indicators, and a structural model that hypothesizes the nature of the relationships among the constructs.

Common Types of SEMs

CONFIRMATORY FACTOR ANALYSIS

In confirmatory factor analysis (CFA), we hypothesize a measurement structure for a set of observed variables and confirm that it fits the data. In Figure 21.7, we have hypothesized that the 17 items of the Abbreviated Affect Regulation Scale (Keiley, Liu, Moon, & Sprenkle, 2004) are indicators of three latent variables or factors (Tolerance, Monitoring, and Flexibility).[4] In addition, we have hypothesized that these three latent variables are related to each other (i.e., that they are not completely orthogonal). Data

---

[4] In CFA, the underlying constructs or latent variables are often referred to as "factors." We use that term in this section on CFA.

were collected from 207 male and female adolescents between the ages of 12 and 17. The respondents took part in a measurement study to determine the factor structure of the scale items. Although 70% of the sample was labeled as gifted, no differences existed in any of the analyses between the gifted and nongifted adolescents. The hypotheses were (1) that adolescents' tolerance of affect (latent, unseen variable) would determine the adolescents' self-reported abilities to tolerate their affect (observed variables: X_{1p} to X_{5p}); (2) that their monitoring of affect (latent, unseen variable) would determine their self-reported abilities to monitor affect (observed variables: X_{6p} to X_{12p}); and (3) that their flexibility in managing affect (latent, unseen variable) would determine their self-reported flexibility (observed variables: X_{13p} to X_{17p}). The full Affect Regulation Scales include 53 items, but for purposes of this chapter, we only include the abbreviated scale of 17 items illustrated in Figure 21.7. For reports on the full instrument, please see Keiley, Moon, and Sprenkle (1999) and Keiley, Moon, Sprenkle, and Liu (2000).

After drawing the path diagram, we have used Mplus to fit the hypothesized model. The nonstandardized and standardized parameter estimates are presented in Figure 21.8. Although we have a significant χ^2 statistic ($\chi^2 = 172.59$, $df = 115$, $p = .000$), our RMSEA statistic is nonsignificant and close to 0 (RMSEA = .05, $p = .55$), and the CFI is .90. Therefore, we can conclude that our model fits the data. Before we examine the factor loadings, we should examine how much variance exists in each of our latent factors. In order for significant variance to exist in underlying latent factors, two conditions must be met. First, the observed variables that we have used to indicate the construct must contain variance themselves. As one of the first steps in any measurement study, the researcher should examine the univariate distributions of all the items. Each item should have a fairly normal distribution of responses across the scale that is being used. If the distribution of an item's responses is very narrow (e.g., only 4's and 5's on a Likert 5-point scale), the item will not contain much variation. In other words, this item will not be useful in discriminating differences among respondents on the behaviors being measured. This lack of variation may occur because differences really do not exist in those behaviors, or because the item is just a poorly constructed item. The second condition is that once measurement error is removed from the observed variables by fitting the CFA, the underlying "true" latent construct itself must have variance. When the latent construct does contain significant variance, we have determined that in the population from which a sample is drawn, differences do exist in the construct that drives the behaviors measured by items. In our study, the estimated variances for the Monitoring and Flexibility factors are significantly different from 0 ($\sigma^2_M = .297$, $p < .001$, and $\sigma^2_F = .382$, $p < .001$), while the variance for the Tolerance factor is only marginally different from 0 ($\sigma^2_T = .157$, $p < .08$). We suspect that tolerance of affect in adolescence is not an easily measured construct, or that our items did not measure tolerance of affect well enough.

When interpreting the estimates from a fitted CFA model, we should pay attention to three essential components. The first two essential components are related to the measurement part of the CFA model, the third to the structural part of the model. First, we should present a description of the psychometric properties of the indicators (see Table 21.3). In this table we have presented the observed variance of each indicator, the estimated error variance of each indicator, and the resulting true variance (observed variance minus error variance). From these variances, we can calculate the estimated reliability of that observed indicator and the factor–indicator correlation of that

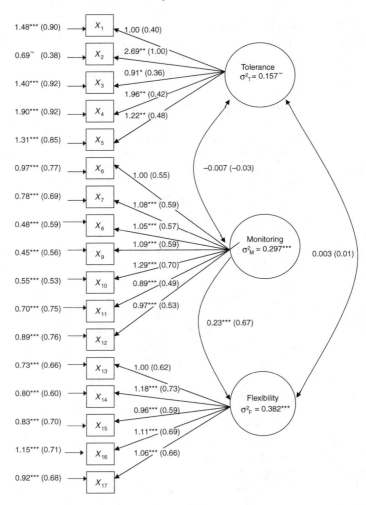

FIGURE 21.8. Fitted CFA model for the 17 items of the Abbreviated Affect Regulation Scale as indicators of three latent variables, Tolerance, Monitoring, and Flexibility, with the unstandardized and standardized parameter estimates ($n = 207$). *Note.* $\sim p < .10$; $*p < .05$; $**p < .01$; $***p < .001$.

indicator with its latent factor. In addition, we have listed both the unstandardized and standardized factor loadings from the fitted model shown in Figure 21.8. In our data, the Tolerance item T6 (X_2 in Figure 21.8), "I'm comfortable with intense anger," has the highest reliability (.625) for that factor. The remaining items on the Tolerance factor are not very reliable. This unreliability may be what is determining the lack of variance in the Tolerance construct noted above. The items for the other two factors are fairly reliable, with estimated reliabilities ranging from .237 to .470 for the Monitoring factor and .289 to .298 for the Flexibility factor. As a side issue, the reader will note in Table 21.3 and in Figure 21.8 that the unstandardized factor loading for the first indicator of each latent construct is 1.00. One of the problems we face in SEM is that the latent constructs are unobserved; therefore, we do not know their natural metric. One of the ways that we define the true score metric is by setting one scaling factor loading to 1.00 from each group of items.

The second component of interpreting the estimates from a fitted CFA model is interpreting the unstandardized factor loadings (see Table 21.3). Each unstandardized factor loading can be interpreted as a regression coefficient; that is, for a 1-unit difference in the latent factor Flexibility (which would be 1 unit of the indicator that we have used to set the metric of the latent factor), we have a 1.060 difference in indicator F14 (X_{17}). Using the unstandardized factor loadings, we can compare factor loadings within each factor. In our CFA, when we compare the unstandardized factor loadings for the Tolerance factor, T6 (X_2) is clearly the most prominent item, with an unstandardized loading of 2.694; M20 (X_{10}) is the most prominent item for the Monitoring factor, with an unstandardized loading of 1.290; and F9 (X_{14}) is the most prominent item for the Flexibility factor, with an unstandardized loading of 1.176. To compare factor loadings across factors, we must use the standardized factor loadings listed in the final column. Across the 17 items, T6 (X_2) is the item with the largest standardized loading, 0.998, followed by M20 (X_{10}) and F9 (X_{14}).

Third, we should interpret the factor-to-factor relationships seen in Figure 21.8. These relationships are the structural part of this CFA. The standardized solution provides the factor–factor correlations. Interestingly, in our fitted model, the estimated

TABLE 21.3. Estimated Psychometric Properties and Factor Loadings from the Fitted Oblique Three-Factor Model of Responses to the Abbreviated Affect Regulation Scale, by Item Number

	Psychometric properties of indicator						
Indicator	Observed variance, σ^2_X	Error variance, σ^2_δ	True variance, $\sigma^2_X - \sigma^2_\delta$	Reliability (true/obs.), $\rho(X)$	Factor–indicator corr., $\sqrt{\rho(X)}$	Unstd. factor loading	Std. factor loading
T2	1.634	1.483	0.151	.092	.303	1.000	0.397
T6	1.828	0.686	1.142	.625	.790	2.694	0.998
T10	1.532	1.402	0.130	.085	.291	0.907	0.360
T12	2.076	1.901	0.175	.084	.290	1.060	0.421
T13	1.541	1.310	0.231	.150	.387	1.216	0.482
M9	1.276	0.974	0.302	.237	.486	1.000	0.545
M10	1.131	0.783	0.348	.308	.555	1.083	0.590
M18	0.805	0.475	0.330	.410	.640	1.051	0.573
M19	0.801	0.450	0.351	.438	.662	1.089	0.594
M20	1.043	0.553	0.490	.470	.685	1.290	0.703
M24	0.944	0.699	0.245	.260	.509	0.892	0.486
M25	1.164	0.886	0.278	.239	.489	0.968	0.528
F8	1.110	0.733	0.377	.340	.583	1.000	0.618
F9	1.330	0.800	0.530	.398	.631	1.176	0.727
F10	1.177	0.826	0.351	.298	.546	0.959	0.593
F13	1.621	1.153	0.468	.289	.537	1.109	0.685
F14	1.352	0.924	0.428	.317	.563	1.060	0.655

correlation of the Tolerance factor with either the Monitoring factor (unstandardized factor loading = -0.007, $\hat{r} = -.03$, p = n.s.) or the Flexibility factor (unstandardized factor loading = 0.003, $\hat{r} = .01$, p = n.s.) is 0, suggesting that no relationship exists between Tolerance and either of these two remaining factors. This lack of correlation could be the result of the Tolerance construct having very little variance, or it could mean that no correlation really does exist in the population among these latent factors. However, the estimated correlation between Monitoring and Flexibility is quite high (unstandardized factor loading = 0.23; $\hat{r} = .67$, $p = .001$), suggesting that these two factors may represent just one underlying factor. We could fit several different models, depending on our hypotheses about the nature of the underlying factors; for pedagogic purposes, however, we will fit a second-order factor analysis.

SECOND-ORDER FACTOR ANALYSIS

In the development of instruments in the field of family research, we often hypothesize a "superfactor" or second-order factor that subsumes or underlies the first-order factors. In our CFA (see Figure 21.9), we might hypothesize an overarching factor of Affect Regulation on which the three subscale factors, Monitoring, Flexibility, and Tolerance, load. In other words, a "superfactor" of Affect Regulation drives the true scores on the three subscales we have already distinguished. In this case, we are treating the second-order factor as an exogenous construct (predictor) of the first-order factors, the endogenous or outcome constructs. This second-order factor may not be entirely successful in predicting the three first-order factors. Therefore, each of these three first-order factors will have variation that is not predicted. Hence each of the first-order factors will have a residual, denoted by the short, slanted arrow pointing toward each of the latent constructs. We then fit our hypothesized second-order factor model to the data.

    Our second-order factor model fits the data, but not as well as previously. The χ^2 statistic ($\chi^2 = 199.17$, $df = 118$, $\chi^2/df = 1.7$, $p = .000$)[5] and the RMSEA statistic (RMSEA = $.06$, $p = .18$) indicate good model fit, but the CFI is $.86$, less than the usual cutoff of $.90$. The measurement model of this second-order CFA model is very similar to the first-order CFA model; we have presented it on the fitted path diagram, but we will not discuss it here. There are some fluctuations, but in general, measurement models are often quite robust when SEMs are fitted with different sets of paths between the latent factors. That is, the relationships among the latent factors can be altered without altering the basic measurement properties of the factors. What we would like to note on the fitted diagram in Figure 21.9 is that the second-order Affect Regulation factor contains significant variance ($\sigma^2_{AR} = .134$, $p < .001$) and is highly correlated with each of the first-order factors ($\hat{r}_{AR-T} = .47$, $\hat{r}_{AR-F} = .72$, and $\hat{r}_{AR-M} = .78$). In addition, the estimates of the reliabilities of our three factors confirm what we found in our first-order factor model; the estimated reliability of Tolerance is $.22$ (fairly low), of Flexibility is $.52$, and of Monitoring is $.60$. Only the Monitoring factor appears to have adequate reliability. Our conclusions based on our CFA might be that the Abbreviated Affect Regulation Scale's subscales have less than adequate psychometric properties.

---

[5] SEMs are deemed to fit the data if the ratio of the estimated χ^2 statistic to the degrees of freedom is less than 5 (Wheaton, Muthen, Alwin, & Summers, 1977) or 3 (Carmines & McIver, 1981).

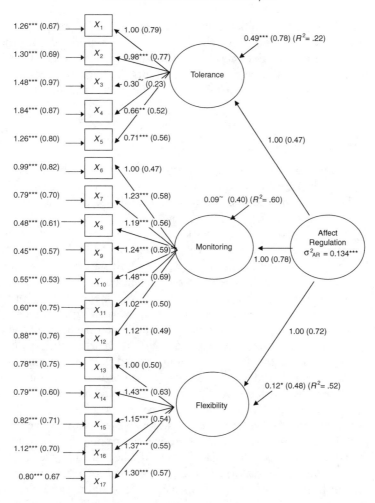

FIGURE 21.9. Fitted second-order CFA model with the unstandardized and standardized parameter estimates for the 17 items of the Abbreviated Affect Regulation Scale as indicators of three latent variables, Tolerance, Monitoring, and Flexibility, and a superorder factor of Affect Regulation (n = 207). *Note.* p = values as in Figure 21.8.

CAVEATS ABOUT SEMS

Before we move on to fitting another SEM, we want to highlight a few important caveats. First, most SEM programs will provide modification indices upon request. These indices are commonly used when researchers are intent on increasing the goodness of fit of their SEM. For example, had we requested modification indices in our second-order CFA discussed above, Mplus would have given us a set of parameters; if we had estimated these as well as the ones we were already estimating, we could have increased the fit indices, such as the CFI. Often the parameters that the statistical programs suggest can be freed to be estimated are the covariances between error terms. The fact is that if enough covariances among error terms are freed, almost all models will fit extremely well. This leads to our second major caveat about SEMs. That is, in developing excellent SEMs as in developing excellent regression models, the researcher should determine based upon research questions and hypotheses the models that should be fit. Therefore, the first steps in developing any SEM are to have a research question and to draw a path diagram that represents the hypothesized set of relations among your observed and latent variables in the population in which you are interested.

SEMs of More Complex Sets of Relationships

In our CFA example, we have presented both a measurement and structural model. However, in other SEMs, we can hypothesize even more complex sets of relationships. To illustrate the use of such SEMs, we present a small section of a larger secondary data analysis (Dankoski & Keiley, 2004), conducted on data originally collected by Glueck and Glueck (1950) for their book *Unraveling Juvenile Delinquency*. These data were initially collected between 1940 and 1948 on 438 white males ages 10–17 who were living in the Boston, Massachusetts area and had juvenile delinquency records. The determination of delinquency status was based on official criminal records, and the participants were recruited through their involvement with one of two correctional facilities in the city. There were two follow-up waves: Time 2 data collection occurred between 1948 and 1956, when the participants were an average age of 25, and Time 3 data collection occurred between 1954 and 1963, when the participants were an average age of 31. Data for this study were obtained from many sources, including medical records; criminal and correction facility records; psychological tests; and semistructured interviews with the boys and their parents, teachers, police officers, social workers, and recreational leaders. All subjects were born between 1924 and 1935, and their ages at Time 1 ranged from 11 years to 17 years, with an average age of 14 years. Over 60% of the sample were children of immigrants, mostly from Italy, England, and Ireland. It should be noted that the period when the data were first collected, the 1940s, was an interesting historical time during which many immigrants settled in ethnic enclaves in large cities (Mindel, Habenstein, & Wright, 1998). The families in this study were also largely of low socioeconomic status (SES), and 95% were from neighborhoods in which gangs and crime were present. Furthermore, the mean education level of the parents was a grade school education.

MEASURES

The outcome construct was based on official criminal records from the two follow-up waves (Times 2 and 3). Violent crimes perpetrated between ages 17 and 25 were coded at Time 2, and violent crimes committed over 25 years of age were coded at Time 3. The items were summed together across time, such that high scores indicated more violent crimes perpetrated as an adult. The log of this variable was used to reduce skewness. This outcome construct, Later Violence against Women, had only one observed variable. Therefore, we have had to set the error variance of that variable to 0 and assume that it was measured without error. Since the measure of Later Violence against Women was based on official criminal records, for our purposes this might be a reasonably safe assumption.

An Externalizing scale (13 items) and an Internalizing scale (9 items) were constructed from teacher-reported items corresponding to the Externalizing and Internalizing scales of the Child Behavior Checklist (CBCL; Achenbach, 1994). Both of the created scales had adequate reliability. The scores on these two scales (observed variables) constituted the latent factor of Affect Dysregulation. The log of both these scales was used to reduce skewness.

Three observed scales (Family Delinquency, Family Alcoholism, and Family Emotional Disorders) composed the latent factor of Family Chaos. These three scales were based on items obtained from both official records and reports by family members. The items constituting the scales were dichotomous (yes–no) variables indicating the presence or absence of each separate condition (i.e., delinquency, alcoholism, or emotional disorders) in (1) Father's Family of Origin, (2) Mother's Family of Origin, (3) Father, and (4) Mother. For each of these scales, the items were summed such that high scores indicated more delinquency, alcoholism, and emotional disorders in a boy's family. The reliability of these three scales was adequate.

STEP 1: RESEARCH QUESTION AND FIRST HYPOTHESIZED PATH DIAGRAM

The question we have investigated is whether Affect Dysregulation in childhood mediates the relationship between Family Chaos and Later Violence against Women in adulthood. Following the procedures outlined in Baron and Kenny (1986), we have fitted three models to determine our mediation hypothesis (see Dankoski & Keiley, 2004, for details). The first model has determined whether the mediator is predicted by the exogenous variable. Figure 21.10 represents this first step in a mediation analysis. We have fitted the model to data and obtained a χ^2 statistic (364.17, $df = 9$, $p < .001$) indicating that the model does not fit the data. Because the sample was fairly large, however, we feel that the GFI of .99 and the SRMR of .01 indicate good model fit (GFI > .90 and SRMR < .05).

INTERPRETING THE PARAMETER ESTIMATES

We present the unstandardized and the completely standardized parameter estimates for our fitted model in Figure 21.10.[6] The parameter estimates that will help us to answer our research question are in the structural part of the model—the paths among the latent variables. However, we first need to check the measurement model to ensure that our latent variables indeed do underlie the observed variables. We follow the steps discussed previously in the section about interpreting CFA models to determine the psychometric properties of the latent factors. From our fitted model, we can see that the estimated-factor–observed-variable correlations of the Externalizing and Internalizing indicators are quite high [$\sqrt{\hat{\rho}(\text{Ext})} = .81$, $\sqrt{\hat{\rho}(\text{Int})} = .77$]. Since the reliability of these measures is the factor–indicator correlation squared, we see that the reliabilities

---

[6] Most SEM programs provide standardized solutions in which the variances of the latent variables are standardized to 1.00, but the variances of the observed variables remain unstandardized. In these solutions, the paths between the factors can be interpreted as correlations, but the paths between the factors and the observed variables are standardized only within each factor, not across factors. In a completely standardized solution, presented here, the variances of the factors and of the observed scores are standardized to 1.00. In these solutions, the path between the factors can still be interpreted as correlations, but now so can the paths from the factors to the observed variables. Those paths are now the factor–indicator correlations.

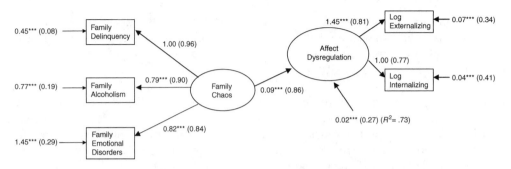

FIGURE 21.10. Step 1 in investigating mediation: Regressing the mediator on the exogenous variable. Fitted SEM with unstandardized and completely standardized (in parentheses) coefficients (*n* = 438). *Note.* ***p < .001, χ^2 (9) = 364.17, *p* < .001; GFI = .99, adjusted GFI = .99, SRMR = .01.

of Externalizing and Internalizing are also adequate [$\hat{\rho}$(Ext) = .66, $\hat{\rho}$(Int) = .60)]. For the Family Chaos factor, the factor–indicator correlations are even higher [$\sqrt{\hat{\rho}}$(Fam Del) = .96, $\sqrt{\hat{\rho}}$(Fam Alc) = .90, and $\sqrt{\hat{\rho}}$(Fam Emot Dis) = .84], indicating that the reliabilities for the three observed variables are also quite good [$\hat{\rho}$(Fam Del) = .92, $\hat{\rho}$(Fam Alc) = .81, and $\hat{\rho}$(Fam Emot Dis) = .71]. When we examine the parameter estimates in the structural part of this model, we see that Family Chaos is significantly related to Affect Dysregulation ($\hat{r}$ = .86). Furthermore, 73% of the variance in Affect Dysregulation is predicted by Family Chaos.

STEP 2: REGRESSING THE OUTCOME VARIABLE ON THE EXOGENOUS VARIABLE

Figure 21.11 represents Step 2 in a mediation analysis. Once again, we have fitted the model to data and obtained a χ^2 statistic (346.34, *df* = 6, *p* < .001) indicating that the model does not fit the data. However, a GFI of .99, and a SRMR of .01 indicate good model fit (GFI > .90 and SRMR < .05). As we have mentioned previously, the estimates of the measurement model of an SEM are fairly robust, and the estimates do not fluctuate much over different fitted models. In this case, the item–construct correlations and item reliabilities are very similar to the ones we have discussed above. In looking at the structural model, we see that Family Chaos is related to the outcome variable, Later Violence against Women ($\hat{r}$ = .48); in fact, Family Chaos predicts 23% of the variance in the outcome.

STEP 3: REGRESSING THE OUTCOME VARIABLE ON BOTH THE MEDIATOR VARIABLE AND EXOGENOUS VARIABLE

Figure 21.12 represents the final step in mediation analysis. After fitting the model, we obtain a GFI of .99 and a SRMR of .01; the model fits the data in the population. Once again, few changes exist in the measurement model. Controlling for all else in the model, Affect Dysregulation does predict Later Violence against Women ($\hat{r}$ = .23) at the *p* = .07 level. Family Chaos is still highly related to Affect Dysregulation ($\hat{r}$ = .86), predicting 74% of the variance in that latent variable (which is similar to the

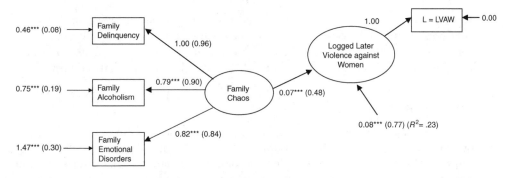

FIGURE 21.11. Step 2 in investigating mediation: Regressing the outcome variable on the exogenous variable. Fitted SEM with unstandardized and completely standardized (in parentheses) coefficients ($n = 438$). *Note.* ***$p < .001$, χ^2 (6) = 346.34, $p < .001$; GFI = .99, adjusted GFI = .99, SRMR = .006.

model in Figure 21.10). However, Family Chaos is less strongly related to Later Violence against Women ($\hat{r} = .23$) than it is in the model in Figure 21.11 ($\hat{r} = .48$). In addition, Affect Dysregulation and Family Chaos predict 24% of the variance in Later Violence against Women, which is not much more than in the model in Figure 21.10, in which only Family Chaos predicts Later Violence against Women. Based on this information, we would say, preliminarily, that Affect Dysregulation may not mediate the relationship between Family Chaos and Later Violence against Women. Because we do not have a series of nested models in the analysis we have presented above, we have not been able to conduct $\Delta\chi^2$ tests. To conduct this test, we would need to fit one more model, similar to the model in Figure 21.12, but with the path between Family Chaos and Later Violence against Women constrained to be 0. Then we could conduct a $\Delta\chi^2$

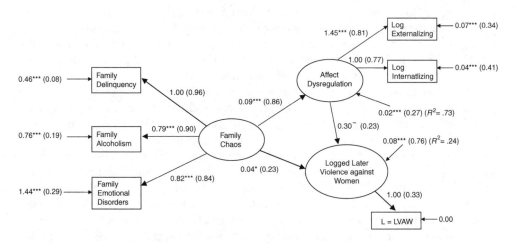

FIGURE 21.12. Step 3 in investigating mediation: Regressing the outcome variable on both the mediator variable and exogenous variable. Fitted SEM with unstandardized and completely standardized (in parentheses) coefficients ($n = 438$). *Note.* ~$p < .07$; *$p < .05$; **$p < .001$. $\chi^2(13)$ = 365.88, $p < .001$; GFI = .99, adjusted GFI = .99, SRMR = .01.

test to determine whether that path is indeed 0 in the population when the effect of Family Chaos on Later Violence against Women is forced to exist only through its effect on Affect Dysregulation and Affect Dysregulation's effect on Later Violence against Women. If we cannot reject that null hypothesis, then mediation exists.

Multiple-Group SEMs

Another advantage of SEM is that we can compare hypothesized covariance structures across groups of respondents. For example, in our path analysis investigating the relationships among emotional support, sexual communication, sexual satisfaction, and marital satisfaction, we could hypothesize that the model will fit differently for the men and women in the population. We might think that the path from sexual satisfaction to marital satisfaction will be stronger for males than for females, controlling for all else in the model. By fitting a multiple-group model and comparing the fit across the two groups, we could determine whether that is true or not. In other words, multiple-group CSA allows for the testing of certain types of interactions. By fitting the multiple-group model for the path analysis, we would be examining the interaction of gender with the path between sexual satisfaction and marital satisfaction to determine whether it is equal across the groups. In that analysis, we would first examine the fit across the two groups without constraining any parameters to be equal. Then we would constrain that one parameter to be equal across the two groups and conduct a $\Delta\chi^2$ test to determine whether the effect of sexual satisfaction on marital satisfaction is equal across the groups. In like manner, we could examine the interaction of gender with any other path of interest in the model.

To illustrate multiple-group analysis, let us examine the SEM that we have fitted in Figure 21.12 and fit this model to two separate groups of respondents: children of U.S. citizens ($n = 176$) and children of immigrants ($n = 262$). What we are interested in detecting is whether the pattern of relationships fitted in Figure 21.12 is different or identical across these two groups of children. Usually, the first model to be fitted would be the one in which we are merely hypothesizing that the pattern of relationships among the constructs is the same across the groups. In that model, no parameters would be constrained to be equal in the two groups, but the pattern of relationships would be the same. If the model fits the data, we would say that the relationships modeled in Figure 21.12 exist in each of the populations.

The next steps depend upon your research questions, your hypotheses, and the particular study in which you are involved. If you feel that the measurement models across the two groups may be different (e.g., different item–construct correlations, different reliabilities), you would constrain those elements to be equal in the two groups and conduct a $\Delta\chi^2$ test. If they are the same, you would retain those constraints in the model as you test the next set of constraints that you are interested in testing. For example, perhaps you feel the variances of the constructs may be different across the two groups (i.e., that the two groups have different variances on these underlying constructs). In that case, you would test those similarly, by constraining them to be equal (either all at once or one at a time), and conduct another $\Delta\chi^2$ test or tests. Again, if the variances are the same, you would retain those constraints as you test the next set of parameters. If they are not the same, you would leave the ones that are not invariant across the groups free to be estimated differently in the two groups. Of course, one of the sets of relationships you would be most interested in would be whether differences exist across the groups in terms of the paths between the constructs (the structural model). Once more, you would constrain them (one at a time or all at once) to be equal, and perform the appropriate $\Delta\chi^2$ test(s). We have done this with our multigroup model and present the unstandardized and standardized parameter estimates in Figure 21.13. The top figure is for the children of U.S. citizens, and the bottom figure is for children of immigrants. Bold parameters vary across groups; all others are constrained to be equal across the two groups.

In the fitted measurement model, we can see that the item Family Emotional Disorders is measured with less error variance ($\sigma^2_{\delta3 \text{ for immigrants}} = .24$) for immigrant children than is the same item for children of U.S. citizens ($\sigma^2_{\delta3 \text{ for nonimmigrants}} = .36$). But the item Family Alcoholism is more highly correlated to Family Chaos for children of U.S. citizens ($\hat{r} = .96$) than for children of immigrants ($\hat{r} = .84$). In fact, Family Alcoholism is the highest-loading item for children of U.S. citizens, while Family Delinquency is the highest-loading item for children of immigrants. We might conclude that delinquency was related most strongly to the overall experience of chaos in the immigrant families studied by Glueck and Glueck (1950), whereas alcoholism was related most strongly to overall chaos for the nonimmigrant families.

In Figure 21.13, what draws our interest the most are the differences that exist in the paths between the latent variables for children of U.S. citizens and for those of immigrants. For children of U.S. citizens, Family Chaos is highly related to Affect Dysregulation ($\hat{r} = .73$), controlling for all else in the model; that is, children of U.S. citizens whose families were highly chaotic evidenced more externalizing and internalizing symptoms than did children of immigrants ($\hat{r} = .25$), and vice versa. However, for the children of immigrants, Affect Dysregulation is very highly related to Later Violence against Women ($\hat{r} = .99$), controlling for all else in the model; in other words, the children of immigrants who showed fewer externalizing and internalizing symptoms also showed much less violence toward women later in their lives than did those who were children of U.S. citizens ($\hat{r} = -.05$). Conversely, those who were highly dysregulated showed greater violence toward women in later life. However, the estimated path between Affect Dysregulation and Later Violence against Women is not significant at all in the model for children of U.S. citizens. In other words, whether they were dysregulated or not early in childhood had no effect on their later violence against women. As would be expected as a result of the degree of relatedness and the level of significance of the paths between Family Chaos and Later Violence against Women and between Affect Dysregulation and Later Violence against Women, more variance is predicted in the outcome of Later Violence against Women for the children of immigrants ($R^2 = .86$) than for the children of U.S. citizens ($R^2 = .25$). Perhaps the immigrant children's encounters with the institutions of school (the Affect Dysregulation variables were teacher-reported) and the juvenile justice system were complicated by discrimination related to such issues as language barriers and cultural differences, which the children of U.S. citizens did not face. This may have caused the children of immigrants to be labeled and "tracked" as troublemakers by such institutions, perhaps creating a greater likelihood that they would remain on the path toward violence as adults. However, for the children of U.S. citizens, who may not have faced such institutional discrimination, their adult perpetration of violence may have been related to family chaos and something other than dysregulated affect reported by teachers.

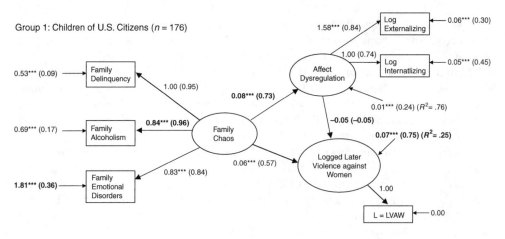

Group 1: Children of U.S. Citizens (*n* = 176)

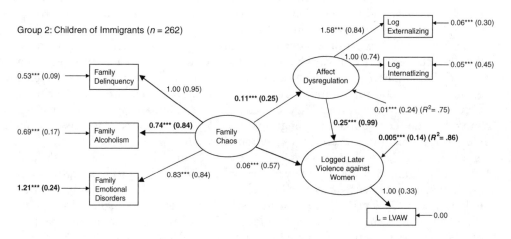

Group 2: Children of Immigrants (*n* = 262)

FIGURE 21.13. Multigroup model comparing children of U.S. citizens (*n* = 176) to children of immigrants (*n* = 262). *Note.* Parameters in parentheses are from the within-group, common-metric, completely standardized solution. Bold parameters vary across groups; all others are constrained across groups. ***p < .001. $\chi^2(34)$ = 404.05, p < .001; GFI = .97, SRMR = .02.

Examples of Other Research Questions That Can Be Investigated with CSA

To illustrate further the usefulness of CSA for family researchers, we present two proposed research studies in which the research questions and hypotheses can be investigated with CSA. For both of these examples, we have focused on areas of family research that have not yet been empirically explored as fully as other areas of family research: grandparents raising grandchildren, and the relationship between family processes and health outcomes. As is our custom, we have developed our research questions and hypotheses prior to designing each study. The questions that we ask determine the methodologies that we should use to answer those questions. For example, if we were interested in grandparents raising grandchildren and wanted to find out what might influence grandparents' depression and level of satisfaction within their role as custodial grandparents, our first step would be to examine the literature to see what is already known about role satisfaction and depression among grandparents raising grandchildren. Once we have this information, we would delineate our research questions and then create a hypothesized model that is substantively tied to our review of the literature of existing theory, research findings, and clinical experience, if appropriate. In this example, our research question is whether grandparents' coping skills and parenting skills, as well as behavior problems displayed by grandchildren (our three predictors), predict grandparents' levels of depression and role satisfaction (our two outcomes). This question is easily answered by conducting a path analysis. Thus, we propose a hypothesized path diagram (Figure 21.14). To actually answer this question, our next step would be to gather data from custodial grandparents. Finding reliable and valid instruments to use would be of great importance. For example, we might use the CBCL (Achenbach, 1994) to measure the observed variable of grandchildren's behavior problems. We might measure the observed variable of grandparents' depression with the Center for Epidemiological Studies Depression scale (Radloff, 1977). Once we have gathered our data and conducted the preliminary analyses, we would fit our hypothesized model and assess its fit. If the fit is acceptable, we could then interpret the parameter estimates and draw conclusions about our hypothesized model and our research question.

In the area of health outcomes, our research question is whether adult attachment style and affect regulation predict health status, after controlling for SES and race (two predictors of health that are well established in the literature). Because we are collecting multiple reliable and valid measures of all of the constructs (health status, adult at-

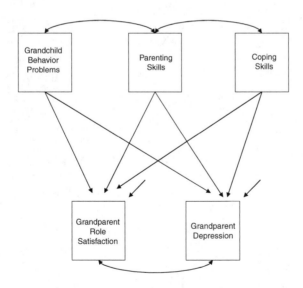

FIGURE 21.14. Hypothesized model of grandparents' coping skills and parenting skills, and behavior problems displayed by grandchildren, predicting grandparents' levels of depression and role satisfaction.

tachment, affect regulation, and SES) except race, our question could easily be answered by conducting a CSA with SEM. Our hypothesized model is presented in Figure 21.15. The literature also shows that the health-protective effects of marital relationships are different for men and women (Kiecolt-Glaser & Newton, 2001), and because women are socialized to be managers of emotional closeness in relationships (Walters, Carter, Papp, & Silverstein, 1988) as well as family health managers (Candib, 1995), we have hypothesized that the model in Figure 21.15 will fit differently for men and women. Therefore, after answering our first question of whether these hypothesized relationships fit our data by fitting the SEM, we would test this second question through fitting a series of nested multiple-group SEMs to test whether this set of relationships is different across men and women. These are just two examples; however, many other research questions and hypotheses in family research can be investigated by using the techniques presented in this chapter.

SUMMARY AND CONCLUSIONS

CSA has much to contribute to family research. Because family relationships are complex and multifaceted, family researchers need complex statistical techniques to best answer their questions. The various tools in the CSA toolkit, such as path analysis, CFA, and SEM, provide sophisticated means of investigating such complex relationships. As a result, though these methods are somewhat difficult to learn, the long-term "payoff" is great for family researchers.

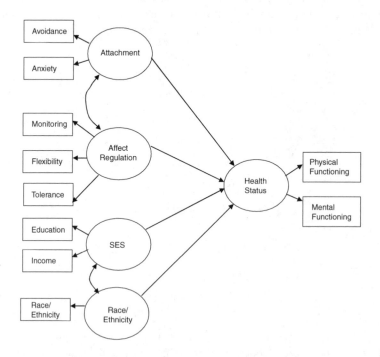

FIGURE 21.15. Hypothesized model of adult attachment, affect regulation, SES, and race predicting health status.

One of the greatest strengths of these statistical methods is the necessity of having a theory-driven hypothesized path model, prior to fitting models to the data. In other words, CSA might better be thought of as "confirmatory" structure analysis. CSA works best as a methodology to answer specific questions and to test specific hypotheses. Of course, all research should be done this way, but in reality, theory does not always clearly drive analyses. However, in CSA, theory is of necessity the starting point. Researchers may be tempted to go on "fishing expeditions" for better fit based on modification indices, but they should avoid this temptation and stick with what makes the most theoretical sense. When this is kept in mind, CSA has the potential to make substantial contributions to the advancement of the family therapy fields through theory-driven, methodologically sophisticated research.

EXEMPLARS

Keiley, M. K., Lofthouse, N., Bates, J., Dodge, K., & Pettit, G. (2003). Differential risks of covarying and pure components of mother and teacher reports of externalizing and internalizing behaviors across ages 5 to 14. *Journal of Abnormal Child Psychology*, 31, 267–283.

Mistry, R. S., Vandewater, E. A., Huston, A. C., & McLoyd, V. C. (2002). Economic well-being and children's social adjustment: The role of family process in an ethnically diverse low-income sample. *Child Development*, 73, 935–951.

O'Farrell, T. J., Murphy, C. M., Stephan, S. H., Fals-Stewart, W., & Murphy, M. (2004). Partner violence before and after couples-based alcoholism treatment for male alcoholic patients: The role of treatment involvement and abstinence. *Journal of Clinical and Consulting Psychology*, 72, 202–217.

Rueter, M. A., & Conger, R. D. (1998). Reciprocal influences between parenting and adolescent problem-solving behavior. *Developmental Psychology*, 34, 1470–1482.

REFERENCES

Achenbach, T. M. (1994). Child Behavior Checklist and related instruments. In M. E. Maruish (Ed.), *The use of psychological testing for treatment planning and outcome assessment* (pp. 517–549). Hillsdale, NJ: Erlbaum.

Baron, R. M., & Kenny, D. A. (1986). The moderator–mediator variable distinction in social psychological research: Conceptual, strategic, and statistical considerations. *Journal of Personality and Social Psychology*, 51(6), 1173–1182.

Bentler, P. M. (1995). *EQS: Structural equations program manual*. Encino, CA: Multivariate Software.

Bollen, K. A. (1989). *Structural equations with latent variables*. New York: Wiley.

Candib, L. M. (1995). *Medicine and the family: A feminist perspective*. New York: Basic Books.

Carmines, E., & McIver, J. (1981). Analyzing models with unobserved variables: Analysis of covariance structures. In G. Bohrnstedt & E. Borgatta (Eds.), *Social measurement: Current issues* (pp. 65–115). Beverly Hills, CA: Sage.

Dankoski, M. E., & Keiley, M. K. (2004). *Affect regulation and the cycle of violence against women: New directions for understanding the process*. Manuscript submitted for publication.

Dolbin-MacNab, M., & Keiley, M. K. (2004). *Emotional support and the prediction of marital and sexual satisfaction*. Manuscript in preparation.

Glueck, S., & Glueck, E. (1950). *Unraveling juvenile delinquency*. New York: Commonwealth Fund.

Joreskog, K. G., & Sorbom, D. (1996). *LISREL 8: User's reference guide*. Chicago: Scientific Software International.

Keiley, M. K., Liu, T., Moon, S., & Sprenkle, D. (2004). *Development of the Affect Regulation Scales for the Gifted*. Manuscript in preparation.

Keiley, M. K., Moon, S., & Sprenkle, D. (1999, August). *Development of the Affect Regulation Scales for the Gifted*. Paper presented at the annual meeting of the American Psychological Association, Boston.

Keiley, M. K., Moon, S. M., Sprenkle, D., & Liu, T. (2000, August). *Affect Regulation Scales for the Gifted: Scale development and testing*. Paper presented at the annual meeting of the American Psychological Association, Washington, DC.

Kiecolt-Glaser, J. K., & Newton, T. L. (2001). Marriage and health: His and hers. *Psychological Bulletin, 127*, 472–503.

Lawrance, K., & Byers, E. S. (1992). Development of the interpersonal exchange model of sexual satisfaction in long term relationships. *Canadian Journal of Human Sexuality, 1*, 123–128.

Lawrance, K., & Byers, E. S. (1995). Sexual satisfaction in long term heterosexual relationships: The interpersonal exchange model of sexual satisfaction. *Personal Relationships, 2*, 267–285.

Lawrance, K., & Byers, E. S. (1998). Interpersonal Exchange Model of Sexual Satisfaction Questionnaire. In C. Davis, W. L. Yarber, R. Bauserman, G. Schreer, & S. Davis (Eds.), *Sexuality related measures* (2nd ed., pp. 514–519). Thousand Oaks, CA: Sage.

Mindel, C. H., Habenstein, R. W., & Wright, R., Jr. (1998). *Ethnic families in America: Patterns and variations* (4th ed.). Upper Saddle River, NJ: Prentice Hall.

Muthen, L. K., & Muthen, B. O. (1998). *Mplus user's guide*. Los Angeles: Muthen & Muthen.

Neale, M. C., Boker, S. M., Xie, G., & Maes, H. H. (1999). *Mx: Statistical modeling*. Richmond, VA: Medical College of Virginia, Department of Psychiatry.

Pierce, G. R. (1994). The Quality of relationships Inventory: Assessing the interpersonal context of social support. In B. R. Burleson, T. L. Albrecht, & I. G. Sarason (Eds.), *Communication of social support: Messages, interactions, relationships, and community* (pp. 247–266). Newbury Park, CA: Sage.

Radloff, L. S. (1977). The CES-D Scale: A self-report depression scale for research in the general population. *Applied Psychological Measurement, 1*, 385–401.

Schumm, W. R., Scanlon, E. D., Crow, C. L., Green, D. M., & Buckler, D. L. (1983). Characteristics of the Kansas Marital Satisfaction Scale in a sample of 79 married couples. *Psychological Reports, 53*, 583–588.

Timm, T. M., & Keiley, M. K. (2004). *The effects of differentiation of self, adult attachment, and sexual communication on sexual and marital satisfaction: A path analysis*. Manuscript in preparation.

Walters, M., Carter, B., Papp, P., & Silverstein, O. (1988). *The invisible web*. New York: Guilford Press.

Wheaton, B., Muthen, B., Alwin, D., & Summers, G. (1977). Assessing reliability and stability in panel models. In D. Heise (Ed.), *Sociological methodology* (pp. 84–136). San Francisco: Jossey-Bass.

Wheeless, L. R., Wheeless, V. E., & Baus, R. (1984). Sexual communication, communication satisfaction, and solidarity in the developmental stages of intimate relationships. *Western Journal of Speech Communication, 48*, 217–230.

Index